CLINICAL
NEUROSURGERY

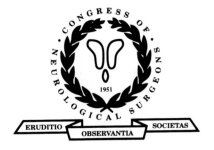

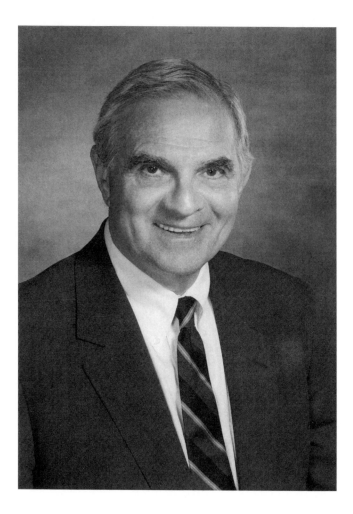

PETER J. JANNETTA, M.D., D.Sci.

CLINICAL NEUROSURGERY

Proceedings

OF THE
CONGRESS OF NEUROLOGICAL
SURGEONS

Montreal, Quebec, Canada
1996

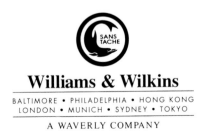

Williams & Wilkins

BALTIMORE • PHILADELPHIA • HONG KONG
LONDON • MUNICH • SYDNEY • TOKYO

A WAVERLY COMPANY

Accurate indications, adverse reactions, and dosage schedules for drugs are provided in this book, but it is possible that they may change. The reader is urged to review the package information data of the manufacturers of the medications mentioned.

Printed in the United States of America   97 98 99
(ISBN 0-683-18313-3)   1 2 3 4 5 6 7 8 9 10

Reprints of Chapters may be purchased from Williams & Wilkins in quantities of 100 or more. Contact Vicki Vaughn, telephone (800) 882-0483 or (410) 528-4374 or fax (410) 361-8016.

Preface

The 46th Annual Meeting of the Congress of Neurological Surgeons was held in Montreal, Quebec at the Montreal Convention Center from September 28–October 3, 1996. Volume 44 of Clinical Neurosurgery represents the official compendium of the platform presentations at that meeting. The Annual Meeting Chairman, Steven Papadopoulos and the Scientific Program Chairman, Mitchel Berger, organized and led an outstanding meeting. Local Arrangements Chairman, Gerard Mohr, coordinated the superb venue for the meeting.

The scientific program featured Dr. Peter J. Jannetta as the honored guest of the Congress. He was hard at work during the entire meeting with contributions at each of the general scientific sessions. These can be found in Chapters 7, 13, 21, and 30. Dr. Stephen Haines, the President of the Congress, directed that the meeting be organized under a general theme of "Outcomes Assessment" and this is reflected in his Presidential Address. Accordingly, General Scientific Sessions I–III comprise a specific component of that theme as follows: General Scientific Session I: Criteria for Patient Selection; General Scientific Session II: How The Operation is Done and General Scientific Session III: Analysis of Outcome. Speakers for each of these sessions were tasked with providing strong supporting arguments for their perspectives using literature-based criteria. This reflects Dr. Haines own interest and education in clinical trails methodology as applied to surgery. The fourth general scientific session changes format and focuses on Treatment of Posterior Fossa Tumors, assembling an internationally recognized panel to address this topic.

Dr. Haines' careful and critical approach on surgical outcomes is developed in his Presidential Address in Chapter 1. In keeping with the Congress' long standing commitment to education, the CNS Resident Award, given to Dr. David Pincus, can be found in Chapter 2.

The weather cooperated and the members of the Congress were treated to an outstanding scientific and social program in a marvelous city. All of the participants of the multiple annual meeting committees should be congratulated on their work. I would like to thank the contributors to Clinical Neurosurgery for their cooperation and timeliness in submitting their manuscripts, and to my associate editors for their prompt and thorough editing of the manuscripts. I would also like to express my gratitude to Trudy Rutherford and Vicki Vaughn at

Williams & Wilkins who have ensured that this volume of *Clinical Neurosurgery* is available for the 1997 meeting. Finally, I would like to acknowledge the efforts of my secretary at the University of Washington, Rosetta Marx, for the organization and drive that are required to assemble such a text.

M. Sean Grady, M.D.
Editor-in-Chief

Editorial Board

Honored Guests

1952—Professor Herbert Olivecrona, Stockholm, Sweden
1953—Sir Geoffrey Jefferson, Manchester, England
1954—Dr. Kenneth G. McKenzie, Toronto, Canada
1955—Dr. Carl W. Rand, Los Angeles, California
1956—Dr. Wilder G. Penfield, Montreal, Canada
1957—Dr. Francis C. Grant, Philadelphia, Pennsylvania
1958—Dr. A. Earl Walker, Baltimore, Maryland
1959—Dr. William J. German, New Haven, Connecticut
1960—Dr. Paul C. Bucy, Chicago, Illinois
1961—Professor Eduard A. V. Busch, Copenhagen, Denmark
1962—Dr. Bronson S. Ray, New York, New York
1963—Dr. James L. Poppen, Boston, Massachusetts
1964—Dr. Edgar A. Kahn, Ann Arbor
1965—Dr. James C. White, Boston, Massachusetetts
1966—Dr. Hugh A. Krayenbühl, Zurich, Switzerland
1967—Dr. W. James Gardner, Cleveland, Ohio
1968—Professor Normal M. Dott, Edinburgh, Scotland
1969—Dr. Wallace B. Hamby, Cleveland, Ohio
1970—Dr. Barnes Woodhall, Durham, North Carolina
1971—Dr. Elisha S. Gurdjian, Detroit, Michigan
1972—Dr. Francis Murphey, Memphis, Tennessee
1973—Dr. Henry G. Schwartz, St. Louis, Missouri
1974—Dr. Guy L. Odom, Durham, North Carolina
1975—Dr. William A. Sweet, Boston, Massachusetts
1976—Dr. Lyle A. French, Minneapolis, Minnesota
1977—Dr. Richard C. Schneider, Ann Arbor, Michigan
1978—Dr. Charles G. Drake, London, Ontario, Canada
1979—Dr. Frank H. Mayfield, Cincinnati, Ohio
1980—Dr. Eben Alexander, Jr., Winston-Salem, North Carolina
1981—Dr. J. Garber Galbraith, Birmingham, Alabama
1982—Dr. Keiji Sano, Tokyo, Japan
1983—Dr. C. Miller Fisher, Boston, Massachusetts
1984—Dr. Hugo V. Rizzoli, Washington, DC
      Dr. Walter E. Dandy (posthumously), Baltimore, Maryland
1985—Dr. Sidney Goldring, St. Louis, Missouri
1986—Dr. M. Gazi Yasargil, Zurich, Switzerland
1987—Dr. Thomas W. Langfitt, Philadelphia, Pennsylvania

1988—Professor Lindsay Symon, London, England
1989—Dr. Thoralf M. Sundt, Jr., Rochester, Minnesota
1990—Dr. Charles Byron Wilson, San Francisco, California
1991—Dr. Bennett M. Stein, New York, New York
1992—Dr. Robert G. Ojemann, Boston, Massachusetts
1993—Dr. Albert L. Rhoton, Jr., Gainesville, Florida
1994—Dr. Robert F. Spetzler, Phoenix, Arizona
1995—Dr. John A. Jane, Charlottesville, Virginia
1996—Dr. Peter J. Jannetta, Pittsburgh, Pennsylvania

Editors-in-Chief
Clinical Neurosurgery

Volume	Date	Editor-in-Chief
1	1953	Raymond K. Thompson, M.D.
2	1954	Raymond K. Thompson, M.D. & Ira J. Jackson, M.D.
3	1955	Raymond K. Thompson, M.D. & Ira J. Jackson, M.D.
4	1956	Ira J. Jackson, M.D.
5	1957	Robert G. Fisher, M.D.
6	1958	Robert G. Fisher, M.D.
7	1959	Robert G. Fisher, M.D.
8	1960	William H. Mosberg, Jr., M.D.
9	1961	William H. Mosberg, Jr., M.D.
10	1962	William H. Mosberg, Jr., M.D.
11	1963	John Shillito, Jr., M.D. & William H. Mosberg, Jr., M.D.
12	1964	John Shillito, Jr., M.D.
13	1965	John Shillito, Jr., M.D.
14	1966	Robert G. Ojemann, M.D. & John Shillito, Jr., M.D.
15	1967	Robert G. Ojemann, M.D.
16	1968	Robert G. Ojemann, M.D.
17	1969	Robert G. Ojemann, M.D.
18	1970	George T. Tindall, M.D.
19	1971	George T. Tindall, M.D.
20	1972	Robert H. Wilkins, M.D.
21	1973	Robert H. Wilkins, M.D.
22	1974	Robert H. Wilkins, M.D.
23	1975	Ellis B. Keener, M.D.
24	1976	Ellis B. Keener, M.D.
25	1977	Ellis B. Keener, M.D.
26	1978	Peter W. Carmel, M.D.
27	1979	Peter W. Carmel, M.D.
28	1980	Peter W. Carmel, M.D.
29	1981	Martin H. Weiss, M.D.
30	1982	Martin H. Weiss, M.D.
31	1983	Martin H. Weiss, M.D.
32	1984	John R. Little, M.D.
33	1985	John R. Little, M.D.
34	1986	John R. Little, M.D.
35	1987	Peter McL. Black, M.D., Ph.D.
36	1988	Peter McL. Black, M.D., Ph.D.
37	1989	Peter McL. Black, M.D., Ph.D.
38	1990	Warren R. Selman, M.D.
39	1991	Warren R. Selman, M.D.
40	1992	Warren R. Selman, M.D.
41	1993	Christopher M. Loftus, M.D.
42	1994	Christopher M. Loftus, M.D.
43	1995	Christopher M. Loftus, M.D.
44	1996	M. Sean Grady, M.D.

Officers of the Congress
of
Neurological Surgeons
1996

STEPHEN J. HAINES, M.D.
President

MARC R. MAYBERG, M.D.
President-Elect

MARK H. CAMEL, M.D.   H. HUNT BATJER, M.D.
Vice-President   *Secretary*

WILLIAM A. FRIEDMAN, M.D.
Treasurer

EXECUTIVE COMMITTEE

ISSAM A. AWAD, M.D.   STANLEY PELOFSKY, M.D.

DANIEL BARROW, M.D.   RICHARD G. PERRIN, M.D.

MITCHEL S. BERGER, M.D.   RICHARD A. ROSKI, M.D.

KEITH L. BLACK, M.D.   MASATO SHIBUYA, M.D.

CURTIS A. DICKMAN, M.D.   LINDA L. STERNAU, M.D.

MARK N. HADLEY, M.D.   RICHARD TOSELLI, M.D.

PAUL MCCORMICK, M.D.   JACK E. WILBERGER, M.D.

STEPHEN M. PAPDOPOULOS, M.D.

Contributors

JOSEPH T. ALEXANDER, M.D., Department of Neurosurgery, Emory University School of Medicine, Atlanta, Georgia (Chapter 19)

OSSAMA AL-MEFTY, M.D., Department of Neurosurgery, University of Arkansas for Medical Sciences, Little Rock, Arkansas (Chapter 26)

PAUL J. APOSTOLIDES, M.D., Division of Neurological Surgery, Barrow Neurological Institute, St. Joseph's Hospital and Medical Center, Phoenix, Arizona, (Chapter 11)

ROY A. E. BAKAY, M.D., Department of Neurosurgery, Emory University School of Medicine, Atlanta, Georgia (Chapter 14)

JOSEPH BARRY, B.S., Department of Neurology, Cornell University Medical College, New York, New York (Chapter 2)

MITCHEL S. BERGER, M.D., Department of Neurological Surgery, University of California, San Francisco, California (Chapter 12)

MARK BERNSTEIN, M.D., F.R.C.S.C., Division of Neurosurgery, Toronto Hospital, University of Toronto, Toronto, Ontario, Canada (Chapter 20)

CHARLES S. COBBS, M.D., Department of Neurological Surgery, University of California, San Francisco, California (Chapter 29)

G. REES COSGROVE, M.D., F.R.C.S.(C), Departments of Neurosurgery and Neurology, Massachusetts General Hospital, Harvard Medical School, Boston, Massachusetts (Chapter 18)

CARLOS A. DAVID, M.D., Division of Neurological Surgery, Barrow Neurological Institute, St. Joseph's Hospital and Medical Center, Phoenix, Arizona (Chapter 27)

MAHLON R. DELONG, M.D., Department of Neurosurgery, Emory University School of Medicine, Atlanta, Georgia (Chapter 14)

CURTIS DICKMAN, M.D., Division of Neurological Surgery, Barrow Neurological Institute, St. Joseph's Hospital and Medical Center, Phoenix, Arizona (Chapter 11)

RICHARD G. FESSLER, M.D., PH.D., Professor of Neurosurgery, Director of Spine Surgery, Department of Neurosurgery, University of Florida School of Medicine, Gainesville, Florida (Chapter 18)

ROBERT A. R. FRASER, M.D., Department of Neurosurgery, Cornell University Medical College, New York, New York (Chapter 2)

AMAR GAJJAR, M.D., Division of Neuro/Oncology, Assistant Member, Department of Hematology/Oncology, St. Jude Children's Research Hospital, Memphis, Tennessee (Chapter 32)

BRUCE J. GANTS, M.D., Department of Otolaryngology, University of Iowa Hospitals & Clinics, Iowa City, Iowa (Chapter 28)

STEVEN A. GOLDMAN, M.D., Ph.D., Department of Neurology, Cornell University Medical College, New York, New York (Chapter 2)

REGIS W. HAID, JR., M.D., Department of Neurosurgery, Emory University School of Medicine, Atlanta, Georgia (Chapter 19)

STEPHEN J. HAINES, M.D., Professor and Chairman, Department of Neurosurgery, Medical University of South Carolina, Charleston, South Carolina (Chapter 1)

CATHERINE HARRISON, B.A., Department of Neurology, Cornell University Medical College, New York, New York (Chapter 2)

MICHAEL J. HARRISON, M.D., Department of Neurosurgery, University of Arkansas for Medical Sciences, Little Rock, Arkansas (Chapter 26)

HAROLD J. HOFFMAN, M.D., B.Sc. (MED.), F.R.C.S.C., F.A.C.S., Division of Neurosurgery, Hospital for Sick Children; Professor, Department of Surgery, University of Toronto, Toronto, Ontario, Canada (Chapter 31)

PETER J. JANNETTA, M.D., D.Sci., Professor and Chairman, Department of Neurological Surgery, University of Pittsburgh School of Medicine, Pittsburgh, Pennsylvania (Chapters 7, 13, 21, 30)

DEAN G. KARAHALIOS, M.D., Division of Neurological Surgery, Barrow Neurological Institute, St. Joseph's Hospital and Medical Center, Phoenix, Arizona (Chapter 10)

JOHN LANGFITT, Ph.D., Departments of Neurosurgery and Neurology, University of Rochester Medical Center, Rochester, New York (Chapter 23)

NICHOLAS S. LITTLE, M.D., Department of Neurological Surgery, Mayo Clinic, Rochester, Minnesota (Chapter 9)

CHRISTOPHER M. LOFTUS, M.D., F.A.C.S., Professor of Surgery, Division of Neurological Surgery, University of Iowa College of Medicine, Iowa City, Iowa (Chapter 16)

PAUL G. MATZ, M.D., Department of Neurosurgery, University of California, San Francisco, California (Chapter 17)

MARC R. MAYBERG, M.D., Professor of Neurological Surgery, Department of Neurological Surgery, University of Washington, Seattle, Washington (Chapter 24)

PAUL C. MCCORMICK, M.D., Associate Professor of Neurological Surgery, Columbia University, College of Physicians & Surgeons, New York, New York (Chapter 3)

TIMOTHY M. MCCULLOCH, M.D., Department of Otolaryngology, University of Iowa Hospitals and Clinics, Iowa City, Iowa (Chapter 28)

ARNOLD H. MENEZES, M.D., Division of Neurosurgery, University of Iowa Hospitals & Clinics, Iowa City, Iowa (Chapter 28)

FREDERIC B. MEYER, M.D., Department of Neurological Surgery, Mayo Clinic, Rochester, Minnesota (Chapter 9)

MAIKEN NEDERGAARD, Ph.D., Department of Cell Biology, New York Medical College, New York, New York (Chapter 2)

GEORGE A. OJEMANN, M.D., Professor of Neurological Surgery, Department of Neurological Surgery, University of Washington, Seattle, Washington (Chapter 8)

ANDRE OLIVIER, M.D., Ph.D., (Chapter 15)

JOHN PENNEY, M.D., Department of Neurosurgery and Neurology, Massachusetts General Hospital, Harvard Medical School, Boston, Massachusetts (Chapter 22)

JOSEPH M. PIEPMEIER, M.D., Department of Neurosurgery, Yale University School of Medicine, New Haven, Connecticut (Chapter 5)

WEBSTER H. PILCHER, M.D., Ph.D., Departments of Neurosurgery and Neurology, University of Rochester Medical Center, Rochester, New York (Chapter 23)

DAVID W. PINCUS, M.D., Department of Neurosurgery, Neurological Institute, Columbia University College of Physicians and Surgeons; Department of Neurology, Cornell University Medical College, New York, New York (Chapter 2)

LAWRENCE H. PITTS, M.D., Department of Neurological Surgery, University of California, San Francisco, California (Chapters 17, 29)

JAMES T. RUTKA, M.D., Ph.D., Division of Neurosurgery, Hospital for Sick Children, University of Toronto, Toronto, Ontario, Canada (Chapter 33)

ROBERT A. SANFORD, M.D., Chief of Pediatric Neurosurgery, Professor of Neurosurgery, Semmes-Murphey Clinic, University of Tennessee, Memphis, Tennessee (Chapter 32)

LESLIE SHINOBU, M.D., Departments of Neurosurgery and Neurology, Massachusetts General Hospital, Harvard Medical School, Boston, Massachusetts (Chapter 22)

VOLKER K. H. SONNTAG, M.D., Division of Neurological Surgery, Barrow Neurological Institute, St. Joseph's Hospital and Medical Center, Phoenix, Arizona (Chapter 10)

ROBERT F. SPETZLER, M.D., Division of Neurological Surgery, Barrow Neurological Institute, St. Joseph's Hospital and Medical Center, Phoenix, Arizona (Chapter 27)

PHILIP A. STARR, M.D., Ph.D., Fellow, Department of Neurosurgery, Emory University School of Medicine, Atlanta, Georgia (Chapter 14)

RONALD R. TASKER, M.D. (Chapter 6)

VINCENT C. TRAYNELIS, M.D., Associate Professor of Neurosurgery, Department of Surgery, Division of Neurosurgery, University of Iowa Hospitals and Clinics, Iowa City, Iowa (Chapter 4, 28)

JERROLD L. VITEK, M.D., Ph.D., (Chapter 14)

JACK E. WILBERGER, JR., M.D., Professor of Neurosurgery, Vice-Director, Division of Neurosurgery, Senior Associate Dean for Student Affairs and Medical Education, Medical College of Pennsylvania, Hahnemann University School of Medicine, Allegheny University of the Health Sciences, Pittsburgh, Pennsylvania (Chapter 25)

CHARLES B. WILSON, M.D., Department of Neurological Surgery, University of California, San Francisco, California (Chapter 29)

Biography of Peter J. Janetta, M.D., D.Sci

Dr. Jannetta received an A.B. degree in 1953 and an M.D. degree in 1957, both from the University of Pennsylvania. He was an intern at the Hospital of the University of Pennsylvania, where he also trained as a surgical resident from 1958 to 1963. During those same years, Dr. Jannetta was a Fellow at the University of Pennsylvania, Harrison Department of Surgical Research and an NIH Fellow in Neurophysiology. After completing a residency in neurosurgery (1963–1966) at UCLA Center for Health Sciences, he was named Associate Professor and Chairman of the Section of Neurological Surgery, Department of Surgery at Louisiana State University Medical Center, later being appointed Professor and Chairman. In 1971, Dr. Jannetta moved to the University of Pittsburgh School of Medicine to the Division of Neurological Surgery as Professor and Director. When the Division of Neurological Surgery at the University of Pittsburgh became the Department of Neurological Surgery in 1973, Dr. Jannetta was made Professor and Chairman, a position which he holds to the present. He is a recognized pioneer in the treatment of cranial nerve compression syndromes, especially those related to facial pain.

Among his many honors, Dr. Jannetta has received an honorary Doctor of Science degree from Washington and Jefferson College. In 1990, he was selected as Vectors/Pittsburgh Man of the Year in the Sciences, and, as one of the recipients of the 1990 Horatio Alger Award, he became a member of the Horatio Alger Association. He was the first W. Eugene Stern Visiting Professor of Neurosurgery at UCLA School of Medicine in 1987 and in 1983 received the Herbert Olivacrona Award. From 1976 to 1978 he was the Frances Sargent Cheever Distinguished Professor at the University of Pittsburgh School of Medicine.

Active in more than 30 professional organizations, he is the Chief of the Medical Advisory Board of the newly formed Trigeminal Neuralgia Association. He also serves on the Medical Advisory Board of the Acoustic Neuroma Association and the boards of several neurosurgical societies. He is former president of the Pennsylvania Neurological Society, the Society of Neurological Anesthesia and Neurologic Supportive Care, and the Pittsburgh Neuroscience Society. In 1994, he was elected to the position of Second Vice-President-at-large of the World Federation of Neurosurgical Societies, and to active membership in the

American Academy of Neurological Surgery. His more than 250 publications include books, book chapters, and refereed articles. He is the subject of Mark L. Shelton's book, *Working in a Very Small Place: The Making of A Neurosurgeon.*

In 1992, the University of Pittsburgh acknowledged the caliber of Dr. Jannetta's contributions to the field of neurosurgery and his stature in the world of medicine by naming him the Walter E. Dandy Professor in Neurological Surgery, and establishing the Peter J. Jannetta Chair in Neurological Surgery.

He was named Secretary of Health of the Commonwealth of Pennsylvania by Governor Tom Ridge in March 1995. Senate confirmation of the nomination occured on May 2, 1995. Dr. Jannetta served one year in that position.

Bibliography of Peter J. Jannetta, M.D., D.Sci.

PUBLICATIONS

Refereed Articles (172)

JANNETTA PJ, ROBERTS B: Sudden complete thrombosis of an aneurysm of the abdominal aorta. **N Engl J Med** 264 (9):434–436, 1961.

PENDERGRASS HP, TRISTAN TA, BLAKEMORE WS, SELLERS AM, JANNETTA PJ, MURPHY JJ: Roentgen technics in the diagnosis and localization of pheochromocytoma. **Radiology** 78 (5):725–737, 1962.

JANNETTA PJ, BLAKEMORE WS: Fractional collection of urine for catecholamine determination in pheochromocytoma. **Surgery** 56 (4): 706–710, 1964.

JANNETTA PJ, WHAYNE TF JR: Formaldehyde-treated, regenerated collagen film and film-laminate as a substitute for dura mater. **Surg Forum** 16:435–437, 1965.

RAND RW, BAUER RO, SMART CR, JANNETTA PJ: Experiences with percutaneous stereotaxic cryocordotomy. **Bull Los Angeles Neurol Soc** 30 (3):142–147, 1965.

WEIDNER W, JANNETTA PJ, SAUL R, HANAFEE W: The neuroradiology of tumors of the corpus callosum. **Neurology** 15 (11):1071–1077, 1965.

JANNETTA PJ, HANAFEE W, WEIDNER W, ROSEN L: Pneumoencephalographic findings suggesting aneurysm of the vertebral-basilar junction. Differentiation of cases simulating mass lesions. **J Neurosurg** 24 (2):530–535, 1966.

JANNETTA PJ, RAND RW: Transtentorial retrogasserian rhizotomy in trigeminal neuralgia by microneurosurgical technique. **Bull Los Angeles Neurol Soc** 31 (3):93–99, 1966.

ERULKAR SD, SPRAGUE JM, WHITSEL BL, DOGAN S, JANNETTA PJ: Organization of the vestibular projection to the spinal cord of the cat. **J Neurophysiol** 29 (4):626–664, 1966.

HANAFEE W, JANNETTA PJ: Aneurysm as a cause of stroke. **Am J Roentgenol Radium Ther Nucl Med** 98 (3):647–652, 1966.

JANNETTA PJ: Anatomy of trigeminal ganglia. Gross (mesoscopic) description of the human trigeminal nerve and ganglion. **J Neurosurg** 26 (1-Suppl):109–111, 1967.

JANNETTA PJ: Structural mechanisms of trigeminal neuralgia. Arterial compression of the trigeminal nerve at the pons in patients with trigeminal neuralgia. **J Neurosurg** 26 (1, Pt. 2):159–162, 1967.

RAND RW, JANNETTA PJ: Micro-neurosurgery for aneurysms of the vertebral-basilar artery system. **J Neurosurg** 27 (4):330–335, 1967.

JANNETTA PJ: The surgical binocular microscope in neurological surgery. **Am Surg** 34 (1):31–34, 1968.

RAND RW, JANNETTA PJ: Microneurosurgery. Application of the binocular surgical microscope in brain tumors, intracranial aneurysms, spinal cord disease, and nerve reconstruction. **Clin Neurosurg** 15:319–342, 1968.

JANNETTA PJ: Microsurgical exploration and decompression of the facial nerve in hemifacial spasm. **Curr Top Surg Res** 2:217–220, 1970.

JANNETTA PJ, HACKETT ER, RUBY JR: Electromyographic and electron microscopic correlates in hemifacial spasm treated by microsurgical relief of neurovascular compression. **Surg Forum** 21:449–451, 1970.

JANNETTA PJ: Trigeminal and glossopharyngeal neuralgia. **Curr Diagn** 3:849–851, 1971.

BERLIN CI, LOWE-BELL SS, JANNETTA PJ, KLINE DG: Central auditory deficits after temporal lobectomy. **Arch Otolaryngol** 96 (1):4–10, 1972.

CRICHLOW RW, SELTZER MH, JANNETTA PJ: Cholecystitis in adolescents. **Am J Dig Dis** 17 (1):68–72, 1972.

JANNETTA PJ: Pain problems of significance in the head and face, some of which often are misdiagnosed. **Curr Probl Surg** (Feb):47–53, 1973.

JANNETTA PJ, KRIEGER AJ: Treatment of pain due to malignancy in the head and neck. **Curr Probl Surg** (Feb):43–47, 1973.

DUNN DK, JANNETTA PJ: Evaluation of chronic pain in children. **Curr Probl Surg** (Feb):64–68, 1973.

KRIEGER AJ, JANNETTA PJ: Pain in the back and lower extremities. **Curr Probl Surg** (Feb):32–43, 1973.

MAROON JC, JANNETTA PJ: Pain following peripheral nerve injuries. **Curr Probl Surg** (Feb):20–32, 1973.

SELKER RG, JANNETTA PJ: Central pain and central therapy of pain. **Curr Probl Surg** (Feb):59–64, 1973.

LEBLANC HJ, JANNETTA PJ, MCGARRY P: Intracranial atypical teratoma. **South Med J** 66 (4):507–508, 1973.

MCCALLUM JE, TENICELA R, JANNETTA PJ: Closed external drainage of cerebrospinal fluid in treatment of postoperative CSF fistulae. **Surg Forum** 24:465–467, 1973.

ALBIN MS, BUNEGIN L, MASSOPUST LC JR, JANNETTA PJ: Ketamine-induced postanesthetic delirium attenuated by tetrahydroaminoacridine. **Exp Neurol** 44 (1):126–129, 1974.

KENNERDELL JS, JANNETTA PJ, JOHNSON BL: A steroid-sensitive solitary intracranial plasmacytoma. **Arch Ophthalmol** 92 (5):393–398, 1974.

JANNETTA PJ: The cause of hemifacial spasm. Definitive microsurgical treatment at the brainstem in 31 patients. **Trans Am Acad Ophthal Otolaryngol** 80 (3, Pt. 1):319–322, 1975.

JANNETTA PJ: Trigeminal neuralgia and hemifacial spasm. Etiology and definitive treatment. **Trans Am Neurol Assoc** 100:53–55, 1975.

JANNETTA PJ: Neurovascular cross-compression in patients with hyperactive dysfunction symptoms of the eighth cranial nerve. **Surg Forum** 26:467–469, 1975.

ALBIN MS, BUNEGIN L, JANNETTA PJ, MASSOPUST LC JR: Tetrahydroaminoacridine (THA). I. Effect on postanesthetic emergence responses and anesthesia sleep-time after ketamine, phencyclidine and thiamylal in animals. **Excerpta Medica Int Cong Series** no. 347, 143–146, 1975.

ALBIN MS, JANNETTA PJ, MAROON JC, TUNG A, MILLEN JE: Anesthesia in the sitting position. **Excerpta Medica Intl Cong Series** no. 347, 775–778, 1975.

ALBIN MS, BUNEGIN L, DUJOVNY M, BENNETT MH, JANNETTA PJ, WISOTZKEY HM: Brain retraction pressure during intracranial procedures. **Surg Forum** 26:499–500, 1975.

DUJOVNY M, VAS R, OSGOOD CP, MAROON JC, JANNETTA PJ: Automatically irrigated bipolar forceps. Technical note. **J Neurosurg** 43 (4):502–503, 1975.

DUJOVNY M, OSGOOD CP, MAROON JC, JANNETTA PJ: Penetrating intracranial foreign bodies in children. **J Trauma** 15 (11):981–986, 1975.

HUNG TK, ALBIN MS, BROWN TD, BUNEGIN L, ALBIN R, JANNETTA PJ: Biomechanical responses to open experimental spinal cord injury. **Surg Neurol** 4 (2):271–276, 1975.

MCCALLUM JE, MAROON JC, JANNETTA PJ: Treatment of postoperative cerebrospinal fluid fistulas by subarachnoid drainage. **J Neurosurg** 42 (4):434–437, 1975.

REIGEL DH, DALLMANN DE, SCARFF TB, JANNETTA PJ: Transcephalic impedance in neonatal hydrocephalics with myelomeningocele. **Surg Forum** 26:481–482, 1975.

RUBY JR, JANNETTA PJ: Hemifacial spasm. Ultrastructural changes in the facial nerve induced by neurovascular compression. **Surg Neurol** 4 (4):369–370, 1975.

ALBIN MS, BABINSKI M, MAROON JC, JANNETTA PJ: Anesthetic management of posterior fossa surgery in the sitting position. **Acta Anaesthesiol Scand** 20 (2):117–128, 1976.

BUNEGIN L, ALBIN MS, JANNETTA PJ: Catecholamine responses to experimental spinal cord impact injury. I. Intrinsic spinal cord synthesis rates. **Exp Neurol** 53 (1):274–280, 1976.

BUNEGIN L, ALBIN MS, JANNETTA PJ: Catecholamine responses to experimental spinal cord impact injury. II. Fate of intravenous (^{3}H) norepinephrine. **Exp Neurol** 53 (1):281–284, 1976.

ALBIN MS, BUNEGIN L, BENNETT MH, DUJOVNY M, JANNETTA PJ: Clinical and experimental brain retraction pressure monitoring. **Acta Neurol Scand [Suppl]** 64:522–523, 1977.

MORGAN CW, JANNETTA PJ: A nerve stimulator for the cerebellopontine angle. Technical note. **J Neurosurg** 46 (5):688–689, 1977.

BENNETT MH, ALBIN MS, BUNEGIN L, DUJOVNY M, HELLSTROM H, JANNETTA PJ: Evoked potential changes during brain retraction in dogs. **Stroke** 8 (4):487–492, 1977.

JANNETTA PJ: Treatment of trigeminal neuralgia by suboccipital and transtentorial cranial operations. **Clin Neurosurg** 24:538–549, 1977.

JANNETTA PJ, ABBASY M, MAROON JC, MORALES-RAMOS F, ALBIN MS: Etiology and definitive microsurgical treatment of hemifacial spasm. Operative techniques and results in forty-seven patients. **J Neurosurg** 47 (3):321–328, 1977.

LAHA RK, JANNETTA PJ: Glossopharyngeal neuralgia. **J Neurosurg** 47 (3):316–320, 1977.

JANNETTA PJ: Observations on the etiology of trigeminal neuralgia, hemifacial spasm, acoustic nerve dysfunction and glossopharyngeal neuralgia. Definitive microsurgical treatment and results in 117 patients. **Neurochirurgia (Stuttg)** 20 (5):145–154, 1977.

CHANG JL, ABOLA EG, REILLY K, ALBIN MS, JANNETTA PJ: Evaluation of cardiac function during neurosurgical procedure in the sitting position. **Surg Forum** 28:467–469, 1977.

JANNETTA PJ, BISSONETTE DJ: Bell's palsy: A theory as to etiology. Observations in six patients. **Laryngoscope** 88 (5):849–854, 1978.

PAZIN GJ, HO M, JANNETTA PJ: Reactivation of herpes simplex virus after decompression of the trigeminal nerve root. **J Infect Dis** 138 (3):405–409, 1978.

FRANK T, MAY M, JANNETTA PJ: Acoustic neurinoma in a child. A case study. **J Speech Hear Disord** 43 (4):506–512, 1978.

HAINES SJ, MAROON JC, JANNETTA PJ: Supratentorial intracerebral hemorrhage following posterior fossa surgery. **J Neurosurg** 49 (6): 881–886, 1978.

HAINES SJ, MARTINEZ AJ, JANNETTA PJ: Arterial cross compression of the trigeminal nerve at the pons in trigeminal neuralgia. Case report with autopsy findings. **J Neurosurg** 50 (2):257–259, 1979.

HUNG TK, LIN HS, ALBIN MS, BUNEGIN L, JANNETTA PJ: The standardization of experimental impact injury to the spinal cord. **Surg Neurol** 11 (6):470–477, 1979.

SHEPTAK PE, JANNETTA PJ: The two-stage excision of huge acoustic neurinomas. **J Neurosurg** 51 (1):37–41, 1979.

JANNETTA PJ: Microsurgery of cranial nerve cross-compression. **Clin Neurosurg** 26:607–615, 1979.

DEEB ZL, JANNETTA PJ, ROSENBAUM AE, KERBER CW, DRAYER BP: Tortuous vertebrobasilar arteries causing cranial nerve syndromes. Screening by computed tomography. **J Comput Assist Tomogr** 3 (6):774–778, 1979.

WANSKI ZJ, ROBINSON AG, JANNETTA PJ: Selective total removal of a growth-hormone-secreting adenoma. Evidence that acromegaly is a primary pituitary disease. **Metabolism** 28 (6):624–628, 1979.

LUNSFORD LD, BISSONETTE DJ, ZORUB DS, JANNETTA PJ: Anterior cervical operation for spondylotic myelopathy. **Surg Forum** 30:457–459, 1979.

PAZIN GJ, ARMSTRONG JA, LAM MT, TARR GC, JANNETTA PJ, HO M: Prevention of reactivated herpes simplex infection by human leukocyte interferon after operation on the trigeminal root. **N Engl J Med** 301 (5):225–230, 1979.

JANNETTA PJ, GENDELL HM: Clinical observations on etiology of essential hypertension. **Surg Forum** 30:431–432, 1979.

SEGAL R, GENDELL HM, CANFIELD D, DUJOVNY M, JANNETTA PJ: Cardiovascular response to pulsatile pressure applied to ventrolateral medulla. **Surg Forum** 30:433–435, 1979.

JANNETTA PJ, TEW JM JR: Treatment of trigeminal neuralgia. **Neurosurgery** 4 (1):93–94, 1979.

HAINES SJ, JANNETTA PJ, ZORUB DS: Microvascular relations of the trigeminal nerve. An anatomical study with clinical correlation. **J Neurosurg** 52 (3):381–386, 1980.

YONAS H, JANNETTA PJ: Neurinoma of the trigeminal root and atypical trigeminal neuralgia. Their commonality. **Neurosurgery** 6 (3):273–277, 1980.

BENNETT MH, JANNETTA PJ: Trigeminal evoked potentials in humans. **Electroencephalogr Clin Neurophysiol** 48 (5):517–526, 1980.

LUNSFORD LD, BISSONETTE DJ, JANNETTA PJ, SHEPTAK PE, ZORUB DS: Anterior surgery for cervical disc disease. Part 1. Treatment of lateral cervical disc herniation in 253 cases. **J Neurosurg** 53 (1):1–11, 1980.

JANNETTA PJ, ROBBINS LJ: Trigeminal neuropathy. New observations. **Neurosurgery** 7 (4):347–351, 1980.

JANNETTA PJ: Neurovascular compression in cranial nerve and systemic disease. **Ann Surg** 192 (4):518–525, 1980.

MØLLER AR, JANNETTA PJ, BENNETT M, MØLLER MB: Intracranially recorded responses from the human auditory nerve. New insights into the origin of brain stem evoked potentials (BSEPs). **Electroencephalogr Clin Neurophysiol** 52 (1):18–27, 1981.

CHANG GL, HUNG TK, BLEYAERT A, JANNETTA PJ: Stress-strain management of the spinal cord of puppies and their neurological evaluation. **J Trauma** 21 (9):807–810, 1981.

GRUNDY BL, LINA A, PROCOPIO PT, JANNETTA PJ: Reversible evoked potential changes with retraction of the eighth cranial nerve. **Anesth Analg** 60 (11):835–838, 1981.

MØLLER AR, JANNETTA PJ: Compound action potentials recorded intracranially from the auditory nerve in man. **Exp Neurol** 74 (3): 862–874, 1981.

BURSICK DM, WATERMAN PM, JANNETTA PJ: Malignant hyperthermia. A neurosurgical case and a review of the syndrome. **Neurosurgery** 9 (4):421–425, 1981.

MØLLER AR, JANNETTA PJ, MØLLER MB: Neural generators of brainstem evoked potentials. Results from human intracranial recordings. **Ann Otol Rhinol Laryngol** 90 (6, Pt. 1):591–596, 1981.

JANNETTA PJ: Cranial nerve vascular compression syndromes (other than tic douloureux and hemifacial spasm). **Clin Neurosurg** 28: 445–456, 1981.

SEGAL R, GENDELL HM, CANFIELD D, DUJOVNY M, JANNETTA PJ: Hemodynamic changes induced by pulsatile compression of the ventrolateral medulla. **Angiology** 33 (3):161–172, 1982.

MØLLER AR, JANNETTA PJ, MØLLER MB: Intracranially recorded auditory nerve response in man. New interpretations of BSER. **Arch Otolaryngol** 108 (2):77–82, 1982.

MØLLER AR, JANNETTA PJ: Comparison between intracranially recorded potentials from the human auditory nerve and scalp recorded auditory brainstem responses (ABR). **Scand Audiol** 11 (1):33–40, 1982.

GRUNDY BL, PROCOPIO PT, JANNETTA PJ, LINA A, DOYLE E: Evoked potential changes produced by positioning for retromastoid craniectomy. **Neurosurgery** 10 (6, Pt. 1):766–770, 1982.

MØLLER MB, MØLLER AR, JANNETTA PJ: Brainstem auditory evoked potentials in patients with hemifacial spasm. **Laryngoscope** 92 (8, Pt. 1):848–852, 1982.

MØLLER AR, JANNETTA PJ: Evoked potentials from the inferior colliculus in man. **Electroencephalogr Clin Neurophysiol** 53 (6):612–620, 1982.

MØLLER AR, JANNETTA PJ: Auditory evoked potentials recorded intracranially from the brain stem in man. **Exp Neurol** 78 (1):144–157, 1982.

SEGAL R, JANNETTA PJ, WOLFSON SK, DUJOVNY M, COOK EE: Implanted pulsatile balloon device for simulation of neurovascular compression syndromes in animals. **J Neurosurg** 57 (5):646–650, 1982.

GRUNDY BL, JANNETTA PJ, PROCOPIO PT, LINA A, BOSTON JR, DOYLE E: Intraoperative monitoring of brain-stem auditory evoked potentials. **J Neurosurg** 57 (5):674–681, 1982.

SEKHAR LN, JANNETTA PJ: Thoracic disc herniation. Operative approaches and results. **Neurosurgery** 12 (3):303–305, 1983.

JANNETTA PJ: Microvascular decompression for trigeminal neuralgia. **Surg Rounds** 6 (April):24–35, 1983.

MØLLER AR, JANNETTA PJ: Interpretation of brainstem auditory evoked potentials. Results from intracranial recordings in humans. **Scand Audiol** 12 (2):125–133, 1983.

MØLLER AR, JANNETTA PJ: Monitoring auditory functions during cranial nerve microvascular decompression operations by direct recording from the eighth nerve. **J Neurosurg** 59 (3):493–499, 1983.

BENNETT MH, JANNETTA PJ: Evoked potentials in trigeminal neuralgia. **Neurosurgery** 13 (3):242–247, 1983.

MØLLER AR, JANNETTA PJ: Auditory evoked potentials recorded from the cochlear nucleus and its vicinity in man. **J Neurosurg** 59 (6):1013–1018, 1983.

JANNETTA PJ: Hemifacial spasm caused by a venule. Case report. **Neurosurgery** 14 (1):89–92, 1984.

SEKHAR LN, JANNETTA PJ: Cerebellopontine angle meningiomas. Microsurgical excision and follow-up results. **J Neurosurg** 60 (3):500–505, 1984.

SEKHAR LN, JANNETTA PJ, MAROON JC: Tentorial meningiomas. Surgical management and results. **Neurosurgery** 14 (3):268–275, 1984.

JANNETTA PJ, MØLLER MB, MØLLER AR: Disabling positional vertigo. **N Engl J Med** 310 (26):1700–1705, 1984.

NIELSEN VK, JANNETTA PJ: Pathophysiology of hemifacial spasm. Part III. Effects of facial nerve decompression. **Neurology** 34 (7):891–897, 1984.

YONAS H, WOLFSON SK, GUR D, ET AL.: Clinical experience with the use of xenon-enhanced CT blood flow mapping in cerebral vascular disease. **Stroke** 15 (3):443–450, 1984.

KAPOOR WN, JANNETTA PJ: Trigeminal neuralgia associated with seizure and syncope. Case report. **J Neurosurg** 61 (3):594–595, 1984.

SOSO MJ, NIELSEN VK, JANNETTA PJ: Palatal myoclonus. Reflex activation of contractions. **Arch Neurol** 41 (8):866–869, 1984.

MØLLER AR, JANNETTA PJ: On the origin of synkinesis in hemifacial spasm. Results of intracranial recordings. **J Neurosurg** 61 (3):569–576, 1984.

MØLLER AR, JANNETTA PJ: Monitoring auditory nerve potentials during operations in the cerebellopontine angle. **Otolaryngol Head Neck Surg** 92 (4):434–439, 1984.

MØLLER AR, JANNETTA PJ: Preservation of facial function during removal of acoustic neuromas. Use of monopolar constant-voltage stimulation and EMG. **J Neurosurg** 61 (4):757–760, 1984.

COOK BR, JANNETTA PJ: Tic convulsif. Results in eleven cases treated with microvascular decompression of the fifth and seventh cranial nerves. **J Neurosurg** 61 (5):949–951, 1984.

JANNETTA PJ, MØLLER AR, MØLLER MB: Technique of hearing preservation in small acoustic neuromas. **Ann Surg** 200 (4):513–523, 1984.

HO M, PAZIN GJ, ARMSTRONG JA, HAVERKOS HS, DUMMER JS, JANNETTA PJ: Paradoxical effects of interferon on reactivation of oral infection with herpes simplex virus after microvascular decompression for trigeminal neuralgia. **J Infect Dis** 150 (6):867–872, 1984.

JANNETTA PJ, SEGAL R, WOLFSON SK: Neurogenic hypertension: Etiology and surgical treatment. I. Observations in 53 patients. **Ann Surg** 201 (3):391–398, 1985.

MØLLER AR, JANNETTA PJ: Synkinesis in hemifacial spasm. Results of recording intracranially from the facial nerve. **Experientia** 41 (3): 415–417, 1985.

EIDELMAN BH, NIELSEN VK, MØLLER MB, JANNETTA PJ: Vascular compression, hemifacial spasm, and multiple cranial neuropathy. **Neurology** 35 (5):712–716, 1985.

MØLLER AR, JANNETTA PJ: Microvascular decompression in hemifacial spasm. Intraoperative electrophysiological observations. **Neurosurgery** 16 (5):612–618, 1985.

JANNETTA PJ, SEGAL R, WOLFSON SK, DUJOVNY M, SEMBA A, COOK EE: Neurogenic hypertension: Etiology and surgical treatment. II. Observations in an experimental nonhuman primate model. **Ann Surg** 202 (2):253–261, 1985.

JANNETTA PJ: Microsurgical management of trigeminal neuralgia. **Arch Neurol** 42 (8):800, 1985.

JANNETTA PJ, BISSONETTE DJ: Management of the failed patient with trigeminal neuralgia. **Clin Neurosurg** 32:334–347, 1985.

MØLLER AR, JANNETTA PJ: Hemifacial spasm. Results of electrophysiologic recording during microvascular decompression operations. **Neurology** 35 (7):969–974, 1985.

BOSTON JR, DENEAULT LG, KRONK L, JANNETTA PJ: Automated monitoring of brainstem auditory evoked potentials in the operating room. **J Clin Monit** 1 (3):161–167, 1985.

SEGAL R, JANNETTA PJ, WOLFSON SK, DUJOVNY M, COOK EE: La hipertension arterial y el neurocirujano. **Neurocirugia (Flanc-Slen)** 1:137–146, 1985.

MØLLER AR, JANNETTA PJ: Monitoring of facial nerve function during removal of acoustic tumor. **Am J Otol** 10 (Nov. Suppl):27–29, 1985.

MØLLER MB, MØLLER AR, JANNETTA PJ, SEKHAR L: Diagnosis and surgical treatment of disabling positional vertigo. **J Neurosurg** 64 (1):21–28, 1986.

MØLLER AR, JANNETTA PJ: Blink reflex in patients with hemifacial spasm. Observations during microvascular decompression operations. **J Neurol Sci** 72 (2–3):171–182, 1986.

MØLLER AR, JANNETTA PJ, BURGESS JE: Neural generators of the somatosensory evoked potentials. Recording from the cuneate nucleus in man and monkeys. **Electroencephalogr Clin Neurophysiol** 65 (4):241–248, 1986.

SEKIYA T, MØLLER AR, JANNETTA PJ: Pathophysiological mechanisms of intraoperative and postoperative hearing deficits in cerebellopontine angle surgery. An experimental study. **Acta Neurochir (Wien)** 81 (3–4):142–151, 1986.

MØLLER AR, JANNETTA PJ: Physiological abnormalities in hemifacial spasm studied during microvascular decompression operations. **Exp Neurol** 93 (3):584–600, 1986.

JANNETTA PJ, MØLLER MB, MØLLER AR, SEKHAR LN: Neurosurgical treatment of vertigo by microvascular decompression of the eighth cranial nerve. **Clin Neurosurg** 33:645–665, 1986.

MØLLER AR, JANNETTA PJ: Monitoring facial EMG responses during microvascular decompression operations for hemifacial spasm. **J Neurosurg** 66 (5):681–685, 1987.

JHO HD, JANNETTA PJ: Hemifacial spasm in young people treated with microvascular decompression of the facial nerve. **Neurosurgery** 20 (5):767–770, 1987.

MORGAN C, JANNETTA PJ, DEGROAT WC: Organization of corneal afferent axons in the trigeminal nerve root entry zone in the cat. **Exp Brain Res** 68 (2):411–416, 1987.

MORGAN C, DEGROAT WC, JANNETTA PJ: Sympathetic innervation of the cornea from the superior cervical ganglion. An HRP study in the cat. **J Auton Nerv Syst** 20 (2):179–183, 1987.

MØLLER AR, JANNETTA PJ, SEKHAR LN: Contributions from the auditory nerve to the brain-stem auditory evoked potentials (BAEPs). Results of intracranial recording in man. **Electroencephalogr Clin Neurophysiol** 71 (3):198–211, 1988.

MARION DW, JANNETTA PJ: Use of perioperative steroids with microvascular decompression operations. **Neurosurgery** 22 (2):353–357, 1988.

SEKIYA T, MØLLER AR, JANNETTA PJ: [Cochlear nerve injuries caused by manipulations in cerebellopontine angle. Part I. Electrophysiological and morphological study in dogs.] **No Shinkei Geka** 16 (4):359–365, 1988.

SEKIYA T, MØLLER AR, JANNETTA PJ: [Cochlear nerve injuries caused by manipulation in cerebellopontine angle. Part II. An electrophysiological and morphological study in rhesus monkeys.] **No Shinkei Geka** 16 (5 Suppl):671–676, 1988.

POLLACK IF, JANNETTA PJ, BISSONETTE DJ: Bilateral trigeminal neuralgia. A fourteen-year experience with microvascular decompression. **J Neurosurg** 68 (4):559–565, 1988.

POLLACK IF, SEKHAR LN, JANNETTA PJ, JANECKA IP: Neurilemomas of the trigeminal nerve. **J Neurosurg** 70 (5):737–745, 1989.

BLOOM PB, VINER ED, MAZALA M, JANNETTA PJ, STIEBER AC, SIMMONS RL: Treatment of loin pain hematuria syndrome by renal autotransplantation. **Am J Med** 87 (2):228–232, 1989.

MØLLER AR, JANNETTA PJ, JHO HD: Recordings from human dorsal column nuclei using stimulation of the lower limb. **Neurosurgery** 26 (2):291–299, 1990.

AMMAR A, LAGENAUR C, JANNETTA PJ: Neural tissue compatibility of teflon as an implant material for microvascular decompression. **Neurosurg Rev** 13 (4):299–303, 1990.

ALTSCHULER EM, JUNGREIS CA, SEKHAR LN, JANNETTA PJ, SHEPTAK PE: Operative treatment of intracranial epidermoid cysts and cholesterol granulomas. Report of 21 cases. **Neurosurgery** 26 (4):606–614, 1990.

SEKHAR LN, JANNETTA PJ, BURKHART LE, JANOSKY JE: Meningiomas involving the clivus. A six-year experience with 41 patients. **Neurosurgery** 27 (5):764–781, 1990.

LINSKEY ME, JANNETTA PJ, MARTINEZ AJ: A vascular malformation mimicking an intracanalicular acoustic neurilemoma. **J Neurosurg** 74 (3):516–519, 1991.

MØLLER AR, MØLLER MB, JANNETTA PJ, JHO HD: Auditory nerve compound action potentials and brainstem auditory evoked potentials in patients with various degrees of hearing loss. **Ann Otol Rhinol Laryngol** 100:488–495, 1991.

MASON WE, KOLLROS P, JANNETTA PJ: Trigeminal neuralgia and its treatment in a 13-month-old child. A review and case report. **J Craniomandib Disord Facial Oral Pain** 5:213–216, 1991.

ZICCARDI VB, PATTERSON GT, JANNETTA PJ, SOTEREANOS GC: Technical innovation. Transfacial approach for infraorbital nerve exploration and orbital-maxillary surgery. **Oral Surg Oral Med Oral Pathol** 72:655–659, 1991.

PATTERSON GT, ZICCARDI VB, JANNETTA PJ, SOTEREANOS GC: Idiopathic trigeminal neuralgia complicated by lingual nerve dysesthesia. **Oral Surg Oral Med Oral Pathol** 74 (3):282–284, 1992.

MØLLER AR, MØLLER MB, JANNETTA PJ, JHO HD: Compound action potentials recorded from the exposed eighth nerve in patients with intractable tinnitus. **Laryngoscope** 102:187–197, 1992.

JUNGREIS CA, JANNETTA PJ, YONAS H: Timing treatment of a giant intracranial aneurysm by the use of magnetic resonance imaging for the determination of intraluminal clot stability. **Skull Base Surg** 3 (1):32–36, 1993.

MØLLER AR, MØLLER MB, JANNETTA PJ, JHO HD: Vascular decompression surgery for severe tinnitus. Selection criteria and results. **Layrngoscope** 103:421–427, 1993.

ROSSEAU GL, JANNETTA PJ, HIRSCH B, MØLLER MB, MØLLER AR: Restoration of useful hearing after microvascular decompression of the cochlear nerve. **Am J Otol** 14:392–397, 1993.

SCLABASSI RJ, KALIA KK, SEKHAR LN, JANNETTA PJ: Assessing brain stem function. **Neurosurg Clin North Am** 4:415–431, 1993.

SAITO S, MØLLER AR, JANNETTA PJ, JHO HD: Abnormal response from the sternocleidomastoid muscle in patients with spasmodic torticollis. Observations during microvascular decompression operations. **Acta Neurochir (Wien)** 124:92–98, 1993.

MØLLER MB, MØLLER AR, JANNETTA PJ, JHO HD, SEKHAR LN: Microvascular decompression of the eighth nerve in patients with disabling positional vertigo. Selection criteria and operative results in 207 patients. **Acta Neurochir (Wien)** 125:75–82, 1993.

JANNETTA PJ: Vascular compression is the cause of trigeminal neuralgia. **APS Journal** 2 (4):217–227 and 237–238, 1993.

MØLLER AR, JHO HD, JANNETTA PJ: Preservation of hearing in operations on acoustic tumors. An alternative to recording brainstem auditory evoked potentials. **Neurosurgery** 34:688–693, 1994.

MØLLER AR, JANNETTA PJ, JHO HD: Click-evoked responses from the cochlear nucleus. A study in human. **Electroencephalogr Clin Neurophysiol** 92:215–224, 1994.

KONDZIOLKA D, LEMLEY T, KESTLE JR, LUNSFORD LD, FROMM GH, JANNETTA PJ: The effect of single-application topical ophthalmic anesthesia in patients with trigeminal neuralgia. **J Neurosurg** 80:993–997, 1994.

LINSKEY ME, JHO HD, JANNETTA PJ: Microvascular decompression for trigeminal neuralgia caused by vertebrobasilar compression. **J Neurosurg** 81:1–9, 1994.

ZICCARDI VB, JANOSKY JE, PATTERSON GT, JANNETTA PJ: Peripheral trigeminal nerve surgery for patients with atypical facial pain. **J Craniomaxillofac Surg** 22 (6):355–360, 1994.

MØLLER AR, JHO HD, JANNETTA PJ: Preservation of hearing in operation on acoustic tumors. An alternative to recording brain stem auditory evoked potentials. **Neurosurgery** 34:688–693, 1994.

RESNICK DK, JANNETTA PJ, BISSONETTE D, JHO HD, LANZINO G: Microvascular decompression for glossopharyngeal neuralgia. **Neurosurgery** 36:64–69, 1995.

POLLOCK BE, LUNSFORD LD, KONDZIOLKA D, ET AL.: Outcome analysis of acoustic neuroma management. A comparison of microsurgery and stereotactic radiosurgery. **Neurosurgery** 36:215–229, 1995.

BARKER FG II, JANNETTA PJ, BISSONETTE DJ, SHIELDS PT, LARKINS MV, JHO HD: Microvascular decompression for hemifacial spasm. **J Neurosurg** 82:201–210, 1995.

JHO HD, JANNETTA PJ: Microvascular decompression for spasmodic torticollis. **Acta Neurochir (Wien)** 134:21–26, 1995.

MØLLER AR, JHO HD, YOKOTA M, JANNETTA PJ: Contribution from crossed and uncrossed brainstem structures to the brainstem auditory evoked potentials. A study in humans. **Laryngoscope** 105: 596–605, 1995.

BARKER FG, JANNETTA PJ, BISSONNETTE DJ, LARKINS MV, JHO HD: The long-term outcome of microvascular decompression for trigeminal neuralgia. **N Engl J Med** 334 (17):1077–1083, 1996.

BARKER FG, JANNETTA PJ, BABU RP, POMONIS S, BISSONETTE DJ, JHO HD: Long-term outcome after operation for trigeminal neuralgia in patients with posterior fossa tumors. **J Neurosurg** 84:818–825, 1996.

LOVELY TJ, JANNETTA PJ: Technical aspects of microvascular decompression of the cranial nerves. **Contemp Neurosurg** 18 (12): 1996.

COMEY CH, JANNETTA PJ, SHEPTAK PE, JHO HD, BURKHART LE: Staged removal of acoustic tumors. Techniques and lessons learned from a series of 83 patients. **Neurosurgery** 37 (5):915–921, 1996.

RESNICK DK, JANNETTA PJ, LUNSFORD LD, BISSONETTE DJ: Microvascular decompression for trigeminal neuralgia in patients with multiple sclerosis. **Surg Neurol** 46:358–362, 1996.

LOVELY TJ, JANNETTA PJ: Microvascular decompression for trigeminal neuralgia. **Neurosurg Clin North Am** 8 (1):11–29, 1997.

Books (2)

SAMII M, JANNETTA PJ (eds): *The Cranial Nerves: Anatomy, Pathology, Physiology, Diagnosis, Treatment.* Berlin, Springer-Verlag, 1981.

ROVIT RL, MURALI R, JANNETTA PJ (eds): *Trigeminal Neuralgia.* Baltimore, Williams & Wilkins, 1990.

Book Chapters (68)

JANNETTA PJ: Changes in erythrocytes (after burns), in Rhoads JE, Howard JM (eds): *Chemistry of Trauma.* Springfield, IL, C.C. Thomas, 1963, pp 39–47.

JANNETTA PJ, RAND RW: Vascular compression of the trigeminal nerve at the pons in patients with trigeminal neuralgia, in, Donaghy RMP, Yasargil MG (eds): *Micro-Vascular Surgery.* St. Louis, C.V. Mosby, 1966, p 150.

RAND RW, JANNETTA PJ: Microneurosurgery for aneurysms of the vertebral-basilar artery system, in Donaghy RMP, Yasargil MG (eds): *Micro-Vascular Surgery.* St. Louis, C.V. Mosby, 1969, p 148.

JANNETTA PJ, RAND RW: Transtentorial retrogasserian rhizotomy in trigeminal neuralgia, in Rand RW (ed): *Microneurosurgery.* St. Louis, C.V. Mosby, 1969, pp 156–169.

JANNETTA PJ: Neurovascular compression of the facial nerve in hemifacial spasm: Relief by microsurgical technique, in Merei FT (ed): *Reconstructive Surgery of Brain Arteries.* Budapest, Publishing House of the Hungarian Academy of Sciences, 1974, pp 193–199.

JANNETTA PJ: Trigeminal neuralgia, in Archer WH (ed): *Oral and Maxillofacial Surgery, 5th Ed.* Philadelphia, W.B. Saunders, 1975, pp 1697–1699.

JANNETTA PJ, MCCALLUM JE: Assessment of the patient with head injury, in Archer WH (ed): *Oral and Maxillofacial Surgery, 5th Ed.* Philadelphia, W.B. Saunders, 1975, pp 1033–1041.

JANNETTA PJ: Vascular compression of the facial nerve at the brainstem in hemifacial spasm: Treatment by microsurgical decompression, in Morely TP (ed): *Current Controversies in Neurosurgery.* Philadelphia, W.B. Saunders, 1976, pp 435–442.

JANNETTA PJ: Microsurgical approach to the trigeminal nerve for tic douloureux, in Krayenbuhl H, Maspes PE, Sweet WH (eds): *Progress in Neurological Surgery.* Basel, Switzerland, S. Karger, 1976, vol 7, pp 180–200.

JANNETTA PJ: Trigeminal neuralgia, in Conn EF (ed): *1977 Current Therapy.* Philadelphia, W.B. Saunders, 1977, pp 754–756.

JANNETTA PJ, ZORUB DS, BISSONETTE DJ: Cranial neuromuscular disorders, in Altman P, Katz D (eds): *Human Health and Disease, Biological Handbooks—II.* Bethesda, MD, Federation of American Societies for Experimental Biology, 1977, pp 258–268.

JANNETTA PJ: Microneurosurgery of the cranial nerves. *Actas del XVIII Congresso Latinoamericano de Neurocirugia.* 1:229–231, 1979.

JANNETTA PJ, ZORUB DS: Microvascular decompression for trigeminal neuralgia, in Buchheit W, Truex R Jr (eds): *Surgery of the Posterior Fossa.* New York, Raven Press, 1979, pp 143–154.

DUJOVNY M, OSGOOD CP, MAROON JC, JANNETTA PJ: Canine cerebral ischemia, in Fein JM, Reichman OH (eds): *Microvascular Anastomoses for Cerebral Ischemia.* Heidelberg, West Germany, Springer-Verlag, 1979, pp 8–22.

JANNETTA PJ: Hemifacial spasm: Microvascular decompression of the VIIth nerve intracranially, in Symon L (ed): *Operative Surgery-Neurosurgery.* London, Butterworths & Co., 1979, pp 374–381.

JANNETTA PJ: Hemifacial spasm, in Ransohoff J (ed): *Modern Techniques in Surgery.* Mount Kisco, NY, Futura Publishing, 1980, pp 15:1–8.

ZORUB DS, JANNETTA PJ: Microvascular decompression of the trigeminal nerve for tic douloureux: Results in 271 cases, in Silverstein H, Norrell H (eds): *Neurological Surgery of the Ear.* Birmingham, AL, Aesculapius Publishing, 1980, pp 294–298.

ZORUB DS, JANNETTA PJ: Hemifacial spasm: Surgical management by microsurgical techniques, in Silverstein H, Norrell H (eds): *Neurological Surgery of the Ear.* Birmingham, AL, Aesculapius Publishing, 1980, pp 202–207.

JANNETTA PJ: Trigeminal neuralgia. Part 1. Intracranial approach [Editorial introduction by Jannetta PJ, Sweet WH.], in Wilson C, Hoff J (eds): *Current Surgical Management of Neurologic Disease.* New York, Churchill Livingstone, 1980, pp 279–288.

JANNETTA PJ: Hemifacial spasm [Editorial introduction by Jannetta PJ, Sweet WH.], in Wilson C, Hoff J (eds): *Current Surgical Management of Neurologic Disease.* New York, Churchill Livingstone, 1980, pp 300–306.

JANNETTA PJ: Trigeminal neuralgia, in Fruanfelder F, Roy F (eds): *Current Ocular Therapy.* Philadelphia, W.B. Saunders, 1980, pp 228–229.

JANNETTA PJ: Neurovascular cross-compression of the eighth cranial nerve in patients with vertigo and tinnitus, in Samii M, Jannetta PJ (eds): *The Cranial Nerves.* Heidelberg, West Germany, Springer-Verlag, 1981, pp 552–555.

JANNETTA PJ: Hemifacial spasm, in Samii M, Jannetta PJ (eds): *The Cranial Nerves.* Heidelberg, West Germany, Springer-Verlag, 1981, pp 484–493.

JANNETTA PJ: Vascular decompression in trigeminal neuralgia, in Samii M, Jannetta PJ (eds): *The Cranial Nerves.* Heidelberg, West Germany, Springer-Verlag, 1981, pp 331–340.

JANNETTA PJ, BENNETT MH: The pathophysiology of trigeminal neuralgia, in Samii M, Jannetta PJ (eds): *The Cranial Nerves.* Heidelberg, West Germany, Springer-Verlag, 1981, pp 312–315.

JANNETTA PJ: Treatment of trigeminal neuralgia by micro-operative decompression, in Youmans J (ed): *Neurological Surgery.* Philadelphia, W.B. Saunders, vol 6, 1982, pp 3589–3603.

JANNETTA PJ: Cranial rhizopathies, in Youmans J (ed): *Neurological Surgery.* Philadelphia, W.B. Saunders, vol 6, 1982, pp 3771–3884.

JANNETTA PJ: Surgical approach to hemifacial spasm: Microvascular decompression, in Marsden CD, Fahn S (eds): *Movement Disorders Neurology 2.* London, Butterworth & Co., 1982, pp 330–333.

JANNETTA PJ: Microvascular decompression in trigeminal neuralgia and hemifacial spasm, in Brackmann DE (ed): *Neurological Surgery of the Ear and Skull Base.* New York, Raven Press, 1982, pp 49–54.

JANNETTA PJ: Medical treatment of trigeminal neuralgia, in Brackmann DE (ed): *Neurological Surgery of the Ear and Skull Base.* New York, Raven Press, 1982, pp 145–148.

JANNETTA PJ: Microvascular decompression in the treatment of trigeminal neuralgia, in Morgan DH, House LR, Hall WP, Vamvas SJ (eds): *Diseases of the Temporomandibular Apparatus, 2nd Ed.* St. Louis, C.V. Mosby, 1982, pp 580–590.

JANNETTA PJ, YONAS H: Head injuries, in Polk HC, Stone HH, Gardner B (eds): *Basic Surgery, 2nd Ed.* Norwalk, CT, Appleton-Century-Crofts, 1983, pp 551–561.

MØLLER AR, JANNETTA PJ: Neural generators of the brainstem auditory evoked potentials, in Nodar RH, Barber C (eds): *Evoked Potentials II*. Stoneham, MA, Butterworth Publishers, 1984, pp 137–144.

JANNETTA PJ: Posterior fossa neurovascular compression syndromes other than neuralgias, in Wilkins RH, Rengachary SS (eds): *Neurosurgery*. New York, McGraw-Hill Book Co., 1984, pp 1901–1906.

JANNETTA PJ: Trigeminal neuralgia: Treatment by microvascular decompression, in Wilkins RH, Rengachary SS (eds): *Neurosurgery*. New York, McGraw-Hill Book Co., 1984, pp 2357–2363.

MØLLER AR, JANNETTA PJ: Neural generators of the brainstem auditory response, in Jacobson JT (ed): *The Auditory Brainstem Response*. San Diego, College Hill Press, 1985, pp 13–31.

JANNETTA PJ: Cranial nerve and brain neurovascular compression syndromes, in Horwitz O, McCombs PR, Roberts B (eds): *Diseases of Blood Vessels*. Philadelphia, Lea and Febiger, 1985, pp 85–96.

JANNETTA PJ: Neurovascular contact in hemifacial spasm, in Portmann M (ed): *Facial Nerve*. Paris, Masson Publishing, 1985, pp 45–48.

JANNETTA PJ: Cranial rhizopathy, in Long D (ed): *Current Therapy in Neurological Surgery*. Toronto, B.C. Decker, 1985, pp 235–238.

JANNETTA PJ: Microvascular decompression for hemifacial spasm, in May M (ed): *The Facial Nerve*, New York, Thieme, 1986, pp 499–508.

MØLLER AR, JANNETTA PJ: Simultaneous surface and direct brainstem recordings of brainstem auditory evoked potentials (BAEP) in man, in Cracco RQ, Bodis-Wollner I (eds): *Frontiers of Clinical Neuroscience: Evoked Potentials*. New York, Alan R. Liss, 1986, pp 227–234.

JANNETTA PJ: Hemifacial spasm: Etiology and treatment, in English G (ed): *Otolaryngology*. Philadelphia, L.L. Lippincott, 1987, vol I, pp 64:1–10.

JANNETTA PJ: Acoustic neurinomas: Neurosurgical approaches and results, in Sekhar LN, Schramm VL Jr (eds): *Tumors of the Cranial Base: Diagnosis and Treatment*. Mount Kisco, New York, Futura Publishing, 1987, pp 563–586.

JANNETTA PJ: Microvascular decompression of the cochlear nerve as treatment of tinnitus, in Feldmann H (ed): *Proceedings III International Tinnitus Seminar Munster*. Karlsruhe, West Germany, Harsch-Verlag, 1987, pp 348–352.

JANNETTA PJ: The surgical treatment of pain in the face, in Hopkins A (ed): *Headache: Problems in Diagnosis and Management*. London, W.B. Saunders, 1988, pp 141–163.

SEKIYA T, MØLLER AR, JANNETTA PJ: Pathophysiological mechanisms causing intra-operative hearing deficits during cerebellopontine angle operations: An animal experimental study, in Fraysee B, Lazorthes L (eds): *Proceedings of the International Symposium, Acoustic Neuromas, Advances and Controversies.* Toulouse, France, Medicales Pierre Fabre, vol I, 1988, pp 207–218.

JANNETTA PJ: Acoustic neurinomas: Neurosurgical approaches and results, in Fraysee B, Lazorthes L (eds): *Proceedings of the International Symposium, Acoustic Neuromas, Advances and Controversies.* Toulouse, France, Medicales Pierre Fabre, vol II, 1988, pp 43–66.

JANNETTA PJ, MØLLER MB: Evaluation and criteria for preservation of hearing in acoustic neurinoma removal, in Fraysee B, Lazorthes L (eds): *Proceedings of the International Symposium, Acoustic Neuromas, Advances and Controversies Vol. II.* Toulouse, France, Medicales Pierre Fabre, vol II, 1988, pp 105–108.

JANNETTA PJ: Neurovascular conflicts in trigeminal neuralgia, in Montorosi M, Granelli P (eds): *1988 Surgical Updating, Book III.* XXVI World Congress of the International College of Surgeons, Milan, Italy, July 3–9, 1988. Bologna, Italy, Monduzzi, pp 1510–1513.

JANNETTA PJ: Cranial rhizopathies, in Youmans JR (ed): *Neurological Surgery.* London, W.B. Saunders, vol 6, chap 161, 1990, pp 4169–4182.

JANNETTA PJ: Treatment of trigeminal neuralgia by micro-operative decompression, in Youmans JR (ed): *Neurological Surgery.* London, W.B. Saunders, vol 6, chap 144, 1990, pp 3928–3942.

JANNETTA PJ: Microvascular decompression of the trigeminal nerve root entry zone, in Rovit RL, Murali R, Jannetta PJ (eds): *Trigeminal Neuralgia.* Baltimore, Williams & Wilkins, 1990, pp 201–222.

JANNETTA PJ, GILDENBERG PL, LOESER JD, SWEET WH, OJEMANN GA, BONICA JJ: Operations on the brain and brain stem for chronic pain, in Bonica JJ (ed): *The Management of Pain.* Philadelphia, Lea & Febiger, vol II, chap 99, 1990, pp 2082–2103.

JANNETTA PJ: Surgical treatment: Microvascular decompression, in Fromm GH, Sessle BJ (eds): *Trigeminal Neuralgia.* Stoneham, MA, Butterworth Publishers, chap 6, 1991, pp 145–157.

JANNETTA PJ: Intraoperative monitoring of evoked potentials in microvascular decompression operations: Influence on surgical strategy, in Schramm J, Møller AR (eds): *Intraoperative Neurophysiological Monitoring.* Berlin, Springer-Verlag, 1991, pp 277–282.

JANNETTA PJ: Microvascular decompression of the facial nerve for hemifacial spasm, in Wilson CB (ed): *Neurosurgical Procedures: Personal Approaches to Classic Operations.* Baltimore, Williams & Wilkins, chap 12, 1992, pp 154–162.

JANNETTA PJ, HAMM IS, JHO HD, SAIKI I: Essential hypertension caused by arterial compression of the left lateral medulla: A follow-up, in Barrow DL (ed): *Perspectives in Neurological Surgery.* St. Louis, Quality Medical Publishing, vol 3, no 1, 1992, pp 107–125.

MØLLER MB, MØLLER AR, JANNETTA PJ, JHO HD: Results of microvascular decompression (MVD) surgery in patients with disabling positional vertigo (DVP), in Motta G (ed): *The New Frontiers of Otorhinolaryngology in Europe.* Proceedings of the Second European Congress of Oto-Rhino-Laryngology and Cervico-Facial Surgery, Sorrento, June 1992. Bologna, Italy, Monduzzi, 1992, pp I/429–I/432.

SEKHAR LN, JAVED T, JANNETTA PJ: Petroclival meningiomas, in Sekhar LN, Janecka VP (eds): *Surgery of Cranial Base Tumors.* New York, Raven Press, 1993, pp 605–659.

MARION DW, JANNETTA PJ: Head injuries, in Polk HC Jr, Gardner B, Stone HH (eds): *Basic Surgery, 4th Ed.* St. Louis, Quality Medical Publishing, 1993, pp 653–668.

JANNETTA PJ: Trigeminal disorders: Supralateral exposure of the trigeminal nerve in the cerebellopontine angle for microvascular decompression, in Apuzzo MJ (ed): *Brain Surgery: Complications Avoidance and Management.* New York, Churchill Livingstone, 1993, pp 2085–2096 and 2109–2111.

MØLLER MB, MØLLER AR, JANNETTA PJ, JHO HD, SEKHAR LN: Cranial nerve disorders, in Bradley WG, Wilkins RH (eds): *Year Book of Neurology and Neurosurgery.* 1995, pp 535–538 [**Acta Neurochi (Wien)** 125:75–82, 1993].

MØLLER AR, JANNETTA PJ: Foreword, in Ernst A, Marchbanks R, Samii M (eds): *Intracranial and Intralabyrinthine Fluids.* New York, Springer Verlag, 1996.

JANNETTA PJ, RESNICK DK: Cranial rhizopathies, in Youman JR (ed): *Neurological Surgery, 4th Ed.* Philadelphia, W.B. Saunders, 1996.

JANNETTA PJ: Microvascular decompression of the trigeminal nerve for tic douloureux, in Youman JR (ed): *Neurological Surgery, 4th Ed.* Philadelphia, W.B. Saunders, 1996.

JANNETTA PJ: Posterior fossa neurovascular compression syndromes other than neuralgias, in Wilkins RH, Rengachary SS (eds): *Neurosurgery, 2nd Ed.* New York, The MacGraw Hill Companies, vol III, 1996, pp 3227–3233.

JANNETTA PJ: Trigeminal neuralgia: Treatment by microvascular decompression, in Wilkins RH, Rengachary SS (eds), *Neurosurgery, 2nd Ed.* New York, The MacGraw Hill Companies, vol III, 1996, pp 3961–3968.

JANNETTA PJ: Treatment of hemifacial spasm, in Wonsiewicz MJ (ed): *Stereotactic and Functional Neurosurgery.* New York, McGraw-Hill (in press).

Abstracts (77)

BLAKEMORE WS, JANNETTA PJ, DANIELSON G, MURPHY JJ: Selection of patients for the surgical treatment of hypertension. **Circulation** 20 (4, Pt. 2):673, Philadelphia, PA, 1959 (abstr).

DOGAN S, ERULKAR SD, JANNETTA PJ: Response of spinal neurons to vestibular, motor cortex and dorsal root stimulation and their interactions. Proceedings of the International Congress of Physiological Sciences. Leiden, vol II, 1962, p 935 (abstr).

ERULKAR SD, WHITSEL BL, DOGAN S, JANNETTA PJ: Vestibular influences on spinal cord neurons. **Fed Proc** 23:112, 1964 (abstr 68).

JANNETTA PJ, RAND RW: Microanatomy of the trigeminal nerve. **Anat Rec** 154 (2):362, 1966 (abstr).

JANNETTA PJ, BLAKEMORE WS: Fractional collection of urine for catecholamine determination in pheochromocytoma. *Yearbook of Cardiovascular and Renal Diseases.* 1965–1966, pp 247–249 (abstr).

JANNETTA PJ, RAND RW: Transtentorial subtemporal retro-gasserian neurectomy in trigeminal neuralgia by microsurgical technique. *Yearbook of Neurology, Psychiatry and Neurosurgery.* 1966–1967, p 649 (abstr).

JANNETTA PJ: Urea, mannitol and other osmotic diuretics. American Society of Anesthesiologists, Eighteenth Annual Refresher Course Lectures. 1967, p 138 (abstr).

ABBOTT M, JANNETTA PJ: Ultrastructural degeneration in the monkey trigeminal spinal nucleus and tract following trigeminal rhizotomy. **Anat Rec** 160 (2):303–304, New Orleans, LA, 1968 (abstr).

JANNETTA PJ: Microneurosurgery for aneurysms of vertebral basilar artery system. *Yearbook of Neurology, Psychiatry and Neurosurgery.* 1969, pp 433–434 (abstr).

JANNETTA PJ, RAND RW: Transtentorial microsurgical selective retrogasserian rhizotomy in trigeminal neuralgia. *Fourth International Congress of Neurological Surgery.* New York, Excerpta Medica, 1969, 193:92 (abstr).

ALBIN MS, MILLEN JE, HEDDEN M, JANNETTA PJ: Cardiopulmonary responses to positional changes during neurosurgery. American Society of Anesthesiologists Annual Meeting. 1972 (abstr).

ALBIN MS, JANNETTA PJ, BUNEGIN L: Rapid differential brain cooling using cephalic immersion. Proceedings of the Second Annual Meeting Society of Critical Care Medicine, May, 1973 (**Crit Care Med** 1 (2):121, 1973) (abstr).

ALBIN MS, JANNETTA PJ, BUNEGIN L: Attenuation of anesthetic and emergence responses to ketamine hydrochloride (KH) using tetrahydroaminacrine (THA). Proceedings of the 1973 American Society of Anesthesiologists Annual Meeting. October, 1973, pp 241–243 (abstr).

JANNETTA PJ: Microsurgical relief of neurovascular trigeminal nerve in tic douloureux. **J Dent Res** 53 (Special Issue):128, 1974 (abstr 294).

JANNETTA PJ: Microsurgical relief of neurovascular trigeminal nerve compression in tic douloureux. International Association for Dental Research, Atlanta, GA, March, 1974, and the IV European Congress of Anesthesiologists. Madrid, Spain, 1974 (abstr).

BUNEGIN L, ALBIN MS, JANNETTA PJ: Changes in blood-spinal cord barrier permeability to norepinephrine after impact injury to spinal cord. **Anat Rec** 181 (2):321, 1975.

SHEPTAK PE, MAROON JC, JANNETTA PJ: The two stage excision of huge acoustic neurinomas. Proceedings of the Congress of Neurological Surgery. October, 1975, p 134 (abstr).

ALBIN MS, JANNETTA PJ: Physiopathological responses to changes in brain retractor pressure. Society of Neurosurgery, Anesthesiology, and Neurology (Supplemental Care). October, 1975 (abstr).

ALBIN MS, HUNG TK, BROWN TD, JANNETTA PJ, BUNEGIN L, ALBIN R: Experimental spinal cord injury biomechanics. Fifth Annual Meeting Society for Neuroscience. **Society for Neuroscience Abstracts** 1:697, 1975 (abstr 1079).

KENNERDELL JS, JANNETTA PJ, JOHNSON BL: A steroid sensitive solitary intracranial plasmacytoma. **Excerpta Medica** 34:7, 1975 (abstr).

MAROON JC, LUNSFORD LD, JANNETTA PJ, DEEB ZL: Hemifacial spasm due to aneurysmal compression of the facial nerve. **Stroke** 8 (1):12–13, 1977 (abstr).

ALBIN MS, BROWN TD, BUNEGIN L, ET AL.: Experimental obliteration of aneurysm using electromagnetically induced thermoferrous coagulation. Proceedings of the American Association of Neurological Surgery. Toronto, April, 1977 (abstr).

ALBIN MS, BUNEGIN L, BENNETT MH, DUJOVNY M, JANNETTA PJ: Clinical and experimental brain retraction pressure monitoring. **Acta Neurol Scand Suppl** 56 (Suppl 64):522–523, 1977 (abstr).

BENNETT MH, JANNETTA PJ: Evoked potentials in trigeminal neuralgia. Second World Congress on Pain, August, 1978 (**Pain Abstracts** 1:66) (abstr).

JANNETTA PJ: Microsurgery of cranial nerve cross compression syndromes. Congress of Neurological Surgeons. September, 1978 (abstr).

JANNETTA PJ: Microvascular decompression of cranial nerves. Congress of Neurological Surgeons. September, 1978 (abstr).

JANNETTA PJ, GENDELL HM: Neurovascular compression associated with essential hypertension. **Neurosurgery** 2 (2):165, 1978 (abstr).

JANNETTA PJ, ABASSY M, MAROON JC, MORALES-RAMOS F, ALBIN MS: Etiology and definitive microsurgical treatment of hemifacial spasm: Operative techniques and results in 47 patients, in Dejong R, Sugar O (eds): *Yearbook of Neurology and Neurosurgery*. 1979, pp 429–430 (abstr).

GENDELL HM, JANNETTA PJ: Neurovascular compression of the ventrolateral medulla: Theoretical considerations and experimental model. 29th Annual Meeting of the Congress of Neurological Surgeons. October, 1979 (abstr).

HAINES SJ, ZORUB DS, JANNETTA PJ: The arterial lesion in trigeminal neuralgia. Neurosurgical Society of America, Annual Meeting. White Sulphur Springs, WV, 1979, p 27 (abstr).

HEROS RC, JANNETTA PJ: Cerebellar infarction from traumatic vertebral artery occlusion. A neurosurgical emergency. Neurosurgical Society of America, Annual Meeting. White Sulphur Springs, WV, 1979, p 41 (abstr).

JANNETTA PJ, BLACK FO: A systematic technique for preservation of hearing in small acoustic neurilemmomas. Neurosurgical Society of America, Annual Meeting. White Sulphur Springs, WV, 1979, p 71 (abstr).

BENNETT MH, JANNETTA PJ: Evoked potentials in trigeminal neuralgia. American Association of Neurological Surgeons. April 22, 1980 (abstr).

JANNETTA PJ: Neurovascular compression in cranial nerve and systemic disease. Annual Meeting of the American Surgical Association. Atlanta, GA, 1980, p 69 (abstr 26).

HUNG TC, KOWACH R, HAUBOLD AD, MARTIN RR, JANNETTA PJ: Combined effects of ulti carbon surface and shear stress on human leukocytes. American Society for Artificial Internal Organs, Inc. Anaheim, CA, May, 1981 (**Asaio Abstracts** 10:27, 1981) (abstr).

JANNETTA PJ, SEGAL R, DUJOVNY M, *ET AL.*: Neurogenic hypertension. **Clin Res** 29 (2):211A, 1981 (abstr).

JANNETTA PJ, SEGAL R, DUJOVNY M, *ET AL.*: Neurogenic hypertension. 50th Anniversary Meeting of the American Association of Neurological Surgeons. Boston, MA, 1981, p 43 (abstr S-4).

GRUNDY BL, JANNETTA PJ, LINA A, PROCOPIO PT, BOSTON JR: BAEP monitoring during cerebellopontine angle surgery. **Anesthesiology** 55 (3A):A127, 1981 (abstr).

JANNETTA PJ, SEGAL R, DUJOVNY M, *ET AL.*: Vascular compression in essential hypertension. Neurosurgical Society of America, Annual Meeting. Pebble Beach, CA, 1981, p 41 (abstr).

MØLLER AR, JANNETTA PJ: Neural generators of the brainstem auditory evoked potentials. Fifth Midwinter Research Meeting of the Association for Research in Otolaryngology. St. Petersburg Beach, FL, January 18–21, 1982 (abstr).

SEKHAR LN, SCHULZ N, JANNETTA PJ: Cerebellopontine angle meningomas: Microsurgical excision and follow-up results. Proceedings of the American Association of Neurological Surgeons Annual Meeting. Honolulu, HI, April 1982 (abstr T-56).

WOLFSON SK JR, SEGAL R, JANNETTA PJ, COOK EE, KNUTTI J: Chronically implanted telemetry in neurogenic hypertension research. Proceedings of the American Association of Neurological Surgeons Annual Meeting. Honolulu, HI, April 1982 (abstr T-62).

MØLLER AR, JANNETTA PJ, MØLLER MB: Neural generators of the brainstem auditory evoked potentials (BAEP) in man studied in intracranial recordings. Proceedings of the American Association for Neurological Surgery. Honolulu, HI, April, 1982 (paper 58) (abstr).

GRUNDY BL, JANNETTA PJ, BOSTON JR, PROCOPIO PT, DOYLE E: Evoked potential monitoring during neurosurgical operations. The American Association of Neurological Surgeons Annual Meeting. Honolulu, HI, April, 1982 (paper 59) (abstr).

MØLLER AR, JANNETTA PJ: Neural generators of the brainstem auditory evoked potentials (BAEP) in man studied in intracranial recordings. The Second International Evoked Potentials Symposium. Cleveland, OH, October 18–20, 1982), Woburn, MA, Butterworth Publishers, 1984 (abstr).

MORGAN C, DEGROAT WC, JANNETTA PJ: Leucine enkephalin and substance-P identified in trigeminal ganglion neurons innervating the cornea in the cat. **Society for Neuroscience Abstracts** 8:474, 1982 (abstr 129.6).

FRIONI C, MORGAN C, NADELHAFT I, DEGROAT WC, JANNETTA PJ: Identification of neurons in the superior cervical ganglion innervating the cornea of the cat. **Society for Neuroscience Abstracts** 8:553, 1982 (abstr 153.9).

MØLLER AR, JANNETTA PJ, MØLLER MB: Intracranially recorded auditory nerve response in man. **O.R.L. Digest** October, 1982, p 15 (abstr).

NIELSEN VK, JANNETTA PJ: Ectopic excitation and ephatic transmission in hemifacial spasm. **Neurology** 33 (Suppl 2):184, 1983 (abstr 3).

NIELSEN VK, JANNETTA PJ: Hemifacial spasm. Electro-physiologic effects of facial nerve decompression. **Electroencephalogr Clin Neurophysiol** 56 (3):S144, 1983 (abstr F233).

JANNETTA PJ, MØLLER AR, MØLLER MB: Preservation of hearing in acoustic neurinomas. Annual Meeting of the Congress of Neurological Surgeons. New York, NY, 1984, p 212 (abstr).

EIDELMAN BH, JANNETTA PJ, MØLLER MB, NIELSEN VK: A syndrome of hemifacial spasm and multiple cranial neuropathy. **Neurology** 34 (Suppl 1):160, 1984 (abstr 126).

MOSTER M, NIELSEN VK, JANNETTA PJ: Threshold current for ephaptic transmission in hemifacial spasm. **Am Neurol Assn** 16 (1):149, 1984 (abstr P139).

BOSTON JR, JANNETTA PJ, DENEALT LG, KRONK L: Interpeak latency changes during intraoperative monitoring of brainstem auditory evoked potentials. **Electroencephalogr Clin Neurophysiol** 61 (2):31P, 1985 (abstr 59).

JANNETTA PJ: Hemifacial spasm. Fifth International Workshop on Neurological Surgery of the Ear and Skull Base. February, 1985 (abstr).

MARION DW, TAYLOR F, JANNETTA PJ: The use of perioperative steroids in microvascular decompression operations: A prosective series of 145 patients. Annual Meeting of the Congress of Neurological Surgeons. Honolulu, HI, 1985, p 144 (abstr).

JANNETTA PJ, MØLLER MB, MØLLER AR: Neurovascular decompression for vertigo. Fifth International Workshop on Neurological Surgery of the Ear and Skull Base. February, 1985 (abstr).

MØLLER AR, JANNETTA PJ: Monitoring of facial function during removal of acoustic tumors. Fifth International Workshop of Neurological Surgery of the Ear and Skull Base. Sarasota, FL, February, 1985 (abstr).

BOSTON JR, DENAULT LG, KRONK L, JANNETTA PJ: Experience with a continuous monitoring algorithm for BAEP during retromastoid craniectomies. **Electroencephalogr Clin Neurophysiol** 61 (3): S145, 1985 (abstr P21.09).

MØLLER AR, JANNETTA PJ: Monitoring auditory functions during cranial nerve microvascular decompression operations by direct recording from the eighth cranial nerve. *Yearbook of Neurology and Neurosurgery.* 1985, pp 481–483, (abstr).

JHO HD, JANNETTA PJ, COOK EE: Animal models simulating pulsatile vascular compression at facial nerve root entry zone in dogs. Annual Meeting of the American Association of Neurological Surgeons. Denver, CO, 1986, p 203 (abstr 15).

SEGAL R, NADELHAFT I, WOLFSON SK, KUPPEL BA, COOK EE, JANNETTA PJ: Ventrolateral medulla projections to the thoracic spinal cord in the baboon. Annual Meeting of the Congress of Neurological Surgeons. New Orleans, LA, 1986, p 224 (abstr).

JANNETTA PJ, MØLLER AR, MØLLER MB: Evaluation and criteria for preservation of hearing in acoustic neurinoma removal. Annual Meeting of the Neurosurgical Society of America. Point Clear, AL, 1986, p 27 (abstr).

JANNETTA PJ: Trigeminal neuralgia and atypical trigeminal neuralgia. International Symposium on the Surgery of the Lower Cranial Nerves. Ljubljana, Yugoslavia, May, 1987 (abstr).

JANNETTA PJ: Vascular compression of the cranial nerves and brain stem as a concept of disease. International Symposium on the Surgery of the Lower Cranial Nerves. Ljubljana, Yugoslavia, May, 1987 (abstr).

NIELSEN VK, EIDELMAN BH, JANNETTA PJ: Ectopic excitation of the eleventh nerve as a possible cause of spasmodic torticollis. **Neurology** 37 (Suppl 1):369, 1987 (abstr PP581).

SEGAL R, NADELHAFT I, WOLFSON SK, COOK EE, JANNETTA PJ: Ventrolateral medulla projections to the intermediolateral nucleus of the thoracic cord in the baboon. **Am J Hypertens** 1 (3, Pt. 2):29–30A, 1988 (abstr).

JHO HD, JANNETTA PJ: Spasmodic torticollis treated with microvascular decompression of the spinal accessory nerve and the brainstem. Annual Meeting of the American Association of Neurological Surgery. Washington, DC, 1989, p 94 (abstr 15).

SEKHAR LN, JANNETTA PJ, BURKHART LE: Clivus meningiomas. Microsurgical excision and follow-up results. Annual Meeting of the American Association of Neurological Surgeons. Nashville, TN, 1990, p 158 (abstr 733).

NANDA A, JANNETTA PJ, MØLLER AR, MØLLER MB: Hearing preservation in acoustic neurinomas. A review. Annual Meeting of the American Association of Neurological Surgeons. Nashville, TN, 1990, p 226 (abstr 743).

DONG M, KOFKE WA, ACUFF J, POLICARE R, JANNETTA PJ, SEKHAR LN: The effects of anesthetic induction upon cerebral blood flow velocities in neurosurgical patients. Fifth International Intracranial Hemodynamics Symposium. San Francisco, February, 1991 (**J Cardiovasc Tech** 9 (3):308, 1991) (abstr).

LARKINS MV, JANNETTA PJ: Recurrent hemifacial spasm. Re-operative outcome. Annual Meeting of the Congress of Neurological Surgeons. Orlando, FL, 1991, p 55 (abstr).

MØLLER MB, MØLLER AR, JANNETTA PJ, JHO HD: Results of microvascular decompression (MVD) surgery in patients with disabling positional vertigo (DVP). Second European Congress of Oto-Rhino-Laryngology and Cervico-Facial Surgery. Sorrento, Italy, June, 1992. (*Abstract Book,* Bologna, Italy, Monduzzi Editore, p 163) (abstr).

SOSO MJ, JANNETTA PJ, GUILIANI MJ: Touch sensation and blink reflexes in trigeminal neuralgia. American Association of Electrophysiological Monitoring Annual Meeting. **Muscle Nerve** 15:1184, 1992 (abstr).

BARKER FG, JANNETTA PJ, JHO HD, BISSONETTE DJ: Microvascular decompression for typical trigeminal neuralgia. A 20 year experience. 62nd Meeting of the American Association of Neurological Surgeons. San Diego, CA, 1994, p 145 (abstr).

KONDZIOLKA D, LEMLEY T, JANNETTA PJ, LUNSFORD LD, KESTLE JRW, FROMM GH: Double-blind, randomized, placebo-controlled trial of ophthalmic anesthesia (proparacaine hydrochloride) for patients with trigeminal neuralgia. 62nd Meeting of the American Association of Neurological Surgeons. San Diego, CA, 1994, p 210 (abstr).

SOSO MJ, DURANT JD, GIULIANI MJ, LOVELY TJ, JANNETTA PJ: Auditory phenomena in hemifacial spasm (P01.058). **Neurology** 46:A131, 1996 (abstr).

Presentations (2)

JANNETTA PJ: Microvascular decompression for trigeminal neuralgia (videotape). The Video Journal of Neurosurgery. The Professional Information Library. Dallas, Texas, 1984.

JANNETTA PJ: Microvascular decompression for hemifacial spasm (videotape). The Video Journal of Neurosurgery. The Professional Information Library. Dallas, Texas, 1984.

Book Reviews (3)

JANNETTA PJ: **J Neurosurg** 49:773–774, 1978. *Microsurgery for stroke.*

JANNETTA PJ: **Surg Rounds** 8:126–128, 1985. *Operative Neurosurgical Techniques: Indications, Methods and Results.*

JANNETTA PJ: **Psychiatry Digest** 1970, p. 69. *The Hypertensive Vascular Crisis.*

Letters Published (18)

JANNETTA PJ: Tic douloureux and facial spasm (letter). **JAMA** 228 (13):1637–1638, 1974.

JANNETTA PJ: Complications from microsurgical treatment of tic douloureux (letter). **J Neurosurg** 40 (5):675, 1974.

MAROON JC, ALBIN MS, JANNETTA PJ: Air embolism. Diagnosis and treatment (letter). **N Engl J Med** 293 (23):1211, 1975.

JANNETTA PJ: Hemifacial spasm (letter). **J Neurosurg** 48 (2):317–318, 1978.

JANNETTA PJ: Glossopharyngeal neuralgia (letter). **JAMA** 239 (20): 2173, 1978.

HAINES SJ, JANNETTA PJ: Microvascular relationships of the trigeminal nerve (letter). **J Neurosurg** 53 (3):425–426, 1980.

JANNETTA PJ: Response to letter to the editor by Ramamurthi B: Two-stage excision of acoustic neurinomas. **J Neurosurg** 53 (2):273, 1980.

SEGAL R, JANNETTA PJ: Letter concerning "Microsurgical anatomy of the posterior inferior cerebellar artery." **Neurosurgery** 11 (4):581, 1982.

JANNETTA PJ: Hemifacial spasm. Treatment by posterior fossa surgery (letter). **J Neurol Neurosurg Psychiatry** 46 (5):465, 1983.

NIELSEN VK, SOSO MJ, JANNETTA PJ: Hemifacial spasm. Difficulties in locating the lesion electrophysiologically (letter). **Muscle Nerve** 7 (8):682–683, 1984.

JANNETTA PJ, MØLLER MB, MØLLER AR: Disabling positional vertigo (letter). **N Engl J Med** 311 (16):1053–1055, 1984.

MØLLER AR, JANNETTA PJ: Response to the letter to the editor by Prass R, Luders H: Constant-current versus constant-voltage stimulation. **J Neurosurg** 62 (4):623, 1985.

JANNETTA PJ: Trigeminal neuralgia (letter). **Neurosurgery** 18 (5): 677, 1986.

MØLLER AR, JANNETTA PJ: Pathophysiology of hemifacial spasm. Localization of the lesion in hemifacial spasm (letter). **Neurology** 36 (4):591–592, 1986.

MØLLER AR, JANNETTA PJ: Device to locate facial nerve during surgery (letter). **Arch Otolaryngol Head Neck Surg** 112 (6):679, 1986.
JANNETTA PJ: Spasmodic torticollis (letter). **J Neurosurg** 65 (5):725, 1986.
JANNETTA PJ: Hemifacial spasm resolution without vascular decompression (letter). **Neurosurgery** 20 (1):63, 1987.
JANNETTA PJ: Complications of cranial nerve microvascular decompression (letter). **Neurosurgery** 22 (2):352, 1988.

Comments (4)

JANNETTA PJ, HIRSCH BE: **Am J Otol** 14:627, 1993. Comment on: Restoration of useful hearing following microvascular decompression of cochlear nerve.
JANNETTA PJ: **Neurosurgery** 35:1137, 1994. Comment on: Primary intraosseous orbital hemangioma. A case report and review of the literature.
JANNETTA PJ: **Neurosurgery** 36:63, 1995. Comment on: Glossopharyngeal neuralgia with cardiac syncope.
JANNETTA PJ: **Neurosurgery** 35:669–670, 1995. Comment on: Repeat operations in failed micrivascular decompression for trigeminal neuralgia.

Editor's Notes (1)

JANNETTA PJ: In Currier RD (ed): *The Yearbook of Neurology and Neurosurgery.* 1986, p 237.

Other Publications (10)

JANNETTA PJ, FURCHGOTT R: Method. The rabbit aorta bioassay for catecholamines in urine, in Helmer O (ed): *Handbook of Clinical Chemistry.* Vol. III, 1960.
JANNETTA PJ (interview): Taking pressure off facial nerves. *Medical World News,* 1972, p 44.
JANNETTA PJ (interview): Extra cut to cut facial pain. *Medical World News,* 14 (8):28, 1973 (and rebuttal of letter to the editor, *Medical World News,* 14 (21):12, 1973).
JANNETTA PJ (interview): Brain surgery reverses "essential" hypertension. *Medical World News,* 20 (24):12, 1979.
LAHA RK, JANNETTA PJ: Atypical trigeminal neuralgia. **Ann Am Inst Oral Biol** 30:51–59, 1980.
JANNETTA PJ: Hemifacial spasm. *Neurology and Neurosurgery Update Series.* Vol 3, no. 8, 1982.

JANNETTA PJ: Forward, in Sekhar LN, Schramm VL Jr (eds): *Tumors of the Cranial Base: Diagnosis and Treatment.* Mount Kisco, New York, Futura Publishing Co., 1987, pix.

ROVIT RL, MURALI R, JANNETTA PJ: Preface, in Rovit RL, Murali R, Jannetta PJ (eds): *Trigeminal Neuralgia.* Baltimore, Williams & Wilkins, 1990, p vii–viii.

JANNETTA PJ: Forward, in Lang J (ed): *Clinical Anatomy of the Posterior Fossa and Its Foramina.* New York, Thieme Medical Publishers, 1990, p v.

JANNETTA PJ (interview): Thoughts from (and for) our new secretary of health [Interview by David Woods]. **PA Med,** 98:21, 1995.

Selected Invited Lectures

1. April 4–9, 1977. American College of Surgeons. 25th Anniversary Meeting. Santiago, Chile.
2. October 18, 1980. William H. Swanson Memorial Lecture. University of Pittsburgh Dental Alumni Association—Dental Alumni Day. Pittsburgh, Pennsylvania.
3. March 29–April 4, 1981. Fifty-fourth General Scientific Meeting. Royal Australian College of Surgeons. Hobart, Australia.
4. April 27–28, 1981. American Academy of Neurology. Toronto, Ontario.
5. May 8–10, 1981. Sixth Annual Sir William Osler Lecture. Monterey, Mexico.
6. October 5–13, 1981. 40th Annual Meeting of Japanese Neurosurgical Society. Kyoto, Japan.
7. March 24, 1983. Dr. Hayes Agnew Lecture. Agnew Surgical Society of University of Pennsylvania. Philadelphia, Pennsylvania.
8. October 2–5, 1983. 108th Annual Meeting of the American Neurological Association. New Orleans, Louisiana.
9. November 28–30, 1983. Herbert Olivercrona Lecture. Karolinska Institutet. Stockholm, Sweden.
10. September 3–6, 1984. Vth International Symposium on the Facial Nerve. Bordeaux, France.
11. October 23–26, 1984. Forty-Third General Assembly of the Japan Neurosurgical Society. Chiba, Japan.
12. February 18–23, 1985. International Symposium on Surgery in and around the Brain Stem and the Third Ventricle. Hanover, W. Germany.
13. July 7–13, 1985. Eighth International Congress of Neurological Surgery. Toronto, Canada.
14. December 6, 1985. Royal Society of Medicine. London, England.

15. January 23–26, 1986. Neurosurgical Society of the Virginias. Hot Springs, Maryland.
16. September 29–October 7, 1986. International Conference on Controversies in Otology and Otoneurosurgery. Sardinia, Italy.
17. February 23, 1987. Long Beach Surgical Society. Long Beach, California.
18. September 11, 1987. First W. Eugene Stern Visiting Professor of Neurosurgery. University of California at Los Angeles, Los Angeles, California.
19. November 2, 1987. Thomas J. Speakman Memorial Lecture. University of Alberta, Edmonton, Canada.
20. June 12–16, 1988. Rocky Mountain Neurosurgical Society. Lake Tahoe, Nevada.
21. October 1–6, 1988. VI International Symposium on the facial nerve. Rio de Janeiro, Argentina.
22. December 8–10, 1988. Buenos Aires Province Society. Pinamar, Argentina.
23. January 18–21, 1989. Sally Harrington Goldwater Visiting Professor. Phoenix, Arizona.
24. June 1–3, 1989. University of California San Diego, California.
25. November 12–14, 1990. NIH Consensus Development Conference. Bethesda, Maryland.
26. November 15, 1990. The John E. Adams Visiting Professor Lecture. University of California at San Francisco. San Francisco, California.
27. January 15, 1991. William Beaumont Medical Research Society Lecturer. The George Washington University Medical Center. Washington, D.C.
28. March 22–23, 1991. Invited Guest Lecturer. Francis P. Boland Surgical Symposium. Scranton, Pennsylvania.
29. May 31,–June 2, 1991. Franc D. Ingraham Visiting Professor. Harvard Medical School. Boston, Massachusetts.
30. September 27–28, 1991. Visiting Professor. University of Indiana. Indianapolis, Indiana.
31. October 30, 1991. Henry Schmidek Lecture. American Association of Neurological Surgeons/Congress of Neurological Surgeons. Review and Update in Neurobiology for Neurosurgeons. Woods Hole, Massachusetts.
32. November 4–5, 1991. The E. Harry Botterell Professorship in Neurosurgery. University of Toronto. Toronto, Canada.
33. March 27, 1992. Neurosurgery Grand Rounds, Mt. Sinai Medical Center, New York, New York.

34. June 15–16, 1992. Invited Presenter and Moderator. First International Skull Base Congress. Hannover, Germany.
35. November 6–7, 1992. Visiting Professor, Department of Neurosurgery, University of Minnesota, Minneapolis, Minnesota.
36. November 11, 1992. Visiting Professor, Department of Neurosurgery, Wayne State University, Detroit, Michigan.
37. December 3, 1992. Visiting Professor. Section of Neurosurgery, University of Chicago, Chicago, Illinois.
38. February 25, 1993. Visiting Professor, Department of Neurosurgery, Temple University. Philadelphia, Pennsylvania.
39. March 17, 1993. Arthur A. Ward Lecturer. Department of Neurosurgery, University of Washington. Seattle, Washington.
40. March 19–20, 1993. Invited Lecturer. North Pacific Neurology and Psychiatry Society Annual Meeting. Semi-Ah-Moo Resort, Blaine, Washington.
41. March 25, 1993. Invited Lecturer. The Jerusalem Symposium on Surgery of the Skull Base and Adjacent Midline Region. Jerusalem, Israel.
42. June 4, 1993. Invited Lecturer. National Heart, Lung, and Blood Institute Workshop: "Clinical Neurobiology in Blood Pressure Regulation." NIH. Bethesda, Maryland.
43. October 12, 1993. Hugo V. Rizzoli Lecturer.' Decade of the Brain International Conference. George Washington University, Washington, D.C.
44. February 7, 1994. Paul C. Bucy Lecturer. Review Course in Neurological Surgery. The National Center for Advanced Medical Education. Chicago, Illinois.
45. April 29, 1994. Joseph McDonald Lecturer. University of Rochester (NY).
46. March 6, 1996. Horatio Alger National Scholarship Award. Central Cambria High School, Pennsylvania.
47. March 22, 1996. Dr. Loyd C. Megison, Jr. Visiting Professor of Neurosurgery. "The Aging Brain, the Base of the Skull, and the Neurosurgeon" Louisiana State University Medical Center, Shreveport, Louisiana.
48. May 11, 1996. Visiting Professor, Oregon Health Sciences University, Portland, Oregon.

MEMBERSHIPS IN PROFESSIONAL AND SCIENTIFIC SOCIETIES

Acoustic Neuroma Association—Medical Advisory Board
Allegheny County Medical Society
Alpha Omega Alpha, Beta Chapter—University of Pennsylvania
American Academy of Clinical Neurophysiology

American Academy of Neurological Surgery
American Association for the Advancement of Science
American Association of Neurological Surgeons—multiple committees
American College of Surgeons—multiple committees
American Medical Association
American Pain Society—Public Information Committee
American Society of Evoked Potential Monitoring—Advisory Board
American Society of Neurophysiological Monitoring—Advisory Board
American Surgical Association
Congress of Neurological Surgeons
International Association for the Study of Pain
International Association for the Study of Pain
      Eastern USA Regional Chapter
International Skull Base Study Group—1988
International Society of Pediatric Neurosurgery
Mid-Atlantic Neurosurgical Society—Board of Directors
Neurosurgical Society of America—Vice President, 1981–1982
New York Academy of Sciences
North American Skull Base Society—founding member, 1989
Pennsylvania Emergency Health Services Council
Pennsylvania Medical Society
Pennsylvania Neurosurgical Society—Board of Directors, Vice President, 1982, President, 1984
Pittsburgh Academy of Medicine—Board of Directors
Pittsburgh Neuroscience Society—President, 1972–1973
Pittsburgh Surgical Society
Ravdin-Rhoads Surgical Society
Research Society of Neurological Surgeons—Host, 1976
Societe Internationale de Chirurgie—United States Chapter
Society for Neuroscience
Society of Critical Care Medicine
Society of Neurosurgical Anesthesia and Neurologic Supportive Care
      Vice President, 1980–1981
      President-Elect, 1981–1982
      President, 1982–1983
Society of Neurological Surgeons—multiple committees
      Program Chairman, 1978
Society of Neurological Surgeons—Vice President, 1991–1992
Trigeminal Neuralgia Association, Chief of Medical Advisory Board
World Federation of Neurosurgical Societies—Second Vice-President
      at large

HONORS AND AWARDS

1949–1953	Pennsylvania State Senatorial Scholarship
1956 summer	Lederle Student Research Fellowship
1956–1957	National Chairman, Committee on Medical Education Student American Medical Association
1957 June	I.S. Ravdin Prize in Surgery University of Pennsylvania School of Medicine
1960 June	Borroughs Wellcome Traveling Fellow, London, England
1960–1963	NIH Fellow in Academic Surgery (Neurosurgery) University of Pennsylvania School of Medicine
1976–1978	Francis Sargent Cheever Distinguished Professor University of Pittsburgh School of Medicine
Nov. 29, 1983	Herbert Olivecrona Lecturer Karolinska Institutet (Stockholm, Sweden)
Feb. 23, 1987	Long Beach Surgical Society—Honorary Member
Sept. 11, 1987	First W. Eugene Stern Visiting Professor of Neurosurgery University of California at Los Angeles School of Medicine
Nov. 2, 1987	Thomas J. Speakman Memorial Lecturer— University of Alberta School of Medicine
May 24, 1988	York High School—25th Member of the William Penn Senior High School Hall of Fame
1989	Rocky Mountain Neurosurgery Society—Honorary Member
Sept. 1989	Doctor of Science, Honoris Causa Washington and Jefferson College
Oct. 1989	German Society for Plastic and Reconstructive Surgery— Honorary Member
Jan. 27, 1990	Man of the Year in the Sciences, Vectors/Pittsburgh
May 18, 1990	Horatio Alger Association—Member
May 1992	University of Pittsburgh—Walter E. Dandy Professor
May 1993	Deutsche Gesellschaft für Chirurgie—Corresponding Member
Nov. 1993	World Federation of Neurosurgical Societies—Second Vice-President at Large
Nov. 1994	American Academy of Neurological Surgery—elected to active membership
July 1996	Italian-American Man of the Year—Italian Scholarship Fund

LISTED IN

Who's Who in the East
Who's Who in America

Contents

——————————————— I ———————————————

GENERAL SCIENTIFIC SESSION I
CRITERIA FOR PATIENT SELECTION

—————————————— II ——————————————
GENERAL SCIENTIFIC SESSION II
HOW THE OPERATION IS DONE

—————————————— IV ——————————————
GENERAL SCIENTIFIC SESSION IV
TREATMENT OF POSTERIOR FOSSA TUMORS

1

Presidential Address: "How Do You Know?"

STEPHEN J. HAINES, M.D.

Perhaps never in the history of medicine have we been so challenged to answer such a simple sounding question as: "How do you know?" From the daily problems of patient care ("How do you know the right way to do a cervical discectomy?" "How do you know the right treatment for sciatica?") to matters of broader patient-care policy ("How do you know the value of reoperation for glioblastoma?") and new interventions ("How do you know the value of radiosurgery for trigeminal neuralgia?"), from seemingly mundane financial affairs ("How do you know the cost of running your practice?") to weighty considerations of broad scope ("How do you know the value of neurosurgery to the health-care system?"), we are asked to document our beliefs with more objectivity, reliability, and reproducibility than ever before. So today, and for the rest of this meeting, and for the rest of your practicing lives, I ask you to take a journey with me to try to understand how it is that we do know that what we do is the right or best thing to do.

LEARNING TO COUNT

We know that much of the authority of practitioners of healing arts in the past relied on appeals to divine or mystical power. Some of the earliest great observers of human anatomy and physiology had their pronouncements enshrined as dogma that controlled the practice of medicine for centuries. The idea that careful tabulation of the results of treatment might lead to better understanding of the best way to treat patients is relatively new.

Pierre Charles Alexandre Louis promoted a method including:

- careful observation and description of clinical details
- systematic record keeping
- rigorous analysis of multiple cases

Presidential Address delivered at the 44th Annual Meeting of the Congress of Neurological Surgeons, Montreal, Quebec, Canada, September 30, 1996.

- cautious generalizations based solely upon observed facts
- verification through autopsy (1, 3).

In 1825 he published an influential study tabulating the results of treatment of tuberculosis with bleeding and finding no evidence of a beneficial effect (8). This and subsequent studies in typhoid fever refuted the dogmatic reliance on bleeding that dominated medicine at that time.

In 1837 there was a great debate in the French Academy of Sciences between Louis and the defender of the status quo, Monsieur Double (4, 9). Essentially, Double claimed that the individual variation between patients exceeded any tendency toward group similarities, observing that ". . . numerical and statistical calculations, open to many sources of fallacy, [are] in no degree applicable to therapeutics."

Louis' claim was that ". . . a therapeutic agent cannot be employed with any discrimination or probability of success in a given case unless its general efficacy in analogous cases has been previously ascertained . . .. Therefore I conceive that without the aid of statistics nothing like real medical science is possible." In essence, Louis concluded that the effect of the treatment must exceed the variation in effectiveness between patients if the treatment is to be advocated for a specific condition. Many American physicians came to Paris to learn from Louis. Tabulation gradually became a standard approach for determining the value of a treatment.

PARALLEL DEVELOPMENT OF NEUROSURGERY AND BIOSTATISTICS

Neurosurgery was not very far advanced at that time, and one would have expected the new field to take advantage of the opportunity to use the most advanced newly developed tools of evaluation to secure its place in the medical armamentarium. Neurosurgery and biostatistics developed in parallel during the last 150 years, and it is an interesting exercise to apply a developmental assessment to neurosurgery's use of evaluative technology.

Table 1 lists the major advances in neurosurgery and biostatistics during the past 150 years as I see them. It was a bit difficult to construct this table for statistics, but the list comes from an historical work by Gehan and Lemak (5) and from discussions with several practicing statisticians.

Where is neurosurgery on the evaluation time line? I asked this question one way in 1979 (6). Reviewing all clinical articles published in the *Journal of Neurosurgery* up to that point, most of them used the most rudimentary evaluation techniques: tables developed by Louis in the 1820s and statistics from the early 1900s. Only 18 of 4865 at-

TABLE 1.
Advances in Neurosurgery and Biostatistics

Time	(Bio)statistics	(Neuro)surgery
Forever	Appeal to the gods	Appeal to the gods
1st millennium AD	Appeal to dogma	Appeal to dogma
1800–1850	Counting/tabulation	Anesthesia
1850–1900	Probability theory, normal distribution, standard deviation	Antisepsis
1900s	Student's t-test, χ^2 test	Sphygmomanometry
1910s	Maximum likelihood methods	Electrocautery
1920s	Experimental design and ANOVA	Ventriculography
1930s	Multivariate analysis	Angiography
1940s	RCT	Myelography
1950s	Odds ratio/relative risk	Steroids
1960s	Life tables	Microsurgery
1970s	Logistic regression	CT scan
1980s	Meta-analysis	Magnetic resonance imaging (MRI) scan
1990s	Exploratory data analysis	Radiosurgery

tempted to use controls, 10 of these with randomization and just 1 with blinding techniques. In the 1970s we were learning to use computerized tomography (CT) scans in neurosurgery, and we were evaluating them with techniques from the 19th century.

If we look at the major advance of the 1990s, radiosurgery, we find that, despite a smattering of more sophisticated techniques, most of the evaluation is done with ancient and outmoded technology. It is as if we were operating with ether, monopolar cautery, and without steroids or the microscope.

There has been a large paradigm shift in the understanding of how to find the truth that is buried in our observations and interpretations of it: a shift from faith and dogma to repeatable observation and hypothesis testing. Technological advances have dominated changes in neurosurgery over the same period of time. We are just beginning to understand the fallacies of observation and to apply modern techniques to evaluation.

PAVING STONES ON THE ROAD OF GOOD INTENTIONS

Why all the fuss, some will say. Are not advances in surgery self-evident? No—and sometimes our desire to help our patients gets in the way of our understanding how best to do it. Why do we have so much trouble making good evaluations of what we do? Mostly because we want to succeed—to have our patients do well because we have done our jobs well. Those good intentions may lead us to overlook some of the reality checks that we encounter along the way.

I would classify these good intentions that may lead to a distorted view of success as:

- the desire to do good and well
- the *surgeon's* selective memory
- the patient's kindness
- and the old saw, "only time will tell."

Desire to Do Good and Well

Let me tell the extracranial-intracranial (EC-IC) bypass story with a perspective different from what you have probably heard before. Believing that carotid endarterectomy prevented ischemic stroke by restoring normal blood flow, and knowing that some patients suffering ischemic stroke had stenotic lesions beyond the reach of endarterectomy, wise and technically sophisticated neurosurgeons reasoned that restoring intracranial blood flow by bypassing the stenosis should prevent stroke. My first mentor in neurosurgery, Pete Donaghy, and his first microsurgical fellow, Gazi Yasargil, developed and simultaneously performed the first EC-IC bypasses. To many, it was self-evident that this was the correct solution to the problem and when the technical success of the procedure was demonstrated, it was declared the standard of therapy.

Unfortunately, it was another beautiful theory destroyed by a few dirty facts. When applied to a population of patients who accurately represented the population undergoing the operation in actual practice and after the results were carefully and objectively observed, recorded, and analyzed, it was found that the operation had no net benefit over nonoperative therapy.

A few still think the benefit is self-evident. I have heard a distinguished neurosurgeon say that he cannot see one of these patients living with the threat of stroke from inaccessible stenosis and send him home without doing *something* for him. This is a laudable emotion but does not justify an ineffective operation. He says "but I know that the operation works," and I say: "Show me—how do you know?"

The Surgeon's Selective Memory

Another problem with our traditional way of evaluating surgical progress is the (selective) surgical memory. One of my colleagues is fond of telling us of the importance of surgical memory: the ability to remember great results and forget bad ones. He says it is essential to the practice of neurosurgery, for anyone who dwells on poor outcomes soon becomes ineffective. He is as fond of telling us that he has never seen a complication of a certain procedure as we are of reminding him of the last time it happened.

In many ways he is right: in day-to-day practice we must focus on the positive. However, what is good for daily practice may not be good for policy making. Our daily optimism must be based on sound observation or else we will make daily errors. How often do we find that our personal estimate of the rate, say, of postendarterectomy stroke or shunt infection is noticeably lower than what we find when our last 100 cases are carefully reviewed? It is very difficult to accurately estimate low-frequency events from memory and when we do we frequently fool ourselves.

The Patient's Kindness

Our patients also desperately want us to succeed. Many are reluctant to tell us about our failures. I have done a large number of microvascular decompressions for trigeminal neuralgia and hemifacial spasm with what I think are excellent results. I try to be open to patient concerns and encourage comments about less than optimal outcomes.

The patients have been grateful and supportive of the operations. When we hired a nurse-clinician to help care for these patients, we found what seemed to be an unusually high incidence of persistent postoperative headache. It turned out that the patients were so glad to be relieved of their primary symptom (and probably, so happy to be alive after brain surgery) that they simply didn't want to bother me with their headaches.

We've essentially solved the headache problem by doing cranioplasties at the end of the procedures, but we wouldn't have even known about the problem without getting someone other than the surgeon involved with the postoperative follow-up. My point is that what seems self-evident—the success or failure of neurosurgery—isn't, and that this is not just an academic concept but applies to daily practice.

"Only Time Will Tell"

One of the most common approaches to evaluation is simply to keep doing a new operation until the weight of opinion determines its usefulness or lack thereof—"Only time will tell." The statement suggests that there is no other (or at least no better) way of doing the evaluation. This is manifestly not true. Table 2 summarizes data comparing the evaluation of neurosurgical therapy in five content areas using either randomized clinical trials or nonrandomized techniques.

In each content area, the value of the treatment under study was not clear after years of nonrandomized evaluation took place. When the number of patients evaluated in inconclusive nonrandomized studies is

TABLE 2.
Controlled versus Uncontrolled Studies in Neurosurgery

Content Area	Uncontrolled		RCT		Ratio
	No. of Studies	N	No. of Studies	N	Uncontrolled/RCT
Antifibrinolytic therapy	21	3,398	8	479	7.1
Chemonucleolysis	>20	>20,000	3	234	>85.5
Antibiotic prophylaxis	15	13,787	5	2,713	6.3
EC-IC bypass	23	2,662	1	1,377	1.9
Carotid endarterectomy	51	17,484	3	1,626	10.8

compared to the number required to obtain a definitive evaluation in RCTs, the results are stunning. The ratio of inconclusive nonrandomized patients to conclusive randomized patients ranges from 2 to 1 to greater than 85 to 1. Clearly, advanced clinical research techniques can find a result much faster and more efficiently than trusting to the passage of time.

Indeed, the passage of time may obscure the true value of a procedure. A useless procedure may seem beneficial because related therapy has improved. A useful procedure may not seem so because of a change in diagnostic criteria, decline in severity of disease over time, and so on. There are many ways better than the passage of time to evaluate new procedures, such as case-control studies, cohort studies, and clinical trials.

FIFTY-SEVEN WAYS TO FOOL YOURSELF

David Sackett, the first North American physician since Osler to be appointed to the Professorship of Medicine at Oxford, has catalogued many ways of fooling one's self at every stage of studying a clinical phenomenon (11). Table 3 emphasizes that there are a multitude of traps in the process.

TOOLS OF KNOWING

The tools available to us fall into four categories:
- logic
- training
- experience
- experimentation or science

Logic is often the first tool used. Faced with a new situation, for which we have no experience or training, we argue from basic principles to

TABLE 3.

Fifty-Seven Ways to Fool Yourself

Literature review	Compliance
Rhetoric	Therapeutic personality (placebo)
"All's well"	Bogus control
One-sided reference	
Positive results	Outcome measurement
"Hot stuff"	Insensitive measure
	Rumination
Sampling	End digit
Popularity	Apprehension
Centripetal	Unacceptability
Referral filter	Obsequiousness
Diagnostic access	Expectation
Diagnostic suspicion	Substitution
Unmasking	Family information
Mimicry	Exposure suspicion
Previous opinion	Recall
Wrong sample size	Attention
Admission rate	Instrument
Prevalence/incidence	
Diagnostic vogue	Analysis
Diagnostic purity	Post-hoc significance
Procedure selection	Data dredging
Missing data	Scale degradation
Chronology	Tidying-up
Starting time	Repeated peeks
Unacceptability	
Migratory	Interpretation
Membership	Mistaken identity
Nonrespondent	Cognitive dissonance
Volunteer	Magnitude
	Significance
Intervention	Correlation
Contamination	Underexhaustion
Withdrawal	

arrive at a plan of action. This usually requires that we assign different values or weights to the facts available. Often what seems "logical" to one person seems illogical to another because the basic principles used or the weights assigned are different.

For example, when a managed health-care plan sets up shop in a community which has not had one before, it seems logical to some physicians to fight, refuse to participate, and organize against the plan, whereas to others it seems logical to adapt, understand the rules by which they operate, and participate while maintaining as much advantage as possible. Logic is obviously a blunt tool, sometimes the only one available, but is very fallible and leads to inconsistent, frequently ineffective, solutions.

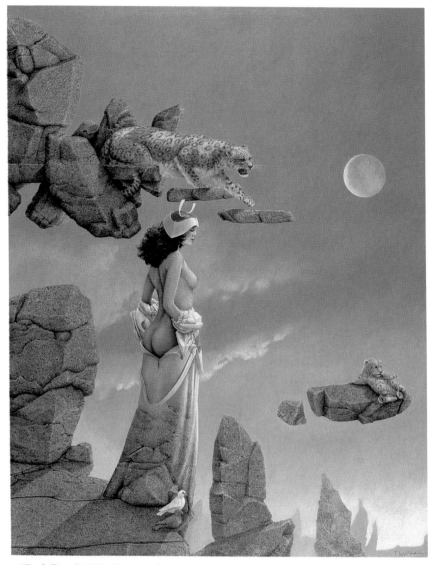

"Rock Dove" 1982 oil on wood 110 × 90 cm © 1996 Michael Parkes/Steltman Galleries New York

The second tool is training. When one wishes to become expert in dealing with a set of situations and there already exists a number of experts in the field, that expertise can be acquired most efficiently by learning from those experts. This is essentially organized experience—learning from others' mistakes.

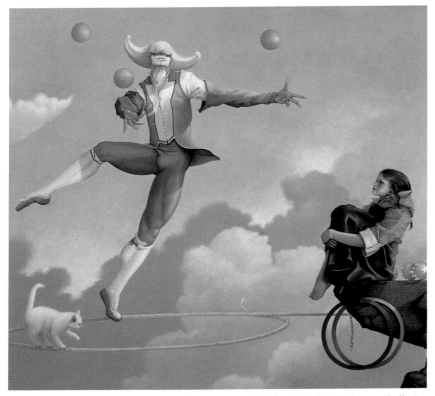

"Juggler" 1981 oil on wood 110 × 90 cm © 1996 Michael Parkes/Steltman Galleries New York

I have had the very good fortune to learn from a number of outstanding neurosurgeons:

- my father, Gerald Haines, from whom I have learned more about the attitude, energy, and discipline needed for the practice of neurosurgery than anyone else could teach me
- Pete Donaghy, the most truly humble pioneer neurosurgery has ever known
- Peter Jannetta, whose ability to create an atmosphere of learning, inquiry, and innovation is unparalleled
- Shelley Chou, a man of patient intelligence, who conquers every problem to which he applies his considerable intellectual skills and inspires respect from all who work with him
- Roberto Heros, who has an unusual ability to guide the hands of those with whom he is operating

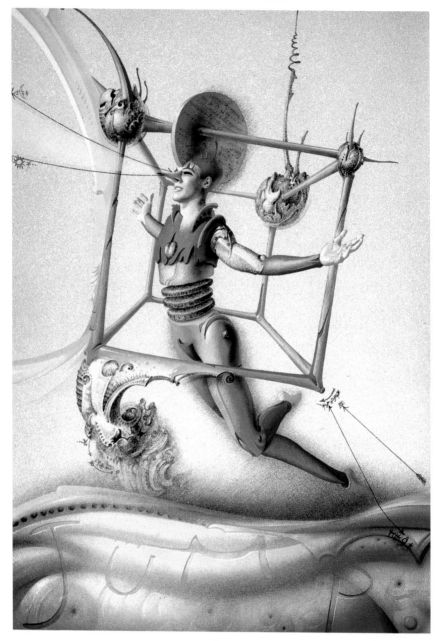

Jump
Gil Bruvel

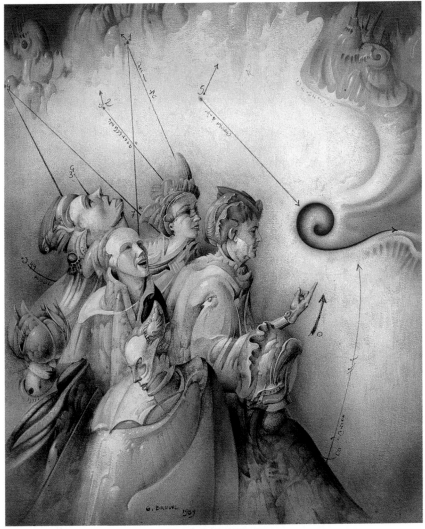

The Spiral of Wisdom
Gil Bruvel

Without the benefit of their experience, distilled through the training process, I could not be a neurosurgeon. We all have a similar story.

Training has the positive value of efficiency. But it is not enough by itself. It may also perpetuate dogma, superstitious behavior, and unrecognized error. What is learned is only as good as the training, experience, and analytic skills of the mentor, filtered by his or her teaching ability.

Experience refines our knowledge, training, and logical deductions and inferences. Positive experience reinforces what we have done, promoting successful behavior but also preserving unnecessary behavior, superstition. For example: an experienced neurosurgeon, call him Harvey, has an extensive and successful experience in lumbar disc surgery. He has always given 10 mg of dexamethasone at the end of the case because he was trained to do so, and he attributes his unusually short average length of stay (for his hospital) of 36 hours to this practice. He associates with an equally experienced neurosurgeon, we will call him Walter, who has never given dexamethasone for routine lumbar discectomy (and, in fact, thinks it's a crazy idea). After 6 months in practice together it is clear that they have identically good results, length of stay, and other indicators of quality.

This suggests to me that the dexamethasone is unnecessary, but perhaps Harvey is so heavy handed that he needs to use the dexamethasone in order to have results as good as his partner. Neither knows if the other is right (although we can assume that each thinks the other wrong). The point, however, is that just because things are going well does not mean that everything being done is necessary to obtain such good results. This wasn't a big problem when resources seemed unlimited, but when the unnecessary expenditure of some resources may result in the unavailability of others, such questions need to be asked. Neither Harvey nor Walter has asked the question, "How do you know?"

Negative experience extinguishes the behavior we blame for the bad result. Unfortunately, unless we analyze things correctly, we may eliminate the wrong behavior. Therefore, experience, while a good teacher, is best at: refining a base of knowledge and skill acquired from more rigorous scientific investigation and adapting general knowledge and skills to our individual abilities. Experience allows us to *artfully interpret* the knowledge and skill we acquire from others to make it most effective when applied by our hands to an individual patient. So each of these tools has an important role, but their true value comes in inverse order to that which we usually employ.

Too often we treat patients based on a logical inference from something passed on to us in training, modifying it as we gain experience (at the expense of our earlier patients), and resort to clinical science only when there is enough controversy to create a political need for scientific results. The bedrock of our actions as a scientifically based profession should be a core of knowledge acquired through rigorous scientific observation and experimentation in the clinical arena. This generates basic principles of care generalizable to many patients. We acquire most of this knowledge through training, through which it is passed on to us with the benefit of avoiding the errors of the past. We refine the application of this general knowledge through our own experience and, when faced with new situations in which we must act before acquiring knowledge, we use logic to develop an action plan from known principles.

VALUE OF THE QUESTION

So what is the value of asking "How do you know?" I hope that it is becoming clearer that it is the best way to have a sound basis for clinical action and make those actions as effective and efficient as possible. With such a high stake in successful outcomes and so many ways to fool ourselves, a little informed skepticism is necessary. Asking the question regularly can improve your daily practice of neurosurgery.

But we are not the only ones in need of some informed skepticism. As resistant as we may be to asking ourselves "How do you know,?" I sense no reluctance on the part of neurosurgeons in asking insurers, HMOs, the Health Care Financing Administration, or the Clintons, "How do you know:

the value of neurosurgical services?"
the need for a certain procedure?"
the right way to deliver health care?"

These are good questions; we should ask them forcefully and demand data to support their decisions that is as good as the data they demand from us. The Congress and the AANS along with the JCSNS are asking these questions regularly and as forcefully as possible through the Joint Washington Committee for Neurosurgery.

There are other good questions, such as: "How do you know that cognitive medicine (thinking about illness and health) is more valuable than procedural medicine (doing something about it)?" or "How do you know that the tort system is the best way to assure quality in the practice of medicine and compensation for losses caused by medical error?" or "How do you know whether you are reimbursing us too much for the expense of running our practices?"

THE SCIENTIFIC LIFE

Where does this leave us? We have chosen a caring and helping profession in which we artfully interpret a body of scientific knowledge for the welfare of our patients. This is what I would call the *scientific life*. The scientific life is one in which we seek to act with predictable outcomes based on careful, valid, and reproducible observations.

However, the science *in* our lives does not eliminate the art *from* our lives. Artful interpretation and application of scientifically derived principles to individual situations is what we do, but we seek to act from a solid base of observed fact. We need to emulate the leopard boldly leaping from the firm base of the mountain into the unknown rather than the juggler balanced in some mysterious way in thin air, sometimes providing a mystically enchanting performance, but too often falling to his death (10). Science and art are inextricably linked as Douglas Hofstadter in his seminal work, *Goedel, Escher and Bach* (7), so elegantly pointed out, or as Gil Bruvel shows in his paintings (2).

Science is indifferent to dogma and authority. Science serves us well as patients, as a profession, and as a society, but only if we are ever skeptical and ask the question, "How do you know?"

It has been a great privilege and responsibility to serve you this year. I have tried to do so on the basis of the best information available, to improve the quality of that information, to artfully interpret and apply it based on my training and experience, and to ask at each critical juncture, "How do you know?" I hope that you all feel the same sense of privilege and responsibility in continuing to seek excellence in providing neurosurgical care to your patients and ask yourselves and those around you, "How do you know?"

REFERENCES

1. Bollet AJ: Pierre Louis: The numerical method and the foundation of quantitative medicine. **Am J Med Sci** 266:92–101, 1973.
2. Bruvel G: The Reality of a Dreamer. Fort Lauderdale, FL, Apropros Art Gallery, 1992, plates "Jump" and "The Spiral of Wisdom."
3. Cassedy JH: *American Medical and Statistical Thinking 1800–1860.* Cambridge, MA, Harvard University Press, 1984, pp 60–64.
4. Double: The inapplicability of statistics to the practice of medicine. **Am J Med Sci** 21:247, 1837.
5. Gehan EA, Lemak NA: *Statistics in Medical Research.* New York, Plenum Medical Book Company, 1994.
6. Haines SJ: Randomized clinical trials in the evaluation of surgical innovation. **J Neurosurg** 51:5–11, 1979.
7. Hofstadter DR: *Goedel, Escher, Bach. An Eternal Golden Braid.* New York, Basic Books, 1980.
8. Louis PCA: Anatomic, pathologic, and therapeutic research on the disease known by the name of gastroenteritis putrid fever, adynamic atoxic typhoid, etc. **Am J Med Sci** 4:403, 1829.

9. Louis PCA: Louis on the application of statistics to medicine. **Am J Med Sci** 21:525, 1837.
10. Parkes M: *Michael Parkes*. Amsterdam, Steltman Editions, 1993, Plates 54 and 95.
11. Sackett DL: Bias in analytic research. **J Chronic Dis** 32:51–63, 1979.

2

In Vitro Neurogenesis by Adult Human Epileptic Temporal Neocortex

DAVID W. PINCUS, MD, PHD; CATHERINE HARRISON-RESTELLI, BA; JOSEPH
BARRY, BS; ROBERT R. GOODMAN, MD, PHD; RICHARD A.R. FRASER, MD;
MAIKEN NEDERGAARD, MD, DMSc; STEVEN A. GOLDMAN, MD, PHD

The adult human brain shows little capacity for self-repair following injury. Terminally differentiated neurons are incapable of mitosis, and compensatory neuronal production has not been observed in any mammalian models of structural brain damage (15, 25). Over the last several years, however, a considerable body of evidence has evolved that suggests a marked degree of cellular plasticity in the adult as well as in the developing central nervous system (CNS). In particular, studies on neural stem cells, both in the embryo and in the adult, have offered strategies for directed neuronal regeneration and structural brain repair (see refs. 1, 6, 9 for reviews). Neural stem cells are the multipotential progenitors of neurons and glia, which are capable of self-renewal (4). Recent evidence indicates that neuronal precursors persist in the adult brain as subependymal cells, and that these may be experimentally directed to resume neuronal production in adulthood (6, 10, 10a, 23, 24). In adult rats, the proliferation of subependymal zone precursor cells, as well as progenitors derived from septum, striatum, and dentate gyrus, is promoted *in vitro* by fibroblast growth factor-2 (FGF-2, or bFGF; refs. 19, 26); thereafter, the survival of their neuronal daughters is supported by brain-derived neurotrophic factor (BDNF; ref. 14).

We have previously demonstrated the presence of neuronal precursors in the temporal subependymal zone (SZ) of the epileptic human brain (14). We now present data suggesting that progenitors may also be derived from temporal neocortex and proliferate in the presence of FGF-2. Furthermore, when exposed to BDNF, neuronal daughter cells survive for prolonged periods in culture and become functionally active.

MATERIALS AND METHODS

Tissue samples

Adult human temporal lobe was obtained during anterior temporal lobectomy, performed for the treatment of medically refractory epilepsy (n = 8, patients; 20–52 years old; 5 males and 3 females). No tissues were obtained from patients known to harbor tumor of any origin, because of the potential danger in confusing proliferating neuroepithelial cells with neoplastic cells *in vitro*. No tumor or macroscopic heterotopias were noted either with preoperative radiography (MRI or CIT) or postoperative histopathology. Tissue pieces were dissected into neocortical and periventricular samples, the latter including the ependyma and subependymal zone (jointly denoted as SZ; Fig. 1).

Culture preparation

Organotypic explant cultures were prepared as described in a previous study (Fig. 2; ref. 14). In brief, tissue samples were cut into roughly 0.3 mm^3 pieces, which were either cultured directly as explants upon laminin, or dissociated for single-cell monolayer culture. Cultures were grown in Dulbecco's modified Eagle's medium/Ham's F-12 with 5% fetal bovine serum and N2 supplement (3). Cultures were grown in control medium or with FGF-2 (20 ng/ml). All cultures were given a complete change to media containing BDNF (20 ng/ml) after 7 days *in vitro* (DIV), with half-volume changes twice weekly thereafter.

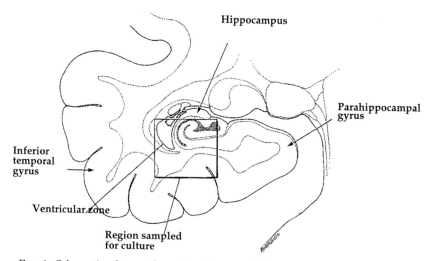

FIG. 1. Schematic of coronal section of temporal lobe showing the region typically sampled for culture (reproduced from ref. 11 with permission).

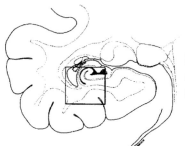

Ventricular zone and cortical samples obtained from operations for intractable seizures.

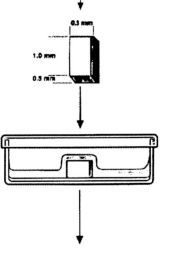

VZ and cortical samples cut into small explants.

Explants plated onto laminin-coated 35mm dishes. Base medium contains 5% serum in DMEM/F12 with N2 and HEPES. Treatment medium contains bFGF and BDNF.

Cellular Outgrowth 5% CO_2 at 37°

FIG. 2. Methods used for *in vitro* studies of human neurogenesis.

Immunocytochemistry

Cultures were incubated for up to 9 weeks, fixed, and probed with antibodies directed against microtubule associated protein-2 (MAP-2; ref. 2). Neurons were defined as those cells with typical multipolar morphology and immunoreactivity for the neuronal protein MAP-2. The protocol used for detecting this antigen was as described previously (8).

^3H-thymidine labeling

The uptake of ^3H-thymidine (0.2 μCi/plate, from 1 mCi/ml stock; 5 Ci/mM, Amersham) by antigenically defined neurons was used as an index of antecedent precursor cell mitosis *in vitro*. Cultures were exposed to ^{3}H-thymidine during their first 7 days *in vitro*, after which a complete media exchange removed residual isotope. Autoradiography was performed as described previously (8). Labeled cells were presumed to have been in S-phase at the time of ^{3}H-thymidine exposure, and to have arisen by the *in vitro* mitosis of parental progenitors.

Calcium imaging

Cells were challenged with a depolarizing stimulus of 60 mM K$^+$, during which their cytosolic calcium levels were observed. Cultures were loaded with 10μM fluo-3 acetomethoxyester (fluo-3 AM, Molecular Probes) for 1 hr at 37°C. A Bio-Rad MRC600 confocal scanning microscope, coupled to an Olympus JMT-2 inverted microscope, was used to image the fluo-3 signal. Excitation was provided by the 488 nm line of a 25 mW argon laser, filtered to <0.1% by neutral density filters. Emission was long pass-filtered (515 nm) and detected with the confocal set to its maximal aperture (7 mm). Images were acquired every 1–5 sec and recorded on a Panasonic TQ-2028F optical disc recorder. Each experiment was carried out at 25°C in HBSS, with 60 mM K$^+$ exchanged for 60 mM Na$^+$ in the potassium-depolarizing solution.

RESULTS

Long-term neuronal survival in vitro

In our initial series of cultures derived from 11 patients, neuronal outgrowth was observed in three. In a follow-up series, cells with neuronal characteristics were observed in SZ outgrowths derived from four of 16 patients (only eight of the 16 were technically viable). These cells were typically isolated in a field of astrocytes and had phase-bright cell bodies with thin processes. Immunocytochemistry and autoradiography were performed in selected cases, verifying the neuronal identity of these cells. The results of this study, which concentrated on the FGF-2 and BDNF-responsiveness of adult SZ-derived progenitors, are reported separately (20, 21). The present report focuses on cultures derived from one patient (a 27-year-old male). Explant cultures derived from this patient's temporal neocortex, as well as from his SZ, generated a profuse neuronal outgrowth *in vitro*. These cells were phase-bright with ramifying, interconnecting processes (Fig. 3). All cultures from this patient were grown in the presence of FGF-2 for the first week and BDNF thereafter. Neurons survived for up to 9 weeks *in vitro*, which was the longest point examined.

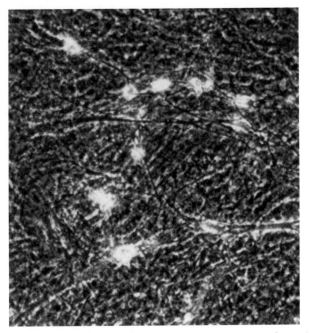

FIG. 3. Long-term neuronal survival in culture. Phase-contrast photomicrograph of adult human temporal neocortex explant culture after 9 weeks *in vitro* reveals field of neurons with interconnecting processes.

Mitotic neurogenesis by neocortical progenitors

A small sample of cortical cultures was exposed to tritiated thymidine in the first week *in vitro*, in order to label those precursor cells dividing in culture. These cultures were switched from FGF-2 to BDNF after a week and maintained in BDNF thereafter. ^{3}H-Thymidine was removed from the media at the time of FGF-2 withdrawal. Three of those cultures that developed significant neuronal outgrowth were followed for 2 months thereafter, then fixed and subjected to combined immunocytochemistry for the neuron-specific antigen MAP-2, and autoradiography for ^{3}H-thymidine. Numerous cells from both SZ and neocortical explants were double-labeled, indicating that these neurons had been generated through *in vitro* mitosis.

Calcium imaging

To confirm the ability of these neuron-like cells to respond in a neuronal fashion to depolarizing stimuli, selected cultures (n = 6) were loaded with the calcium indicator dye fluo-3, and exposed to 60 mM K^+ during confocal microscopy. Glial responses to depolarization were minimal under these culture conditions. In contrast, neuron-like cells verified as such displayed rapid and reversible elevations in cytosolic calcium in response to K^+, consistent with the activity of neuronal voltage-gated calcium channels (data not shown). In a previous study of adult human SZ-derived neurons *in vitro*, we found that neurons displayed a mean calcium increment of >400% to potassium-depolarization, in contrast to an average astrocytic calcium response of <20%, and undetectable oligodendroglial responses (14). On this basis, in the present experiment we defined a 100% calcium increment to depolarization as a necessary condition for assigning neuronal identity. Neurons achieving this criterion were found invariably to express MAP-2 upon fixation and immunocytochemistry.

DISCUSSION

The present study confirms our previous findings of neurogenesis in cultures derived from adult human epileptic temporal lobe. In addition to our previous data, however, in which neurogenesis and neuronal outgrowth were limited to SZ-derived samples and selected subcortical white matter dissociates, we now report evidence of extensive neurogenesis in neocortical tissue derived from a 27-year-old male epileptic.

Verification of neuronal identity

Precursor-derived cells were stained for the neuronal antigen MAP-2 and were functionally active. Only a fraction (<20%) of MAP-2 identified neurons incorporated ^{3}H-thymidine under these culture conditions. In our similar prior study of adult avian brain cultures, only explants derived from neurogenic regions of the brain displayed such neuronal outgrowth (8). Furthermore, prelabeling the mitotic precursor population with ^{3}H-thymidine *in vivo* revealed that most, if not all, of the neurons in these outgrowths were newly generated (10). Similar results have been noted in mammalian systems (16). Thus, it is likely that the majority of neurons observed in these cultures were derived from precursors, that survive to either produce or terminally differentiate as neurons *in vitro*. Were it possible to prelabel mitotic cells *in vivo*, we suspect that a larger proportion of cells would be ^{3}H-thymidine positive.

Nature of cortical progenitor cells in adult animals

Neuronal progenitors in the neocortical parenchyma were at best rare. We have noted neurogenesis by cortical tissue derived from only two of the 27 patients that we have studied thus far in our combined series. These include the patient discussed in the present report, as well as a second patient, from whom functionally active neurons were identified in cortical dissociate cultures (*unpublished data*). Nonetheless, the very existence of such cells is remarkable. Most previous studies found that the source of neural precursors in both adult birds and mammals is the ventricular zone (8, 16, 17), through which they are widely dispersed (13, 18, 27). Yet some precedent for the idea of parenchymal progenitor cells does exist. Neuronal precursors have been reported to reside in parenchymal as well as ventricular sites in the adult rodent brain (19, 24), as have been oligodendrocyte progenitors (7). Whether the adult cortical progenitors identified in this patient are homologous to their counterparts in either the developing cortex (4) or adult subependyma (13, 14) is unknown.

Are cortical neuronal precursors a specific feature of epileptic brain?

Our observations suggest that rare residual neuronal precursors, might persist within adult neocortex. However, the nature of these parenchymal neural precursor cells is confounded by the epileptic pathology of these patients. These cortical progenitors might have derived from cells in microheterotopic foci that were not apparent on routine pathologic examination. An intriguing corollary of this possibility is that the heterotopic cell aggregations associated with several uncommon forms of refractory epilepsy might include inappropriately situated neuronal precursors (12). For instance, the nodular subependymal heterotopias, with their periventricular locales and granule cell predominance, might constitute reservoirs of subependymal cells with precursor potential (5, 11, 22). These heterotopic cell rests may be comprised of aberrant ventricular zone emigrants, which remain functionally quiescent, yet develop into neurons when presented a permissive *in vitro* environment.

Thus, adult epileptic temporal cortex may harbor residual neuronal precursors analogous to those of the SZ. These may be parenchymal precursors, or aberrant migrants with neuronal potential in epileptic subventricular heterotopias. Their source notwithstanding, the proliferation and survival of their neuronal daughter cells suggest the promise of generating new neurons in adult human brain tissue.

REFERENCES

1. Alvarez-Buylla A, Lois C: Neuronal stem cells in the brain of adult vertebrates. **Stem Cells** 13:263–272, 1995.
2. Bernhardt R, Matus A: Light and electron microscopic studies of the distribution of microtubule-associated protein 2 in rat brain: a difference between dendritic and axonal cytoskeletons. **J Comp Neurol** 226:203–221, 1984.
3. Bottenstein JE, Sato GH: Growth of a rat neuroblastoma cell line in serum-free supplemented medium. **Proc Natl Acad Sci U S A** 76:514–517, 1979.

4. Davis AA, Temple S: A self-renewing multipotential stem cell in embryonic rat cerebral cortex. **Nature** 372:263–266, 1994.
5. Dubeau F, Tampieri D, Lee N, *et al*.: Periventricular and subcortical nodular heterotopia. A study of 33 patients. **Brain** 118:1273–1287, 1995.
6. Gage FH, Ray J, Fisher LJ: Isolation, characterization, and use of stem cells from the CNS. **Annu Rev Neurosci** 18:159–192, 1995.
7. Gensert JM, Goldman JE: In vivo characterization of endogenous proliferating cells in adult rat subcortical white matter. **Glia** 17:39–51, 1996.
8. Goldman SA: Neuronal development and migration in explant cultures of the adult canary forebrain. **J Neurosci** 10:2931–2939, 1990.
9. Goldman SA: Neuronal precursor cells and neurogenesis in the adult forebrain. **Neuroscientist** 1:338–350, 1995.
10. Goldman SA, Zaremba A, Niedzwiecki D: In vitro neurogenesis by neuronal precursor cells derived from the adult songbird brain. **J Neurosci** 12:2532–2541, 1992.
10a. Goldman, SA, Kirschenbaum, B, Harrison, C, Thaler, H: Neuronal precursors of the adult rat subependymal zone persist into senescence, with no decline in spatial extent or BDNF-response. **J. Neurobiol.** 32:554–566, 1997.
11. Huttenlocher PR, Taravath S, Mojtahedi S: Periventricular heterotopia and epilepsy. **Neurology** 44:31–55, 1994.
12. Jay V, Becker LE: Surgical pathology of epilepsy: A review. **Pediatr Pathol** 14: 731–750, 1994.
13. Kirschenbaum B, Goldman SA: Brain-derived neurotrophic factor promotes the survival of neurons arising from the adult rat forebrain subependymal zone. **Proc Natl Acad Sci USA** 92:210–214, 1995.
14. Kirschenbaum B, Nedergaard M, Preuss A, *et al*.: In vitro neuronal production and differentiation by precursor cells derived from the adult human forebrain. **Cereb Cortex** 4:576–589, 1994.
15. Korr H: Proliferation of different cell types in the brain. **Adv Anat Embryol Cell Biol** 61:1–72, 1980.
16. Lois C, Alvarez-Buylla A: Proliferating subventricular zone cells in the adult mammalian forebrain can differentiate into neurons and glia. **Proc Natl Acad Sci U S A** 90:2074–2077, 1993.
17. Morshead CM, Reynolds BA, Craig CG, *et al*.: Neural stem cells in the adult mammalian forebrain: A relatively quiescent subpopulation of subependymal cells. **Neuron** 13:1071–1082, 1994.
18. Nottebohm F: Neuronal replacement in adulthood. **Ann N Y Acad Sci** 457:143–161, 1985.
19. Palmer TD, Ray J, Gage FH: FGF-2-responsive neuronal progenitors reside in proliferative and quiescent regions of the adult rodent brain. **Mol Cell Neurosci** 6:474–486, 1995.
20. Pincus DW, Harrison C, Barry J, *et al*.: FGF2/BDNF-responsive neuronal progenitor cells in the adult human subependyma (submitted for publication).
21. Pincus DW, Harrison C, Barry J, Goodman RR, *et al*.: In Vitro Generation of Precursor-Derived Neurons From Adult Human Epileptic Temporal Neocortex. Congress of Neurological Surgeons, 1996 (abstract).
22. Raymond AA, Fish DR, Stevens JM, *et al*.: Subependymal heterotopia: A distinct

neuronal migration disorder associated with epilepsy. **J Neurol Neurosurg Psychiatry** 57:1195–1202, 1994.

23. Reynolds BA, Weiss S: Generation of neurons and astrocytes from isolated cells of the adult mammalian central nervous system. **Science** 255:1707–1710, 1992.

24. Richards LJ, Kilpatrick TJ, Bartlett PF: De novo generation of neuronal cells from the adult mouse brain. **Proc Natl Acad Sci U S A** 89:8591–8595, 1992.

25. Sturrock RR: Changes in cell number in the central canal ependyma and in the dorsal grey matter of the rabbit thoracic spinal cord during fetal development. **J Anat** 135:635–647, 1982.

26. Vescovi AL, Reynolds BA, Fraser DD, *et al.*: bFCF regulates the proliferative fate of unipotent (neuronal) and bipotent (neuronal/astroglial) EGF-generated CNS progenitor cells. **Neuron** 11:951–966, 1993.

27. Weiss S, Reynolds BA, Vescovi AL, *et al.*: Is there a neural stem cell in the mammalian forebrain? **Trends Neurosci** 19:387–393, 1996.

I

General Scientific Session I
Criteria For Patient Selection

3

Selection Criteria for Degenerative Lumbar Spine Instability

PAUL C. McCORMICK, M.D.

Between 1979 and 1990 the annual rate at which lumbar spine fusion was performed in the United States more than doubled, from 18,000 to 38,000 (9). Degenerative conditions of the lumbar spine were by far the most common surgical indication (Table 1). Currently lumbar fusion accounts for about 12%, or 46,000, of the nearly 400,000 lumbar spine surgeries performed annually in the United States (6, 33, 34). Although the rate and percentage of lumbar fusion have stabilized since their peak levels in the late 1980s, there remains a striking ninefold regional variation in the performance of lumbar fusion in the United States (10). Such variation obviously reflects significant uncertainty among surgeons who perform lumbar fusion, particularly with respect to the value of lumbar fusion in the management of degenerative lumbar instability, the definition and diagnostic criteria of lumbar instability, and selection factors for treatment. As a result, we continue to struggle with the central question, what are the indications for lumbar spine fusion? This chapter seeks to address this question specifically as it relates to selection criteria for degenerative lumbar instability. Presentation of the scientific evidence on which these criteria have been developed will serve as the primary focus of discussion.

From a conceptual standpoint, clinical instability defined as "a loss or reduction in the mechanical integrity of a motion segment which is manifested by pain or neurologic symptoms when physiologic loads are applied," is straightforward (26). Note that no specific radiographic criteria nor measurable biomechanical parameter are contained in this definition. That lumbar fusion which "minimizes or eliminates motion and augments the weight-bearing capacity of an injured motion segment," would be an effective treatment of clinical instability so defined seems intuitive (26). Unfortunately, the empiric evidence in support of the efficacy of spinal fusion is much less compelling. There are two reasons for this. The first is the nature of clinical instability and the second is the failure of the physicians who perform lumbar fusion to

TABLE 1
Degenerative Conditions of the Lumbar Spine

Lumbar stenosis
Degenerative spondylolisthesis
Degenerative scoliosis
Facet syndrome
Degenerative disk disease

establish the efficacy of this treatment in a methodologically valid manner.

The aim of this chapter, therefore, is threefold. First, the nature of clinical instability along with its complexities and difficulties with diagnosis and management will be reviewed. Secondly, our scientific evidence in support of lumbar spine fusion, as it appears in our own peer-reviewed literature, will be presented and evaluated. Finally, despite the enormous problems and complexities associated with clinical instability, it will be suggested that the methodologies and measurement instruments now exist which will allow us to address some of the questions regarding lumbar fusion in a scientifically valid manner.

NATURE OF CLINICAL INSTABILITY

The main problem with the diagnosis of clinical instability stems from its nearly uniform clinical presentation as low back pain. So the first challenge is how to identify from a huge and heterogeneous population of patients with low back pain those patients who have clinical instability as its cause and are, therefore, most likely to benefit from lumbar spine fusion. Further, by its nature, pain is a subjective personal experience which is difficult to quantify. Its effect on the various aspects of an individual's life and functioning can vary considerably, largely as a result of psychologic, behavioral, and socioeconomic variables, so that measurable impairment is often not proportional to the resultant disability. Patient selection is made even more difficult by the absence of a consensus of a diagnostic criteria for clinical instability and a lack of any single objective parameter that identifies clinical instability and predicts outcome of treatment. Matters are further complicated by the realization that surgical factors (*i.e.*, selection, performance) and the manner in which we choose to measure outcome can affect outcome independent of selection criteria. So it's not simply a question of who do we fuse but also of how and what to fuse, how to confirm achievement of the surgical objective, and how to define an appropriate outcome. Indeed, it is often difficult to ascertain whether a poor outcome is related to a failure of selection process, surgical choice or performance, or inappropriate outcome measurement.

Despite these complexities, we have tended to consider low back pain rather simplistically as a purely physical disorder (Table 2). In this "physical disease model" we assume that there is a structural cause for low back pain, and our response has been to search for better methods of physical diagnosis. It is further assumed that the patient's pain and functional disability level are proportional to the loss of structural integrity so that surgery, because of its invasive nature, is often considered only for the most functionally disabled patients in order to maximize its perceived benefit. Finally, this model assumes a total resolution of pain and functional disability with structural repair, and, faced with inconsistent results of spinal fusion, more expanded methods of structural repair, such as circumferential fusion and longer segment instrumentation with deformity correction, have become popular.

OBJECTIVE DIAGNOSTIC CRITERIA FOR DIAGNOSIS OF CLINICAL INSTABILITY

In accordance with the physical disease model we have sought to simplify the diagnostic and selection criteria for clinical instability through the identification of an objective, measurable parameter which would comprehensively identify the structural cause of the patient's symptoms, define the operative indications and objectives, and predict a successful outcome with surgery. These objective parameters include specific radiographic abnormalities and the results of clinical tests such as discography, facet injection, or trial bracing (3, 4, 12, 17). The problem with these studies is that many imaged abnormalities are asymptomatic. In addition, there can be an inconsistent relationship between a radiographic abnormality and clinical symptoms, as is seen with spondylolisthesis. Finally, there is often an

TABLE 2.
Physical Disease Model: Low Back Pain

Assumption	Response
1. Structural (physical) basis for low back pain	1. Better methods of physical diagnosis (*e.g.*, MRI, discography)
2. Pain/functional disability level proportional to structural integrity loss	2. Surgery for most disabled
3. Resolution of pain/disability with structural repair (*i.e.*, fusion)	3. Expand fusion methods (*e.g.*, circumferential, deformity correction)

uncertain relationship between symptoms and structural abnormalities. This has become even more problematic as diagnostic imaging methods have become more sensitive. For example, the frequent incidence of MRI abnormalities in asymptomatic individuals is well known (3). Degenerative and/or bulging discs are present in over one-third of asymptomatic individuals (4, 17). Even dynamic flexion-extension studies suffer from a relatively low specificity because of the wide range of angular and translational motion in normal individuals. In the study by Boden and Wiesel (4) for example, 42% of asymptomatic volunteers met the criteria for instability for at least one lumbar level. The sensitivity of dynamic flexion-extension studies is also compromised by defining clinical instability according to the biomechanical criteria of excessive or abnormal motion. Indeed, not all painful joints are excessively mobile. Not only is diagnostic accuracy of specific radiographic abnormalities poor, particularly if uniformly applied to all patients with low back pain for the diagnosis of clinical instability, but they fail to assess nonorganic patient-specific factors which clearly have an impact on patient outcome. Indeed, the correlation of various psychologic characteristics and socioeconomic variables with low back pain, functional disability, and the response to treatment is well known (Table 3) (14, 15, 18, 21, 23, 30, 38). In fact it is now well established that these factors not only contribute to functional disability but are more predictive of long-term chronic low back pain disability than physical factors.

Perhaps more importantly, many of these predictive factors can be objectively quantified (Table 4). Interestingly, many of the factors that predict long-term low back pain disability are also predictive of a poor outcome following surgery. In their study on lumbar disc herniation, Junge et al. (20) correlated a poor surgical outcome with duration of working disability, number of previous lumbar surgeries, number of other painful areas, avoidance behavior, and depression. In the study on lumbar fusion by Riley et al. (31), the patients with a poor outcome

TABLE 3
Patient-Specific Factors That Affect Outcome

Psychologic characteristics
  DSM-III-R
    Axis I—Clinical syndromes (*e.g.*, depression, substance abuse, somatoform disorder)
    Axis II—Personality disorders (*e.g.*, dependent, avoidant)
Socioeconomic variables
  Worker's Compensation
  Personal injury (litigation)
  Job satisfaction

TABLE 4
Factors Associated or Predictive of Chronic Disability and/or Poor Treatment Outcome

· High self-assessed pain and disability scores
· Prolonged (>6 mo) work disability
· Number of previous surgeries
· Worker's compensation/personal injury
· Job factors (level, satisfaction, stress)
· Depression
· Elevated MMPI scales 1 (hysteria) and 3 (hypochondriasis)
· Nonorganic physical signs (*e.g.*, sham sciatic grimacing)
· Nonanatomic pain drawing

had a statistically significant elevation in their Minnesota Multiphasic Personality Inventory (MMPI) scales 1 and 3 (hypochondriasis and hysteria), compared to those with a successful outcome.

Thus it appears that a purely physical disease model for lower back pain is inadequate. Instead, as Gordon Waddell suggests, low back pain is a complex physical and psychosocial phenomenon which is influenced by physical, psychologic, and socioeconomic factors (37).

SCIENTIFIC "EVIDENCE" IN SUPPORT OF LUMBAR FUSION

The literature evidence in support of lumbar fusion has been critically reviewed by Turner *et al.* (35). In their attempted meta-analysis of the literature on lumbar fusion no randomized controlled studies were identified. Only 4 of the identified 47 articles were clearly prospective in nature, 18 were retrospective, and in 25 articles the nature of the study design could not be identified. Independent outcomes assessment was performed in only 17% of the studies. They further noted that there was a 72.6% satisfactory outcome in the retrospective studies, whereas only a 54.1% satisfactory outcome average was noted in the prospective studies. The range of satisfactory outcomes in these studies varied considerably from 16 to 93%. Significant limitations in the literature evidence in support of lumbar fusion were noted by the authors, and in particular poorly identified heterogeneous patient populations, nonstandardized selection criteria, performance assessment bias, and nonstandardized outcomes were common problems in most studies. On the basis of this meta-analysis, these authors concluded that "The literature on spinal fusion is totally inadequate. Meta-analysis is impossible because of the lack of randomized trials, incomplete reporting of data and statistical analysis." Similar findings were noted in the review of the outcomes of lumbar fusion in a workers compensation population from the State of Washington. In this study, Franklin *et al.* (13) reviewed the long-term follow-up of 388 patients who had undergone previous lumbar fusion. After a minimum follow-up of 3 years, 68% of the patients noted that their back pain was worse and 56% stated that the quality of life was no better. More than two-thirds of the patients remained totally work-disabled at 2 years, and 23% of these patients had undergone a repeat surgery within 2 years of their index surgery. Curiously, however, 62% of patients did note satisfaction with their experience with spinal fusion. Based on their review, the authors concluded that "The burden of proof for continuing to perform lumbar spine fusion in the context of the patient with chronic pain in a workers compensation program should fall on the surgeons who perform or advocate the procedure."

The bulk of the empiric or scientific evidence in support of lumbar fusion as it appears in literature consists predominantly of the retrospective case series. Unfortunately, the problems with this study design are so pervasive as to weaken or preclude any meaningful or valid conclusions regarding the efficacy of lumbar fusion. The typical retrospective case series is characterized by small patient numbers, incomplete patient description, nonstandardized outcomes measurements, frequent lack of control groups, biased surgeon or treating physician outcome assessment, and often a high lost follow-up rate. In retrospective case series without controls, the efficacy data are unclear because there is no comparative group from which alternative or no treatments can be compared. It is simply not possible to determine whether patient outcomes reflect treatment effects, placebo effects, or the natural history of the disorder. Even with the presence of a control group, retrospective case series tend to overestimate the benefit of treatment, as noted by Turner et al. (35). Further, the uniform collection of relevant data is unlikely so that patient selection and treatment probably did not produce equivalent treatment groups. Nowhere are the shortcomings of this study design more apparent than in the literature on degenerative disc disease in which discography is utilized as the definitive diagnostic modality and the sole selection criteria for lumbar fusion (5, 7, 16, 22, 24, 27, 28, 39). Degenerative disc disease, or internal disc disruption, has specific diagnostic criteria which includes similar or exact pain reproduction with disc injection, grade II or III disc disruption on postdiscography computerized tomography (CT), and a control disc injection which does not reproduce the patient's pain. Concordant pain is defined as exact pain reproduction on injection of a disrupted disc, whereas discordant pain describes exact pain reproduction on injection of a nondisrupted disc (i.e., false-positive). The reported incidence of false-positive (i.e., discordant pain) responses varies between 10 and 30% (2, 36). For the most part, the literature on lumbar fusion for degenerative disc disease diagnosed with discography consists of retrospective case series in which there is a heterogeneous and poorly defined patient population and retrospective data analysis. Discography as a diagnostic and selection modality is applied in a noncontrolled fashion. Most of these studies then attempt to indirectly validate or discredit the diagnostic accuracy and/or predictive value of discography with nonstandardized, surgeon-assessed, retrospectively determined outcome at variable intervals with significant lost follow-up. It should not be surprising, therefore, that the reported success rates with lumbar fusion are extremely variable and range from 30 to 90% (28).

Because discography is a clinical test, it is also possible that its result may be affected by psychologic characteristics. Indeed, this was addressed in the study by Block et al. (2). In this study, mean MMPI [scales 1 (hypochondriasis (HS)) and 3 hysteria (HY)] were significantly higher in patients who noted discordant positive pain on disc injection. This study clearly demonstrated that discographic results are influenced by psychologic factors and it raises the question of whether pain on injection of an abnormal disc is related to physical factors, psychologic factors, or both. The literature on discography is further limited by the general absence of control groups of patients with concordant discographic pain on injection but in whom no treatment is undertaken. This was addressed in the recent study by Rhyne et al. (30 A). In this study, 25 patients who reported concordant pain on discography but refused surgical intervention were followed. Sixtyeight percent noted significant improvement of their low back pain at 3 years following a discography. Twelve of 15 patients were back at work. Six patients worsened over time, but in four of these six patients, a significant psychiatric disorder existed as a covariate.

Therefore, it is difficult to reach a valid conclusion regarding the diagnostic accuracy or predictive value of discography for the diagnosis of degenerative disease. The current literature is hampered by heterogeneous and poorly described patient populations. The selection criteria for discography is not uniform nor is the discographic technique and assessment. Surgical factors such as choice and performance are also variable. There is a generally nonstandardized outcome assessment bias.

Despite these methodologic and design limitations, the accumulated discography evidence probably does support the following observations. First, it seems likely that discography is probably predictive of outcome in some patients. The strength of correlation varies among patients. Secondly, the correlation may vary individually according to the specific outcome parameter (e.g., pain, functional status, work) measured. Finally, however, the diagnostic accuracy and predictive

value of discography as the single determinant of clinical instability
are unacceptably low. Similar conclusions can probably be applied to
other clinical tests such as facet injection and trial bracing.

DEGENERATIVE SPONDYLOLISTHESIS

The evidence in support of lumbar fusion for a degenerative spondylolisthesis is more convincing. In the meta-analysis by Mardjetko *et
al.* (25),an average of 90% good or excellent clinical outcome was noted
in patients treated with decompression and concomitant fusion as
compared to 69% good or excellent outcome in patients treated with
decompression alone. The predominant retrospective case series nature of the studies included in this meta-analysis, with its inherent
flaws, needs to be emphasized. Similar benefits for lumbar fusion in
the treatment of spondylolisthesis were also identified in the prospective study by Herkowitz and Kurz (19). Although this study was
prospective, it was not randomized. Allocation of the treatment group
of decompression and fusion versus decompression alone was done on
an alternating basis. This introduces some bias because the treating
physician is aware to which treatment group each patient will be
allocated. In this study, 24 of 25 patients who were treated with
decompression and fusion had a good or excellent outcome, whereas
only 11 patients who were managed with laminectomy alone had
similarly successful results. Further questions regarding the validity
of the study were raised by the 39% pseudoarthrosis rate and the
potential bias of treating surgeon-assessed outcomes. No preoperative
or intraoperative factors were identified that would predict which
patients would benefit most from fusion. Therefore, while the evidence
and support of lumbar fusion in the management of degenerative
spondylolisthesis are more convincing, these studies clearly need to be
repeated. Because degenerative spondylolisthesis has relatively uniform diagnostic criteria and homogeneous factors with a relative absence of psychologic or secondarily gained issues, it lends itself well to
a prospective randomized study design. Such a study would not only
serve to strengthen the support of fusion for degenerative spondylolisthesis, but it may also identify factors that predict the patients who
would benefit from concomitant arthrodesis at the time of decompression.

In summary, the scientific evidence as it appears in peer-reviewed
literature in support of lumbar spinal fusion is inconsistent and is
plagued by significant limitations of study design and methodology. If
treatment efficacy is to be established, it needs to be addressed in a
methodically valid manner. This would include complete and rigorous
definitions of the study populations, treatment, and outcome. There

needs to be random allocation and similar treatment of control patients. Measurement instruments which are reliable, valid, and reproducible are required. Fortunately these instruments continue to be developed and have been validated in previous studies on lumbar disc herniation and stenosis (18, 29, 32). Most importantly, however, is to acknowledge the need to establish efficacy in a methodically valid manner. This will most likely require a multicenter collaboration in which there is developed and agreed-upon minimum data set for study comparison. Because of its heterogeneous nature, the patient population must be rigorously defined to identify relevant and predictive variables. The use of validated instruments and techniques to measure pain, functional status, general health status, comorbidities, patient expectations, psychologic characteristics, socioeconomic variables, and clinically relevant, patient referenced multidimensional outcomes is the best method to establish the efficacy of lumbar spinal fusion and to better select the patients for whom lumbar fusion is most likely to be effective (11).

REFERENCES

1. Atlas SJ, Deyo RA, Keeler RB, *et al.*: The Maine lumber spine study, Part III. **Spine** 21:1787–1795, 1996.
2. Block AR, Vanharanta H, Ohnmeiss DD: Discographic pain report: Influence of psychological factors. **Spine** 3:334–338, 1996.
3. Boden SD, Davis DO, Dian TS, *et al.*: Abnormal magnetic resonance scans in asymptomatic subjects. **J Bone Joint Surg Am** 72:403–408, 1990.
4. Boden SD, Wiesel SW: Lumbosacral segmental motion in normal individuals: Have we been measuring instability properly? **Spine** 15:571–576, 1990.
5. Bogduk N, Modic MT: Controversy: Lumbar discography. **Spine** 21:402–404, 1996.
6. Cherkin DC, Deyo RA, Loesser JD, *et al.*: An international comparison of back surgery rates. **Spine** 19:1201–1206, 1994.
7. Colhoun E, McCall IW, Williams L, *et al.*: Provocation discography as a guide to planning operations on the spine. **J Bone Joint Surg Br** 70B:267–271, 1988.
8. Daltroy LH, Cats-Baril WL, Katz JN, *et al.*: The North American Spine Society lumbar spine outcome assessment instrument. **Spine** 21:741–749, 1996.
9. Davis H: Increasing rates of cervical and lumbar spine surgery in the United States. **Spine** 15:1117–1124, 1994.
10. Deyo RA: Non-surgical care of low back pain. **Neurosurg Clin N Am** 2:851–862, 1991.
11. Deyo RA, Anderson G, Bombardier C, *et al.*: Outcome measures for studying patient with low back pain. **Spine** 19:2032S–2036S, 1994.
12. Esses SI, Moro JK: The value of facet joint blocks in patient selection for lumbar fusion. **Spine** 18:183–190, 1993.
13. Franklin GM, Haug J, Heyer NJ, *et al.*: Outcome of lumbar fusion in Washington State Workers' Compensation. **Spine** 19:1897–1904, 1994.

14. Frymoyer JW: Predicting disability from low back pain. **Clin Orthop** 279:101–109, 1992.
15. Gatchel RJ, Polatin PB, Mayer TG: The dominant role of psychosocial risk factors in the development of chronic low back pain disability. **Spine** 20:2702–2709, 1995.
16. Grubb SA, Lipscomb HJ: Results of lumbosacral fusion for degenerative disc disease with and without instrumentation. **Spine** 17:349–355, 1992.
17. Hayes MA, Howard TC, Gruel CR, et al.: Roentgenographic evaluation of lumbar spine flexion-extension in asymptomatic individuals. **Spine** 14:327–331, 1989
18. Hazard RG, Haugh LD, Reid S, et al.: Early prediction of chronic disability after occupational low back injury. **Spine** 21:945–951, 1996.
19. Herkowitz HN, Kurz LT: Degenerative lumbar spondylolisthesis with spinal stenosis. **J Bone Joint Surg Am** 73:802–808, 1991.
20. Junge A, Dvorak J, Ahrens St.: Predictors of bad and good outcomes of lumbar disc surgery. **Spine** 20:460–468, 1995.
21. Klenerman L, Slade PD, Stanley IM, et al.: The prediction of chronicity in patients with an acute attack of low back pain in a general practice setting. **Spine** 20:478–484, 1995.
22. Knox BD, Chapman TM: Anterior lumbar interbody fusion for discogram concordant pain. **J Spinal Disord** 6:242–244, 1993.
23. Lancourt J, Kettelhut: Predicting return to work for lower back pain patients receiving Worker's Compensation. **Spine** 17:630–640, 1992.
24. Lee CK, Vessa P, Lee JK: Chronic disabling low back pain syndrome caused by internal disc derangements. **Spine** 20:356–361, 1995.
25. Mardjetko SM, Connolly PJ, Shott S: Degenerative lumbar spondylolisthesis: A Meta-analysis of literature 1970–1993. **Spine** 19:2256S–2265S, 1994.
26. McCormick PC: The indications and techniques of lumbar spine fusion, in Youmans JR (ed): *Neurological Surgery.* Philadelphia, W.B. Saunders, 1996, ed 4. pp 2461–2492.
27. Newman MH, Grinstead GL: Anterior lumbar interbody fusion for internal disc disruption. **Spine** 17:831–833, 1992.
28. Parker LM, Murrell SE, Boden SD, et al.: The outcome of posterolateral fusion in highly selected patients with discogenic low back pain. **Spine** 21:1909–1917, 1996.
29. Patrick DL, Deyo RA, Atlas SJ, et al.: Assessing health-related quality of life in patient with sciatica. **Spine** 20:1899–1909, 1995.
30. Polatin PB, Kinney RK, Gatchel RJ, et al.: Psychiatric illness and chronic low back pain. **Spine** 18:66–71, 1993.
30A. Rhyne AL, Smith SE, Wood KE. et al.: Outcome of unoperated discogram—positive low back pain. **Spine** 20:1997–2001, 1995.
31. Riley JL, Robinson ME, Geisser ME, et al.: Relationship between MMPI-2. Cluster profiles and surgical outcome in low back pain patients. **J Spinal Disord** 8:213–219, 1995.
32. Stucki G, Daltroy L, Liang MH, et al.: Measurement properties of a self-administered outcome measure in lumbar spinal stenosis. **Spine** 21:796–803, 1996.
33. Taylor VM, Deyo RA, Cherkin DC, et al.: Low back hospitalization; Recent U.S. trends and regional variations. **Spine** 19:1207–1213, 1994.

34. Taylor VM, Deyo RA, Goldberg H, *et al.*: Low back pain hospitalization in Washington State: Recent trends and geographic variations. **J Spinal Disor** 8:1–7, 1995.
35. Turner JA, Ersek M, Herron L.: Patient outcomes after lumbar spinal fusions. **JAMA** 268:907–911, 1992.
36. VAnharanta H, Guyer RD, Ohnmeiss D, *et al.*: Disc deterioration in low back syndromes. **Spine** 13:1349–1351, 1988.
37. Waddell G: A new clinical model for the treatment of low back pain. **Spine** 12:632–643, 1987.
38. Werneke MW, Harris DE, Lichter RL: Clinical effectiveness of behavioral signs for screening chronic low back pain patients in a work-oriented physical rehabilitation program. **Spine** 16:2412–2418, 1993.
39. Wetzel FT, LaRocca SH, Lowery GL, *et al.*: The treatment of lumbar spinal pain syndromes diagnosed by discography. **Spine** 19:792–800, 1994.

CHAPTER

4

Evidence-based Management of Type II Odontoid Fractures

VINCENT C. TRAYNELIS, M.D.

The incidence of spinal trauma in this country exceeds 11,000 cases per annum (7, 17). More than 60% of spinal injuries affect the cervical spine (12, 16), and approximately one-fifth of all cervical injuries involve the axis (15). The most common axis injury is an odontoid fracture, the majority of which have been classically called the type II or dens fracture (3, 5, 15). The nonoperative treatment options for this injury include no treatment, immobilization with a cervical collar, or halo/Minerva immobilization. Additionally, patients may be managed surgically with a posterior fusion or anterior screw fixation. This chapter represents an effort to develop evidence-based guidelines for the treatment of type II odontoid fractures.

Recently, a number of practice guidelines have been developed, using a scientific method. It appears that these have resulted in not only improved patient care but also a reduction in medical time and cost (8, 22). The American Medical Association has suggested that a number of attributes are required for the development of scientifically sound, clinically relevant guidelines (2). The most important of these attributes focuses on the methods by which the literature is reviewed and the evidence is graded. Data may be classified into four categories. Class I evidence includes data collected in prospective trials. These trials may or may not be randomized. Class II evidence consists of data that are collected prospectively as well as retrospective analyses based on reliable data. Class II studies include cohort studies, prevalence studies, and case control studies. Class III evidence is based on retrospectively collected data. Articles that would fall into this category include clinical series, databases, and case reviews. Class IV data consist of single-case reports and anecdotes, testimony, theory, and common sense.

Treatment recommendations for any given disease entity may be weighted according to available evidence (20). Treatment recommendations are generally divided into three groups. Standards reflect a high degree of clinical certainty, and these are based on class I data or very strong class II data. Guidelines reflect a moderate degree of clinical certainty in terms of therapeutic efficacy; they are usually based on class II evidence or a preponderance of class III evidence. Options reflect mild or unclear clinical certainty, and these are usually based on class III data.

A Medline search of the literature from January 1966 to September 1996 was performed using the key terms odontoid process: injury, or surgery. The search was limited to English. One hundred eighty-one articles were detected with this search and the abstract of each reviewed. After the initial review, 40 articles were then selected for more comprehensive examination. This search strategy failed to identify any references before 1980. For that reason, a second search from January 1966 to September 1996 was performed, using only axis as the key word; this search was limited to English. The search yielded 686 articles, and after review of the abstracts of each article, an additional 48 reports were selected for comprehensive examination. Based on the abstract review, those articles that dealt with human patients, appeared to have an appropriate study design, patient number, and adequate follow-up were chosen for comprehensive review.

A number of outcome measures can be used to determine the success of treatment of odontoid fractures. These may include fusion, morbidity, mortality, cost, length of hospitalization, length and degree of disability, etc. For the purpose of this review, fusion was chosen as the only outcome criterion. It has been recognized that the radiographic determination of fusion may be difficult and imprecise and that it may not be congruent with other outcomes, such as pain, disability, and function. However, because medical and/or surgical management of odontoid fractures is aimed at stability and is represented by radiographic fusion, this is a reasonable outcome measure to examine. Generally, evidence of bony radiographic union, such as trabecula crossing the fracture site, as well as absence of abnormal motion on flexion and extension films, is believed to represent a successful fusion. The literature was reviewed with attention to the criteria used to determine fusion.

In summary, the literature was critically assessed, and only reports clearly dealing with type II odontoid fractures were used as evidence. With these restrictions, no class I data were identified. A single article provided class II evidence. Ten articles were chosen for use as class III evidence. Each of these articles clearly documented the long-term course of at least 15 patients treated in a similar manner. The data used are presented in Tables 1–5.

TABLE 1
No Treatment

Author/Ref/Yr	Description of Study	Data Class	Conclusions
Clark/10/1985	Multicenter review of 18 untreated patients Radiographic criteria for fusion: Evidence of trabeculation across the fracture site and absence of movement on lateral flexion/ extension radiographs	III	0/18 successful fusions (0%)

TABLE 2
Traction/Collar

Author/Ref/Yr	Description of Study	Data Class	Conclusions
Govender/14/1988	26 patients; 1 mo in traction (2–4 kg), then rigid collar 6–8 wk. Patients assessed at 3 mo Radiographic criteria for fusion: Bony continuity across fracture site and no movement on flexion/extension tomograms	III	19/26 successful fusion (73%), 2/26 fibrous union (8%), 5/26 nonunion (19%) No mortality Seven halo pin site infections, 3 patients had skin excoriation over chin secondary to halter traction
Anderson/3/1974	22 patients; 6 wk traction, then cervical brace Radiographic criteria for fusion: Not provided	III	14/22 successful fusion (64%) Degree and direction of displacement was not related to fusion outcome

A single article dealt with the course of 18 patients who were not treated (Table 1) (10). This multicenter review compiled the experience of surgeons in the Cervical Spine Research Society. None of the 18 untreated patients went on to fusion; therefore, no treatment should not be considered as a management option.

Two retrospective reviews totaling 48 patients dealt with the treatment of type II odontoid fractures with a cervical collar (Table 2) (3, 14). In both of these studies, patients were first treated for 4–6 weeks with traction and then placed in a cervical brace for a variable period of time. Thirty-three of the forty-eight were found to have a successful fusion, for a rate of 69%. Thus, traction followed by cervical collar immobilization should be considered a treatment option. Such man-

TABLE 3
Halo/Minerva

Author/Ref/Yr	Description of Study	Data Class	Conclusions
Bettini/6/1991	Retrospective review, 17 patients treated with Minerva or halo; minimum follow-up: 1.6 yr	III	12/17 successful fusion (71%)
	Radiographic criteria for fusion: Not specified		Failure was associated with diastasis or displacement >2 mm
Hadley/15/1989	75 patients immobilized 10–25 wk: 65 with halo, 8 SOMI, 2 P-collar. Sixty-eight patients available for long-term follow-up	III	54/68 successful fusion (79%)
	Radiographic criteria for fusion: flexion/extension lateral radiographs		Displacement >6 mm was significant for nonunion; age, neurologic status, direction of displacement not statistically related to fusion outcome
Schweigel/21/1987	28 patients treated with a halo for an average of 8 wk (3–12) Radiographic criteria for fusion: "Evidence of stability and bony healing"	III	25/28 successful fusion (89%) Age and direction of displacement did not effect fusion outcome; displacement greater than 4 mm may have been a negative factor for successful fusion
Clark/10/1985	Multicenter review of 38 patients treated with halo Radiographic criteria for fusion: Evidence of trabeculation across the fracture site and absence of movement on lateral flexion/extension radiographs	III	25/38 Successful fusions (66%) Failure associated with displacement and angular deformity; age not a factor in fusion outcome
Maiman/18/1982	15 patients treated with traction, halo, or Minerva; Average time of immobilization was 10 wk (3.5–24) Radiographic criteria for fusion: Tomographic evidence of avascular necrosis, gross instability with a demonstrable gap at the fracture line, and no evidence of healing	III	0/15 successful fusions (0%)

TABLE 4
Posterior Cervical Fusion

Author/Ref/Yr	Description of Study	Data Class	Conclusions
Bednar/4/1995	Examined mortality in cohort study; one retrospective group consisted of 33 patients treated with halo (includes 4 patients with Type III fractures); the second group consisted of 11 patients over age 50 treated with Brooks fusion and immobilized in a P-collar for 3 mo postoperatively; fusion only assessed for operative cases	II	In-hospital mortality with halo treatment was ~27%; patients >50 yr of age had ~42% mortality; no fusion assessment of halo treatment
	Radiographic criteria for fusion: Continuous trabeculated bone bridging the posterior elements of C1-C2, with no mobility in the C1-C2 segment on flexion/extension radiographs		11/11 successful fusions (100%) for operated patients at 6 mo; no mortality in operated group
			Lack of comorbidity data for halo treated cohort weakens study
Coyne/11/1995	15 patients treated with posterior wire fusion; almost all patients immobilized in P-collar postoperatively; a few with halo; minimum follow-up, 2 yr; mean, 4.7 yr	III	13/15 successful fusions (87%)
	Radiographic criteria for fusion: absence of C1-C2 movement on lateral flexion/extension radiographs and evidence of continuity of trabecular bone formation between C1 and C2 across the graft		No mortality
Clark/10/1985	Multicenter review of 26 posterior fusions	III	24/26 successful fusions (92%)
	Radiographic criteria for fusion: Evidence of trabeculation across the fracture site and absence of movement on lateral flexion/extension radiographs		There were two complications: One fracture displaced and one patient experienced worsening of myelopathy thought to be secondary to wire placement

TABLE 4—*continued*
Posterior Cervical Fusion

Author/Ref/Yr	Description of Study	Data Class	Conclusions
Maiman/18/1982	49 patients: 34 had early posterior wire/graft stabilization; postoperative immobilization with Minerva for average of 5 wk	III	17/49 successful fusions (35%)
	Radiographic criteria for nonfusion: tomographic evidence of avascular necrosis, gross instability with a demonstrable gap at the fracture line and no evidence of healing; fusion results evaluated 6 mo postsurgery		Mortality 4%

agement may be particularly applicable in the setting of the multi-trauma patient who is confined to the intensive care unit for an extended period of time.

Five articles containing class III data accumulated from a minimum of 15 patients each addressed the treatment of type II odontoid fractures with either a halo or Minerva vest (Table 3) (6, 10, 15, 18, 21). In general, patients in these series were immobilized for 8–10 weeks. The overall fusion rate was 70% (116/166); however, the fusion success varied widely, depending on the series. Maiman and Larson had no successful fusions, whereas Schweigel reported an 89% success rate. Most of these articles examined several factors in an attempt to predict which patients will achieve a successful bony union. Age was not found to be a predictor of fusion success in any of these studies. Likewise, the direction of displacement was not a factor for fusion success in any report. The degree of displacement did correlate negatively with fusion success in four of the five studies. In one of these reports, the amount of displacement that had a negative influence on the fusion rate was vague, and in the other three series, displacement greater than 2, 4, and 6 mm was found to be detrimental to a positive outcome. Immobilization should be considered a treatment option. This treatment appears to be most successful in patients with nondisplaced fractures.

Four articles provided appropriate evidence for fusion outcome analysis after a surgical posterior cervical fusion in patients with type II odontoid fractures (Table 4) (4, 10, 11, 18). One of these articles was graded as class II data and the other three as class III evidence. Bednar *et al.* (4) retrospectively reviewed 33 patients treated with halo

TABLE 5
Anterior Screw Fixation

Author/Ref/Year	Description of Study	Data Class	Conclusions
Etter/13/1991	19 patients treated with anterior odontoid screw fixation; there was one early postoperative death; for other patients, minimum follow-up was 1 yr	III	15/19 successful fusions from primary procedure (79%)
	Radiographic criteria for fusion: Not provided		Major complication rate was 17.4%; these included one death, two posterior fracture displacements (one treated with posterior fusion), and a screw fracture culminating in a nonunion
			Minor complication rate was 13%; these included one inconsequential screw fracture and two wound hematomas requiring surgical evacuation

immobilization and found a high mortality within the group; therefore, they altered their management protocol and subsequently collected data prospectively on 11 patients stabilized shortly after injury with a Brooks-Jenkins type fusion (9). Examining only mortality as an outcome, this study demonstrated significantly less mortality in the surgical population, as compared to that of patients treated with a halo. Their conclusion is weakened by the fact that comorbidity data is not provided for the halo group; therefore, there is no way to ascertain whether the two patient populations had equivalent systemic injuries. Fusion was only assessed in the surgical patients, and Bednar *et al.* reported a 100% success rate in this group.

Overall, 65 of 101 patients with a type II odontoid fracture treated with a posterior fusion achieved a successful bony union (64%). The surgical mortality rate was 2%. Major morbidity associated with surgery was difficult to determine in each article, but it appears to be about 2%. The complications associated with this treatment technique included loss of reduction and development of new neurologic deficit. No report dealt with augmentation of internal fixation with posterior C1-C2 transarticular screws. It appears that the atlantoaxial fusion success rate can be improved on with transarticular screw fixation; however, there are no solid data clearly describing the results of this technique in an adequate number of patients with type II odontoid fractures (19).

Only a single paper providing class III data dealing with anterior screw fixation for type II odontoid fractures was detected (Table 5) (13). This manuscript updated a previous report on the same subject published earlier by this group (1). Etter *et al.* (13) retrospectively reviewed 19 patients and reported that 15 individuals developed a successful fusion after their primary procedure (79%). The major complication rate was 17.4%, and these complications included one death shortly after surgery and two fracture displacements. Thirteen percent of the operated patients suffered minor morbidity, which included two urgent reoperations for evacuation of wound hematomas as well as a late screw fracture.

This review indicates that currently there are no treatment standards available to guide the care of type II odontoid fractures. Likewise, no treatment guidelines can be determined based on an appropriate review of the available literature. Four treatment options do exist. These include traction followed by immobilization in a cervical collar, immobilization with a halo or Minerva vest, posterior cervical fusion, or anterior screw fixation. In general, the fusion success rate with each of these management techniques is similar, with the exception of the anterior screw fixation, which appears to have a slightly higher fusion success rate. This is offset, however, by its increased complication rate.

More data are necessary to determine treatment standards and/or guidelines for the management of type II odontoid fractures. Although such data could be accumulated through prospective trials, cohort studies and case control studies would probably provide welcome information in a more timely fashion. Such studies should deal not only with fusion as an outcome measure but also address issues such as mortality, morbidity, length of hospitalization, and cost. Finally, it would also be pertinent to examine patient quality of life after treatment of these injuries. Although every surgeon treating odontoid fractures believes maintenance of normal spinal mobility correlates positively with quality of life, only class IV data exist to support this notion.

ACKNOWLEDGMENT

Invaluable advice, guidance, and criticism were graciously provided by Beverly C. Walters, M.D.

REFERENCES

1. Aebi M, Etter C, Coscia M: Fractures of the odontoid process: Treatment with anterior screw fixation. **Spine** 14:1065–1070, 1989.
2. AMA Office of Quality Assurance and Health Care Organizations: *Attributes to Guideline Development of Practice Parameters.* Chicago, American Medical Association, 1990.
3. Anderson LD, D'Alonzo RT: Fractures of the odontoid process of the axis. **J Bone Joint Surg Am** 56:1663–1674, 1974.
4. Bednar DA, Parikh J, Hummel J: Management of type II odontoid process fractures in geriatric patients: A prospective study of sequential cohorts with attention to survivorship. **J Spinal Disord** 8:166–169, 1995.
5. Benzel EC, Hart BL, Ball PA, et al.: Fractures of the C2 vertebral body. **J Neurosurg** 81:206–212, 1994.
6. Bettini N, Cervellati M, DiSilvestre M, et al.: The nonsurgical treatment of fractures of the dens epistrophe. **Chir Organi Mov** 76:17–24, 1991.
7. Bracken MB, Freeman DH, Hellenbrand K: Incidence of acute traumatic hospitalized spinal cord injury in the United States, 1970–1977. **Am J Epidemiol** 113:615–622, 1981.
8. Brain Trauma Foundation: *Guidelines for the Management of Severe Head Injury.* American Association of Neurological Surgeons, Park Ridge, IL, 1995.
9. Brooks AL, Jenkins EB: Atlanto-axial arthrodeses by the wedge compression method. **J Bone Joint Surg Am** 60A:279–283, 1978.
10. Clark CR, White AA III: Fractures of the dens: A multicenter study. **J Bone Joint Surg Am** 67:1340–1348, 1985.
11. Coyne TJ, Fehlings MG, Wallace MC, et al.: C1-C2 posterior cervical fusion: Long-term evaluation of results and efficacy. **Neurosurgery** 37:688–692, 1995.
12. Ersmark H, Lowenhielm P: Factors influencing the outcome of cervical spine injuries. **J Trauma** 28:407–410, 1988.
13. Etter C, Coscia M, Jaberg H, et al.: Direct anterior fixation of dens fractures with a cannulated screw system. **Spine** 16:S25–S32, 1991.
14. Govender S, Grootboom M: Fractures of the dens—The results of non-rigid immobilization. **Injury** 19:165–167, 1988.
15. Hadley MN, Dickman CA, Browner CM, et al.: Acute axis fractures: A review of 229 cases. **J Neurosurg** 71:642–647, 1989.
16. Huelke DF, O'Day J, Mendlesohn RA: Cervical injuries suffered in automobile crashes. **J Neurosurg** 54:316–322, 1981.
17. Kraus JF, Franti CE, Riggins RS, et al.: Incidence of traumatic spinal cord lesions. **J Chronic Dis** 28:471–492, 1975.
18. Maiman DJ, Larson SJ: Management of odontoid fractures. **Neurosurgery** 11:471–476, 1982.
19. Marcotte P, Dickman CA, Sonntag VKH, et al.: Posterior atlantoaxial facet screw fixation. **J Neurosurg** 79:234–237, 1993.
20. Rosenberg J, Greenberg MK: Practice parameters: Strategies for survival into the nineties. **Neurology** 42:1110–1115, 1992.
21. Schweigel JF: Management of the fractured odontoid with halo-thoracic bracing. **Spine** 12:838–839, 1987.
22. Woolf SH: Practice guidelines: A new reality in medicine. **Arch Intern Med** 153:2646–2655, 1993.

CHAPTER

5

Criteria for Patient Selection:
Low-Grade Gliomas

JOSEPH M. PIEPMEIER, M.D.

The typical adult patient with a low-grade glioma is a male or female about 35 years of age with the new onset of epilepsy found to have a nonenhancing cerebral mass lesion with low signal on T1-weighted MRI and high signal on T2-weighted scans (7–9, 13–16, 18, 21, 22, 26). These patients frequently have no significant neurological deficits on routine examination. Although most neurosurgeons would agree that this constellation of findings suggests the presence of a low-grade glioma, there are widely divergent opinions regarding the most appropriate management of these patients (1, 2, 7, 10–16, 18, 20, 23–25). The focus of this report is not to reconcile the differences in management strategies but to address the treatment plans most commonly used at our institution. Our selection and management strategies have been developed from review and analysis of our patient population derived from patients with cerebral astrocytomas, oligodendrogliomas, and oligoastrocytomas contained in the Tumor Data Bank, prospectively, collected over the past 14 years (Table 1). Since 1986, patient management decisions also have been directed by the joint collaborative effort of specialists in neurosurgery, neurology, medical oncology, radiation oncology, neuroradiology, and neuropathology on the Neurooncology Tumor Board. This group meets weekly to review imaging studies, pathology slides, and clinical data. The interdisciplinary expertise of this group forms the basis for patient management, including selection of treatment options.

HISTORY AND PREOPERATIVE SYMPTOMS

The most common initial indication of a low-grade glioma is a seizure. The incidence of new onset of epilepsy as the first symptom of the tumor is as high as 80% (7, 13–19, 21, 22, 25, 27, 28). Headache, focal neurological deficits, and cognitive changes also are observed but are less common. Neurological deficits on neurological examination depend on tumor location and size. However, in many patients the

51

TABLE 1
Numbers of Patients with Low-Grade Gliomas in the Yale Neuro-oncology Tumor Data Bank

Yale-Neuro-oncology Tumor Data Bank 1982–1996	
150 Patients	
Astrocytoma	91
Oligodendroglioma	35
Oligoastrocytoma	24

routine examination fails to detect significant problems. More subtle changes in motor skills, memory, or learning often can be found on detailed neuropsychological exam.

In my experience, detailed questioning regarding the patient's past history often can reveal evidence suggestive of chronic problems that frequently remain undetected or appear unrelated to the tumor. For example, episodes of loss of contact, deterioration in performance at work or school, and personality changes may be an indication of chronicity and, perhaps, undetected epilepsy that may have been occurring for many years. These findings may give some indication of the length of time that the tumor has been present and often predate by several years the ictal event that brings the patient to medical attention. This information is important, because it suggests that the natural history of many low-grade gliomas may include a significant period of time before the tumor is identified. Evidence of chronicity gives the physician some indication of the earlier growth rate of the lesion. Chronic epilepsy identifies a unique subgroup of low-grade glioma patients with a distinctly favorable prognosis (18). Because these patients traditionally are treated by epilepsy surgeons and the strategies for management are different than treatment strategies for more typical low-grade glioma patients, this population will not be addressed in this report.

IMAGING

The appropriate use of preoperative imaging is critical in developing selection criteria and treatment strategies for low-grade glioma patients. Magnetic resonance imaging gives the best anatomic definition of low-grade gliomas. Although these imaging studies do not provide adequate information for conclusive diagnosis, the typical findings of a nonenhancing mass lesion in the white matter or cortex are suggestive (5, 7–9, 13, 14, 20, 21). Because other pathologic conditions can have a similar appearance, including high-grade tumors, cortical dysplasia, dysembryoplastic neuroepithelial tumors, and cerebrovascular disease, confirmation of the precise histology of the lesion is commonly recommended (9). In the authors experience, there are a few patients who fit this clinical profile but have not received a diagnostic biopsy. These patients either refused biopsy or had small lesions in critical regions that were considered to be at higher risk for stereotactic biopsy.

In addition to an MRI for anatomic definition of the tumor, we also have used functional MRI (fMRI) to help define primary somatosensory, language, and vision cortex in patients with tumors located in these critical regions and to provide an indication regarding the relative risk of tumor resection. These studies have been useful in demonstrating either infiltration and/or displacement of important cortical regions and have been highly accurate when confirmed by intraoperative cortical mapping. Functional imaging also is helpful in patients who have a history of earlier brain injury, because often there is relocation of function in patients who sustained injuries at an early age.

Because MRI can provide only anatomic information, we have examined patients with suspected low-grade gliomas with [18]fluorodeoxyglucose positron emission tomography (PET) to establish a metabolic profile for the tumor (5). This information can help direct stereotactic biopsies and tumor sampling at surgery for the purposes of correlating histology with tumor metabolism. To date, 80% of all purely low-grade gliomas have been hypometabolic on PET. The significance of hypermetabolism on PET in patients with low-grade gliomas is addressed below.

SURGICAL OPTIONS

The general policy at our institution favors surgical resection of low-grade gliomas. This strategy has been supported by my patient data (Table 2), which indicates that gross total resection of a low-grade glioma carries a 5% risk of tumor recurrence, whereas anything less

TABLE 2

Incidence of Gross Total Resection (GTR): Subtotal/Biopsy for 150 Patients with Low-Grade Gliomas

Histology	% GTR	% Subtotal/Biopsy
Astrocytoma	50 (4)[a]	50 (44)
Oligodendroglioma	57 (5)	43 (53)
Oligoastrocytoma	58 (7)	42 (50)
Total	53 (5)	47 (47)

[a]Numbers in parentheses give percentage of tumor recurrence in each group.

than gross total resection results in a 50% risk of recurrence over a median follow-up period of 8 years (18). The significance of tumor recurrence is critical, because the primary cause of mortality for a patient with a low-grade glioma is tumor recurrence with a high-grade lesion. Consequently, the goal of treatment is to prevent or delay this transition to a more malignant lesion. At first recurrence, more than 50% of patients with low-grade astrocytomas have evolved into high-grade lesions. The relative risk for transition from oligodendrogliomas is significantly less (10% at first recurrence). Oligoastrocytomas carry a 50% incidence of high-grade transition at first recurrence, suggesting that the astrocytic component of the tumor generally is the more aggressive (Table 3). In my experience gross total resection significantly reduces the risk of tumor recurrence and subsequent evolution of a high-grade tumor. Gross total resection has been accomplished in approximately 50% of patients with astrocytomas, oligodendrogliomas, and oligoastrocytomas. Because my data does not include a randomized study population, these findings must be tempered with the understanding that well-demarcated or polar lesions that are more likely to be resected may define a subpopulation of low-grade glioma patients with a lower risk of recurrence and malignant change than those with diffusely infiltrative and unresectable tumors.

The selection process in determining whether a tumor can be resected with acceptable morbidity is dependent on tumor location, invasiveness, comorbidity of the patient's health, and the patient's understanding of relative risks and benefits (1, 2, 4). Well-demarcated tumors that are in surgically resectable regions (*e.g.*, polar tumors) are removed under general anesthesia without evoked potential or motor mapping. The extent of tumor resection is determined by comparing volumes derived from imaging with the resection region and by direct intraoperative findings of changes in texture, color, and vascularity of tumor tissue. The latter is facilitated by the liberal use of the operating microscope for improved illumination and magnification. To facilitate the intraoperative identification of tumor margins, MRI-guided stereotactic localization of predetermined tumor margins and the use of intraoperative ultrasound can facilitate gross total removal.

TABLE 3
Percentage of Tumors Found to Be High-Grade at Recurrence

	High-Grade Tumor at Recurrence
Astrocytoma	50%
Oligodendroglioma	10%
Oligoastrocytoma	50%

Tumors bordering language regions are resected by neuroleptic anesthesia with intraoperative speech mapping (1, 2). Cortical regions that generate speech problems when stimulated are labeled and protected during tumor resection. Somatosensory evoked potentials (SSEP) and direct motor stimulation are used for tumors bordering primary somatosensory cortex, typically using general anesthesia. Recording of SSEP generated from stimulation of the contralateral median nerve localizes primary hand sensory cortex while phase reversal determines the central sulcus. Confirmation of primary motor cortex is achieved by means of bipolar stimulation (6–10 mA) of the cortex anterior to the central sulcus. Further exploration of the precentral gyrus can localize face, arm, and leg (interhemispheric) primary motor regions. Intraoperative stimulation during tumor resection can help map descending motor fibers below the cortical surface.

Histologic confirmation of tumors that can not be resected generally can be confirmed by CT- or MRI-guided stereotactic biopsy (6, 8). Specific areas to be sampled include representative tissue from areas on contrast enhancement, hypermetabolism on PET, surrounding peritumoral tissue, and multiple samples of the main tumor volume. In addition to histology, samples can be used for obtaining a labeling index to establish an estimate of the proliferative activity of the lesion and for determining the topographical and spatial definition of the tumor cells (4).

ILLUSTRATIVE CASES

Figure 1A demonstrates a T2-weighted MRI from a 35-year-old female with new onset of seizures and a normal neurological examination. This nonenhancing tumor appears to arise within the region of the primary somatosensory cortex of the dominant hemisphere. Figure 1B illustrates the fMRI, suggesting that primary motor cortex (black dots anterior to tumor) is displaced anteriorly by the lesion. PET (Fig. 1C) revealed a hypometabolic tumor. At surgery (Fig. 1D) the primary motor cortex (white markers) could be stimulated (bipolar electrode) and was found to be displaced, as suggested by the fMRI. A gross total resection of an oligodendroglioma was accomplished (Fig. 1E).

Figure 2A illustrates a T2-weighted MRI from a 30-year-old male with 6 months of seizures from a nonenhancing tumor originating in the supplementary motor cortex and extending laterally into the region of the primary motor cortex. An fMRI (Fig. 2B) confirmed the tumor's location and suggested that the lateral portion of the tumor infiltrated motor cortex for the hand. A preoperative PET indicates a hypometabolic tumor (Fig. 2C). At surgery, resection was limited to the astrocytoma in the supplementary motor area while stimulation of the

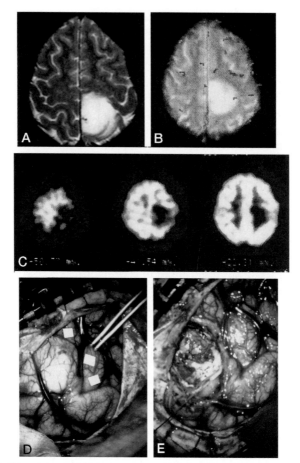

FIG. 1 (**A**) T2-weighted MRI of an oligodendroglioma arising in the region of the primary somatosensory cortex of the dominant hemisphere. (**B**) fMRI of tumor in **A**. Black dots anterior to tumor mark primary motor cortex. (**C**) PET of tumor in **A**, revealing decreased FDG uptake in the region of the tumor. (**D**) Intraoperative photograph of the tumor (*white mass*) and the primary motor cortex (*white markers*) stimulated by a bipolar electrode. (**E**) Intraoperative photograph demonstrating tumor resection with preservation of primary motor cortex.

lateral tumor generated a motor response in the contralateral hand, signifying that the tumor infiltrated the primary motor region. This portion of the tumor underwent biopsy.

PATIENT EDUCATION

An important part of the patient selection process involves patient education regarding the indications for intervention, the options for

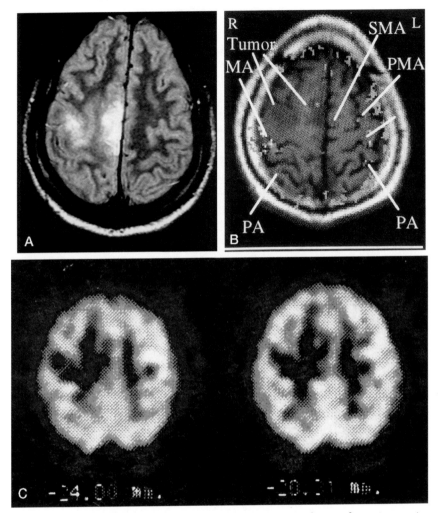

Fɪɢ. 2. (A) T2-weighted MRI of an astrocytoma arising in the supplementary motor cortex of the right hemisphere and extending laterally into the presumed primary motor cortex. (B) fMRI of the tumor in **A**. MA and PMA, primary motor cortex; PA, parietal cortex; SMA, supplementary motor cortex. (C) PET of tumor in **A**, revealing decreased FDG uptake in the tumor region.

treatment, and the anticipated results of the proposed management plan. Obviously, much of this information is dependent on the histology of the lesion and can not be determined before pathologic confirmation of the diagnosis. This author has found it very helpful to include the patient as much as is reasonable in this decision-making process. Although it is unreasonable for the patient to make surgical decisions, the potential neurologic deficits that may result from surgical removal of the tumor need to be addressed so that the patient understands the relative benefits and liabilities of treatment. Because surgical procedures near primary language cortex require the patient to be awake at surgery for speech mapping, preoperative patient education regarding the tasks that will be performed during surgery and formal preoperative testing of language function can be very helpful to the surgeon and educational for the patient. Emotional and educational needs of patients and their families also are addressed by a Neuro-oncology Support Group that includes participation by a neuro-oncology clinical coordinator and nursing and social services. Patients who are willing to share their experiences and emotional and educational support provided by the group offer patients a valuable resource for living with a brain tumor.

SELECTION FOR POSTOPERATIVE THERAPY

The optimal use of postoperative therapy in the management of low-grade gliomas remains to be defined. However, over the past 2 decades the length of survival for patients with low-grade gliomas has been increasing (18). Although there are likely several reasons for this increased survival, this trend is not dependent on any specific method or strategy of treatment. During this same time period, the length of preoperative symptoms has progressively decreased, suggesting that at least part of the survival benefit may be a result of earlier identification of the lesion by better imaging.

Part of the difficulty in selecting the type of therapy and the timing for additional treatment results from significant variability in the growth rate and anaplastic transition in low-grade gliomas. My policy is similar to that of others who consider treatment most beneficial when the tumor is actively growing (3, 18). Consequently, we have sought to try to identify nonmorphologic characteristics that help to classify these lesions. For example, our experience demonstrates that the outcome of patients who receive immediate radiotherapy does not differ from those who receive radiotherapy at recurrence or progression (18). Although our patients have not been randomized, comparison of patients who received immediate radiotherapy with those who had delayed radiotherapy at the time of recurrence/progression shows that there were no differences in the age, neurologic status, or extent of surgery between these two groups. In our patients, immediate radiotherapy (median, 54 Gy) does not reduce the incidence of recurrence, prevent more malignant evolution of the tumor or influence the timing of recurrence (18). In addition, there is no difference in survival between these two groups. Consequently, patients who are neurologically stable with adequate seizure control on medication commonly are observed until their low-grade gliomas have demonstrated clinical or radiographic evidence of progression. This policy necessitates that the patients are instructed regarding the philosophy behind observation rather than intervention. This policy is not to be misinterpreted as a lack of appreciation of the potential for progression, recurrence, or malignant evolution but rather as a result of careful analysis from my patients that shows that in the absence of some indication of progressive tumor growth, earlier postoperative therapy does not influence the course of the disease.

Additional information that helps to characterize the biologic behavior of a low-grade glioma can be helpful in selecting patients for postoperative therapy and the timing of treatment (3, 17). This information can be derived from labeling indices from tumor samples, follow-up PET studies, monitoring with MRI, and neurologic examinations. These additional data points enable the surgeon to plot a growth curve for each patient's tumor and to intervene when evidence of growth or progression is detected. At my institution, this process is considered to optimize therapy for each individual patient.

At this time there is insufficient data from these studies to provide conclusive evidence regarding which, if any of these parameters, will be most helpful in predicting the course of the disease and the response to treatment. However, of the 34 patients with both preoperative PET studies and contrast-enhanced MRI examinations (Table 4), our preliminary findings suggest that either hypermetabolism on PET (20% of patients) or enhancement with contrast on MRI (35% of patients) carry a higher risk of progression or recurrence, compared to that of patients with neither of these findings (Fig. 3**A** and **B**). More importantly, when both hypermetabolism and enhancement are present (12% of patients), all tumor recurrences are high-grade lesions. In contrast, when neither

TABLE 4

PET and Contrast-Enhanced MRI Results from 34 Patients Who Had Both Imaging Studies before Biopsy of a Low-Grade Glioma

Imaging	% Recurrence/Progression	% High-grade
PET+/MRI+[a]	50	100
PET−/MRI−	37	14
PET+/MRI−	75	66
PET−/MRI+	63	40

[a]PET+, hypermetabolic tumor; PET, hypometabolic tumor; MRI+, contrast enhancement; MRI−, no enhancement; % high-grade, incidence of anaplastic tumors at recurrence/progression.

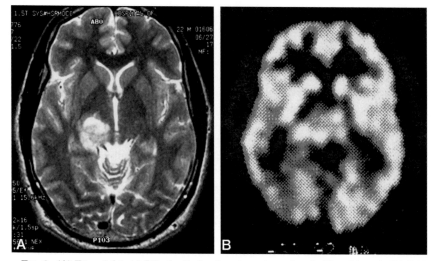

FIG. 3. (**A**) T2-weighted MRI of a thalamic astrocytoma (grade II on biopsy). (**B**) PET of tumor in **A** revealing increased FDG uptake in the tumor.

hypermetabolism nor contrast enhancement were detected (56% of patients), the risk of high-grade evolution at recurrence drops to 14%. When examined separately, hypermetabolism on PET appears to carry a somewhat higher risk of malignant evolution (66%) than contrast enhancement on MRI (40%).

CONCLUSIONS

Based on the literature of the past 2 decades it is apparent that up to two-thirds of the natural history of a low-grade glioma may occur before the patient reaches medical attention. As the length of preoperative symptoms is decreasing and the tumors are identified earlier in the course of the disease, it is increasingly more important to try and adapt treatment policies that conform to the best interests of the patient. My selection process is predicated on the principle that malignant evolution of the tumor is the most significant event in determining survival. As a result, we have adopted a policy of weighing the risks and benefits of aggressive surgery, observation, immediate radiotherapy, and delayed treatment according to the biological behavior of each patient's lesion.

The addition of PET has been helpful in selected cases in which increased 18-fluoro-2-deoxy-D-glucose (FDG) uptake is considered to be sufficient to establish an aggressive low-grade tumor and possibly as an indicator of impending malignant evolution in a tumor that morphologically resembles a low-grade glioma. Although we have tended to treat these patients with aggressive surgery and immediate radiotherapy, we do not have sufficient data to determine whether this policy result in improved outcome.

The most important aspect of our selection process is the joint effort of the Neuro-oncology Tumor Board and the objective assessment of outcome results from the Tumor Data Bank. This process of detailed data collection and collaborative consultation has enabled us to establish outcome results from our patient population and to assess the influence of treatment strategies on this population. As the process continues it is likely that our treatment options and selection criteria will evolve over time. By managing patients in this manner I believe that we can provide optimal care for our patient population, based on objective data and careful assessment.

REFERENCES

1. Berger M: Role of surgery in diagnosis and management, in Apuzzo HJ (ed): *Benign Cerebral Glioma*. Park Ridge, IL, American Association of Neurological Surgeons, 1995, pp 293–307.
2. Berger M, Tucker M, Spence A, *et al.*: Reoperation for glioma. **Clin Neurosurg** 38:172–186, 1991.
3. Cairncross G, Macdonald D: Chemotherapy for oligodendroglioma. **Arch Neurol** 48:225–227, 1991.
4. Daumas-Duport C: Patterns of tumor growth and problems associated with histological typing of low-grade gliomas, in Apuzzo MJ (ed): *Benign Cerebral Glioma*. Park Ridge, IL, American Association of Neurological Surgeons, 1995, pp 125–147.
5. DeWitte O, Levivier M, Violon P, *et al.*: Prognostic value of positron emission tomography with 18-fluoro-2-deoxy-D-glucose in the low-grade glioma. **Neurosurgery** 39:470–477, 1996.
6. Hoshino T, Rodriguez L, Cho K, *et al.*: Prognostic implications of the proliferative potential of low-grade astrocytomas. **J Neurosurg** 69:839–842, 1988.
7. Janny P, Cure H, Mohr M, *et al.*: Low-grade supratentorial astrocytomas: Management and prognostic factors. **Cancer** 73:1937–1945, 1994.
8. Kelly P, Daumas-Duport C, Scheithaur B, *et al.*: Stereotactic histologic correlations of computed tomography and magnetic resonance imaging defined abnormalities in patients with glial neoplasms. **Mayo Clin Proc** 62:450–459, 1987.
9. Kondziolka D, Lunsford D, Martinez J: Unreliability of contemporary neurodiagnostic imaging in evaluating suspected adult supratentorial (low-grade) astrocytoma. **J Neurosurg** 79:533–536, 1993.
10. Kreth F, Faist M, Warnke P, *et al.*: Interstitial radiosurgery of low-grade gliomas. **J Neurosurg** 82:418–429, 1995.
11. Laws E, Taylor W, Clifton M, *et al.*: Neurosurgical management of low-grade astrocytoma of the cerebral hemispheres. **J Neurosurg** 61:665–673, 1984.
12. Leibel S, Sheline G, Wara W, *et al.*: The role of radiation therapy in the treatment of astrocytomas. **Cancer** 35:1551–1557, 1975.

13. Lunsford D, Somaza S, Kondziolka D, et al.: Survival after biopsy and irradiation of cerebral nonanaplastic astrocytoma. **J Neurosurg** 82:523–529, 1995.

14. McCormack B, Miller D, Budzilovich G, et al.: Treatment and survival of low-grade astrocytomas in adults 1977–1988. **Neurosurgery** 31:636–642, 1992.

15. Philipon J, Clemenceau S, Fauchon F, et al.: Supratentorial low-grade astrocytomas in adults. **Neurosurgery** 32:554–559, 1993.

16. Piepmeier J: Observations on the current treatment of low-grade astrocytic tumors of the cerebral hemispheres. **J Neurosurg** 67:177–181, 1987.

17. Piepmeier J: Research strategies for evaluating the biological diversity of low-grade astrocytomas. **Perspect Neurosurg** 4:1–20, 1994.

18. Piepmeier J, Christopher S, Spencer D, et al.: Variations in the natural history and survival of patients with supratentorial low-grade astrocytomas. **Neurosurgery,** 38:872–879, 1996.

19. Piepmeier J, Fried I, Makuch R: Low-grade astrocytomas may arise from different astrocyte lineages. **Neurosurgery** 33:627–632, 1993.

20. Pollack I, Claassen D, Al-Shboul Q, et al.: Low-grade gliomas of the cerebral hemispheres in children: An analysis of 71 cases. **J Neurosurg** 82:536–547, 1995.

21. Recht L, Lew R, Smith T: Suspected low-grade glioma: Is deferring treatment safe? **Ann Neurol** 31:431–436, 1992.

22. Scoffietti R, Chio A, Giordana M, et al.: Prognostic factors in well-differentiated cerebral astrocytomas in the adult. **Neurosurgery** 24:686–692, 1989.

23. Shaw E, Daumas-Duport C, Scheithauer B, et al.: Radiation therapy in the management of low-grade supratentorial astrocytomas. **J Neurosurg** 70:853–861, 1989.

24. Shaw E, Scheithauer B, Gilbertson D, et al.: Postoperative radiotherapy of supratentorial low-grade gliomas. **J Radiat Oncol Biol Phys** 16:663–668, 1989.

25. Steiger H, Markwalder R, Seiler R, et al.: Early prognosis of supratentorial grade 2 astrocytomas in adult patients after resection or stereotactic biopsy. **Acta Neurochir** 106:99–105, 1990.

26. Vecht C: Effect of age on treatment decisions in low-grade glioma. **J Neurol Neurosurg Psychiatry** 56:1259–1264, 1993.

27. Vertosick F, Selker R, Arena V: Survival of patients with well-differentiated astrocytomas diagnosed in the era of computed tomography. **Neurosurgery** 28:496–501, 1994.

28. Westergaard L, Gjerris F, Klinken L: Prognostic parameters in benign astrocytomas. **Acta Neurochir** 123:1–7, 1993.

6

Selection of Patients for Surgery for Parkinson's Disease

R. R. TASKER, M.D.

The surgical treatment of Parkinsonism, particularly for the relief of tremor, originally consisted of interrupting the corticospinal tract at various levels in the central nervous system, substituting a certain degree of paralysis for tremor relief. When Russell Meyers (9) discovered that movement disorders could be ameliorated by operations on the basal ganglia, a new era in neurosurgery began. However, the morbidity and mortality of such operations done by open craniotomy would have proven prohibitive; fortunately at this time, Spiegel *et al.* (13) introduced the human stereotactic technique, wherein stereotactic pallidotomy became the surgical treatment of choice for Parkinson's disease. Probably chance events, both in the United States and Europe, then led to the discovery that so-called ventrolateral thalamotomy was superior to pallidotomy, at least for the treatment of tremor, and rather abruptly interest in pallidotomy waned. The introduction of L-dopa therapy then greatly reduced the referral of parkinsonian patients for any kind of surgery until relatively recently. In the last few years the increased sophistication of imaging, of stereotactic instruments and of a growing knowledge of the pathophysiology of Parkinson's disease has led to a renewed interest in the surgical treatment of the disease (4).

CURRENT SURGICAL PROCEDURES FOR PARKINSON'S DISEASE

Although a large number of different operations have been proposed over the years for the treatment of Parkinson's disease, at the present time it is likely that most patients are treated by means of pallidotomy or thalamotomy, the thalamic target of choice being Hassler's nucleus ventralis intermedius (Vim) (11, 12). Although adrenal medullary grafting has proven disappointing, fetal mesencephalic grafting is effective and is being actively investigated as an experimental procedure. In addition, the technology developed for the treatment of chronic pain by so-called deep brain stimulation (DBS) has been applied to the treatment of Parkinson's disease (1, 3). Curiously, DBS and lesion making in the same target sites in globus pallidus internus (GPi) and Vim appear to achieve exactly the same results. Thus far, experience with DBS in GPi is limited and will not be reviewed in detail whereas bilateral chronic stimulation of the subthalamic nucleus of Luys (STN) is being investigated (7). This chapter will deal mainly with pallidotomy, Vim thalamotomy, and Vim DBS.

PERSONAL OUTCOME DATA

Our conclusions concerning choice of surgery in Parkinson's disease are based on various reviews (5, 6, 8, 14–17) of our own surgical experience over the years, as summarized in Table 1. These studies were retrospective and not originally designed to compare outcome after the various procedures, so they should be considered descriptive. The GPi data are based on the CAPIT (2) Assessment and are only partly comparable to the other data. In a direct comparison of outcome data in 13 Vim DBS implants in Parkinson's disease and 3 in essential tremor with 23 Vim thalamotomies in Parkinson's disease and 2 in essential tremor during the same time frame (16), 62.5% of implants abolished or left only insignificant contralateral tremor whereas 63.7% of thalamotomies did so. The difference between the groups was that none of the implants were repeated because any breakthrough of tremor was overcome by adjustment of the stimulation parameters

TABLE 1.
Comparison of Vim Thalamotomy and DBS and Pallidotomy

	% Patients Improved		
	Vim DBS (16)	Vim Thalamotomy	GPi Pallidotomy (6)[a]
Total relief of contralateral tremor	62.5	49 (15)	21% reduction overall
Significant or total relief of contralateral tremor	93.8	92 (15)	
Significant relief of contralateral rigidity	50	56 (15)	28% reduction overall
Relief of contralateral dopa dyskinesia	20	36 (15)	90% reduction overall
Significant improvement contralateral dexterity	64	29.9 (17)	50% improvement overall
Significant improvement in gait and stance	0	0.9 (17) worse	Slightly worse
Significant improvement in speech	0	Net worsening (17)	Not recorded

[a] "Off" contralateral performance 12 months postoperatively; tends to induce hypophonia.

whereas 27.3% of the thalamotomies were repeated in an effort to control significant recurrent tremor. This high repetition rate (we normally repeat about 15% of procedures) reflects the small number of cases studied, two of whom, operated on bilaterally, proved particularly resistant to tremor abolition.

CHOICE OF PROCEDURE

Once the decision has been made that surgical intervention is indicated in Parkinson's disease, it must be understood that Vim thalamotomy, Vim DBS, and GPi pallidotomy each play a distinct role and that none of them is capable of altering the course of Parkinson's disease. Hopefully, in the future mesencephalic fetal grafting or implantation of engineered cells may accomplish this. Table 2 summarizes the author's opinion as to the choice of operative procedures for different features of Parkinson's disease. For the relief of tremor, procedures performed on Vim are most effective. It is the author's opinion that rigidity by itself is seldom a disabling problem for the patient; bradykinesia is, and the bradykinetic patient often looks rigid. In those rare patients in whom rigidity is a problem, in the author's experience the most effective lesion is in the thalamus just rostral to the ideal lesion for relief of tremor in Hassler's nucleus ventralis oralis anterior and posterior (Voa Vop) or in GPi. Although pallidotomy may reduce tremor and rigidity, particularly contralaterally to the lesion, the effects are not as striking as those obtained by means of thalamic lesions or DBS. On the other hand, although thalamic lesions may reduce dopa dyskinesia (10), GPi lesions do so dramatically and far more successfully, and they are the preferred treatment for dopa dyskinesia. For the relief of bradykinetic features, such as clumsiness and slowness in hand movement and abnormalities of gait, GPi pallidotomy stands apart as the only procedure known at this time that offer the possibility of some degree of amelioration of these features.

Whereas bilateral DBS STN and fetal mesencephalic grafts are also effective for the relief of bradykinetic features, these are still experi-

TABLE 2.
Choice of Surgical Procedures in the Treatment of Parkinson's Disease

Chief Disabling Feature	Preferred Procedure
Tremor	Vim thalamotomy or DBS
Bradykinetic features	GPi pallidotomy
Dopa-induced dyskinesia	GPi pallidotomy
Rigidity[a]	Ventral oral (Voa, Vop) thalamotomy
	GPi pallidotomy

[a] Rarely a disability in itself.

mental procedures and will not be discussed further. None of these procedures improve speech deficits.

The next issue concerns the choice between destructive lesions and DBS. Table 3 lists the author's views on this question, with the comments concerning DBS GPi very preliminary. Before discussing details it must be recognized that DBS entails the cost of the implanted equipment ($5000–7000), the continuing medical care necessary to manage the equipment, the risk of infection or of equipment failure, and the need to replace a battery-powered device in time. Lesion making, on the other hand, is a once-only procedure that entails none of these disadvantages. The advantage of DBS over lesion making in Vim only becomes apparent as one follows the patient postoperatively. If tremor recurs after a lesion, the only recourse is to reoperate; if it recurs after DBS, tremor relief can nearly always be recaptured by simply adjusting the parameters of stimulation. If ataxia, dysarthria, or gait disturbance (the "cerebellar" complications) (18) appear after thalamotomy, one must wait for time and physiotherapy to correct them; when they appear with Vim DBS they can usually be avoided by parameter adjustments. It may be that DBS presents less risk in elderly or ill patients than making a lesion, but no published evidence addresses this issue. However, it is clear that, because bilateral Vim thalamotomy carries a 25–35% risk of aggravating dysarthria and, in our experience, bilateral GPi pallidotomy carries the risk of inducing cognitive dysfunction, possibly related to the size of the lesions made (and larger lesions may be needed to improve bradykinesia), DBS is preferred in each case to lesion making for second-side surgery. The author is unaware of outcome data for combined GPi and Vim lesions on the same side or for GPi lesions on one side, with Vim lesions on the other.

TABLE 3.
Lesions versus *DBS in Surgery for Parkinson's Disease*

Site	Lesion	DBS
GPi	First side	Second side to minimize cognitive dysfunction ?High risk patients
Vim	First side if patient prefers lesion to DBS or other factors prevent DBS	First side to enhance success and reduce complication rate
		Second side to minimize risk of worsening dysarthria ?High-risk patients

REFERENCES

1. Benabid AL, Pollack P, Gao D, et al.: Chronic electrical stimulation of the ventralis intermedius nucleus of the thalamus as a treatment of movement disorders. **J Neurosurg** 84:203–214, 1996.
2. CAPIT Committee: Langston WJ, Widner H, Goetz CG, et al.: Core Assessment Program for Intracerebral Transplantations (CAPIT). **Mov Disord** 7(1):2–13, 1992.
3. Galvez-Jimenez N, Lang AE, Lozano A, et al.: Deep brain stimulation in Parkinson's disease: New methods of tailoring functional surgery to patient needs and response. **Neurology** 46:A402, 1996.
4. Laitinen LV, Bergenheim AT, Hariz MI: Leksell posteroventral pallidotomy in the treatment of Parkinson's disease. **J Neurosurg** 76:53–61, 1992.
5. Lang AE, Lozano A, Duff J, et al.: Posteroventral medial pallidotomy in Parkinson's disease. **Mov Disord** 10:691, 1995.
6. Tasker R, Miyasaki J, Galvez-Jimenez N, Hutchison W, Dostrovsky J. Medial pallidotomy in late-stage Parkinson's disease and striatonigral degeneration. **Adv Neurol** 1997 (in press).
7. Limousin P, Pollack P, Benazzouz A, et al.: Effect on parkinsonian signs and symptoms of bilateral subthalamic nucleus stimulation. **Lancet** 345:91–95, 1995.
8. Lozano AM, Lang AE, Galvez-Jiminez N, et al.: GPI pallidotomy improves motor function in patients with Parkinson's disease. **Lancet** 346:1383–1386, 1995.
9. Meyers R: A surgical procedure for the alleviation of postencephalitic tremor with notes on the physiology of the premotor fibres. **Arch Neurol Psychiatry** 44:455–459, 1940.
10. Narabayashi H, Yokochi F, Nakajima Y: Levodopa-induced dyskinesia and thalamotomy. **J Neurol Neurosurg Psychiatry** 47:831–839, 1984.
11. Schaltenbrand G, Bailey P: *Introduction to Stereotaxis with and Atlas of the Human Brain*. Stuttgart, Germany, Thieme, 1959.
12. Schaltenbrand G, Wahren W: *Atlas for Stereotaxy of the Human Brain*. Stuttgart, Germany, Thieme, 1977.
13. Spiegel EA, Wycis HT, Freed H, et al.: Stereoencephalotomy. **Proc R Soc Exp Biol Med** 69:175–177, 1948.
14. Tasker RR: The outcome of thalamotomy for tremor, in PL Gildenberg, RR Tasker (eds): *Textbook of Stereotactic and Functional Neurosurgery*. New York, McGraw-Hill, in press, 1997.
15. Tasker RR, De Carvalho GC, Li CS, et al.: Does thalamotomy alter the course of Parkinson's disease? 69:563–583, 1996.
16. Tasker RR, Munz M, Junn FSCK, et al.: DBS and thalamotomy for tremor compared. **Acta Neurochir**, submitted for publication, 1996.
17. Tasker RR, Siqueira J, Hawrylshyn P, et al.: What happened to Vim thalamotomy for Parkinson's disease? **Appl Neurophysiol** 46:68–83, 1983.
18. Yasui N, Narabayashi H, Kondo T, et al.: Slight cerebellar signs in stereotactic thalamotomy and subthalamotomy for Parkinsonism. **Appl Neurophysiol** 39:315–320, 1976/77.

CHAPTER

7

Selection Criteria for the Treatment of Cranial Rhizopathies by Microvascular Decompression (Honored Guest Lecture)

PETER J. JANNETTA, M.D., D.SCI.

Although once considered a preposterous and dangerous treatment, microvascular decompression (MVD) has become an accepted, and, in fact, preferred treatment for a number of cranial nerve rhizopathies. Dandy was first to propose that vascular compression of the trigeminal root caused trigeminal neuralgia (TN) (1). In 1959, Gardner and Milkos were first to report on the successful treatment of TN by mobilizing an artery off the trigeminal nerve in the cerebellopontine angle (2). Since 1966, with the utilization of the operating microscope, much has been published on the safety and efficacy of MVD (3).

All of the cranial rhizopathies for which MVD is effective in treating are, essentially the same disease process; *i.e.*, nonfascicular nerve stimulation causing hyperactive syndromes variably accompanied by loss of function. The syndromes include TN, hemifacial spasm (HFS), disabling positional vertigo (DPV), Ménière's disease, disequilibrium, tinnitus, glossopharyngeal neuralgia (GPN), spasmodic torticollis, and "essential" (neurogenic) hypertension (HTN). All of the cranial nerves and the brainstem are subject to the forces of vascular compression, dependent mainly upon vascular deterioration (arteriosclerosis), sagging of the brain, and congenital factors affecting the configuration of the posterior fossa and its contents. In all patients in whom MVD is contemplated, brain imaging is mandatory to eliminate other causes, *e.g.*, tumors, aneurysms, arteriovenous malformations, and multiple sclerosis.

In patients with these syndromes, most often the clinician is managing a problem that is affecting quality of life, not one that is itself life-threatening. (An exception to this is hypertension, which is clearly a major source of morbidity and mortality worldwide.) Once the patient reaches the point that his or her life is being ruined by pain or other dysfunction, and medication is not effective or is causing significant side effects, MVD is a reasonable option. The most important aspect of the preoperative evaluation for MVD is the history and physical examination. Patients with "typical" as opposed to "atypical" syndromes have better results. Age by itself is not a contraindication to MVD. A healthy 80-year-old will tolerate the procedure well.

Some of these syndromes are very common. The age-adjusted prevalence of HTN is 20% (4), and over 40 million Americans suffer from tinnitus (5). As we get older, these syndromes become even more common. In the elderly, nearly everyone manifests VIIIth nerve dysfunction with hearing loss, tinnitus, and balance difficulties. For this reason, it is important for the physician and neurosurgeon to recognize these syndromes and to be aware of the treatment options.

SELECTION CRITERIA FOR SPECIFIC SYNDROMES

Trigeminal Neuralgia

The patient with intermittent sharp, lancinating pain in the distribution of the trigeminal nerve who has had some response to medication (phenytoin, carbamazepine, or baclofen) and is now refractory to medication or is suffering from medication side effects is an excellent candidate for MVD. Other features of this symptom complex, *i.e.*, typical TN, include a memorable onset of the original pain, trigger points, and exacerbating factors like wind against the face, eating, and talking. Other facial pain syndromes include atypical trigeminal neuralgia, nervus intermedius neuralgia, cluster headaches, myofacial pain syndrome, temporomandibular joint disease, and dental neuromas.

Precise correlation between symptoms and the point of vascular compression seen *intraoperatively* is the rule: rostral compression of V at the brainstem causes V_3 pain; medio-lateral compression causes V_2 pain; the rare caudal compression causes V_1 pain; and atypical trigeminal neuralgia is caused by compression of the motor-proprioceptive fibers (portio minor) distally. After starting with a V_3 pain syndrome, patients will frequently progress to include V_2 and V_1 pain as the offending vessels move caudally on the trigeminal nerve.

VIIth Nerve Disorders

HEMIFACIAL SPASM

Hemifacial spasm (HFS) is disabling and very distressing to patients. Although painless, these involuntary spasms are disfiguring, and can interfere with reading, driving, speaking, *etc.* The syndrome is uncommon, with a prevalence of 7/100,000 population (6). In typical HFS (>90% of cases), contractions first affect the orbicularis oculi muscle and then progress caudally to affect the cheek, corner of the mouth, and platysma. In atypical HFS, the onset of spasms is in the buccal musculature with progression up through the face. Sustained contracture (tonus phenomenon) is common in both typical and atypical cases with hemifacial eye closure and pulling of the corner of the mouth over to the side. Virtually all healthy patients with tonus phenomenon have mild facial weakness. *All* patients with hemifacial spasm are candidates for MVD and should expect a good result (84% excellent; 10% good results at 10 years follow-up) (7). Medication is useless, and botulinum toxin injection with some exceptions is usually short-lasting with diminishing returns after each injection.

Acute vascular stretch/compression of VII by shifted arterial loops is associated with loss of function, which is manifested as Bell's palsy. Facial nerve ischemia, viral infection, and genetic factors are purported causes of this syndrome; however, each theory has its shortcomings. We have noted and reported stretching of the facial nerve by an arterial loop in patients with a remote diagnosis of Bell's palsy. With MVD of the facial nerve, facial function improved (8). The clinical characteristics of rapid, unilateral loss of facial nerve function combined with the observation of vascular compression of the facial nerve have led us to perform MVD in cases of Bell's palsy (9).

VIIIth Nerve Disorders

Disabling positional vertigo (vertigo and/or disequilibrium with or without nausea and vomiting) (DPV), Ménière's disease, decreased vestibular function (stumbling, *etc.*), tinnitus, and hearing loss are all caused by vascular compression of the vestibular-cochlear nerve. Once again, the history and physical examination are the most important tools in selecting patients for MVD. A nearly constant sensation of true vertigo, *i.e.*, spinning, associated with nausea is characteristic of DPV. Symptoms may be made worse by changes in position of the head or body, and may be improved by lying on the contralateral side, hence the term positional. On physical examination, the patient with DPV may drift toward the affected side when walking and may have nystagmus. As opposed to vestibular neuronitis, DPV becomes progressively worse with the passage of time and usually does not improve with vestibular suppressant medications (Antivert, Dramamine). In contrast to patients with benign paroxysmal positional vertigo (BPPV), the patient with DPV is rarely without symptoms. As noted previously, the differential diagnosis in patients with DPV includes BPPV, vestibular neuronitis, and perilymphatic fistula (10, 11). Ménière's disease is nothing more than a specific subset of vascular compression of VIII and is relieved by MVD. The criteria for the diagnosis of Ménière's disease have changed over the years as the testing procedures have changed.

Preoperative assessment includes brain imaging and brainstem and auditory evoked responses (BSERS). Abnormalities in BSERS are present in 50% of patients with DPV (Møller, MB, personal communication). These abnormalities include mile to moderate unilateral hearing loss, an increase in latency between peaks I and III ipsilaterally, and/or between peaks III and V on the contralateral side. Symptoms and signs of vascular compression of adjacent cranial nerves (GPN, HFS, and TN) may also accompany the symptoms of VIIIth nerve compression. Precise correlation between symptoms and the point of vascular compression is the rule: vertigo/compression of the superior vestibular nerve at the brainstem; nausea/compression of the inferior vestibular nerve at the brainstem; disequilibrium without vertigo/compression of the superior vestibular nerve just distal to the brainstem; hearing loss and tinnitus/compression of the cochlear nerve at any point along its course; and decreased vestibular function/compression and stretch of the vestibular nerves anywhere.

Disorders of the glossopharyngeal and vagus nerves with or without autonomic dysfunction

Glossopharyngeal neuralgia is characterized by intermittent, lancinating pain involving the posterior tongue, pharynx, and deep ear structures. It is an uncommon but disabling disorder. Once head and neck pathology is eliminated as a cause of the pain, patients with the symptoms described above are excellent candidates for MVD of IX and X, with 79% of patients completely relieved of pain (12).

Pathologic processes affecting cranial nerves IX, X, and the brainstem can present in various ways. Commonly, the clinician elicits a combination of cranial nerve dysfunction and long tract signs. It is also possible for pathologic processes affecting the brainstem to manifest with autonomic dysfunction and sleep apnea, as these processes are regulated in brainstem centers. Over the years, we have encountered patients with unusual manifestations of brainstem dysfunction that can be attributed to vascular compression of the brainstem and lower cranial nerves. The pathophysiology of such disorders is straightforward: stimulation or dysfunction of cranial nerves IX, X, brainstem autonomic centers, and long tracts. The resulting symptoms and syndromes that have been ameliorated and/or relieved with MVD include sleep apnea (13), syncope, intractable and seemingly unexplainable vomiting and diarrhea, hemiparesis, ataxia, and neurogenic ("essential") hypertension. The latter disorder will be discussed separately.

XIth Nerve Dysfunction, Spasmodic Torticollis

Spasmodic torticollis is characterized by involuntary tonic or clonic contractions of the cervical musculature resulting in rotation and/or flexion or extension of the head and neck. Lesions of the striatum, labyrinthine dysfunction, and neuromuscular disease have been implicated as causes of torticollis, but with no evidence. Once head and neck trauma and tumors have been eliminated, we can attribute spasmodic torticollis to vascular compression of cranial nerve XI and the upper cervical rootlets and opt for MVD as the treatment of choice for this disorder (14).

Essential or Neurogenic Hypertension

Any patient with essential hypertension(HTN) who has demonstrated good compliance with a medical regimen of weight loss, exercise, and medication and is still hypertensive or is suffering from medication side effects is a candidate for left lateral medullary MVD. A vast and growing amount of data based on neurophysiologic studies, animal experiments, epidemiologic data, radiologic studies, and clinical series supports the hypothesis that vascular compression of the left medulla oblongata is the cause, the underlying "common soil" of HTN.

NEUROPHYSIOLOGIC DATA

Reis et al. reviewed the anatomy and neurophysiology of brainstem cardiovascular control (15). The reticlaris rostroventrolateralis nucleus in the medulla is the site of the brainstem cardiovascular center. It contains a set of adrenergic neurons high in phenyl ethanolamine N-methyl transferase (PNMT) activity, the C1 group. The C1 area, in turn, receives input from baroreceptors, chemoreceptors, and cardiac afferent fibers via the nucleus tractus solitarius. The C1 group then provides excitatory input to the intermedio-lateral cell column of the spinal cord from which sympathetic outflow to the body originates.

ANIMAL STUDIES

Animal studies have demonstrated that compression of the left lateral medulla can produce cardiovascular stimulation and/or HTN in formerly normotensive animals. In 1982, Segal et al. demonstrated in cats that pulsatile compression of the left lateral medulla results in increased cardiac stroke volume and cardiac output (16). A neurovascular compression simulator (NCS) for use in animal models of HTN was described by Segal et al. in 1982 (17, 18). This device consists of an intra-aortic balloon, a smaller cephalic balloon, and a connecting tube. With each cardiac systole, the rise in intra-aortic pressure is transmitted to the cephalic balloon, which is surgically implanted against the left lateral medulla. In 10 baboons studied by Jannetta *et al.* in 1985, HTN developed in five with the NCS, whereas no changes in blood pressure or pulse were found in five controls with NCS deflated. Unrestrained baboons with NCS's showed significant long-term HTN that normalized after deflation of the NCS (19). Utilizing a canine model, Yamamoto *et al.* found that compression of the left medulla lateral to the inferior olive caused HTN, while right-sided compression did not (20), verifying the earlier baboon work. Granata and Reis demonstrated that bilateral microinjection of an α-adrenergic agonist or histamine into the C1 area produces a dose-dependent decrease in blood pressure and pulse (21). In a similar study, Chida *et al.* found that bilateral lesions of the medulla in the rat abolished elevations in blood pressure and pulse (22).

EPIDEMIOLOGIC DATA

Van Ouwerkerk *et al.* examined the frequency of "essential" HTN in patients with TN or HFS (23). Patients with TN on either side or right-sided HFS had the same prevalence of HTN as the control population. Patients with left-sided HFS, however, had nearly twice the prevalence of HTN as controls. Katusic *et al.* found the prevalence of HTN in patients with GPN to be twice that of a control population (24). In a similar study, the same group found that patients with HFS and TN had an increased prevalence of HTN (25).

RADIOLOGIC DATA

Naraghi *et al.* examined the brainstems of 55 patients postmortem (26); 24 were diagnosed with "essential" hypertension, 10 were diagnosed with "renal" hypertension, and 21 patients with normal blood pressures during life served as controls. After perfusion and microsurgical inspection, the authors found no case of neurovascular compression of the left VLM in controls or in patients with "renal" hypertension, whereas all patients with essential hypertension had "definite" compression of the left VLM. Unfortunately, this was not a blinded evaluation. Kleineberg *et al.* determined the post of the root entry zone (REZ) of the left glossopharyngeal and vagus nerves in 10 cadavers and created a template delineating the REZ in standard angiographic projections (27). Angiograms of 107 hypertensive and 100 normotensive patients were compared retrospectively. In 80% of hypertensive patients, an artery crossed the REZ of cranial nerves IX and X, whereas this occurred in only 35% of normotensive patients. Naraghi *et al.* subsequently published a properly controlled study that further corroborated the prior work and our work (28).

CLINICAL DATA

In 1973, we operated on a 55-year-old woman with GPN who suffered a hypertensive stroke 2 hours after an uneventful MVD of cranial nerves IX and X (29). Another patient that same year had severe HTN for several days following MVD for GPN. These events directed our attention to vascular compression of the medulla as the cause of essential hypertension. In 1979, Jannetta and Gendel described the first clinical report on vascular compression as the etiology of HTN: 16 consecutive hypertensive patients had vascular compression of the VLM; 11 by the VA, and five by the PICA. The patients with VA compression had the more severe HTN. No VLM compression was seen in over 30 normotensive patients who underwent MVD for other reasons. Microvascular decompression was performed in five patients with HTN. One patient had normal blood pressure for 10 months; one had a significant decrease in blood pressure; and three had a gradual return to normal (29). A study of 52 patients by Jannetta *et al.* showed similar results. Hypertensive patients had arterial compression of the left lateral medulla, and 88.6% were relieved by MVD, half on no medication and the others with significant decrease postoperatively. At long-term follow-up in 30 patients, 26 have remained normotensive or have had significant improvement (30, 31). Others have reported similar encouraging results.

The more refractory the hypertension, the worse the patient does with surgery. Again, all patients with "essential" HTN having difficulty with medications or in controlling their blood pressure are candidates for MVD.

Other problems of aging are caused by vascular compression of the cranial nerves and brainstem: in short, by pulsatile compression of nonfascicular nervous tissue. We inherit our parents' blood vessels in various combinations. This is the genetic relationship of these occasionally to frequently familial "diseases." As other problems are synthesized and the clinical pathological correlations and operative techniques are developed, a brave new world of neurosurgery dependent on a growing concept of disease will emerge, a great opportunity for patients and their well-prepared neurosurgeons.

ACKNOWLEDGMENTS

The author wishes to thank Kamal Kalia, M.D., for his assistance with preparation of the manuscript.

REFERENCES

1. Dandy WE: Treatment of trigeminal neuralgia by the cerebellar route. **Ann Surg** 787:96, 1932.
2. Gardner WJ, Milkos MV: Response of trigeminal neuralgia to "decompression" of sensory root. **JAMA** 170:1773–1776, 1959.
3. Barker FG II, Jannetta PJ, Bissonette DJ, et al.: **N Engl J Med** 334(17):1077–1089, 1996.
4. Burt VL, Culter JA, Higgins M, et al.: Trends in the prevalence, awareness, treatment, and control of hypertension in the adult US population. Data from the health examination surveys, 1960 to 1991. **Hypertension** 26(1):60–69, 1995.
5. Van Ouwerkerk WJR, Samii M, Ammirati M: Essential hypertension in patients with hemifacial spasm or trigeminal neuralgia, in Frowein RA, Brock M, Klinger M, (eds): Advances in Neurosurgery, Vol 17. Berlin, Springer Verlag, 1988, pp 188–193.
6. Auger RG, Whisnant JP: Hemifacial spasm in Rochester and Olmstead County, Minnesota, 1960 to 1984. **Arch Neurol** 47:1233–1234, 1990.
7. Barker FG, Jannetta PJ, Bissonette DJ, et al.: Microvascular decompression for hemifacial spasm. **J Neurosurg** 82:201–210, 1995.
8. Jannetta PJ, Resnick D: Cranial rhizopathies, in Youmans JR (ed) Philadelphia: WB Saunders, 1996, pp 3563–3574. **Neurological Surgery** Fourth Edition
9. Jannetta PJ, Bissonette DJ: Bell's palsy: A theory as to etiology. Observations in six patients. **Laryngoscope** 88:849–854, 1978.
10. Møller MB, Møller AR, Jannetta PJ: Microvascular decompression of the eighth nerve in patients with disabling positional vertigo: selection criteria and operative results in 207 patients. **Acta Neurochir** 125:75–82, 1993.
11. Møller MB, Møller AR, Jannetta PJ, et al.: Diagnosis and surgical treatment of disabling positional vertigo. **J Neurosurg** 64:21–28, 1986.
12. Resnick DK, Jannetta PJ, Bissonette DB, et al.: Microvascular decompression for glossopharyngeal neuralgia. **Neurosurgery** 36:64–99, 1995.
13. Hoffman RM, Stiller RA: Resolution of obstructive sleep apnea after microvascular brainstem decompression. **Chest** 107(2):570–572, 1995.
14. Jho HD, Jannetta PJ: Spasmodic torticollis treated with microvascular decompression of the spinal accessory nerves, the upper cervical nerve roots and the brainstem. **Acta Neurochir** (in press).
15. Reis DJ, Ruggiero DA, Morrison SF: The C1 area of the rostral ventrolateral medulla oblongata. **Am J Hypertens** 2:363S–374S, 1989.
16. Segal R, Jannetta PJ, Wolfson SK, et al.: Implanted pulsatile balloon device for simulation of neurovascular compression syndromes in animals. **J Neurosurgery** 57:646–650, 1982.
17. Segal R, Gendell HM, Canfield D, et al.: Hemodynamic changes induced by pulsatile compression of the ventrolateral medulla. **Angiology** 33(3):161–172, 1982.
18. Segal R, Jannetta PJ, Wolfson SK, et al.: Implanted pulsatile balloon device for simulation of neurovascular compression syndromes in animals. **J Neurosurg** 57(5):646–650, 1982.
19. Jannetta PJ, Segal R, Wolfson SK, et al.: Neurogenic hypertension: etiology and surgical treatment. II. Observations in an experimental nonhuman primate model. **Ann Surg** 202(2):253–261, 1985.

20. Yamamoto I, Yamada S, Sato O: Microvascular decompression for hypertension. Clinical and experimental study. **Neurol Med Chi** (Tokyo) 31:1–6, 1991.

21. Granata AR, Reis DJ: Hypotension and bradycardia elicited by histamine into the C1 area of the rostral ventrolateral medulla. **Eur J Pharmacol** 136:157–162, 1987.

22. Chida K, Iadecola C, Reis DJ: Lesions of rostral ventrolateral medulla abolish some cardio- and cerebrovascular components of the cerebellar fastigial pressor and depressor responses. **Brain Res** 508:93–104, 1990.

23. van Ouwerkerk WJR, Samii M, Ammirati M: Essential hypertension in patients with hemifacial spasm or trigeminal neuralgia. **Adv Neurosurg** 17:188–193, 1989.

24. Katusic S, Williams DB, Beard CM, *et al.:* Incidence and clinical features of glossopharyngeal neuralgia, Rochester, Minnesota 1945–1984. **Neuroepidemiology** 10: 266–275, 1991.

25. Katusic S, Williams DB, Beard CM, *et al.:* Epidemiology and clinical features of idiopathic trigeminal neuralgia and glossopharyngeal neuralgia: Similarities and differences, Rochester, Minnesota, 1945–1984. **Neuroepidemiology** 10:276–281, 1991.

26. Naraghi R, Gaab MR, Walter GF, *et al.:* Arterial hypertension and neurovascular compression at the ventrolateral medulla. A comparative microanatomical and pathological study. **J Neurosurg** 77:103–112, 1992.

27. Kleineberg B, Becker H, Gaab MR: Neurovascular compression and essential hypertension. An angiographic study. **Neuroradiology** 33:2–8, 1991.

28. Naraghi R, Geiger H, Crnac J, *et al.:* Posterior fossa neurovascular anomalies in essential hypertension. **Lancet** 344:1466–1470, 1994.

29. Jannetta PJ, Gendel HM: Clinical observations on etiology of essential hypertension. **Surg Forum** 30:431–432, 1979.

30. Jannetta PJ, Segal R, Wolfson SK: Neurogenic hypertension: Etiology and surgical treatment. I. Observations in 53 patients. **Ann Surg** 201(3):391–398, 1985.

31. Jannetta PJ, Hamm IS, Jho HD, *et al.:* Essential hypertension caused by arterial compression of the left lateral medulla: A follow-up. **Perspectives in Neurological Surgery** 3:107–125, 1992.

—

8

Temporal Lobe Epilepsy

GEORGE A. OJEMANN, M.D.

Four issues important in selection of patients with temporal lobe epilepsy (TLE) for surgical therapy are considered in this chapter: (*a*) Are there surgical procedures that result in a higher probability of control of seizures than would be expected from antiepileptic drug therapy and, if so, will this make a difference in the patient's quality of life? (*b*) When should the patient be considered refractory to antiepileptic drug therapy? (*c*) If the surgical option is a resective operation, what diagnostic studies identify the focal site of seizure origin? (*d*) What studies establish that this focus can be resected with a low risk of new neurologic deficits?

ARE THERE SURGICAL PROCEDURES THAT RESULT IN A HIGHER PROBABILITY OF SEIZURE CONTROL THAN ANTIEPILEPTIC DRUG THERAPY? DOES THIS MAKE A DIFFERENCE IN QUALITY OF LIFE?

Our group addressed this issue in a study by Dodrill, L. Ojemann, Batzel, and Fraser (none of them surgeons) that compared patients with partial (focal) epilepsies, mostly temporal, who underwent surgical resection between 1982 and 1987, to a matched series of patients with similar epilepsy who had been concurrently medically managed. Outcome was assessed for seizure frequency in the 4th and 5th years after operation or entry into the study, by several objective quality of life measures administered before operation or entry and five years later, and by changes in vocational status over that interval. The surgical series consisted of 109 consecutive patients undergoing temporal lobe resection who were also given quality-of-life and other neuropsychologic measures preoperatively. They were matched to a series of 82 patients with similar partial seizure disorders who had been managed medically over the same period, and also administered the same measures before entry into the study. This matched group is similar in age and duration of seizures (17 years) but has a slightly lower seizure frequency than the surgical group. At entry into the study, the medically managed group was similar to the surgical group in terms of vocational measures such as hours worked and average earnings. The matched medical group was vigorously managed, many in specialized epilepsy centers, on an average of 4.7 antiepileptic drugs, with 28% participating in experimental drug evaluations. Although this study antedates the development of modern magnetic resonance imaging (MRI) techniques now used in case selection and does not reflect the most modern surgical techniques or outcomes, with the present more aggressive use of surgical therapy for epilepsy, no such matched control group could now be assembled. Indeed, many of the control patients have been operated on subsequently.

Seizure control was significantly better in the surgical group, with 54 of the 109 patients (50%) seizure-free in the 4th and 5th postoperative years, compared to 4 of 82 (5%) in the medically managed group ($P < .0001$) (14). On using the two objective measures of the patient's perception of their quality of life, the Washington Psychosocial Review and Washington Psychosocial Seizure Inventory (8), 5 years after surgery or entry into the study, the members of the surgical group showed significantly better overall adjustment and adjustment to seizures on both measures and better emotional and vocational adjustment on the latter measure (3). Vocationally, at the end of the study, the surgical group also showed significantly more improvement than the medically managed group. Average earnings and hours worked were significantly greater for the surgical group, with the somewhat unexpected finding that the medically managed group lost ground vocationally over the study period, working fewer hours at the end of the study than on entry and experiencing changes in average earnings that did not keep pace with inflation (Fraser and Dodrill, unpublished data). In one subset of patients, those who were students at the time of surgery or entry into the study who subsequently entered the workforce, the vocational benefits of surgery were particularly evident. Ninety percent of the patients in this group who had undergone surgical therapy were working, compared to 47% of similar patients managed medically (3). This finding indicates the importance of surgical therapy in younger patients, before the patient has settled into a dependent lifestyle. The conclusion from this study is that, even with case selection and surgical techniques of a decade ago, in patients with epilepsy that had been refractory to previous management, resective surgery is more likely to achieve seizure control, an improved quality of life based on the patient's own perception, and better vocational outcome than that achieved with continued medical management (as assessed 5 years after operation or entry into the study).

WHEN SHOULD THE PATIENT BE CONSIDERED REFRACTORY TO
ANTIEPILEPTIC DRUG MANAGEMENT?

Antiepileptic drugs represent the initial management of patients with epilepsy. For the majority of patients they control seizures. However, in a general practice survey from Great Britain, 38% of all epileptics were still having seizures on medical management in the 5th year after diagnosis (17). Patients with complex partial seizures are more likely to be refractory to medical management, with only about one-half controlled by antiepileptic drug therapy (28). After the initial 2 years of therapy, only an additional 10% or less of patients become seizure-free with further medical management (36, 38, 39). Indeed, this has also been the experience with the new antiepileptic drugs that have recently come onto the market; only 5–10% of patients refractory to standard antiepileptic drugs became seizure-free with the addition of any of the new drugs (41, 50). It is of interest that the outcome criterion used for surgical therapy of epilepsy (seizure-free) is so different from that used for the evaluation of new antiepileptic drugs (the proportion of patients with a 50% reduction in seizures).

Most patients with epilepsy thus fall into one of two groups: those with seizures readily controlled with the standard antiepileptic drugs, phenytoin, carbamazepine, and valproate, alone or in combination at therapeutic levels, or those who will not be completely controlled on any combination of any tolerated drugs (refractory patients). Depending on seizure frequency, it will usually be evident within 2 years of therapy in which group a patient belongs. Surgical therapy is usually only considered for the refractory patients. Occasionally, surgical therapy will also be considered in patients who will not take antiepileptic drugs because of what the patient considers to be intolerable side effects, for these patients too are refractory to medical management, although because of toxicity, not efficacy. In such patients it is often worth trying one of the newer antiepileptic drugs, gabapentine, lamotrigine, or vigabitron, for these drugs will sometimes provide the same degree of control as standard drugs but with less toxicity. The refractory group includes a high proportion of patients with complex partial seizures arising from the temporal lobe, one of the reasons for the emphasis on temporal lobe operations in the surgical management of epilepsy. The group of refractory patients is not small. Epilepsy is thought to occur in 0.5–1.0% of the population. If only 20% of patients are considered refractory (probably an underestimate) and 40% of them are surgical candidates, there are about 100,000 surgical candidates in the United States (30). Of these patients, 60–80% will have TLE. The recent growth in epilepsy surgery seems warranted.

Both the quality of life studies and considerations of medical management discussed above have emphasized having a seizure-free patient as the therapeutic goal. There are additional biologic and psychosocial reasons for this. Uncontrolled generalized seizures are associated with an increased mortality rate (26), and there is some evidence that uncontrolled partial seizures are associated with ongoing neuronal degeneration (16). Only when a patient is seizure-free can a driver's license be obtained and epilepsy no longer be an issue in employment. Having a seizure-free patient as the therapeutic goal has a major effect on which surgical options to consider for patients with refractory epilepsy. For among the procedures in use today, callosal section, vagal nerve stimulation, and multiple subpial transections or resections, only resective surgery results in a high proportion of patients who are subsequently seizure-free. Thus, the initial evaluation of refractory patients should be directed at establishing whether they are candidates for a resection.

WHAT DIAGNOSTIC STUDIES IDENTIFY THE SITE OF SEIZURE ORIGIN?

There is general agreement that the site of seizure origin is most accurately identified by convergence of findings from several different sources onto a single brain site. For TLE, the most important findings are derived from an EEG and high-resolution MRI. There are a number of EEG techniques used to identify the site of seizure origin. Those in general use include the location of interictal epileptiform activity, the interictal spike (IIS), on routine outpatient scalp EEGs; the site of seizure onset on scalp EEG recordings obtained on inpatient continuous video-EEG monitoring; and the location of seizure onsets on intracranial EEG recordings obtained through depth or subdural electrodes. The site of a "focal functional deficit," where the usual EEG fast activity induced by barbiturates or diazepines is absent, has also been related to the site of seizure onset (27). The value of ambulatory EEG recording, and of magnetoencephalographic localization of IIS, has not been established.

High-resolution MRI-oriented perpendicular to the axis of hippocampus demonstrates the internal anatomy of that structure (18). The presence of atrophy, to quantitative measures (22) or visual inspection correlates well with the pathologic changes of medial temporal sclerosis (MTS). There are a large number of other imaging techniques that have been used to identify the focus in TLE. Decreased glucose metabolism on positron emission tomography (PET) with fluorodeoxyglucose (FDG) has been used to identify the side of onset in TLE, but the changes are too widespread to establish the site of onset within a hemisphere (10). PET with appropriate ligands demonstrates loss of benzodiazepine receptors in the medial temporal lobe on the side of the focus, a change that often correlates with the presence of MTS (19). That change, in combination with PET demonstration of increased μ-opiate receptors in the temporal neocortex, is believed to lateralize the side of seizure onset reliably (29). Single-photon emission tomography (SPECT) has been used to identify changes in blood flow in the focus, with the focus characterized by decreased flow present between seizures, and in increased flow with seizures (25, 40). However, interictal SPECT has been unreliable, whereas ictal SPECT is technically difficult to use. Changes in MR spectroscopy have also been used to identify the focus in TLE. They include decreased n-acetylaspartate concentration in the focus, a change that also correlates with presence of MTS (24). Changes in pH and phosphate concentrations have also been described in the focus (23). Evidence pointing to the location of the focus has also been derived from neuropsychologic assessment and the changes in memory measures after intracarotid amobarbital perfusion (56).

A major challenge in evaluating patients with refractory TLE is deciding which combinations of these diagnostic studies provides a cost-effective identification of the focus. Some of these tests involve substantial investment of resources, especially scalp and intracranial seizure recording, PET, and the intracarotid amobarbital perfusion test. Some also expose the patient to additional risks. It is quite easy to invest many more resources in the diagnostic evaluation of a patient with TLE than are required for the resective surgery (31). Appropriate selection of diagnostic tests to identify a focus remains a controversial area, although a few areas of consensus have developed in the past decade. Perhaps the clearest consensus is that many patients with TLE can be selected for resective surgery *without* the need for intracranial recording of seizure onsets.

At the University of Washington Epilepsy Center, we use a series of steps in the evaluation of patients with TLE, with criteria for proceeding with a resection at each step (35). The first step involves routine scalp EEG recordings obtained over at least 3–6 months, and high-resolution MRI. When these studies demonstrate exclusively unilateral temporal IIS and unilateral MR changes in hippocampus on the same side and the clinical characteristics of the seizures are compatible with that localization, the patient is considered a surgical candidate. Patients with unilateral temporal interictal foci have a high probability of being seizure-free after resection, and scalp seizure monitoring does not provide additional information that improves the outcome in these patients (21). Patients with unilateral hippocampal atrophy on high-resolution MR are also likely to be seizure-free after a resection (22). In the 77 of our patients undergoing initial temporal resections for nontumoral refractory epilepsy since the development of high-resolution MR who had been followed prospectively for 1 year after operation, of those with this combination of findings 72% were completely seizure-free, and another 12% had only a single seizure in that first postoperative year (G. Ojemann, unpublished data). In this patient group, there is no justification for expending further resources on diagnostic evaluation; specifically, there is no need for such resource-intensive studies as scalp seizure monitoring or PET scans. Although it has been suggested that MR changes alone may be adequate to select patients for temporal lobe resections, this has not been our experience. We have had cases in which the imaging change and EEG change were on opposite sides and the patient was seizure-free after a temporal resection on the side of the EEG changes (51), as well as cases in which the EEG changes suggested bilateral involvement but there were MR changes only on one side, where a temporal resection on the side of the MR changes was ineffective. Thus, it is the combination of unilateral EEG and MR changes on the same side that predicts a favorable outcome after a temporal resection. The presence of neuropsychologic test findings suggest that intact brain function also increases the chance of becoming seizure-free after a resection (7).

Unfortunately, only a minority of patients with refractory TLE (40% of our 77 patients) meet these initial criteria. A typical patient not meeting the initial criteria is one with bitemporal IIS, even when there is preponderance of these discharges on one side. The next step in the diagnostic evaluation of these remaining patients is admission to an inpatient unit equipped for continuous EEG-video monitoring, with recording of the EEG changes at onset of the patient's habitual seizures. This is usually facilitated by reducing the patient's antiepileptic drugs but never by using seizure-inducing drugs, as the seizures induced by those agents may not be localized to the site of origin of the patient's habitual seizures (48). When these recordings demonstrate all seizure onsets on the same side as MR changes, the patient is a surgical candidate, with a relatively high probability of becoming seizure-free (68% at 1-year follow-up in our 77 patient series; G. Ojemann, unpublished data). In the absence of an imaging change the probability of being seizure-free after a resection is less, even when all recorded interictal or ictal activity comes from one side. In our series only 40–50% of these patients are seizure-free 1 year after operation (G. Ojemann, unpublished data). It is in patients with obscure seizure onsets on scalp EEG or in whom those recordings show seizures beginning on either side that additional diagnostic studies such as PET, SPECT, and the specialized MR techniques are indicated. When the scalp seizure recordings show an origin on only one temporal lobe, and none of these studies points to an origin elsewhere, we will proceed with a temporal resection, recognizing that the probability of becoming seizure-free is only about one-half of that of patients with MR and EEG changes in the same temporal lobe.

There remains a group of patients with refractory TLE who have not had a focal origin established by the previous evaluation. A typical patient has bitemporal interictal activity and either obscure onset on scalp seizure monitoring (most seizures from one side but a few seemingly arising in the other temporal lobe) or a lack of convergence of findings from previous diagnostic studies. These patients are candidates for recording of seizure onsets from intracranial electrodes. They represent a minority of patients with refractory TLE. There are a variety of techniques for intracranial electrode placement in these patients. These include depth electrodes placed from a lateral approach or posteriorally (46), as well as subdural electrodes usually placed on basal and lateral temporal surfaces through burr holes (55). We prefer to use subdural electrodes. Although they are somewhat less sensitive than depth electrodes, they rarely provide misleading lateralization, and they have a slightly lower incidence of major complications. Whether the orbital frontal cortex needs to be sampled in intracranial recordings in TLE is controversial. It has been suggested that seizures seemingly of temporal lobe origin rather often arise in orbital frontal cortex (52). However, this has not been our experience. Most of our cases with complex partial seizures and temporal epileptic events on EEG arise in the temporal lobe. We reserve recording from orbital frontal cortex for those patients with atypical EEG or clinical features. Outcome in patients who require subdural recordings is generally not as good as in those who can be selected on scalp EEG criteria. When all recorded seizures arise in one temporal lobe, about one-half of the patients were seizure free at 1-year follow-up (G. Ojemann, unpublished data). When one or a few seizures appeared to arise from the other side but were subclinical or the onset was questionable, patients still did relatively well, with 40% seizure-free at 1 year. However, if there were unquestionably clinical seizures with onsets from either side, even when most seemed to come from one side, resection of that temporal lobe resulted in only 18% seizure-free at 1 year.

WHAT STUDIES ESTABLISH THAT THIS FOCUS CAN BE RESECTED WITH A LOW RISK OF NEW NEUROLOGIC DEFICIT?

In TLE, the major functional concerns relate to whether language is present in the temporal lobe that will be operated on and especially to whether resection of that temporal lobe will worsen recent memory.

Approximately 9% of these patients will have bilateral and 5% right hemisphere language representation; there is a rare patient who is righthanded, has a right temporal focus, and has right hemisphere language. We use the intracarotid amobarbital perfusion test (47, 53) to establish language lateralization in each patient and intraoperative mapping of language in planning dominant hemisphere resections (34). However, one study of successive series of cases suggests that there is only a small increase in postoperative language deficits with dominant temporal resections done without language mapping, compared to those done with mapping (2, 20). Many Epilepsy Centers reserve intracarotid amobarbital perfusion assessment of language for cases where odd dominance is suspected, such as in left-handed patients. However, our data indicate that once patients who are left-handed because of a right hemiparesis are excluded, there is no statistical relation between handedness and language lateralization (53).

In the past, the intracarotid amobarbital test was also the standard method for establishing the risk to recent memory of a temporal resection (4). Patients who "failed" this test during perfusion of the side of proposed operation were not considered for operation, for fear of producing an amnestic syndrome from resecting the one working medial temporal lobe (37, 43). Unfortunately, the validity of this method for predicting memory loss after temporal resections was little assessed. Recent studies of that issue have indicated several problems: different instruments for measuring memory during the intracarotid amobarbital perfusion give different results, and no memory measure predicts the postoperative occurrence of the verbal memory loss that patients complain of with sufficient reliability that is useful in an individual patient (9). The author's current view of assessing the risk of memory loss with a temporal resection is that no patient should be denied operation based solely on failing an arbitrary criterion for performance on a memory measure during intracarotid amobarbital perfusion of the side of proposed operation. Rather, memory risk should be assessed from the multiple factors that have been associated with loss after operation. These include: (a) age of onset of seizures, with onset after age 5 (42) or after age 18 (C. B. Dodrill, unpublished data) increasing the probability of a loss; (b) preoperative verbal memory (those with relatively intact verbal memory are much more likely to have a loss after a temporal resection); (c) absence of imaging changes of MTS, and associated with that, a lower chance of being seizure-free after an operation (the combination of a temporal resection and persisting seizures is especially likely to be associated with postoperative recent memory loss); (d) Female patients; (e) Older-aged patients and (f) in loss with ipsilateral and no loss with contralateral intracarotid amobarbital perfusion but only on certain memory measures (9). The relative weightings of these different factors in predicting postoperative memory loss has not been determined. However, consideration of all these factors will identify a group at high risk for memory loss; whether to proceed with the operation in those patients depends on the importance of facile recent verbal memory to their function (6). Intraoperative factors contribute some to reducing the risk to memory. Surprisingly, medial extent of the resection often has not correlated with memory loss (33, 54), whereas lateral extent has done so in some studies (33). Intraoperative mapping of lateral neocortical sites related to memory may be useful in reducing the risk of memory loss in patients at high risk based on preoperative evaluation (32).

CASE SELECTION AND INTRAOPERATIVE TECHNIQUE

There are a large number of techniques for resecting temporal lobe in refractory TLE. These fall into two large classes. One class includes anatomically uniform operations, such as measured anterior temporal lobectomy (5, 11), amygdalohippocampectomy (49), or radical hippocampectomy (45). The other class are operations tailored to individual patient's pathophysiology, using either intraoperatively derived data (44) or extraoperative data (1). There are few comparative studies of the different techniques and little evidence of large differences in outcome. Indeed, favorable outcomes have been reported with temporal lobe resections that remove only neocortex (15), only neocortex and amygdala (12), only neocortex and hippocampus and not amygdala (13), and only amygdala and hippocampus and not neocortex (49), although there is suggestive evidence that outcome is better with removal of at least some hippocampus. The reality, however, is that case selection has a greater impact on outcome from resective surgery in refractory TLE than the technique used for the operation.

REFERENCES

1. Arroyo S, Lesser RP, Awad IA, et al.: Subdural and epidural grids and strips, in Engle J Jr (ed): Surgical Treatment of the Epilepsies. New York, Raven Press 1993, pp 377–386.
2. Barbaro N, Walker J, Laxter KD: Temporal lobectomy and language functions. **J Neurosurg** 75:830, 1991.
3. Batzel L, Fraser R: Resection surgery for epilepsy: Outcome and quality of life. **Neurosurg Clin N Am** 4:345–352, 1993.
4. Branch C, Milner B, Rasmussen T: Intracarotid sodium amytal for the lateralization of cerebral speech dominance. **J Neurosurg** 21:399–405, 1964.
5. Crandall P: Cortical resections, in Engle J Jr (ed): Surgical Treatment of the Epilepsies. New York, Raven Press, 1987, pp 377–404.

6. Delgado-Escueta A, Treiman O, Walsh G: The treatable epilepsies. **N Engl J Med** 308:1576–1584, 1983.

7. Dodrill C, Wilkus R, Ojemann G, et al.: Multidisciplinary prediction of seizure relief from cortical resection surgery. **Ann Neurol** 20:2–12, 1986.

8. Dodrill CB, Batzel LW, Queisser HR, et al.: A objective method for the assessment of psychological and social problems among epileptics. **Epilepsia** 21:123–135, 1980.

9. Dodrill CB, Ojemann GA: Exploratory comparison of three methods of memory assessment with the intracarotid amobarbital procedure. **Brain Cogn**, 33:210–223, 1997.

10. Engle J Jr, Kuhl DE, Phelps ME, et al.: Interictal cerebral glucose metabolism in partial epilepsy and its relation to EEG changes. **Ann Neurol** 12:510–517, 1982.

11. Falconer M: Anterior temporal lobectomy for epilepsy, in Logue V (ed): *Operative Surgery, Neurosurgery.* London, Butterworth, 1971, vol 14, pp 142–149.

12. Feindel W, Rasmussen T: Temporal lobectomy with amygdalectomy and minimal hippocampal resection: Review of 100 cases. **Can J Neurol Sci** 18(suppl 4):603–605, 1991.

13. Golding S, Edward I, Harding GW, et al.: Temporal lobectomy that spares the amygdala for temporal lobe epilepsy. **Neurosurg Clin N Am** 4:263–272, 1993.

14. Haglund M, Ojemann LM: Seizure outcome in patients undergoing temporal lobe resections for epilepsy. **Neurosurg Clin N Am** 4(2):337–344, 1993.

15. Hardiman O, Burke T, Phillips J, et al.: Microdysgenesis in resected temporal neocortex: Incidence and clinical significance in focal epilepsy. **Neurology** 38:1041–1047, 1988.

16. Harris AB: Degeneration from experimental seizures (abstr.). **Soc Neurosci** 2:246, 1976.

17. Hart Y, Sanders J, Johnson A: Remission of seizures in early epilepsy: Results of a population-based study. **Epilepsia** 33:68–69, 1992.

18. Hayes CE, Tsuruda JS, Mathis CM: Temporal lobes: Surface MR coil phased array imaging. **Radiology** 189:918–920, 1993.

19. Henry TR, Frey RA, Sackellares JG, et al.: In vivo cerebral metabolism and central benzodiazepine—receptor binding in temporal lobe epilepsy. **Neurology** 43:1998–2006, 1993.

20. Herman B, Wyler A, Somes G: Language function following anterior temporal lobectomy. **J Neurosurg** 74:560–566, 1991.

21. Holmes M, Dodrill C, Wilensky A, et al.: Unilateral focal preponderance of interictal epileptiform discharges as a predictor of seizure origin. **Arch Neurol** 53:228–232, 1996.

22. Jack CR, Sharbrough FW, Cascino GD, et al.: Magnetic resonance image-based hippocampal volumetry: Correlation with outcome after temporal lobectomy. **Ann Neurol** 31:138–146, 1992.

23. Laxer KD, Hubesch B, Sappey-Marinier D, et al.: Increased pH and inorganic phosphate in temporal seizure foci, demonstrated by ^{31}PMRS. **Epilepsia** 33:618–623, 1992.

24. Layer G, Traber F, Mueller LU, et al.: "Spectroscopic imaging": A new MR technique in the diagnosis of epilepsy? **Radiology** 33:178–184, 1993.

25. Lee BI, Markand ON, Siddiqui AR, et al.: Single photon emission computed tomog-

raphy (SPECT) brain imaging using HIPDM: Intractible complex partial seizures. **Neurology** 36:1471–1477, 1986.

26. Leetsma JE, Kalehar MS, Teas SS, *et al.*: Sudden unexpected death associated with seizures: Analysis of 66 cases. **Epilepsia** 25:84–88, 1984.

27. Leib JP, Babb TL, Engel J Jr: Quantitative comparison of cell loss and thiopental-induced EEG changes in human epileptic hippocampus. **Epilepsia** 30:147–156, 1989.

28. Mattson RH, Cramer JA, Collins JF, *et al.*: Comparison of carbamazepine, pheno-barbital, phenytoin and primidone in partial and secondary generalized tonic-clonic seizures. **N Engl J Med** 313:145–151, 1985.

29. Mayberg H, Sadzot B, Meltzer C, *et al.*: Quantification of mu and non-mu opiate receptors in temporal lobe epilepsy using positron emission tomography. **Ann Neurol** 30:3–11, 1991.

30. NIH Consensus Conference: Surgery for epilepsy. **JAMA** 264:729–733, 1990.

31. Ojemann GA: Different approaches to resective surgery: Standard and tailored, in Theodore W (ed): *Surgical Treatment of Epilepsy*. Amsterdam, Elsevier, 1992, pp 169–174.

32. Ojemann GA, Dodrill C: Verbal memory deficits after temporal lobectomy for epilepsy: Mechanism and intraoperative prediction. **J Neurosurg** 62:101–107, 1985.

33. Ojemann GA, Dodrill CB: Intraoperative techniques for reducing language and memory deficits with left temporal lobectomy. **Adv Epileptol** 16:327–330, 1987.

34. Ojemann GA, Ojemann J, Lettich E, *et al.*: Cortical language localization in left, dominant hemisphere: An electrical stimulation mapping investigation in 117 patients. **J Neurosurg** 71:316–326, 1989.

35. Ojemann GA, Silbergeld DL: Approaches to epilepsy surgery. **Neurosurg Clin N Am** 4:183–191, 1993.

36. Ojemann LM, Dodrill CB: Natural history of drug resistant seizures: Clinical aspects. *Epilepsy Res Suppl* 5:13–17, 1992.

37. Penfield W, Mathieson G: Memory: Autopsy findings and comments on the role of hippocampus in experimental recall. **Arch Neurol** 31:145–154, 1974.

38. Porter R, Perry J, Lacy J: Diagnostic and therapeutic reevaluation of patients with intractable epilepsy. **Neurology** 27:1006–1011, 1977.

39. Reynolds EH: Early treatment and prognosis of epilepsy. **Epilepsia** 28:97–106, 1987.

40. Rowe CC, Berkovic SF, Austin MC, *et al.*: Visual and quantitative analysis of interictal SPECT with technetium-99m-HMPAO in temporal lobe epilepsy. **J Nucl Med** 32:1688–1694, 1991.

41. Sander J, Duncan JS: Vigabatrin, in Shorvon S, Dreifus F, Fish D, et al (eds): *The Treatment of Epilepsy*. Oxford, England, Blackwell Science, 1996, pp 491–499.

42. Saykin A, Gur R, Sussman N: Memory deficits before and after temporal lobectomy: Effect of laterality and age of onset. **Brain Cogn** 9:191–200, 1989.

43. Scoville W, Milner B: Loss of recent memory after bilateral hippocampal lesions. **J Neurol Neurosurg Psychiatry** 20:11–21, 1957.

44. Silbergeld DL, Ojemann GA: The tailored temporal lobectomy. **Neurosurg Clin N Am** 4:273–281, 1993.

45. Spencer D, Spencer S, Mattson R, *et al.*: Access to the posterior medial temporal lobe

structures in the surgical treatment of temporal lobe epilepsy. **Neurosurgery** 15:667–671, 1984.

46. Spencer SS, So NK, Engel J Jr, *et al.:* Depth Electrodes, in Engle J Jr (ed): *Surgical Treatment of the Epilepsies.* New York, Raven Press, 1993, ed 2, pp 359–376.

47. Wada J, Rasmussen T: Intracarotid injection of sodium amytal for the lateralization of cerebral speech dominance: Experimental and clinical observations. **J Neurosurg** 17:266–282, 1960.

48. Weiser HG, Bancaud J, Talairach J, *et al.:* Comparative value of spontaneous and chemically and electrically induced seizures in establishing the lateralization of temporal lobe seizures. **Epilepsia** 20:47–49, 1979.

49. Weiser HG, Yasargil M: Selective amygdalohippocampectomy as a surgical treatment of mesiobasal limbic epilepsy. **Surg Neurol** 17:445–457, 1982.

50. Wilensky A: History of focal epilepsy and criteria for medical intractability. **Neurosurg Clin N Am** 4:193–198, 1993.

51. Wilensky AJ, Holmes MD, Ojemann GA, *et al.:* Hippocampal abnormalities on high-resolution magnetic resonance imaging do not necessarily indicate site of seizure onset. **Epilepsia** 36 (suppl 3):S9, 1995.

52. Williamson PD, Spencer DD, Spencer SS, *et al.:* Complex partial seizures of frontal lobe origin. **Ann Neurol** 18:497–504, 1985.

53. Woods R, Dodrill C, Ojemann G: Brain injury, handedness and speech lateralization in a series of amobarbital studies. **Ann Neurol** 23:510–518, 1988.

54. Wyler AR, Hermann BP, Somes G: Extent of medial temporal resection on outcome from anterior temporal lobectomy: A randomized prospective study. **Neurosurgery** 37:982–991, 1995.

55. Wyler AR, Ojemann GA, Lettich E, *et al.:* Subdural strip electrodes for localizing epileptogenic foci. **J Neurosurg** 60:1195–1200, 1984.

56. Wylie E, Naugle R, Chelune G, *et al.:* Intracarotid amobarbital procedure. II. Lateralizing value in evaluation for temporal lobectomy. **Epilepsia** 32:865–869, 1991.

CHAPTER

9

Indications for Carotid Endarterectomy

NICHOLAS S. LITTLE, M.D., AND FREDRIC B. MEYER, M.D.

After the first published successful report in 1954 (16), carotid artery endarterectomy emerged as the most common vascular procedure performed in the United States in the 1980s (62). During this time, the surgery was performed often without clear indications, and the morbidity/mortality reported by many institutions was alarmingly high, leading to a reappraisal of the operation. More recently, prospective clinical investigations have standardized, to some degree, the management of both symptomatic and asymptomatic carotid disease.

Several large multicenter trials have helped to define certain indications for surgery (2, 3, 5, 45, 46). However, controversy still exists over the indications in patients who fall outside of the categories as defined by these studies. Confounding factors that considerably change the decision algorithm include the patient's general health, with emphasis on comorbid cerebral and cardiovascular pathology, and imaging characteristics of the carotid stenosis. Many studies have attempted to address these issues individually and at times have produced conflicting results. To add to these difficulties there has been a desire to move away from conventional contrast angiography, with its attendant morbidity, and replace it with duplex ultrasound and magnetic resonance angiography (MRA). These have been inherently less accurate at revealing factors of presumed increased risk, such as intracranial pathology, plaque ulcers, and intraluminal thrombus.

The aim of this chapter is to address the currently accepted indications for surgery and to highlight those aspects that continue to generate controversy. However, there will always remain a significant role for individualized surgical judgment.

SYMPTOMATIC CAROTID ARTERY DISEASE

Three large multicenter trials—NASCET, ECST, and the VA trial— all demonstrated an improvement in outcome in symptomatic carotid stenoses >70% (2, 5, 45). The 30-day risk of major stroke or death in operated cases was 2.1, 3.7 and 6.5%, respectively. Longer-term risks for any stroke in these operated groups was 9 (2 years), 10.3 (3 years), and 7.7% (1 year), respectively. The risk faced in the medically treated groups for the same time period was 26% (2 years), 16.8% (3 years), and 19.4% (1 year), respectively. The VA trial, which was terminated early, also included crescendo transischemic attack (TIA) in its analysis, and if they were excluded, then the risk of stroke was not significantly different (7.7% *versus* 7.1%) between the medical and surgical groups (Table 1).

For NASCET and ECST the benefit of surgery was apparent at 3 and 6 months, respectively. The VA trial noted a benefit for stenoses >50%, whereas the other two major trials only found definite benefit for stenoses >70%. For moderate stenoses (30–69%) there was no clear benefit in either NASCET or ECST. In patients with stenosis <30% ECST found no benefit. Because of differences in measurement, a stenosis of 70% as determined by means of ECST criteria was equivalent to 45% stenosis as determined by means of NASCET. This is because ECST compared the degree of stenosis to the presumed dimension of the carotid bulb, whereas NASCET used the internal carotid diameter distal to the stenosis as the reference.

Risk for perioperative stroke is thought by most to be related to the clinical situation. In cases of surgery for previous TIA, the rate of perioperative ipsilateral stroke is lower than that for previous stroke. Therefore, even in clinical situations in which the 30-day morbidity is 6–7%, there is still a long-term benefit with surgery in patients with symptomatic severe stenosis (>70%). In the less common patient with a symptomatic moderate stenosis (50–69%), it is likely that there would be a benefit only if the perioperative complication rate was very low. Indicators of increased risk of stroke, such as ulceration and contralateral occlusion, if not treated surgically may, when present, enhance the potential benefits of surgery.

TABLE 1

Comparison of Results of Major Symptomatic Carotid Endarterectomy Trials

Symptomatic Trial	Death/Stroke Rate (30-day) (%)	Late Death/Stroke Rate (Surgical/Medical)	Time to Benefit (mo)
NASCET	2.1	9% /26% (2 yr)	3
ECST	3.7	10.3% /16.8% (3 yr)	6
VA	6.5%	7.7% /19.4%[a] (1yr)	2

[a] Note that the VA trial included crescendo TIAs in their major morbidity outcome data. If these were excluded, then the difference was not significant 7.7% (7.1%).

ASYMPTOMATIC CAROTID ARTERY DISEASE

Early trials of endarterectomy for asymptomatic carotid stenosis failed to show a significant benefit (6, 45, 70). This was the result of several factors, including flawed design and inadequate numbers. The ACAS (4) study revealed a significant benefit of surgery in men with stenoses >60% (as measured by NASCET criteria). A benefit in women was not demonstrated. Over the course of 5 years the stroke rate in the surgical group was 5.1%, compared to that in the medically treated group, which was 11.0%. A large proportion of the risk in the surgical group was attributable to angiography (1.2% stroke rate). The medical group did not undergo angiography. Women in the study showed less benefit, largely because of increased angiographic and perioperative complications. Stroke risk reduction over 5 years was 17% for women. With exclusion of these factors it was 56%. Overall, the benefit of surgery was apparent at 10 months and statistically significant at 3 years. However, the 30-day morbidity/mortality for the surgical group was 2.3%, significantly less than the morbidity in other trials of symptomatic patients. Without angiography this complication rate was 1.5%.

The ACAS study raised several questions, including whether the excellent surgical results reported in this study could be extrapolated to most surgeons and centers and whether the risk/benefit ratio of angiography was favorable in this group. Despite these results the Stroke Prevention Patient Outcome Research Team (42) concluded that widespread ultrasound screening is not cost-effective. In ACAS 75% of the studied arteries were associated with a bruit. It has also been noted that the cost-effectiveness of prophylactic endarterectomy for asymptomatic stenosis has not been proven (78) despite the ACAS findings.

Obviously, the benefit of a prophylactic procedure is related to the age of the patient, operative risk, and patient tolerance to immediate versus long-term risks. In various studies the risk of ipsilateral stroke in those with asymptomatic stenosis ranged from 2–5%/year (7, 26, 56, 57). Using a Markov decision analysis model, Sarasin et al. (66) found that the surgical risk must be less than 2% in an 85-year-old patient and 5% in a 55-year-old patient to provide the likelihood of benefit.

As with symptomatic stenoses of <69%, other risk factors, such as plaque ulceration, stenosis progression, and radiologic evidence of infarction, may identify subsets that will benefit from surgery (10, 48, 80). Plaque ulceration has been considered by many to be a risk factor for stroke, with a risk rate of up to 7.5% for large ulcers >40 mm^2 (7, 26). The contribution of smaller ulcers to risk is less well-defined.

Although the overall risk of operation is lower in asymptomatic patients (20, 53), it is likely not acceptable in the older or medically unwell patient. Limits for operative risk were set by the *ad hoc* committee of the AHA stroke council. These were 3% for asymptomatic patients, 5% for patients with TIA, 7% for patients with previous stroke, and 10% for recurrent stenosis (52). The status of surgery on women remains controversial; however, most would agree that in a middle-aged, otherwise healthy female with severe stenosis, surgery should be considered.

SPECIFIC SURGICAL SITUATIONS AFFECTING DECISION ANALYSIS

Contralateral Stenosis

Results from the NASCET trial of patients with diseased, nonoccluded carotid arteries revealed little difference between risk with mild-to-moderate contralateral stenosis and severe contralateral stenosis. There was no significant difference in either the medical or surgical groups. Ipsilateral stroke risk was 29.3% and 26.2% in the medical group and 9.3% and 8.3% in the surgical group for severe and mild-to-moderate contralateral stenosis, respectively. Results from the asymptomatic VA trial showed that in these patients, bilaterality of stenosis >50% significantly increased the risk of stroke or death in both medical and surgical groups. Therefore, the presence of bilateral disease, especially in an asymptomatic patient, is a potential positive influence on surgical decision making.

Contralateral Occlusion

The NASCET trial confirmed the results of several previous studies with the reporting of a marked increase in morbidity and mortality in this group (21, 37, 63). They found that over 2 years the risk of stroke in the medical group was 69% and in the surgical group 22%. Perioperative risk of stroke or death was 4.0%. Most studies support these figures; however, some have found no increased risk of perioperative events (59, 65). In series looking at EEG changes and/or selective shunting required with cross-clamping there is a significant increase of both with contralateral occlusion (38, 63, 79). As with general studies of carotid endarterectomy, good results have been reported with no shunting, universal shunting, or selective shunting (49, 63, 65). Therefore, it would seem reasonable to proceed with the usual protocol of the particular surgeon recognizing the increased risk and dealing with it appropriately. In summary, the presence of a contralateral occlusion would be an indication to consider a prophylactic endarterectomy in an asymptomatic ipsilateral carotid stenosis.

Tandem Lesions

The presence of intracranial occlusive disease has been thought by some to be a contraindication to extracranial carotid surgery. Increased likelihood of slow flow and thrombus formation at the endarterectomy site is one cited concern. Some recent reviews have not supported this and other concerns, either in the immediate perioperative period or over the long term (40, 43, 64). Other studies have reported reversal of siphon stenosis in some patients after endarterectomy (14, 36). Perhaps not surprisingly, the evidence of more diffuse atherosclerotic disease has been associated with increased long-term cardiac morbidity and mortality (43). Unfortunately, in the NASCET trial, patients were excluded if their siphon stenosis exceeded their proximal internal carotid stenosis. Therefore, it is reasonable to proceed with surgery in these cases with symptomatic carotid lesions unless the intracranial stenosis is severe and is markedly greater than the extracranial stenosis.

Plaque Ulceration

The presence of ulcers in the atherosclerotic plaque, seen best on standard angiography, is considered by many to be a significant risk factor. The size of the ulcer determined by multiplying the width and length is proportional to risk (52). Large ulcers >40 mm^2, independent of percent stenosis, may have a stroke risk of up to 7.5% per year (7, 26). Smaller ulcers are considered at less risk. Results from NASCET indicate that the combination of severe stenosis and plaque ulceration more than doubles the risk for stroke in asymptomatic patients (17).

A study by Valton *et al.* (77) of ultrasonically detectable middle cerebral artery, high-intensity transient signals (HITS) that putatively represent emboli found that these emboli occurred in 63% with concomitant ulceration, compared to 23% with no ulceration. Even though carotid angiography is the "gold standard" imaging procedure, the sensitivity for ulcer detection is only on the order of 50% (19, 76). With ultrasound and MRA this modest sensitivity is reduced, with current resolution only able to detect a minority of surgically observed ulcers. A recent article, however, claims a >90% sensitivity rate with ultrasound (30), illustrating the high variance in imaging resolution reported in the literature. In patients with moderately (<70%) severe symptomatic stenosis and asymptomatic severe stenosis, the presence of ulcers is likely to be a positive surgical influence on surgical decision analysis.

Heterogeneous Plaque/Intraplaque Hemorrhage

The significance of intraplaque characteristics, as determined by Duplex scanning, is less clear. Two studies have claimed an increased risk for stroke in subsets of patients with plaque heterogeneity, whereas others found no increased risk (34, 74, 75). A study by Sitzer *et al.* (69) found a strong association between plaque ulceration and intraluminal thrombus with downstream emboli but no correlation with intraplaque hemorrhage or fissuring. Further data is needed to determine the influence of plaque hemorrhage on decision making.

Intraluminal Thrombus

There is little doubt that the presence of intraluminal thrombus is an indicator of increased risk for stroke or TIA. The major source of ongoing controversy is the appropriate management of these patients. As with the detection of ulceration, ultrasound and MRA have significant decreased sensitivity for the detection of thrombus (31). This may be offset by the potential of ultrasound to detect emboli, which are more prevalent in cases of intraluminal thrombus (69, 77).

All symptomatic patients with intraluminal thrombus should be immediately heparinized. For those with a high-grade stenosis in association with an intraluminal thrombus, surgery should be performed carefully with no manipulation of the carotid artery and branches during exposure. In those patients with an intraluminal thrombus without an associated stenosis, heparinization followed by coumadin for 3 months is the appropriate treatment (8, 9, 27, 39).

Internal Carotid Artery (ICA) Occlusion

Early studies of thromboendarterectomy of occluded ICAs reported perioperative morbidity/mortality rates of 15–16% (29, 46, 54). Since then, few have advocated revascularization in the chronically occluded group. Sporadic studies have advocated operations in subsets of these patients (24, 46). The annual risk of ipsilateral stroke in both asymptomatic and symptomatic patients is 4–5% (22), indicating that if it can be performed safely, then revascularization may yet play a role in the symptomatic chronically occluded artery.

Patients with an acute occlusion and fixed or progressive neurologic deficit may benefit from emergency surgery. As expected, time to reperfusion is critical in outcome. In one study (50) of 34 (33 inpatient occlusions) 38.8% had significant improvement from preoperative deficits, and the mortality rate was 20.6%. This compares with the natural history reports of 2–12% of patients with good recovery and 16–55% mortality in patients with an acute carotid occlusion and acute neurologic deterioration (50).

The *ad hoc* committee of the AHA (52) declared that there was insufficient data to make recommendations but thought it likely that in selected cases of acute occlusion, rapid surgical intervention might be of benefit. In those with severe deficits from occlusion, the outcome is poor in both surgical and medical groups. Poor prognostic factors of acute occlusion include severe neurologic deficit, decreased level of consciousness, and intracerebral hemorrhage. Studies that exclude these patients have improved outcomes (24, 28, 32, 46).

So-called stump syndromes or embolic events related to a chronically occluded ICA is another possible indication for exploration and/or repair, only if the patient has failed anticoagulation. Some advocate thromboendarterectomy where possible and ICA stumpectomy and ECA/CCA endarterectomy in unsalvageable cases (38, 46).

Recent Stroke

Patients with a fixed severe deficit or depressed level of consciousness are unlikely to be candidates for emergency surgery. Surgery in the context of an evolving stroke or fluctuating neurologic condition is controversial, and there is no doubt that perioperative risk is greater (35, 52, 60, 61).

The risk of dysautoregulation and hyperperfusion syndromes leading to hemorrhage and edema is greater in those with significant stroke (38). For this reason many surgeons defer operations for 3–6 weeks in stroke patients. In contrast some studies have demonstrated no increased risk for early surgery in cases of recent stroke, compared to those for TIA patients (35, 60, 62).

In stroke patients, EEG monitoring may be unreliable. Therefore, for surgeons who selectively shunt, consideration must be given to empiric shunt placement (38). Strict blood pressure control perioperatively must be maintained to avoid complications of dysautoregulation. There is no convincing evidence that delay of surgery has any significant benefit in those with small area infarction. In this situation early but not emergency surgery would be most appropriate.

Coexistent Intracranial Aneurysm/Arteriovenous Malformation (AVM)

Most surgeons recommend treatment of the symptomatic lesion (33, 73). In cases in which both are asymptomatic, relative risks must be weighed. Subsequent rupture of an intracranial aneurysm has rarely been reported after repair of extracranial ICA stenosis (1). In the majority of cases the carotid stenosis is symptomatic, and the intracranial abnormality found on preoperative imaging is not.

Concurrent Carotid and Coronary Disease

Because of the diffuse nature of atherosclerotic disease, significant carotid stenoses are commonly encountered in both carotid and coronary arteries in the same patient. Cardiac morbidity rates are higher than cerebral morbidity in studies of patients with asymptomatic carotid disease (4), and cardiac causes are responsible for mortality in 25–50% of those undergoing carotid surgery (2, 11, 12, 47, 55).

In a meta-analysis by the AHA they found that in cases of coexisting symptomatic coronary disease and symptomatic or asymptomatic carotid artery disease, perioperative stroke rate was similar with combined procedures or if carotid surgery preceded coronary bypass surgery. Frequency of stroke was increased if coronary bypass preceded carotid endarterectomy, and frequency of myocardial infarction was increased if endarterectomy preceded coronary bypass.

Recent studies separating asymptomatic and symptomatic carotid disease groups found that the perioperative risk of stroke in asymptomatic patients is low enough not to justify either prophylactic or concurrent endarterectomy (23, 68). With symptomatic carotid disease and severe unstable coronary disease, both requiring surgery, the answer is not clear. Some surgeons would prefer to operate on the symptomatic carotid lesion initially with second-stage coronary bypass (38). However, the relative merits of this approach, compared to those of combined surgery, remain undefined (52), and the majority of surgeons presently would favor combined carotid and cardiac revascularization.

Evaluation of Carotid Stenosis—Imaging

The three most commonly used imaging modalities are contrast angiography, duplex ultrasound, and MRA/MRI. Because of the morbidity of cerebral angiography, efforts have been made to replace it with the other noninvasive techniques. Permanent neurologic morbidity from angiography in most series is in the order of 1–2% (4, 25); however, it remains the gold standard, with most surgeons continuing to use it (2, 4, 52).

Others advocate the use of ultrasound or MRA, either alone or in combination, on the basis of decreased morbidity and improved cost-effectiveness (31, 51). They think that the advantages resulting from these factors outweigh the disadvantages in resolution of imaging intracranial disease, plaque characteristics, intraluminal thrombi, and occlusion *versus* high-grade stenosis.

Ultrasound is widely used as a screening test in both symptomatic patients and others with asymptomatic bruits. Angiography is mostly used in cases in which a surgical lesion has been suggested on ultrasound and the patient is being considered for surgery. Various ultrasound techniques, such as color-assisted Doppler, transcranial Doppler, and oculoplethysmography, have increased the accuracy for predicting occlusion, siphon disease, ulceration, plaque hemorrhage, intracranial disease, and embolization (18, 72, 77). In general the sensitivity of ultrasound is significantly higher than the specificity, with the greatest imaging difficulty occurring in occluded vessels. Similarly, MRA has increased sensitivity, compared to specificity. The combination of the two noninvasive tests greatly enhances accuracy when there is concordance (31, 58).

Both MRA and ultrasound tend to overread the degree of stenosis. This would most commonly be a problem in asymptomatic patients, occasionally leading to unnecessary operations without angiography. MRA has some advantages over ultrasound in that it is less operator-dependent, has high interobserver agreement, and has the ability to visualize intracranial vessels (51). A standard MRI may be done at the same time to screen for evidence of infarction, which may indicate increased risk in asymptomatic patients (4). MRA is by far the least accurate in assessment of plaque morphology and thrombosis.

A difficulty arises in the assessment of asymptomatic stenoses in situations in which risk assessment is crucial. Factors as mentioned that are seen best with current technology by angiography, such as plaque ulcers, thrombi, and distal intracranial vascular disease, are not as well-defined with the noninvasive techniques. This, along with the oversensitivity of these tests, means that decision making may not be optimal. However, this is offset by the extra 1% risk (higher in some centers (13) of major morbidity incurred by the test. If the surgeon believes the contribution of these potentially occult imaging factors is not critical and the institution has high-quality noninvasive imaging systems, then they may choose to operate without angiography. Many surgeons believe endarterectomy should be performed, regardless of occlusive intracranial disease (41, 64, 67), and that ulceration *per se* is not an indication for surgery (5, 31).

CT angiography is another of the noninvasive modalities that is becoming increasingly available. It is unlikely in the near future to replace ultrasound as a screening procedure; however some reports claim increased accuracy for detection of plaque ulcers, calcification, loops, and aneurysms (15, 71). As with MRA there is the potential to screen for intracranial abnormalities and may be more accurate for determining critical stenosis *versus* occlusion (71). More comparison studies need to be performed to validate its potential against the other more established tests.

TABLE 2
Relative Accuracy of Imaging to Detect Factors for Increased Risk of Stroke

Imaging Modalities	MRA/MRI	Ultrasound	Angiography
Contralateral stenosis	+++	+++	++++
Contralateral occlusion	+++	+++	++++
Plaque ulceration	+/−	++	+++
Plaque hemorrhage	−	+++	−
HITS/emboli	−	++	−
Tandem/intracranial stenosis	+++	−	++++
Thrombus	+/−	++	++++
Recent stroke	++++	−	−
Intracranial malformation	+++	−	++++
Silent infarction	++++	−	−

TABLE 3
Influence of Clinical and Radiological Factors on Surgical Decision Making

Factor	Stroke Risk	Likelihood of Surgical Benefit
Symptomatic >70%	+++++	+++++
Symptomatic 50–69%	++	+++
Symptomatic <50%	−	−
Asymptomatic >69%	++	+++
Contralateral stenosis	+	++
Contralateral occlusion	++	+++
Plaque ulceration	+++	+++
Plaque hemorrhage	+/−	+/−
HITS/emboli	+	+
Tandem/intracranial stenosis	+	+/−
Thrombus	+++	−
Recent stroke	++	+/−
Intracranial malformation	−	+/−
Silent infarction	+	+

The current position on the use of angiography is not clear. There is no doubt that in the future it will be replaced by increasingly sophisticated noninvasive techniques. At this time, most surgeons use angiography, at least for cases in which there are ultrasound and MRA discordance, and many use it in all cases (31, 51, 58). As with recommendations for asymptomatic surgery the real answer is likely to be reliant on individual institutional expertise and morbidity (Table 2).

CONCLUSION

In this chapter we have attempted to review the guidelines for operative therapy of carotid occlusive disease. Each surgeon must compare his or her own morbidity and mortality figures to the predicted natural history of the patient's carotid stenosis. As described, the factors involved in the decision analysis are numerous, and the significance of each is naturally given different weight by the surgeon secondary to experience and interpretation of the literature (Table 3). The direction of future imaging strategies is clearly moving away from angiography on the basis of cost-effectiveness and improved morbidity of ultrasound and MRA (and possibly CT-angio). One of the dangers of abandonment of angiography is that information available to make a decision on borderline cases will be limited. Hopefully, in the near future inherent problems of noninvasive tests, such as interobserver variability and resolution, will improve to the point at which these concerns are no longer valid.

REFERENCES

1. Adams HP Jr: Carotid stenosis and coexisting ipsilateral intracranial aneurysm: A problem in management. **Arch Neurol** 34(8):515–516, 1977.
2. Anonymous: Beneficial effect of carotid endarterectomy in symptomatic patients with high-grade carotid stenosis. North American Symptomatic Carotid Endarterectomy Trial Collaborators (see comments). **N Engl J Med** 325(7):445–453, 1991.
3. Anonymous: Carotid surgery versus medical therapy in asymptomatic carotid stenosis. The CASANOVA Study Group (see comments). **Stroke** 22(10):1229–1235, 1991.
4. Anonymous: Endarterectomy for asymptomatic carotid artery stenosis. Executive Committee for the Asymptomatic Carotid Atherosclerosis Study (see comments). **J Am Med Assoc** 273(18):1421–1428, 1995.
5. Anonymous: MRC European Carotid Surgery Trial: Interim results for symptomatic patients with severe (70–99%) or with mild (0–29%) carotid stenosis. European Carotid Surgery Trialists' Collaborative Group (see comments). **Lancet** 337(8752): 1235–1243, 1991.
6. Anonymous: Results of a randomized controlled trial of carotid endarterectomy for asymptomatic carotid stenosis. Mayo Asymptomatic Carotid Endarterectomy Study Group (see comments). **Mayo Clin Proc** 67(6):513–518, 1992.
7. Autret A, Pourcelot L, Saudeau D, et al.: Stroke risk in patients with carotid stenosis. **Lancet** 1(8538):888–890, 1987.
8. Biller J, Adams HP Jr, Boarini D, et al.: Intraluminal clot of the carotid artery: A clinical-angiographic correlation of nine patients and literature review. **Surg Neurol** 25(5):467–477, 1986.
9. Buchan A, Gates P, Pelz D, et al.: Intraluminal thrombus in the cerebral circulation: Implications for surgical management. **Stroke** 19(6):681–687, 1988.
10. Caplan LR: Brain embolism, revisited. **Neurology** 43(7):1281–1287, 1993.
11. Chimowitz MI, Weiss DG, Cohen SL, et al.: Cardiac prognosis of patients with carotid stenosis and no history of coronary artery disease. Veterans Affairs Cooperative Study Group 167. **Stroke** 25(4):759–765, 1994.
12. Cohen SN, Hobson RWD, Weiss DG, et al.: Death associated with asymptomatic carotid artery stenosis: Long-term clinical evaluation. VA Cooperative Study 167 Group. **J Vasc Surg** 18(6):1002–1009; discussion, 1009–1011, 1993.

13. Davies KN, Humphrey PR: Complications of cerebral angiography in patients with symptomatic carotid territory ischaemia screened by carotid ultrasound. **J Neurol Neurosurg Psychiatry** 56(9):967–972, 1993.

14. Day AL, Rhoton AL, Quisling RG: Resolving siphon stenosis following endarterectomy. **Stroke** 11(3):278–281, 1980.

15. Dillon EH, van Leeuwen MS, Fernandez MA, et al.: CT angiography: application to the evaluation of carotid artery stenosis. **Radiology** 189(1):211–219, 1993.

16. Eastcott HHJ, Pickering GW, Rob CG: Reconstruction of internal carotid artery in a patient with intermittent attacks of hemiplegia. **Lancet** 2:994–996, 1954.

17. Eliasziw M, Streifler JY, Fox AJ, et al.: Significance of plaque ulceration in symptomatic patients with high-grade carotid stenosis. North American Symptomatic Carotid Endarterectomy Trial. **Stroke** 25(2):304–308, 1994.

18. Erickson SJ, Mewissen MW, Foley WD, et al.: Stenosis of the internal carotid artery: assessment using color Doppler imaging compared with angiography. AJR. 152(6): 1299–1305, 1989.

19. Estol C, Claasen D, Hirsch W, et al.: Correlative angiographic and pathologic findings in the diagnosis of ulcerated plaques in the carotid artery. **Arch Neurol** 48(7):692–694, 1991.

20. Fode NC, Sundt TM Jr, Robertson JT, et al.: Multicenter retrospective review of results and complications of carotid endarterectomy in 1981. **Stroke** 17(3):370–376, 1986.

21. Friedman SG, Riles TS, Lamparello PJ, et al.: Surgical therapy for the patient with internal carotid artery occlusion and contralateral stenosis. **J Vasc Surg** 5(6):856–861, 1987.

22. Gasecki AP, Eliasziw M, Ferguson GG, et al.: Long-term prognosis and effect of endarterectomy in patients with symptomatic severe carotid stenosis and contralateral carotid stenosis or occlusion: Results from NASCET. North American Symptomatic Carotid Endarterectomy Trial (NASCET) Group. **J Neurosurg** 83(5):778–782, 1995.

23. Gerraty RP, Gates PC, Doyle JC: Carotid stenosis and perioperative stroke risk in symptomatic and asymptomatic patients undergoing vascular or coronary surgery. **Stroke** 24(8):1115–1118, 1993.

24. Hafner CD, Tew JM: Surgical management of the totally occluded internal carotid artery: A ten-year study. **Surgery** 89(6):710–717, 1981.

25. Hankey GJ, Warlow CP, Sellar RJ: Cerebral angiographic risk in mild cerebrovascular disease. **Stroke** 21(2):209–222, 1990.

26. Hennerici M, Hulsbomer HB, Hefter H, et al.: Natural history of asymptomatic extracranial arterial disease: Results of a long-term prospective study. **Brain** 110(Part 3):777–791, 1987.

27. Heros RC: Carotid endarterectomy in patients with intraluminal thrombus (editorial). **Stroke** 19(6):667–668, 1988.

28. Hugenholtz H, Elgie RG: Carotid thromboendarterectomy: A reappraisal. Criteria for patient selection. **J Neurosurg** 53(6):776–783, 1980.

29. Hunter JA, Julian OC, Dye WS: Emergency operation for acute cerebral ischemia due to carotid artery obstruction: Review of 26 cases. **Ann Surg** 162:901–904, 1965.

30. Kagawa R, Moritake K, Shima T, et al.: Validity of B-mode ultrasonographic findings

in patients undergoing carotid endarterectomy in comparison with angiographic and clinicopathologic features. **Stroke** 27(4):700–705, 1996.

31. Kent KC, Kuntz KM, Patel MR, *et al.:* Perioperative imaging strategies for carotid endarterectomy: An analysis of morbidity and cost-effectiveness in symptomatic patients. **JAMA** 274(11):888–893, 1995.

32. Kusunoki T, Rowed DW, Tator CH, *et al.:* Thromboendarterectomy for total occlusion of the internal carotid artery: A reappraisal of risks, success rate and potential benefits. **Stroke** 9(1):34–38, 1978.

33. Ladowski JS, Webster MW, Yonas HO, *et al.:* Carotid endarterectomy in patients with asymptomatic intracranial aneurysm. **Ann Surg** 200(1):70–73, 1984.

34. Lennihan L, Kupsky WJ, Mohr JP, *et al.:* Lack of association between carotid plaque hematoma and ischemic cerebral symptoms. **Stroke** 18(5):879–881, 1987.

35. Little JR, Moufarrij NA, Furlan AJ: Early carotid endarterectomy after cerebral infarction. **Neurosurgery** 24(3):334–338, 1989.

36. Little JR, Sawhny B, Weinstein M: Pseudo-tandem stenosis of the internal carotid artery. **Neurosurgery** 7(6):574–577, 1980.

37. Littooy FN, Halstuk KS, Mamdani M, *et al.:* Factors influencing morbidity of carotid endarterectomy without a shunt. **Am Surg** 50(7):350–353, 1984.

38. Loftus CM, Quest DO: Technical issues in carotid artery surgery 1995 (see comments). **Neurosurgery** 36(4):629–647, 1995.

39. Lopez-Bresnahan MV, Kearse LA, Jr, Yanez P, *et al.:* Anterior communicating artery collateral flow protection against ischemic change during carotid endarterectomy. **J Neurosurg** 79(3):379–382, 1993.

40. Lord RS, Raj TB, Graham AR: Carotid endarterectomy, siphon stenosis, collateral hemispheric pressure, and perioperative cerebral infarction. **J Vasc Surg** 6(4):391–397, 1987.

41. Mackey WC, O'Donnell TF Jr, Callow AD: Carotid endarterectomy in patients with intracranial vascular disease: Short-term risk and long-term outcome. **J Vasc Surg** 10(4):432–438, 1989.

42. Matchar DB, Duncan PW, Samsa GP, *et al.:* The Stroke Prevention Patient Outcomes Research Team: Goals and methods. **Stroke** 24(12):2135–2142, 1993.

43. Mattos MA, van Bemmelen PS, Hodgson KJ, *et al.:* The influence of carotid siphon stenosis on short- and long-term outcome after carotid endarterectomy. **J Vasc Surg** 17(5):902–910; discussion 910–911, 1993.

44. Mayberg MR, Wilson SE, Yatsu F, *et al.:* Carotid endarterectomy and prevention of cerebral ischemia in symptomatic carotid stenosis. Veterans Affairs Cooperative Studies Program 309 Trialist Group (see comments) JAMA 266(23):3289–3294, 1991.

45. Mayberg MR, Winn HR: Endarterectomy for asymptomatic carotid artery stenosis: Resolving the controversy (editorial; comment). JAMA 273(18):1459–1461, 1995.

46. McCormick PW, Spetzler RF, Bailes JE, *et al.:* Thromboendarterectomy of the symptomatic occluded internal carotid artery. **J Neurosurg** 76(5):752–758, 1992.

47. McCrory DC, Goldstein LB, Samsa GP, *et al.:* Predicting complications of carotid endarterectomy. **Stroke** 24(9):1285–1291, 1993.

48. Meissner I, Wiebers DO, Whisnant JP, *et al.:* The natural history of asymptomatic carotid artery occlusive lesions. JAMA 258(19):2704–2707, 1987.

49. Meyer FB, Fode NC, Marsh WR, et al.: Carotid endarterectomy in patients with contralateral carotid occlusion. **Mayo Clin Proc** 68(4):337–342, 1993.

50. Meyer FB, Sundt TM Jr, Piepgras DG, et al.: Emergency carotid endarterectomy for patients with acute carotid occlusion and profound neurological deficits. **Ann Surg** 203(1):82–89, 1986.

51. Mittl RL Jr, Broderick M, Carpenter JP, et al.: Blinded-reader comparison of magnetic resonance angiography and duplex ultrasonography for carotid artery bifurcation stenosis (see comments). **Stroke** 25(1):4–10, 1994.

52. Moore WS, Barnett HJ, Beebe HG, et al.: Guidelines for carotid endarterectomy: A multidisciplinary consensus statement from the Ad Hoc Committee, American Heart Association. **Circulation** 91(2):566–579, 1995.

53. Moore WS, Vescera CL, Robertson JT, et al.: Selection process for surgeons in the Asymptomatic Carotid Atherosclerosis Study (see comments). **Stroke** 22(11):1353–1357, 1991.

54. Murphey F, Maccubbin DA: Carotid endarterectomy: A long term follow-up study. **J Neurosurg** 23:156–168, 1965.

55. Musser DJ, Nicholas GG, Reed JFR: Death and adverse cardiac events after carotid endarterectomy. **J Vasc Surg** 19(4):615–622, 1994.

56. Norris JW, Zhu CZ, Bornstein NM, et al.: Vascular risks of asymptomatic carotid stenosis. **Stroke** 22(12):1485–1490, 1991.

57. O'Holleran LW, Kennelly MM, McClurken M, et al.: Natural history of asymptomatic carotid plaque: Five year follow-up study. **Am J Surg** 154(6):659–662, 1987.

58. Patel MR, Kuntz KM, Klufas RA, et al.: Preoperative assessment of the carotid bifurcation: Can magnetic resonance angiography and duplex ultrasonography replace contrast arteriography? **Stroke** 26(10):1753–1758, 1995.

59. Perler BA, Burdick JF, Williams GM: Does contralateral internal carotid artery occlusion increase the risk of carotid endarterectomy? **J Vasc Surg** 16(3):347–352; discussion 352–353, 1992.

60. Piotrowski JJ, Bernhard VM, Rubin JR, et al.: Timing of carotid endarterectomy after acute stroke. **J Vasc Surg** 11(1):45–51; discussion 51–52, 1990.

61. Pokras R, Dyken ML: Dramatic changes in the performance of endarterectomy for diseases of the extracranial arteries of the head. **Stroke** 19(10):1289–1290, 1988.

62. Pritz MB: Carotid endarterectomy after recent stroke: Preliminary observations in patients undergoing early operation. **Neurosurgery** 19(4):604–609, 1986.

63. Redekop G, Ferguson G: Correlation of contralateral stenosis and intraoperative electroencephalogram change with risk of stroke during carotid endarterectomy (see comments). **Neurosurgery** 30(2):191–194, 1992.

64. Roederer GO, Langlois YE, Chan AR, et al.: Is siphon disease important in predicting outcome of carotid endarterectomy? **Arch Surg** 118(10):1177–1181, 1983.

65. Sachs SM, Fulenwider JT, Smith RBD, et al.: Does contralateral carotid occlusion influence neurologic fate of carotid endarterectomy? **Surgery** 96(5):839–844, 1984.

66. Sarasin FP, Bounameaux H, Bogousslavsky J: Asymptomatic severe carotid stenosis: Immediate surgery or watchful waiting? A decision analysis. **Neurology** 45:2147–2153, 1995.

67. Schuler JJ, Flanigan DP, Lim LT, et al.: The effect of carotid siphon stenosis on

stroke rate, death, and relief of symptoms following elective carotid endarterectomy. **Surgery** 92(6):1058–1067, 1982.

68. Schwartz LB, Bridgman AH, Kieffer RW, et al.: Asymptomatic carotid artery stenosis and stroke in patients undergoing cardiopulmonary bypass. **J Vasc Surg** 21(1): 146–153, 1995.

69. Sitzer M, Muller W, Siebler M, et al.: Plaque ulceration and lumen thrombus are the main sources of cerebral microemboli in high-grade internal carotid artery stenosis. **Stroke** 26(7):1231–1233, 1995.

70. Solis MM, Ranval TJ, Barone GW, et al.: The CASANOVA study: Immediate surgery versus delayed surgery for moderate carotid artery stenosis? (letter, comment). **Stroke** 23(6):917–919, 1992.

71. Steger W, Vogl TJ, Rausch M, et al.: [CT angiography in carotid stenosis: Diagnostic value compared to color-coded duplex ultrasonography and MR angiography]. **Rofo Fortschr Geb Rontgenstr Neuen Bildgeb Verfah** 162(5):373–380, 1995.

72. Steinke W, Kloetzsch C, Hennerici M: Carotid artery disease assessed by color Doppler flow imaging: Correlation with standard Doppler sonography and angiography. AJNR 11(2):259–266, 1990.

73. Stern J, Whelan M, Brisman R, et al.: Management of extracranial carotid stenosis and intracranial aneurysms. **J Neurosurg** 51(2):147–150, 1979.

74. Sterpetti AV, Schultz RD, Feldhaus RJ, et al.: Ultrasonographic features of carotid plaque and the risk of subsequent neurologic deficits. **Surgery** 104(4):652–660, 1988.

75. Gomez CR: Carotid plaque morphology and risk for stroke. **Stroke** 21(1):148–151, 1990.

76. Streifler JY, Eliasziw M, Fox AJ, et al.: Angiographic detection of carotid plaque ulceration: Comparison with surgical observations in a multicenter study. North American Symptomatic Carotid Endarterectomy Trial. **Stroke** 25(6):1130–1132, 1994.

77. Valton L, Larrue V, Arrue P, et al.: Asymptomatic cerebral embolic signals in patients with carotid stenosis: Correlation with appearance of plaque ulceration on angiography. **Stroke** 26(5):813–815, 1995.

78. Warlow C: Endarterectomy for asymptomatic carotid stenosis? (see comments). **Lancet** 345(8960):1254–1255, 1995.

79. Whittemore AD, Kauffman JL, Kohler TR, et al.: Routine electroencephalographic (EEG) monitoring during carotid endarterectomy. **Ann Surg** 197(6):707–713, 1983.

80. Zukowski AJ, Nicolaides AN, Lewis RT, et al.: The correlation between carotid plaque ulceration and cerebral infarction seen on CT scan. **J Vasc Surg** 1(6):782–786, 1984.

II

General Scientific Session II
How The Operation Is Done

10

Degenerative Lumbar Spinal Instability: Technical Aspects of Operative Treatment

DEAN G. KARAHALIOS, M.D., PAUL J. APOSTOLIDES, M.D., AND VOLKER K. H. SONNTAG, M.D.

This chapter focuses on detailed descriptions of specific operative treatments for degenerative lumbar spinal instability. Selection criteria and indications for treatment of degenerative lumbar spinal instability are covered in two separate chapters in this volume.

Frymoyer and Selby (13) have defined spinal instability as a "symptomatic condition in which, in the absence of new injury, a physiological load induces abnormally large deformations at the vertebral joint." There are a number of causes of spinal instability, including trauma, neoplasm, infection, congenital malformation, iatrogenic causes, and degenerative processes. Degenerative lumbar spinal instability can be divided into a number of categories: degenerative spondylolisthesis, degenerative segmental instability (abnormal movement on dynamic radiographic studies), "mechanical" back pain from micromotion, iatrogenic segmental instability (from the treatment of degenerative spondylosis), degenerative scoliosis, and degenerative/osteoporotic fractures.

Whatever the etiology, patients chosen for treatment should be selected carefully. Without proper selection, a high failure rate can be expected. We base our decision to treat patients both on clinical and radiographic evidence of instability. Clinically, patients complain of back pain, and a radicular component is often present as well. The L5 is the most commonly involved nerve root, because the degenerative slippage or instability most commonly occurs at the L4-L5 segment. Patients' symptoms tend to be exacerbated by movement and relieved by immobility. A trial in an external brace, such as a thoracolumbar spinal orthosis (TLSO), may resolve or improve the patient's symptoms, a finding that further supports the presence of instability. Radiographically, patients may have evidence of instability based on spondylolisthesis. The treatment of a grade I spondylolisthesis by fusion and fixation remains controversial and should be considered carefully on a case-by-case basis. Patients with grade II slips usually benefit from treatment, and patients with grade III or IV slips who are symptomatic greatly benefit. Patients with symptoms consistent with instability but who do not demonstrate spondylolisthesis on static radiographs should undergo flexion-extension (dynamic studies) radiography to uncover occult instability. Patients with more than 4 mm of movement or 10° of angulation on these studies may be considered having symptoms of instability and are good candidates for treatment. In such cases, the argument for treatment is strengthened if the patient experiences some relief with external immobilization as well.

The goals of treatment should be the relief of pain, functional or neurologic improvement, and correction and/or control of the patients' structural deformity. Treatment options include decompression of the spinal canal and neural foramina alone, with fusion, or with fusion and fixation/instrumentation. There has been considerable debate regarding the appropriate approach. The following section of the chapter is a detailed description of our anterior and posterior operative approaches to this problem.

POSTERIOR OPERATIVE APPROACH FOR TRANSPEDICULAR SCREW FIXATION

Indications

A posterior approach with decompression and transpedicular screw fixation is the procedure of choice for most cases of degenerative lumbar spinal instability. This approach allows for adequate decompression of the spinal canal, lateral recess, and neural foramina. It also allows for the placement of bone graft for a facet joint and/or posterolateral fusion. When there is significant anterior compressive pathology, this approach may be inadequate, and an anterior approach, which is described later, may be the best choice.

Preoperative Planning

Preoperatively, radiographic studies are obtained and may include magnetic resonance imaging (MRI), myelograms, and computed tomography (CT) scans to evaluate the extent of decompression needed. Axial CT images are necessary to ascertain the suitability of the pedicles to be instrumented for the placement of screws. In general, the pedicle diameter should be at least 5 mm in the lumbar region for the placement of screws (Fig. 1). A rule of thirds is used for preoperative planning for transpedicular screw fixation; that is, the pedicle screw diameter should be no greater than two-thirds the width of the pedicle to be instrumented, and the pedicle screw length should not extend further than two-thirds the length of the body.

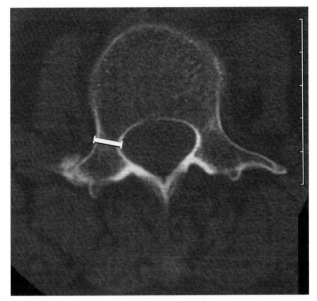

FIG. 1 Axial CT scan of a lumbar vertebra through the level of the pedicle. The diameter of the pedicle through which a screw is to be placed should be measured preoperatively so that an appropriately sized pedicle screw can be placed. In general, the diameter of the pedicle screw should be no larger than two-thirds the diameter of the pedicle to prevent the pedicle from fracturing. (Reproduced with permission from the Barrow Neurological Institute®)

Anesthesia, Patient Positioning, and Monitoring

A general anesthetic is administered, and the patient is positioned in the prone position on the operating-room table. The patient is placed on chest rolls with the knees slightly bent. Pressure points are padded appropriately, and leads are attached for somatosensory-evoked potential (SSEP) monitoring. The C-arm is brought into position for intraoperative fluoroscopy. The patient is prepared and draped, and the C-arm is used to obtain a lateral fluoroscopic image to confirm the location of the pathology and to plan the incision.

Exposure

A dorsal midline incision is used. The dissection is carried down to the fascial level, using electrocautery. Once the level of the fascia is reached, the dissection proceeds laterally on either side to obtain bone graft material from the iliac crest. (The details of this procedure are described later.) Once the bone graft has been obtained, the midline dissection is continued, and the paraspinous musculature is dissected off of the spinous processes and lamina, using the bovie extracautery. It is usually necessary to expose one to two levels above and below the intended level of decompression to obtain an exposure that is sufficiently lateral over the transverse processes. At this point in the dissection, it is often useful to switch self-retaining retractors from the D'Errico retractors (Codman, Raynham, MA) to the Karlin crankframe spinal retractor (Codman, Raynham, MA). Dissection then continues laterally over the facets and transverse processes when one uses the bovie electrocautery. It may be necessary to reduce the energy of the cautery to avoid transmitting unnecessary heat to the spinal nerve roots exiting below the transverse processes. One also must be cautious not to dissect ventrally to the transverse processes, because the nerve roots that lie there may be injured. Also, the transverse processes should not be exposed above or below the intended fusion site, so as to avoid unintended fusion of adjacent levels. However, there should be general caudal extension of the exposure if S1 is involved in the fusion.

Decompression

A bone cutter is used to remove the spinous processes of the levels to be decompressed, and a double-action rongeur is used to thin the lamina. Sharp curettes may then be used to dissect through the ligamentum flavum. The laminectomy is performed with a series of Kerrison punches (2–5 mm). It may be necessary to perform a facetectomy or to thin the hypertrophied facets laterally using the Midas Rex drill with an AM-8 dissecting tool (Midas Rex Pneumatic Tools, Inc., Fort Worth, TX). Under microscopic magnification, the lateral recesses are decompressed with Kerrison punches and microcurettes. Once an adequate level of exposure has been obtained (usually when the medial aspect of the pedicle is flush with the decompression), the involved nerve roots are identified. The nerve roots are followed out under each pedicle and through their respective foramina. A dental tool (Woodson) is used to explore the foramina. If pathologic stenosis is present, a foraminotomy is performed with 2- and 3-mm Kerrison punches until the dental instrument is easily placed through the foramen. Once the foraminotomy has been completed, the disc spaces are examined for any herniated discs or prominent bulges. Bulging discs are not treated unless they are significantly compressing the thecal sac. However, after a posterior decompression it would be unlikely that a disc bulge would cause any significant compression. Herniated disc fragments, however, are removed using a microdissectomy technique.

Transpedicular Screw Fixation

A number of universal/pedicle screw-based systems have been developed for posterior fixation of the thoracolumbar and sacral spine (Table 1). No system appears to have a clear-cut advantage over the others, and each has relative advantages and disadvantages, compared to the others. Therefore, surgeons should choose a familiar system that they have used successfully.

The first step in placement of the pedicle screws is to identify important pedicle landmarks. The pedicle is identified by visual, tactile, and radiographic means. The external landmarks are visualized over the dorsal surface of the lumbar spine (Fig. 2A). The point of intersection of a line drawn through the axial plane of the transverse process and the sagittal plane through the lateral superior facet marks the center of the pedicle. Using a dental instrument and/or a Penfield dissector from within the canal, the surgeon can define the superior, inferior, and medial borders of the pedicle, thus gaining tactile information (Fig. 2B). Occasionally, with very wide decompressions, the pedicle can be visualized directly. Next, radiographic confirmation of the location of the pedicle can be obtained. Anteroposterior (AP) fluoroscopy may be performed to identify the "target" sign (Fig. 2C). Lateral fluoroscopy may be used to identify the superior and inferior margins of the pedicle and the relative positions of the disc space and neural foramina (Fig. 2D).

The same overall process is used for pedicle identification at the level of the sacrum. On visual inspection of the dorsal sacrum, one may

TABLE 1
Spinal Screw Fixation Systems

AMSET R-F
AO dynamic compression plates
Cotrel-Dubousset (CD)
Danek plate and screws
Edwards modular system
Fixateur Interne
ISOLA
Moss Miami
PWB system
Rogzinski
Roy-Camille posterior screw plate
Simmons plating system
Texas Scottish Rite Hospital (TSRH)
Vermont spinal fixateur
Variable screw–plate fixation systems (VSP)
Wiltse
Zielke

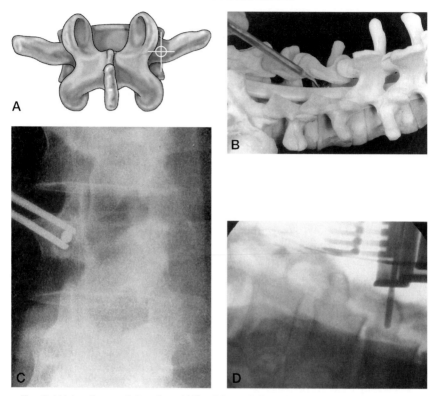

FIG. 2 (**A**) A point overlying the middle of the pedicle is found by determining the point of intersection of a line drawn through the axial plane of a transverse process and the sagittal plane through the lateral superior facet. (Reproduced with permission from the Barrow Neurological Institute.) (**B**) After decompression, the pedicle may be palpated with a dental instrument, thus defining its superior, inferior, and medial borders. (**C**) Anteroposterior and (**D**) lateral fluoroscopic images may be used to confirm the location of the pedicle. (Reproduced with permission from the Barrow Neurological Institute®)

identify certain external landmarks—the first dorsal sacral foramen and the sacral recession. The point overlying the pedicle is usually near the inferolateral portion of the S1 facet (Fig. 3**A**). After a decompression,tactile information may also be obtained, as the superior and medial aspects of the pedicle may be palpated within the canal using a dental instrument. Once again fluoroscopy may be used to identify the pedicle both in the sagittal and coronal planes (Fig. 3**B**).

Once an entry point has been chosen, the bone is decorticated using a high-speed drill (Fig. 4**A**). Then under fluoroscopic guidance, a T-handled probe is manually advanced through the cancellous center of the pedicle into the vertebral body (Fig. 4**B**). The mediolateral

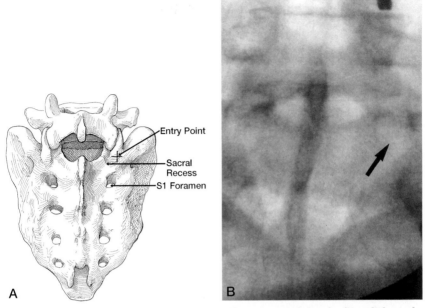

FIG. 3 Localization of the sacral pedicle. (**A**) The point overlying the S1 pedicle on the dorsal surface of the sacrum is usually near the inferolateral portion of the S1 facet. (**B**) As in the lumbar region, fluoroscopy may be used to identify the pedicle. (Reproduced with permission from the Barrow Neurological Institute®)

orientation in the axial plane depends on the level. These angles have been well described by Zindrick *et al.* (5, 38) (Table 2).

The rostrocaudal orientation through the pedicle is determined by the lateral fluoroscopic image. The goal is to maintain a projectory that is parallel to the endplate. As the T-handled probe is being advanced through the pedicle, if possible, the pedicle should be palpated from within the canal with an instrument to confirm that the medial, superior, and inferior borders are not being breached. An appropriate-sized hole tap is then advanced through the pedicle under fluoroscopic guidance along the same trajectory as the T-handle (Fig. 4**C**). Once the hole has been tapped, a ball-tipped pedicle probe is inserted into the hole. The walls of the hole are examined to ensure that the cortex has not been breached (Fig. 4**D**). An appropriate-sized pedicle screw is advanced into the pedicle and body along the predetermined trajectory under lateral fluoroscopic guidance. The length of the pedicle screw selected depends on the depth of the hole, as measured by the T-handle. Again, the screw tip can be advanced at least halfway but no more than two-thirds through the vertebral body (Fig. 4**E**). Once the

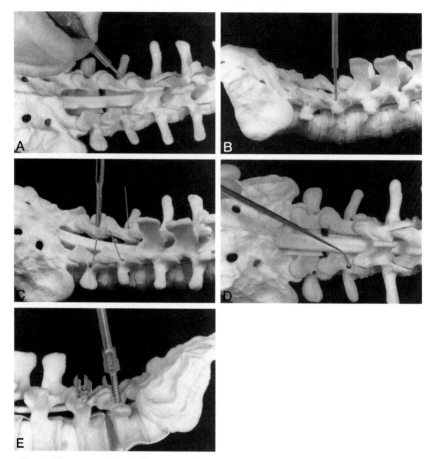

FIG. 4 Placement of pedicle screws. (**A**) A high-speed drill may be used to place a hole through the cortical bone overlying the pedicle entry point. (**B**) The T-handled probe is advanced through the cancellous center of the pedicle into the vertebral body. (**C**) The hole tap is then advanced along the same trajectory as the T-handle. (**D**) A ball-tipped pedicle probe is inserted into the hole made by the T-handle and tapped to ensure that the cortex adjacent to the spinal canal and neural foramen has not been breached. (**E**) Pedicle screws are advanced through the pedicle and into the body along the predetermined trajectory. If any questions remain regarding the proper placement of the hole for the pedicle screw, Steinmann pins may be placed within the holes before screw placement, and an anteroposterior fluoroscopic image may be obtained to confirm that the pins are within the appropriate "target" area. (Reproduced with permission from the Barrow Neurological Institute®)

screws are in place, an AP fluoroscopic image may be obtained to confirm that the pedicle screws have been properly placed within the pedicle "targets" and that the screw tips are oriented appropriately medially. An alternative to this approach is to place Steinmann pins

TABLE 2
Pedicle Width and Angulation[a]

Spinal Level	Mean Transverse Pedicle Width (mm)[b]	Mean Transverse Pedicle Angles (°)[b]
T-10	6.3 (3.1–8.5)	4.6 (0.0–13.5)
T-11	7.8 (3.1–12.0)	1.2 (−6.0–9.5)
T-12	7.1 (3.0–11.0)	−4.2 (−17–14.5)
L-1	8.7 (4.5–13.0)	10.9 (6.5–14.5)
L-2	8.9 (4.0–13.0)	12.0 (5.0–17.5)
L-3	10.3 (5.3–16.0)	14.4 (8.0–23.5)
L-4	12.9 (9.1–17.0)	17.7 (5.5–27.5)
L-5	18.0 (9.1–29.0)	29.8 (19–44)

[a]Modified from analysis by Zindrick *et al.* (38). Reprinted with persmission from Lippincott-Raven Publishers.
[b]Numbers in parentheses indicate the range for each mean value.

within the holes made before screw placement and to obtain an AP fluoroscopic image (Figs. 4C and 5).

A malleable endotracheal tube stylet is used as a template for the rod. This maneuver is useful for determining both the length of the rod and its contour, should it need to be bent. The rod is then cut and bent to match the template (Fig. 6A). The pedicle screw is attached to the rods using connectors. The surgeon may be able to partially reduce a deformity using the distractor or compressor (Fig. 6B) and/or the corkscrew device (Fig. 6C). Once reduction is acceptable, the bolts are tightened provisionally. A torque wrench may be used for the final tightening of the screw (Fig. 6D). Crosslinking should be added if an element of rotational instability is present; however, if the fixation is between L5 and S1, there is seldom enough room for crosslinking.

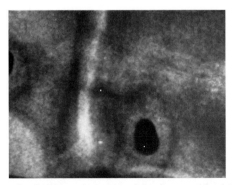

FIG. 5 Anteroposterior fluoroscopic image of lumbar vertebral body demonstrating "target site" with a Steinmann pin in the center, demonstrating successful localization of the pedicle. (Reproduced with permission from the Barrow Neurological Institute®)

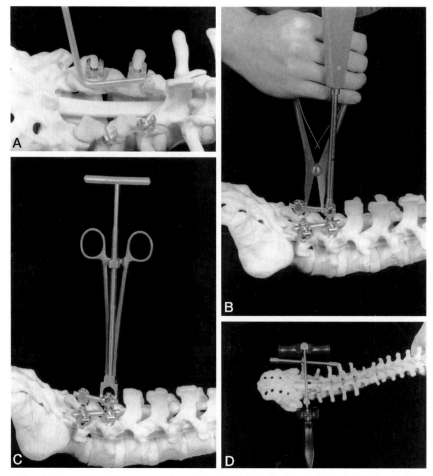

Fig. 6 Assembling the screw rod construct. (**A**) A malleable endotracheal tube stylet is used to measure the distance between the pedicle screws and then as a template to cut and contour the rod appropriately. (**B**) Distraction, as depicted here, or compression may be used to reduce a deformity. (**C**) The corkscrew device is used to properly seat the rod and eyebolt connector onto the pedicle screw. It can also be used for reduction. (**D**) The torque wrench is used for final tightening. (Reproduced with permission from the Barrow Neurological Institute®)

Bone Graft Harvesting

As discussed previously, all decompressions for degenerative lumbar spinal instability should be followed with instrumentation and bone grafting for fusion. Instrumentation alone is insufficient to maintain long-term stabilization. The instrumentation is intended only to act as interim stabilization while bony fusion takes place. As described earlier, before one dissects through the dorsal lumbar fascia, a lateral exposure is performed to expose the posterior iliac crest. The fascia overlying the posterior iliac crest may be incised with the bovie electrocautery device. This exposure should not extend more than 8 cm anteriorly to avoid injuring the superior cluneal nerves. The gluteal musculature is reflected off the posterior aspect of the iliac crest using the bone electrocautery. It is often helpful to use a Taylor retractor to expose the dorsal surface of the iliac crest once the musculature has been dissected free. Unicortical strips are obtained by chiseling through the outer dorsal cortex of the iliac crest with a narrow straight osteotome, that is, creating a series of matchsticks. A series of bone gouges may then be used to remove cancellous material (Fig. 7). Bone wax or Gelfoam can be used for hemostasis. The graft site should be irrigated copiously with an antibiotic saline solution. The overlying fascia is closed primarily, and there is usually no need for drainage (33). If possible, a separate incision for bone graft harvesting should be avoided. With instrumentation of upper lumbar segments, however, it may not be practical to extend the incision caudally enough to harvest graft from the same incision. In this instance, separate incisions are appropriate.

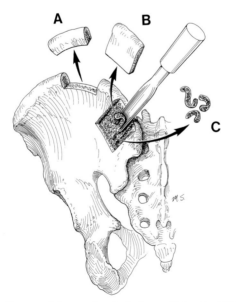

FIG. 7 Iliac crest. Bone graft harvesting techniques. Tricortical (**A**), unicortical (**B**) or cancellous (**C**) bone graft material can be harvested from the posterior iliac crest. (Reproduced with permission from the Barrow Neurological Institute®)

Fusion Techniques

The most common technique for fusion via the posterior approach is the posterolateral fusion. It is important to have adequate lateral exposure of the transverse processes for this technique. The bone surfaces of the transverse processes should be decorticated with a pituitary forceps or a drill. Cancellous bone obtained from the iliac crest is packed over the decorticated surfaces of the transverse processes. Next, cortical strips obtained from the iliac crest are packed over the cancellous graft material (Fig. 8A). Finally, the bone removed from the decompression can be added if the soft tissue is adequately removed. Again, care must be taken to avoid exposing adjacent segments to prevent unwanted extension of the fusion.

A facet-joint fusion may also be performed. A liberal facetectomy for decompression may be performed if fusion and instrumentation are planned at the same level. The joint capsule may be entered with a sharp rongeur or drill. The cartilage is removed, and the cancellous

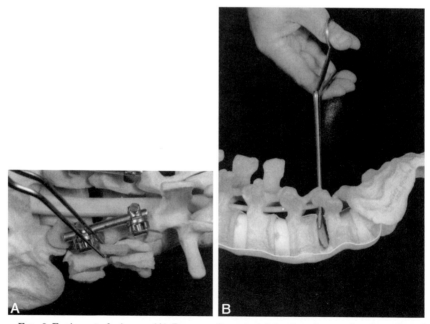

Fig. 8 Fusions techniques. (**A**) Bone graft material is placed over the decorticated surfaces of the transverse processes for a posterolateral fusion. (**B**) With retraction of the thecal sac and nerve root medially and after discectomy, a posterolateral interbody fusion (PLIF) may be performed by wedging bone graft material into the disc space. (Reproduced with permission from the Barrow Neurological Institute®)

bony surfaces are exposed. The joint may be packed tightly with cancellous bone graft obtained from the iliac crest.

Another fusion technique that may be performed via the posterior approach is the posterior lateral interbody fusion (PLIF). This technique involves extensive medial retraction of the thecal sac and nerve roots to create a window through which bone may be packed into the disc space after discectomy (Fig. 8B). Because of the excessive retraction on the thecal sac and nerve roots necessary for this procedure, there is an associated high neurologic complication rate. Consequently, we do not perform this procedure on a routine basis. Additional fusion techniques after a posterior approach for fixation may include the anterior interbody fusion or corpectomy, followed by vertebral body reconstruction. These techniques require a second anterior approach that we believe is excessive and unnecessary unless anterior compressive pathology is present or the anterior load-bearing capability of the spine is lost.

ANTERIOR APPROACH FOR SCREW-PLATE FIXATION

Indications

Our primary indication for proceeding anteriorly requires the presence of significant anterior compressive pathology. This criterion implies bony compression, because in the lumbar spine a herniated or severely bulging disc may be easily approached posteriorly. When there is significant anterior bony compression, as might be encountered in a degenerative/osteoporotic fracture with subsequent instability, we advocate an anterior approach with corpectomy and discectomy for decompression, followed by reconstruction with a cage and/or graft and rigid anterior fixation with a screw-plate system. Rarely, an anterior approach may also be considered if the pedicles are not suitable for posterior fixation, or if an anterior approach is warranted for diagnostic purposes (biopsy) in the absence of spinal canal compromise. For anterior stabilization after decompression, we usually use the Z-Plate System (Sofamor-Danek, Memphis, TN).

Preoperative Planning

Axial CT images through the vertebral bodies adjacent to the corpectomy site are analyzed. The lateral distance across the vertebral body adjacent to the spinal canal is measured to determine the length of the bolt (Fig. 9A–C). The measurement is performed at the superior aspect of the body above (at the level of the pedicle) and at the inferior aspect of the body below. Bicortical purchase, which should be attempted with bolt and screw placements, should be considered when

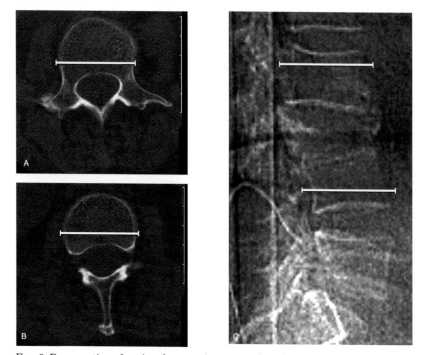

FIG. 9 Preoperative planning for anterior screw-plate fixation. The lateral distance across the vertebral body adjacent to the spinal canal is measured to determine bolt length. This measurement is performed at the (**A**) superior aspect of the body, above (**B**), and at the inferior aspect of the body below. (**C**) Sagittal reconstruction demonstrating the location of the axial images chosen for measurement and their relationship to the pedicles and corpectomy site. (Reproduced with permission from the Barrow Neurological Institute®)

the measurements are made. The distances measured are compared to the scale on the CT scan. In general, it is better to round up to the next 5-mm length so that bicortical purchase can be ensured. The screw should be 5 mm longer than the bolt.

Anesthesia, Patient Positioning, and Monitoring

A general anesthetic is administered, and the patient is intubated. If fixation is to involve the upper lumbar segments and it is anticipated that the diaphragm may need to be traversed and a thoracotomy performed, a double-lumen endotracheal tube should be placed for ventilation of one lung. The patient is placed on the operating room table in the lateral decubitus position with the left side up. Typically, the left side exposure is more desirable, because the aorta is more easily manipulated than the vena cava. Furthermore, the Z-plate screw system described is designed for a left-sided approach. If a right-sided approach is desired, the plate must be turned upside down to ensure that the trajectory of the bolt/screw is appropriate.

Exposure

A retroperitoneal and, for higher exposures, a combined retroperitoneal and transthoracic approach is needed. A multidisciplinary approach and the assistance of a thoracic surgeon is required during this approach. Ribs may be removed and used later for graft material. After it is exposed, the psoas muscle can be followed superiorly to its insertion point along the inferolateral border of L1. The psoas muscle is dissected from the lateral surface of the lumbar spinal column using a combination of sharp and blunt dissection. The segmental vessels at the midportion of the vertebral body must be divided. These vessels are identified, tied or clipped, and then divided with the cautery. This dissection proceeds caudally to expose the entire lateral surface of the inferior vertebral body to be instrumented. The entire exposure should allow identification of the vertebral body that is to be decompressed and reconstructed, as well as the disc spaces between this vertebral body and those above and below. It is also necessary to expose fully the vertebral bodies above and below the corpectomy site to the extent of the next adjacent disc spaces. C-arm fluoroscopy may be used for localization.

Decompression

The pedicles at each level should be identified. Partial removal of the pedicle may be necessary to determine the location of the spinal canal. It is helpful to expose the dura in this region to confirm the location of the spinal canal (Fig. 10**A**). Discectomies are then performed above and below the planned corpectomy site. The annulus is cut with a scalpel, and the disc material is removed with a combination of curettes and disc space rongeurs (Fig. 10**B**). This maneuver allows for visualization of the superior and inferior boundaries of the corpectomy. A U-shaped defect in the vertebral body is created, leaving bone along the spinal canal (dorsally), ventrally, and along the contralateral (lateral) margin (Fig. 10**C**). The spinal canal is decompressed by pulling the remaining margin of bone along the canal surface into the corpectomy defect using a curette (Fig. 10**D**).

Reconstruction of Corpectomy Site

Once a corpectomy has been performed for anterior compressive pathology, it becomes necessary to reconstruct the defect to restore the load-bearing capabilities of the spinal column. A high rate of failure

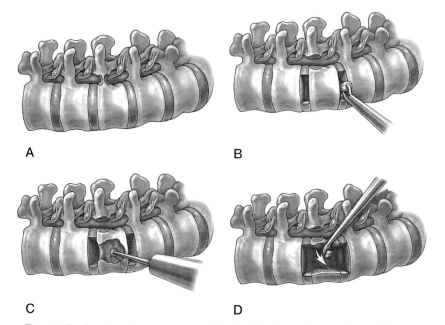

A B

C D

FIG. 10 Performing the corpectomy. (**A**) Partial dissection of the pedicles using Kerrison punches allows for identification of the thecal sac. Once the spinal canal is located, the discectomies and corpectomy may be performed safely. (**B**) Discectomies are performed above and below the corpectomy site. (**C**) A U-shaped defect is created in the vertebral body using a double-action rongeur, followed by a high-speed drill to complete the corpectomy. (**D**) The thin shell of cortical bone remaining within the canal is pulled into the corpectomy defect using a curette, thus completing the decompression. (Reproduced with permission from the Barrow Neurological Institute®)

can be expected for both anterior and posterior fixation systems if a corpectomy is performed without reconstruction, because the stress on the instrumentation becomes excessive.

There are many options for reconstructing corpectomy sites. Our preference is to use a Harm's cage packed with morcellated graft material obtained from the corpectomy site itself, from resected rib, or from the iliac crest. Alternatively, a tricortical iliac crest bone graft from the patient can be used for reconstruction. Other alternatives include the use of allograft, specifically, tricortical iliac crest from cadaveric specimens, or long bone strut grafts packed with morcellated autograft material. Nonbiologic materials such as methylmethacrylate can also be used for reconstruction (33).

Screw-Plate Fixation

A number of anterior screw-plate systems are available (Table 3). The technique described below pertains to the Z-plate screw system. As described previously, preoperative determination of the lengths of the bolts and screws that are to be placed is paramount, and the adjacent disc spaces and the spinal canal must be identified. The bolt is placed 8–10 mm from the next disc space above and below the corpectomy and 8–10 mm from the spinal canal (Fig. 11). The entry points are marked with a bone awl or cautery. Bolt holes are then made using a straight awl with a bolt-positioning guide (Fig. 12**A**). The awl is advanced parallel next to the adjacent disc space, angling 10° away from the spinal canal. Once the hole is made, the bolt is advanced along the same trajectory as the bone awl (Fig. 12**B**). The next step is to distract the bolts and thus the adjacent vertebral bodies with the distractor to reduce the deformity properly. An appropriately sized graft-filled cage may be placed to reconstruct the corpectomy defect (Fig. 12**C**). The cage may be repositioned as necessary using an impactor (Fig. 12**D**). Once the cage is positioned as necessary, an appropriately sized plate may be placed over the bolts. Nuts are placed onto the bolts with the starter shaft in place while compression is applied. Final tightening of the nuts is performed in compression (Fig. 12**E**). The torque wrench is then used to tighten the nuts to 80 in-lbs. The next step is placement of the screws. The holes for the screws in the vertebral body are made using the straight awl and screw-positioning guide. The awl is advanced parallel to the disc space angling 10° toward the spinal canal (Fig. 12**F**). An appropriately sized screw (as previously determined on the preoperative studies) is advanced along the same trajectory (Fig. 12**G** and **H**). Once the final construct is achieved, the length and position of the bolts and screws are rechecked with AP and lateral fluoroscopy. The surgeon must also visually inspect the position of the cage to ensure that it does not encroach upon the spinal canal.

TABLE 3
Anterior Fixation Systems

Anterior locking plate system (ALPS)
Anterior TSRH
Armstrong CASP
ASIF T plate
KANEDA anterior spinal instrumentation
Kostuik-Harrington
Yuan plate
Zielke-Slot
Z-plate anterior thoracolumbar instrumentation

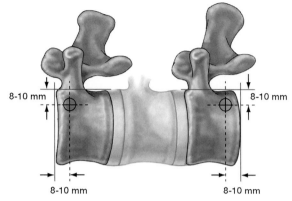

8-10 mm   8-10 mm

8-10 mm   8-10 mm

FIG. 11 Location of the bolt placement sites. The bolt is placed 8–10 mm from the next disc space above and below the corpectomy and 8–10 mm from the spinal canal. (Reproduced with permission from the Barrow Neurological Institute®)

CASE EXAMPLES

Case 1

A 74-year-old woman presented with severe long-standing back and leg pain. Radiographic studies demonstrated an L4-L5 spondylolisthesis (Fig. 13**A**). The patient was placed in a TLSO for a 2-week trial of immobilization, and her symptoms markedly improved. She was thus considered an appropriate candidate for posterior decompression followed by transpedicular screw fixation and posterolateral fusion. The procedure was performed, and there were no perioperative complications (Fig. 13**B**). The patient remained in her TLSO, and at 6 weeks the posterolateral bone graft appeared to be fusing. At 10 weeks, her flexion-extension studies demonstrated no abnormal movement, and she was removed from the TLSO. Her symptoms had completely resolved.

Case 2

A 59-year-old man presented after experiencing lower back pain and left lower extremity radiculopathy for several years. His pain worsened with movement. Plain radiographs revealed decreased disc space height at L3-L4, and multilevel malalignment with a mild level rotatory scoliosis. MR imaging demonstrated stenosis at multiple levels with a left-sided herniated disc at L3-L4, malalignment over multiple levels, and evidence of movement based on endplate changes (Fig. 14**A**). Dynamic studies demonstrated movement at L2-L3, L3-L4, and L4-L5. The patient underwent a decompressive laminectomy, multi-

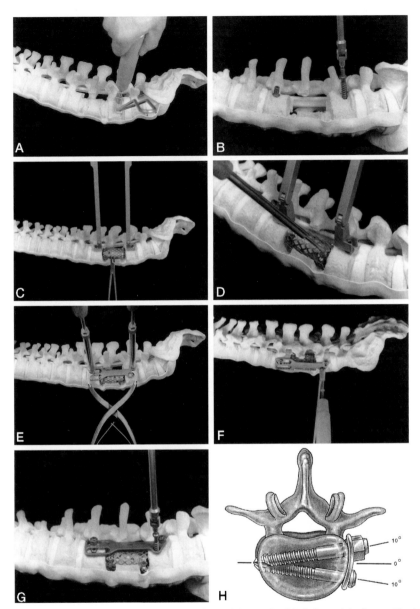

FIG. 12 Bolt placement. (**A**) The straight awl is used with bolt-positioning guide to make the bolt holes. (**B**) The awl is advanced parallel to the adjacent disc space, angling 10° away from the spinal cord. (**C**) A distractor may be used to reduce the deformity. A bone graft-filled cage may be placed within the defect for reconstruction. (**D**) Once in place, the cage may be repositioned using a specially designed impactor and mallet. (**E**) An appropriately sized plate is placed over the bolts. Nuts are placed onto the bolts and provisionally tightened with the starter shafts. The starter shafts are left in place, compression is applied, and final tightening of the nuts is performed in compression. (**F**) The straight awl and screw-positioning guide are used to place screw holes angling 10° toward the spinal canal. (**G**) An appropriately sized screw is advanced along the awl's trajectory. (**H**) Proper screw bolt orientation in vertebral body. (Reproduced with permission from the Barrow Neurological Institute®)

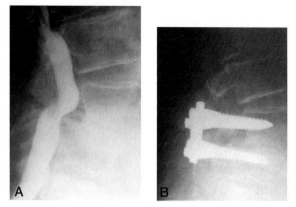

FIG. 13 *Case 1:* (**A**) Myelogram demonstrating significant thecal sac compression from grade II spondylolisthesis at the L4-L5 level. (**B**) Lateral plain radiograph of the lumbosacral spine after posterior decompression and placement of pedicle screw-rod fixation system to immobilize L4-L5. (Reproduced with permission from the Barrow Neurological Institute®)

level pedicle screw fixation (from L2 to L5), and posterolateral fusion (Fig. 14**B** and **C**). Postoperatively, his symptoms resolved.

Case 3

A 74-year-old woman presented with severe back and leg pain. Radiographic studies showed a compression fracture associated with a degenerative osteoporotic fracture (Fig. 15**A**). Conservative treatment with external bracing was attempted. The patient's symptoms improved, but she demonstrated progressive kyphosis. A methylmethacrylate vertebroplasty worsened her condition (Fig. 15**B**). She thus underwent an anterior/retroperitoneal approach with corpectomy for decompression, reconstruction with a Harm's cage and bone graft, and fixation with an anterior screw-plate system (Fig. 15**C** and **D**). There were no complications. She was maintained in a TLSO for about 3 months after surgery and was then weaned from the brace. Dynamic studies at that time demonstrated no abnormal movement. Her progressive kyphosis appeared to be arrested, and her symptoms were markedly improved.

Case 4

A 57-year-old woman presented with severe incapacitating back pain. Preoperative studies demonstrated angulation/kyphosis and endplate changes at L1-L2 (Fig. 16**A**). However, there was no significant compromise of the spinal canal. A workup for osteomyelitis, including

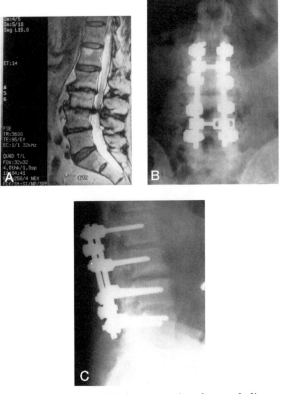

FIG. 14 *Case 2:* (**A**) Preoperative MRI demonstrating abnormal alignment at multiple levels in the lumbar region. Also evident are endplate changes at multiple levels consistent with pathologic movement. The herniated disc at L3-L4 significantly compromises the spinal canal. (**B**) AP and (**C**) lateral plain radiographs demonstrating immobilization of the involved levels. Partial reduction and realignment were achieved. The bone graft laid down for posterolateral fusion is evident on the AP view. (Reproduced with permission from the Barrow Neurological Institute®)

biopsy, was negative. The patient's symptoms were relieved with external immobilization in a TLSO. She was thus considered an appropriate candidate for instrumentation and fusion. Typically, we would have proceeded with a posterior approach, including pedicle screw fixation and posterolateral fusion, because there was no anterior compressive pathology. In this case, however, an anterior approach was selected for better access to pathologic areas for biopsy. The patient tolerated the anterior approach with anterior interbody fusion and screw plate fixation (Fig. 16**B**), and her symptoms were markedly improved after surgery.

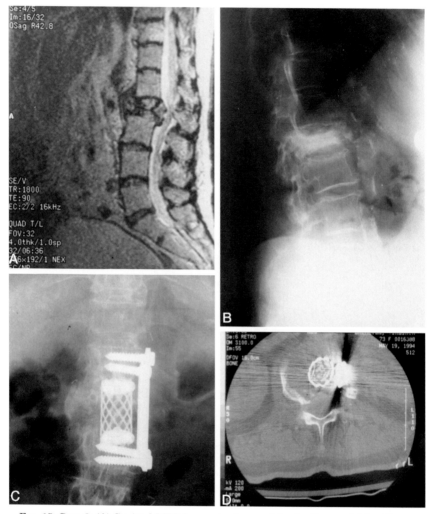

FIG. 15 *Case 3:* (**A**) Sagittal MRI demonstrating vertebral collapse at L2 with retropulsed fragments compromising the spinal canal. (**B**) Continued vertebral collapse and progressive kyphosis despite vertebroplasty. (**C**) Postoperative AP radiograph demonstrating Harm's cage and anterior screw-plate system in place after decompression. (**D**) Axial CT scan confirming adequate decompression and proper positioning of the instrumentation. (Reproduced with permission from the Barrow Neurological Institute®)

DISCUSSION

The literature opposing routine fusion and/or fixation after lumbar decompression (2, 10, 16, 20, 26, 28, 32) has been convincingly countered by contemporary studies, suggesting that instrumentation and

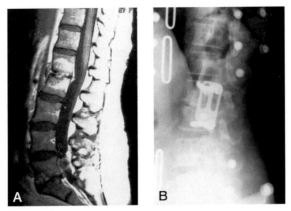

FIG. 16 *Case 4:* (**A**) Sagittal MRI of lumbar spine demonstrating endplate changes at L1-L2 level consistent with movement as well as anterior angulation and kyphosis. There is, however, no significant compromise of the spinal canal from anterior compressive pathology. (**B**) Postoperative lateral plain radiograph after an anterior/retroperitoneal approach with anterior interbody fusion and screw-plate fixation. (Reproduced with permission from the Barrow Neurological Institute®)

fusion are beneficial to selected patients (3, 4, 9, 14, 15, 18, 21, 24, 25, 34, 35). A prospective randomized study by Zdeblick (35) demonstrated that fusion rates were higher with rigid pedicle screw-rod fixation systems, compared to those of fusion without instrumentation. Instrumentation with fusions was also associated with improved overall clinical outcomes. A meta-analysis of the literature performed by Mardjetko *et al.* (25) demonstrated that patients with degenerative lumbar spondylolisthesis fared better if they were fused after decompression, and fusion rates were enhanced by an adjunctive spinal instrumentation. There was, however, no significant difference between the results achieved by control devices, such as Harrington rods and Luque rectangle fixations, and pedicle screw devices. A recent cohort study of pedicle screw fixation (34) concluded that pedicle screw fixations for degenerative spondylolisthesis were associated with a statistically significantly higher rate of fusion than noninstrumented procedures. Furthermore, patients treated with pedicle screw systems had better clinical outcomes, including less pain, improved function, and greater neurologic recovery than the control patients treated with noninstrumented fusion. The rate of nondevice morbidity was similar between the two groups. The Cohort Study Scientific Committee concluded that the potential benefits of pedicle screw fixation greatly outweighed the potential risks associated with implant breakage or intra- and postoperative complications. These carefully performed studies indicated that pedicle screw fixation is the "industry standard" for the treatment of degenerative lumbar spinal instability with few exceptions. With this technique, a 93% fusion rate and an 86% patient satisfaction rate are possible (25).

With pedicle screw-fixation systems, a stable construct can always be expected, because three-column fixation is obtained by design. As a result, fewer segments need to be fused. With proper placement, there is no compromise of the spinal canal or foramina—an unlikely situation with systems consisting of hooks and claws or sublaminar wires. Because of the rigid fixation, patients may also be mobilized rapidly to minimize postoperative complications. Pedicle screw-base systems, however, also have potential disadvantages. These disadvantages include the increased technical difficulty in placing the devices, the potential for a 10% rate of instrument-related complications (25), and the potential for neurologic injury from improper placement.

Anterior approaches for degenerative lumbar spinal instability are performed less frequently than posterior approaches. However, anterior interbody fusions without fixation have been associated with a 94% fusion rate and an 86% rate of patient satisfaction (19, 25, 29, 31). As stated, our indications for an anterior approach for the treatment of degenerative lumbar spinal instability require the presence of significant anterior compressive pathology, necessitating decompression, or the contraindication of a posterior fixation/fusion. Such a decompression usually implies that a corpectomy must be performed. After the corpectomy, the load-bearing capabilities of the spine must be restored, and thus a reconstruction also is required. Because the nonunion rate without fixation can be high (1, 7, 8, 11, 12, 27), we believe that anterior fusions/reconstruction should be augmented with rigid fixation. If we extrapolate from our experience with posterior instrumentation to augment fusion, we can expect that patients with anterior fixation augmenting anterior reconstruction can be mobilized more rapidly and will have higher rates of fusion. This has been confirmed by modern clinical and animal studies (17, 22, 23, 37). Anterior fixation after anterior decompression usually eliminates the need for an additional posterior approach for stabilization (6, 7, 17, 22, 23, 30, 36).

A number of anterior fixation systems have been devised and tested rigorously (36). An anterior fixation system should provide rigid fixation with high pull-out strength. The constructs should have a low profile and be easy to place. It is also helpful if the system permits distraction for the reduction of deformities and compression for bone grafts. Perhaps the most important factor, however, is that surgeons should choose a system that is familiar and that has been used successfully in the past.

CONCLUSIONS

In the treatment of degenerative lumbar spinal instability, the selection of patients with appropriate indications for fixation and fusion is probably of greater significance than the actual type of procedure that is performed. In the patient with clear evidence of instability, the literature favors the use of instrumentation to augment fusion. The issue then becomes how to determine the best way to instrument or fixate the lumbar spine. The literature suggests that for posterior approaches, any fixation system that immobilizes the involved segments will tend to augment fusion and to improve patient satisfaction. In experienced hands, however, pedicle screw-base systems offer theoretical advantages over other systems with no significantly increased rates of morbidity. A consensus on the best pedicle screw-fixation system is lacking. We recommend that surgeons use familiar systems that they have used successfully in the past. The best way to fuse the lumbar spine for posterior approaches is controversial. The posterolateral type, which is the most popular, is associated with a high rate of fusion and is easily performed with the posterior exposure needed for pedicle-screw fixation. We recommend that anterior approaches be reserved for the rare patient who has anterior compressive pathology or contraindications for a posterior approach. The vertebral body should always be reconstructed to restore the load-bearing capabilities of the spinal column. Rigid fixation, using an anterior screw-plate system, should then be performed to reduce and stabilize the spine and to augment fusion. This strategy can obviate the need for a second posterior approach to fixate and stabilize the lumbar spine.

REFERENCES

1. Benzel EC, Larson SJ: Functional recovery after decompressive operation for thoracic and lumbar spine fractures. **Neurosurgery** 19:772–778, 1986.

2. Bernhardt M, Swartz DE, Clothiaux RL, et al.: Posterolateral lumbar and lumbosacral fusion with and without pedicle screw internal fixation. **Clin Orthop** 284:109–115, 1992.

3. Bolesta MJ, Bohlman HH: Degenerative spondylolisthesis. **AAOS Instructional Course Lecture** 35:11989.

4. Bridwell KH, Sedgewick TA, O'Brien MF, et al.: The role of fusion and instrumentation in the treatment of degenerative spondylolisthesis with spinal stenosis. **J Spinal Disord** 6:461–472, 1993.

5. Dickman CA, Fessler RG, MacMillan M, et al.: Transpedicular screw-rod fixation of the lumbar spine: Operative technique and outcome in 104 cases. **J Neurosurg** 77:860–870, 1992.

6. Dickson JH, Harrington PR, Erwin WD: Results of reduction and stabilization of the

severely fractured thoracic and lumbar spine. **J Bone Joint Surg Am** 60:799–805, 1978.

7. Dunn HK: Anterior stabilization of thoracolumbar injuries. **Clin Orthop** 189:116–125, 1984.

8. Dunn HK, Goble EM, McBride GG, et al.: An implant system for anterior spine stabilization. **Orthop Trans** 5:433–434, 1981.

9. Feffer HL, Wiesel SW, Cuckler JM, et al.: Degenerative spondylolisthesis: To fuse or not to fuse? **Spine** 10:287–289, 1985.

10. Fitzgerald JA, Newman PH: Degenerative spondylolisthesis. **J Bone Joint Surg Br** 58:184–192, 1976.

11. Flynn JC, Hoque MA: Anterior fusion of the lumbar spine: End-result study with long-term follow-up. **J Bone Joint Surg Am** 61:1143–1150, 1979.

12. Freebody D, Bendall R, Taylor RD: Anterior transperitoneal lumbar fusion. **J Bone Joint Surg Br** 53:617–627, 1971.

13. Frymoyer JW, Selby DK: Segmental instability: Rationale for treatment. **Spine** 10:280–286, 1985.

14. Hanley EN Jr.: Decompression and distraction-derotation arthrodesis for degenerative spondylolisthesis. **Spine** 11:269–276, 1986.

15. Herkowitz HN, Kurz LT: Degenerative lumbar spondylolisthesis with spinal stenosis: A prospective study comparing decompression with decompression and intertransverse process arthrodesis. **J Bone Joint Surg Am** 73:802–808, 1991.

16. Herron LD, Trippi AC: L4-5 degenerative spondylolisthesis: The results of treatment by decompressive laminectomy without fusion. **Spine** 14:534–538, 1989.

17. Kaneda K, Abumi K, Fujiya M: Burst fractures with neurologic deficits of the thoracolumbar-lumbar spine: Results of anterior decompression and stabilization with anterior instrumentation. **Spine** 9:788–795, 1984.

18. Kaneda K, Kazama H, Satoh S, et al.: Follow-up study of medial facetectomies and posterolateral fusion with instrumentation in unstable degenerative spondylolisthesis. **Clin Orthop** 203:159–167, 1986.

19. Kim NH, Kim HK, Suh JS: A computed tomographic analysis of changes in the spinal canal after anterior lumbar interbody fusion. **Clin Orthop** 286:180–191, 1993.

20. Kim SS, Denis F, Lonstein JE, et al.: Factors affecting fusion rate in adult spondylolisthesis. **Spine** 15:979–984, 1990.

21. Knox BD, Harvell JC Jr, Nelson PB, et al.: Decompression and luque rectangle fusion for degenerative spondylolisthesis. **J Spinal Disord** 2:223–228, 1989.

22. Kostuik JP: Anterior spinal cord decompression for lesions of the thoracic and lumbar spine, techniques, new methods of internal fixation results. **Spine** 8:512–531, 1983.

23. Kostuik JP: Anterior fixation for fractures of the thoracic and lumbar spine with or without neurologic involvement. **Clin Orthop** 189:103–115, 1984.

24. Lombardi JS, Wiltse LL, Reynolds J, et al.: Treatment of degenerative spondylolisthesis. **Spine** 10:821–827, 1985.

25. Mardjetko SM, Connolly PJ, Shott S: Degenerative lumbar spondylolisthesis: A meta-analysis of literature 1970–1993. **Spine** 19:S2256–S2265, 1994.

26. Reynolds JB, Wiltse LL: Surgical treatment of degenerative spondylolisthesis (abstr.). **Spine** 4:148–149, 1979.
27. Riska EB, Myllynen P, Bostman O: Anterolateral decompression for neural involvement in thoracolumbar fractures: A review of 78 cases. **J Bone Joint Surg Br** 69:704–708, 1987.
28. Rosenberg NJ: Degenerative spondylolisthesis: Surgical treatment. **Clin Orthop** 117:112–120, 1976.
29. Satomi K, Hirabayashi K, Toyama Y, et al.: A clinical study of degenerative spondylolisthesis: Radiographic analysis and choice of treatment. **Spine** 17:1329–1336, 1992.
30. Schmidek HH, Gomes FB, Seligson D, et al.: Management of acute unstable thoracolumbar (T11-L1) fractures with and without neurological deficit. **Neurosurgery** 7:30–35, 1980.
31. Takahashi K, Kitahara H, Yamagata M, et al.: Long-term results of anterior interbody fusion for treatment of degenerative spondylolisthesis. **Spine** 15:1211–1215, 1990.
32. Wiltse LL, Kirkaldy-Willis WH, McIvor GW: The treatment of spinal stenosis. **Clin Orthop** 115:83–91, 1976.
33. Yonemura KS: Bone grafts: Types of harvesting and their complications, in Menezes AH, Sonntag VKH (eds): *Principles of Spinal Surgery.* New York, McGraw-Hill, 1996, pp 151–156.
34. Yuan HA, Garfin SR, Dickman CA, et al.: A historical cohort study of pedicle screw fixation in thoracic, lumbar and sacral spinal fusions. **Spine** 19:S2279–S2296, 1994.
35. Zdeblick TA: A prospective, randomized study of lumbar fusion: Preliminary results. **Spine** 18:983–991, 1993.
36. Zdeblick TA: Z-plate anterior thoracolumbar instrumentation, in Hitchon PW, Traynelis VC, Rengachary S (eds): *Techniques in Spinal Fusion and Stabilization.* New York, Thieme, 1995, p 279.
37. Zdeblick TA, Shirado O, McAfee PC, et al.: Anterior spinal fixation after lumbar corpectomy: A study in dogs. **J Bone Joint Surg Am** 73:527–534, 1991 (Published erratum appears in **J Bone Joint Surg Am** 73(6):952, 1991.)
38. Zindrick MR, Wiltse LL, Doornik A, et al.: Analysis of the morphometric characteristics of the thoracic and lumbar pedicles. **Spine** 12:160–166, 1987.

11

Surgical Techniques for Upper Cervical Spine Decompression and Stabilization

CURTIS A. DICKMAN, M.D., PAUL J. APOSTOLIDES, M.D.,
AND DEAN G. KARAHALIOS, M.D.

Rigid internal fixation of the craniovertebral junction or upper cervical spine remains a challenging problem for spinal surgeons because of the complex anatomy, biomechanics, and kinematics of this region. The goals of treatment are to preserve neurologic function, decompress the neural elements, reduce pathologic subluxations, restore immediate stability, promote osseous union for long-term stability, and preserve normal motion segments whenever possible.

The criteria for patient selection and the analysis of outcome after upper cervical spine trauma are reviewed in separate chapters in this volume by different authors. This chapter focuses on the various surgical techniques that we use for decompression and stabilization of the craniovertebral junction and upper cervical spine.

All procedures are performed under general anesthesia, and all patients receive routine perioperative antibiotics. Continuous intraoperative somatosensory-evoked potential monitoring and brainstem auditory-evoked potential monitoring are used to assess the physiologic status of the spinal cord and brainstem during these procedures.

TRANSORAL APPROACH TO THE CRANIOVERTEBRAL JUNCTION

A transoral approach (5, 6, 10, 25, 29–31, 38–40, 42) occasionally may be needed to decompress trauma patients who have a hypertrophic nonunion of a C2 fracture (Fig. 1A and **B**). More commonly, however, patients with upper cervical trauma who require surgery will need only internal fixation without decompression. The patient is positioned supine on the operating table with the head in a neutral position and the neck slightly extended. The head is secured to the operating table with a Mayfield headholder or modified Mayfield fixation device (Durr-Fillauer Medical, Inc., Chattanooga, TN) if a halo brace was placed preoperatively. The anterior bars of the halo brace

137

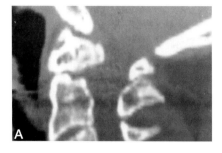

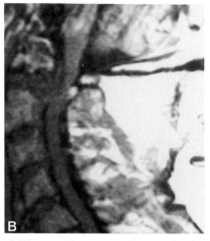

FIG. 1 Sagittal (**A**) computed tomography and (**B**) magnetic resonance images showing a chronic hypertrophic nonunion of a traumatic type II odontoid fracture causing significant brainstem compression.

can be removed to allow room for retractors and to bring the surgeon's hands closer to the patient's mouth.

A self-retaining transoral retractor system (Spetzler-Sonntag, Aesculap, San Francisco, CA) is used to facilitate wide exposure of the posterior oropharynx (Fig. 2**A** and **B**). The retractor frame has a very low profile to improve lighting and operative exposure. It rigidly attaches to the operating room table via crossbars to stabilize the retractors intraoperatively and to allow rotation of the table during the procedure. The tongue and endotracheal tube are retracted caudally

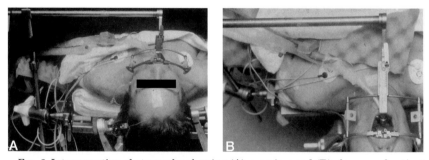

FIG. 2 Intraoperative photographs showing (**A**) overview and (**B**) close-up of patient positioning and the low-profile, self-retaining retractor system (Spetzler-Sonntag, Aesculap, San Francisco, CA), which provides a wide exposure of the posterior oropharynx for transoral odontoidectomy.

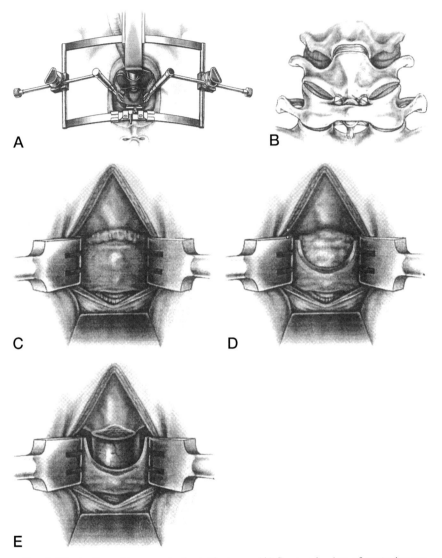

FIG. 3 Illustration of transoral odontoidectomy. (**A**) Surgeon's view of posterior oro-pharynx after placement of self-retaining retractor system. (**B**) Anatomic relationships of anterior aspects of C1-C2 underlying posterior oropharynx mucosa and muscles. The C1 tubercle is a key landmark that verifies the position of the midline. (**C**) A vertical midline incision is made in the median raphé of the posterior oropharynx to expose the anterior arch of C1 and the body of C2. (**D**) The inferior portion of the anterior C1 arch is resected to expose the base of the odontoid process. (**E**) The dens is detached from its ligamentous attachments, transected at the base, and removed en bloc if possible. (Reproduced with permission from the Barrow Neurological Institute®.)

with a rigid wide-blade retractor. The soft palate and uvula are retracted superiorly with a malleable-blade retractor. Teeth guards attached to the retractor frame cover and protect the patient's teeth. The patient's tongue should be inspected after the retractor system is positioned to ensure that it is not pinched between the wide-blade retractor and the teeth to avoid severe swelling or necrosis. Routine tracheostomy is rarely necessary unless severe, preoperative bulbar or respiratory disturbances exist.

The oropharynx and retractors are sterilized with Betadine solution. An intraoperative radiograph is obtained to judge the spinal alignment after positioning and to confirm the extent of the cephalad and caudal exposure provided by the retractor system. A Trendelenburg position of the table is often used to provide the best perspective of the craniovertebral junction. The surgeon sits above the patient's head and has a direct view of the patient's mouth and oropharynx (Fig. 3**A** and **B**). The surgical microscope is used immediately to improve lighting, to provide variable magnification, and to allow the cosurgeon to observe and assist during the procedure.

The C1 tubercle is palpated to verify the position of the midline. A vertical midline incision is made in the median raphé of the posterior pharyngeal wall mucosa, pharyngeal muscles, and the anterior longitudinal ligament using either a monopolar cautery or a scalpel (Fig. 3**C**). A palatal incision is avoided if possible because it can cause nasal regurgitation, dysphagia, and a nasal tone of voice. The layers of the posterior oropharynx are maintained as a single thick layer to facilitate a strong tissue closure. Periosteal elevators are used to dissect the anterior longitudinal ligament subperiosteally and to separate the tissue flap from the anterior surfaces of the C1 arch, the C2 vertebral body, and the inferior clivus. Adjustable, telescoping tooth-bladed retractors are inserted to retract the pharyngeal flaps laterally to maintain a wide exposure.

Curettes and periosteal elevators are used to define the boundaries of the clivus, the base of the odontoid process, the anterior C1 arch, and the C2 vertebral body. The inferior one- to two-thirds of the anterior C1 arch is resected to expose the base of the odontoid process using a combination of high-speed air drill with small cutting and diamond burrs and various Kerrison rongeurs (Fig. 3**D**). As much of the anterior C1 arch as possible should be left intact to preserve the structural integrity of the C1 ring. However, enough bone needs to be removed to expose the dens satisfactorily.

After the anterior C1 arch is partially resected, the lateral margins of the odontoid process are defined. The alar and apical ligaments are detached sharply with curved curettes. The base of the dens is partially transected with a cutting burr; the osteotomy is completed by removing the posterior cortex of the dens with a 1-mm Kerrison rongeur or a diamond burr. The dens is grasped with a toothed rongeur and removed en bloc if possible (Fig. 3**E**). The dens can also be removed in a piecemeal fashion, but it is often more difficult to access its apex.

Soft tissue pathology often must be resected to decompress the neural elements adequately. The transverse ligament and tectorial membrane may also need to be removed to visualize the dura and normal pulsation of the thecal sac. However, the surgeon must beware of attenuated dura and ligaments that adhere to the dura. Meticulous microsurgical techniques are necessary to avoid a cerebrospinal fluid (CSF) leak from inadvertent intradural entry. Intradural entry is associated with a high risk of postoperative morbidity and mortality. If an intraoperative CSF leak occurs, a fascial patch is placed directly over the dura and secured with fibrin glue (24). A lumbar drain is inserted postoperatively, and appropriate antibiotic coverage and the lumbar drain are maintained for at least 1 week.

The boundaries of the decompression can be assessed intraoperatively by placing iodinated contrast material into the decompression site and obtaining a lateral cervical radiograph. Once the brainstem and spinal cord have been decompressed adequately, the wound is irrigated with antibiotic solution, and hemostasis is achieved. The wound is closed with interrupted or running 2-0 vicryl suture in a single layer that includes the mucosa, pharyngeal muscles, and ligaments. Multilayer closures are more difficult to perform and can attenuate the tissue layers and weaken the incision line.

A nasogastric feeding tube is inserted intraoperatively while directly visualizing the oropharyngeal incision to avoid inadvertent malpositioning of the tube. The patient receives postoperative enteral nutrition via the feeding tube for at least 3 days and remains intubated until postoperative swelling of the tongue subsides. The patient also remains in an external orthosis until spinal stability can be restored (11, 15).

THREADED STEINMANN PIN FUSION OF THE CRANIOVERTEBRAL JUNCTION (4, 13, 16, 35–37)

The patient is positioned prone with the head secured to the operating table using a Mayfield headholder or a modified Mayfield fixation device (Durr-Fillauer Medical, Inc., Chattanooga, TN) if a halo brace was placed preoperatively (Fig. 4**A**). The posterior bars and vest plate of the halo brace are removed to access the neck and iliac crest. After positioning, an intraoperative lateral radiograph is obtained to assess the alignment of the craniovertebral junction.

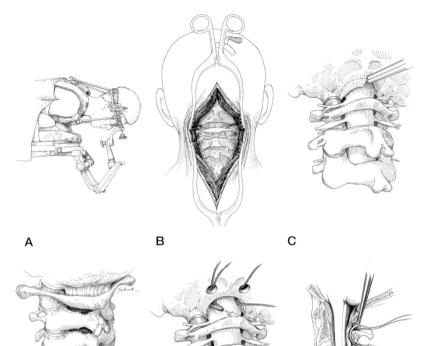

A   B   C

D   E   F

FIG. 4 Illustration of occipitocervical fusion using a threaded Steinmann pin. (**A**) A modified Mayfield fixation device for the halo brace facilitates stabilization of the patient to the operating room table. (**B**) A posterior cervical skin incision provides access to the craniovertebral junction. (**C**) The posterior rim of the foramen magnum is enlarged. (**D**) The cervical laminae are notched medially as close to the spinous processes as possible to facilitate passage of the sublaminar wires. (**E**) Suboccipital wires are passed carefully from burr holes to the foramen magnum. (**F**) Passage of sublaminar wires is facilitated by carefully placing the blunt end of a large needle attached to the suture under each laminae to be fused. (**G**) The suture is tied to the end of the wire and carefully passed under the lamina using a simultaneous two-handed feeding and pulling technique. (**H**) Primary and (**I**) secondary curvatures are made in the pin using a custom rod-bending tool. (**J**) The threaded Steinmann pin is secured to the craniovertebral junction with braided cable. (**K**) A unicortical plate of bone can be used to provide a template for the fusion mass to develop in patients who have undergone a previous posterior decompression. (**A–G, J, K** reproduced with permission from the Barrow Neurological Institute®.)

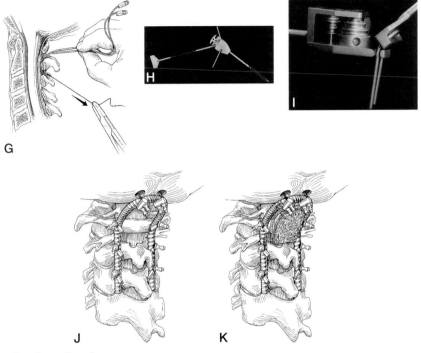

G

H

I

J   K

FIG. 4–continued

A midline skin incision is made from the inion to the spinous process of C7. The nuchal fascia is divided in a midline sagittal plane. Sharp subperiosteal dissection is used to expose the occipital squamosa, foramen magnum, and dorsal arches and facet joints of the upper cervical vertebra to be fused (Fig. 4**B**). Meticulous care should be taken to avoid dislocation of unstable vertebral segments, injury to the vertebral arteries, and exposure of nonfused segments. The spinal canal should be decompressed before reduction and internal fixation.

The posterior occipitoatlantal membrane is detached from the rim of the foramen magnum and C1. The posterior rim of the foramen magnum is then enlarged using Kerrison rongeurs (Fig. 4**C**). Two or three burr holes are placed into the thick portion of the occipital bone approximately 5–10 mm superior to the enlarged rim of the foramen magnum. The burr holes are waxed, and the dura is dissected away from the inner table of the skull toward the foramen magnum.

The soft tissue, interspinous ligaments, and ligamentum flavum are removed completely from the vertebrae to be fused. The superior and inferior laminae of these vertebrae are often notched medially as close to the spinous processes as possible with a Kerrison rongeur to facilitate passage of the sublaminar wires (Fig. 4D). If facets are to be wired, drill holes are placed through the inferior facets into the joints. Sublaminar wires are preferred over facet wires for fixation because they provide more secure stabilization and are stronger than the facets in resisting wire pullout. Suboccipital wires and sublaminar or facet wires are then placed.

Wiring is performed with either stainless steel or titanium braided cable. Suboccipital wires are passed from the occipital burr holes to the foramen magnum after the tip of the wire has been bent into a blunt loop to help avoid dural penetration and injury to the cerebellum and dural venous sinuses (Fig. 4E). Sublaminar wires are passed under the laminae as medial as possible to minimize the risks of dural penetration and neurologic injury. Sublaminar wire placement can be facilitated by carefully passing the blunt end of a large needle attached to a 2-0 vicryl or silk suture under each lamina (Fig. 4F). The suture is tied to the end of the wire, and both are carefully passed under the lamina using a simultaneous two-handed feeding and pulling technique (Fig. 4G). Sublaminar wires are positioned at the most lateral aspects of the laminae during fixation.

A wide (5/32-inch) diameter, stainless-steel threaded Steinmann pin or grooved titanium rod is bent into a "U"-shape with a custom rod-bending tool (BendMeister Rod Bender; Sofamor Danek, Inc., Memphis, TN) (Fig. 4H). Smooth secondary curves are fashioned to match the contour of the craniovertebral junction (Fig. 4I). The curves of the pin need to be smooth because sharp angles may create stress risers that could encourage the pin to break.

Precise shaping of the pin is required to seat the implant flushly against all fixated bone surfaces to create the most stable occipitocervical construct. A sterile, malleable endotracheal tube stylet may be used as a template for contouring the pin. When placed into the wound, the pin should lie flush against the occiput and laminae. Gaps between the pin and the bone surfaces may loosely fixate the vertebrae and allow excessive motion. The pin length is measured, and the ends are cut so that they do not extend beyond the lowest segment to be fused.

The pin is wired against the occiput and cervical laminae or facets (Fig. 4J). The threads of the pin prevent vertical settling of the construct. The occiput, facet joints, and posterior arches of the cervical levels to be fused are decorticated segmentally using currettes and a high-speed air drill to maximize the surface area for bone incorporation. Generous amounts of autologous iliac crest cancellous bone grafts are compressed against the levels to be fused. If a suboccipital craniectomy or cervical laminectomy is required to decompress the neural

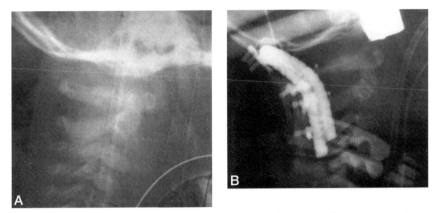

FIG. 5 (**A**) Preoperative and (**B**) postoperative lateral radiographs of a child with a traumatic occipitoatlantal dislocation treated with threaded Steinmann pin fusion of the craniovertebral junction.

elements, a unicortical plate of iliac crest bone can be sutured or wired to the central portion of the Steinmann pin to facilitate fusion and preserve the decompression (Fig. **4K**). A routine multilayered wound closure is performed (Fig. **5A** and **B**).

Postoperatively, patients are usually treated with a Philadelphia collar. A halo brace may be considered to augment the fixation if the patient has a traumatic occipitocervical dislocation, widespread bony destruction, or extremely soft bone. Coexistent rheumatoid arthritis or other severely degenerative disease process may limit the rigidity of the fixation and the development of a solid osseous union.

INTERSPINOUS FUSION (16, 18, 35)

Patients are often placed in a halo brace perioperatively to satisfactorily control C1-C2 motion and optimize the fusion rate. The patient is positioned prone with the halo brace secured to the operating table using a modified Mayfield fixation device (Durr-Fillauer Medical, Inc., Chattanooga, TN). The posterior bars and vest plate of the halo brace are removed to access the neck and iliac crest. After positioning, an intraoperative lateral radiograph is obtained to assess spinal alignment.

A midline skin incision is made from the midocciput to the spinous process of C3. Sharp subperiosteal dissection is used to expose the C1 and C2 posterior arches and facet joints (Fig. **6A**). The soft tissue, posterior occipitoatlantal membrane, interspinous ligaments, and ligamentum flavum of the atlas and axis are removed completely. Care is taken to preserve the pericranium of the occiput and skull base to

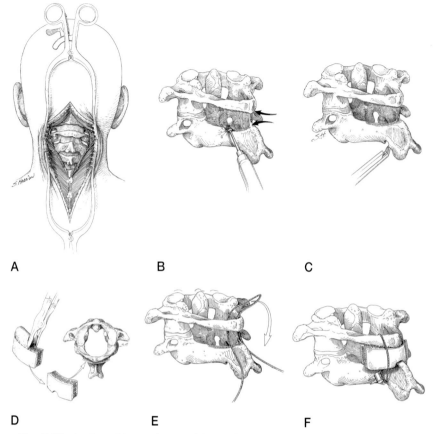

FIG. 6 Illustration of interspinous wiring technique. (**A**) A posterior cervical incision provides access to the upper cervical spine. (**B**) The fusion site is prepared by decorticating the inferior edge of the posterior C1 arch and the superior edges of the C2 spinous process and the posterior arch of C2. (**C**) Bilateral notches in the inferior surfaces of the C2 lamina help seat the wires. (**D**) Curved bicortical strut graft is sized and fitted to recreate the normal anatomic distance between the C1 and C2 arches. (**E**) A braided cable wire is placed in a U-shaped loop and passed beneath the posterior arch of C1. (**F**) The cable is tightened and crimped to trap the bone graft between the wires and to compress it between the posterior arches of C1 and C2. (Reproduced with permission from the Barrow Neurological Institute®.)

prevent an inadvertent occipitocervical fusion. However, if the posterior C1 arch is displaced upwardly against the occiput, the posterior rim of the foramen magnum may need to be enlarged to facilitate wire passage under the posterior ring of the atlas.

The fusion site is prepared by decorticating the inferior edge of the posterior C1 arch and the superior edges of the C2 spinous process and posterior C2 arch with a high-speed drill or Kerrison rongeurs (Fig. 6**B**). The decortication exposes cancellous bone in the fusion bed for apposition with cancellous bone of the graft to promote fusion. Bilateral notches are made in the inferior surfaces of the C2 laminae to seat the wires where they join the C2 spinous process (Fig. 6**C**).

An autologous, curved, tricortical bone graft (approximately 4 cm long × 3 cm high) is obtained from the posterior iliac crest. The rounded upper cortical edge of the graft is removed with a Lexsell rongeur to create a bicortical curved strut graft (Fig. 6**D**). The strut graft is fitted precisely between the posterior arches of C1 and C2 to recreate the normal height of the C1-C2 complex. The curve of the graft approximates the curve of the posterior C1 ring. The inferior margin of the bone graft is notched in the midline to match the contour of the C2 spinous process. The graft is removed temporarily to permit the wire to be placed.

A loop of braided wire cable is passed beneath the posterior C1 arch in the midline (Fig. 6**E**). Sublaminar wire placement can sometimes be facilitated by carefully passing the blunt end of a large needle attached to a 2-0 vicryl or silk suture under the posterior C1 arch. The suture is tied to the loop of the cable, and both are passed carefully under the C1 arch using the simultaneous feeding-and-pulling technique. The graft is repositioned between the atlas and axis. The loop of wire is passed over the posterior C1 ring, behind the graft, and is secured in the notch beneath the base of the C2 spinous process. The free ends of the cable are positioned anteriorly to the graft and are also passed beneath the notch in the C2 spinous process. The cable is tightened and crimped to trap the bone graft between the wires and to compress it between the posterior C1 and C2 arches (Fig. 6**F**).

The surfaces of the posterior C1-C1-C2 arches and bone graft are decorticated with currettes and a high-speed air drill. Additional morcellized, cancellous bone graft from the iliac crest is compressed against the fusion surfaces. C1-C2 wiring techniques allow substantial C1-C2 motion to occur in the destabilized spine (12, 22). Therefore, supplemental rigid fixation, either internally with C1-C2 screws or externally with a halo brace, is recommended to maximize the fusion of the unstable segments. Postoperatively, the patient usually remains in a halo brace 10–12 weeks until evidence of fusion is documented radiographically.

POSTERIOR ATLANTOAXIAL TRANSARTICULAR FACET SCREW FIXATION
(14, 17, 23, 27, 28, 41)

Meticulous preoperative planning and precise operative techniques are required to achieve success with this technique. Preoperative plain radiographs are used to assess the alignment of C1-C2 and to verify that the C1-C2 complex can be reduced adequately. Preoperative computed tomography (CT) scans with sagittal reconstructions are used to define the position of the vertebral arteries and architecture of the C1 lateral masses and C2 facets (33). An anomalous vertebral artery or comminuted fractures of the C1 lateral masses or C2 pars preclude screw placement.

The patient is positioned prone. If possible, controlled flexion of the patient's neck is performed to obtain the proper trajectory for insertion of the drill and screws. The patient's head is secured to the operating table using a Mayfield headholder. A modified Mayfield fixation device (Durr-Fillauer Medical, Inc., Chattanooga, TN) is used if a halo brace was placed preoperatively, and the posterior bars and vest plate of the halo brace are removed to access the neck, back, and iliac crest. Lateral fluoroscopic monitoring is used intraoperatively to assess spinal alignment during positioning, drilling, and screw insertion. The skin preparation should extend down to the upper thoracic spine for percutaneous placement of the transarticular facet screws.

We prefer a technique using cannulated screws for C1-C2 screw and odontoid screw insertion (14). The technique uses a long thin Kirschner (K)-wire to drill the initial path into the bone. This strategy permits the trajectory to be repositioned, fixates adjacent unstable segments, and guides the screws into the bones.

A midline posterior cervical incision is made to access the atlas and axis. Sharp subperiosteal dissection is performed to expose the posterior C1-C2 arches and the C1-C2 articular surfaces. The ligamentum flavum is removed from the C1-C2 laminae and C2 pars interarticularis. The pars is exposed medially to allow the mediolateral trajectory of the screws to be adjusted through its central axis. The screw entry point is located approximately 2–3 mm above the caudal edge of the C2 inferior facet and approximately 2–3 mm lateral to the medial border of the C2-C3 facet (Fig. 7**A**). Occasionally, this entry point must be adjusted 1–2 mm to compensate for altered anatomic relationships. A high-speed drill or bone awl is used to penetrate the cortical bone at the entry point to help direct the insertion of the K-wire and to prevent it from migrating as drilling is initiated.

A trajectory between 0 and 10° medially is required to place the K-wire and screw through the central axis of the C2 pars in the sagittal orientation (Fig. 7**B**). A lateral trajectory must be avoided to prevent injury of the vertebral artery. A no. 4 Penfield dissector is placed directly along the upper surface of the C2 pars into the atlantoaxial facet joint and retracted upward to displace the C2 nerve root and its surrounding venous plexus superiorly (Fig. 7**C**). Retraction of the C2

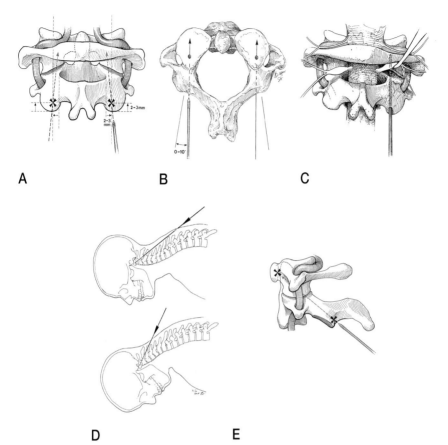

A   B   C

D   E

FIG. 7 Illustrations demonstrating (**A**) screw entry point, (**B**) trajectory of screw placement through central axis of C2, and (**C**) elevation of the C2 nerve root and its surrounding venous plexus during screw placement. (**D**) Proper screw trajectory may require percutaneous screw placement (*top*) or direct screw placement through the incision (*bottom*). (**E**) Lateral view of C1-C2 showing proper screw trajectory. [**A, C,** and **E,** reproduced with permission from the Barrow Neurological Institute; **B** and **D,** modified from (28).]

nerve root provides direct visualization of the C2 pars and the C1-C2 facet joint and protects the C2 root during K-wire and screw placement. Bleeding from the venous plexus around the C2 root is controlled with gentle Surgicel packing and bipolar cauterization.

The atlas and axis are realigned by manual reduction before the screw is placed. The surgeon must then decide whether the proper screw trajectory can be achieved directly through the incision or whether a percutaneous method is needed (Fig. 7**D**). Percutaneous screw placement is often needed because the patient's neck usually cannot be flexed sufficiently during positioning without dislocating C1-C2. Long tools, drill bits, and a tissue sheath are required for percutaneous screw insertion. Percutaneous drilling should not be performed without prior subperiosteal exposure of C1 and C2 because it is crucial to place the K-wire and screw while directly visualizing the C2 pars to ensure the proper mediolateral screw trajectory.

The position of the percutaneous tunnel is judged by holding a long instrument adjacent to the patient's neck and thorax and imaging the trajectory with fluoroscopy. Bilateral paramedian stab incisions are made in the skin in the upper thoracic region. The tunneler and tissue sheath are tunneled carefully through the soft tissues of the neck. The tip of the tissue sheath is positioned adjacent to the C2-C3 facet. A handle on the tissue sheath is used to manipulate the sheath to alter the trajectory of the drills and screws.

The tunneler is removed, and the K-wire drill guide is inserted into the tissue sheath. A 50-cm long, 1.2-mm diameter K-wire is used to drill the initial screw trajectory. The sharp tip and threads along the distal 1 cm of the K-wire help cut a path into the bone. The K-wire is attached to a reversible pneumatic drill, passed through the drill guide to the entry point, and drilled through the C2 pars interarticularis, across the posterior edge of the C1-C2 facet joint, and into the lateral mass of C1 (Fig. 7**E**). Once the K-wire begins to engage the bone, the position and trajectory of the drill guide and sheath should not be altered or the K-wire will bend, creating excessive torque that will break the K-wire. If the trajectory of the K-wire is suboptimal and needs to be repositioned, the K-wire should be removed completely by reversing the drill direction. The K-wire is then reinserted in a new entry point on the bone surface along a new tract. Lateral fluoroscopic monitoring is used to adjust the trajectory of the K-wire so that its tip is positioned at the posterior cortex of the C1 anterior arch (Fig. 8**A**). Screws ventral to this cortical rim can penetrate through C1 anteriorly and enter the pharynx; screws cephalad to the superior aspect of the anterior C1 arch may cross the occipitoatlantal joint.

After the K-wire is positioned satisfactorily in the bone, the screw length is measured. The screw length (*i.e.*, length of the K-wire within the bone) is measured by inserting a second K-wire of identical length (50 cm) into the tissue sheath until it contacts the bone surface. The difference between the ends of the K-wires is then measured with a ruler. The screw length should be 1 or 2 mm shorter than the measured length if a gap between the bone surfaces will be reduced with the screw using a lag effect. The widest diameter screw should be used to fixate C1-C2 because its minor diameter is the primary determinant of

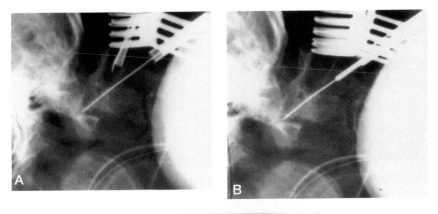

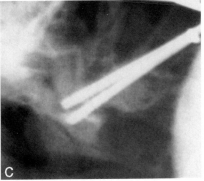

FIG. 8 Lateral fluoroscopic images showing (**A**) the K-wire entering the C2 inferior facet, crossing the pars interarticularis, entering the C1 lateral mass, and being positioned at the posterior cortex of the C1 anterior arch; (**B**) the hollow screw being inserted over the K-wire into the bone; and (**C**) the final position of two cannulated screws from Dickman CA, Foley KT, Sonntag VKH, Smith MM. Cannulated screws for odontoid screw fixation and atlantoaxial transarticular screw fixation. [Reproduced with permission from (14).]

its bending strength. A 3.5- or 4.0-mm diameter screw that averages 40 mm (range, 35–50 mm) in length is usually appropriate.

A self-tapping, end-threaded cannulated screw is placed over the K-wire and inserted into the bone using a hollow screw driver. The hollow screw and hollow screwdriver are inserted over the K-wire within the tissue sheath. The end of the K-wire should protrude beyond the end of the screwdriver to allow the surgical assistant to anchor it with a needle holder and prevent it from advancing.

As the screw is advanced into the bone, the position of the K-wire and screw is periodically checked fluoroscopically (Fig. 8**B**). Once the screw has crossed the fracture line or the articular surface and is

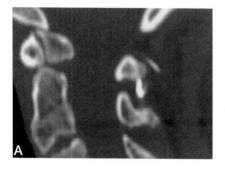
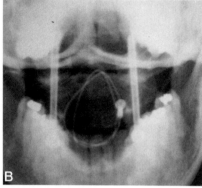
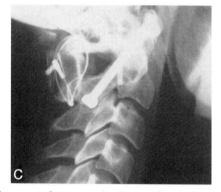

FIG. 9 (**A**) Lateral computed tomography image of a chronic nonunion of a type II odontoid fracture after failed posterior wiring. (**B**) Anteroposterior and (**C**) lateral plain postoperative radiographs after C1-C2 transarticular facet screw fixation and interspinous wiring.

satisfactorily seated within the distal bone fragment, the K-wire is removed using the reversible drill. The final position of the screw is verified with fluoroscopy (Fig. 8C). A tap may be needed to cross the bicortical C1-C2 facet joints prior to screw insertion if the patient's bone is very dense. However, one should avoid using unnecessary tools (especially power tools) over the K-wire because they can bind the K-wire and inadvertently advance it intradurally.

As the screw crosses the joint space into C1, the surgeon can feel the atlas and axis lock together with a characteristic stiffness. The screw head is positioned flushly against the bone surfaces or recessed slightly into the bone to prevent the screw from levering against the C2-C3 joint space. The screw should not be overtightened because it will shear through the cortex of the C2 pars and C2 facet, destroying its

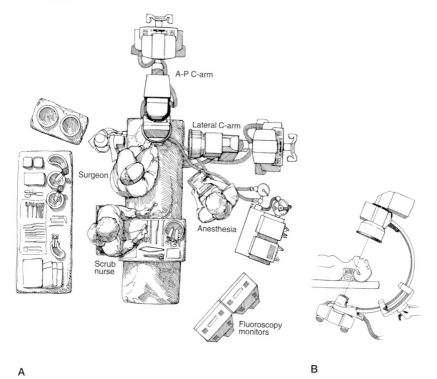

A

B

FIG. 10 Illustration showing (**A**) the organization of the surgical suite and the relative positions of the patient, personnel, and equipment. (**B**) The patient is positioned with the neck extended and the anteroposterior C-arm is positioned to provide an open-mouth view of the dens. (Reproduced with permission from the Barrow Neurological Institute.)

purchase in the bone. The contralateral screw is then inserted with identical techniques. A midline, autologous, bicortical interspinous strut graft from the iliac crest is subsequently wired to C1 and C2 to promote fusion and to provide immediate rigid three-point fixation that obviates the need for routine postoperative halo immobilization (Fig. 9A–C). Patients are placed in a soft cervical collar or a Philadelphia collar until fusion is documented radiographically.

ODONTOID SCREW FIXATION (1–3, 7–9, 14, 17, 20, 21, 26, 32)

Patient positioning and setup of the C-arms are critical for the success of this procedure and often take longer than the surgical insertion of the screw (Fig. 10A). The patient is placed in the supine position. The head and neck are extended to provide the proper screw trajectory into the tip of the dens. Extension is performed carefully under fluoroscopic monitoring to avoid distraction or subluxation of the fracture. The head is positioned on a radiolucent headrest and supported on a doughnut. Alternatively, the patient can be kept in a halo brace until screw fixation is achieved.

Precise imaging using simultaneous anteroposterior (AP) open-mouth and lateral plane fluoroscopy with two C-arms is mandatory to visualize C2 intraoperatively and to accurately guide the screw trajectory. The AP C-arm is positioned above the head of the operating table, and the mouth is propped open widely with cloth, gauze, or other radiolucent materials (Fig. 10**B**). The lateral C-arm is positioned on the patient's left side. The anesthesiologist is positioned on the left side near the patient's torso, and the surgeon stands on the patient's right side.

The fracture must be reduced into anatomic alignment by head positioning or intraoperative manipulation before the screw is inserted. Ideally, the dens should be reduced preoperatively and its alignment verified with fluoroscopy after the patient is positioned on the operating table. However, it is not always possible to restore C1-C2 alignment preoperatively. A posteriorly displaced dens can be reduced intraoperatively by pushing the C2 body posteriorly with a curette. An anteriorly displaced dens can be reduced by pushing the anterior C1 arch posteriorly with a curette and by further extending the patient's head and neck.

A transverse incision is made in the neck over the C4 or C5-C6 level (Fig. 11**A**). This lower-neck incision facilitates a drill trajectory parallel to the anterior border of the cervical spine. The platysma muscle is identified, divided, and undermined widely to allow adequate soft-tissue retraction. The deep cervical fascia is dissected to separate the sternocleidomastoid muscle and carotid sheath from the trachea and esophagus. The dissection is deepened to the level of the prevertebral fascia and then extended superiorly over the anterior surface of the spine to expose the C2-C3 interspace. The longus colli muscles adjacent to the C2-C3 disc space are coagulated at their medial borders and dissected laterally using the subperiosteal technique. Operative exposure is maintained with either a Hardy self-retaining transphenoidal retractor, Apfelbaum retractors (Fig. 11**B**; Aesculap, San Francisco, CA), Caspar retractors, or hand-held retractors. The proper exposure and screw trajectory often cannot be achieved in individuals with barrel-shaped large chests, short necks, or fixed cervical flexion deformities, and these patients should undergo posterior atlantoaxial arthrodesis.

A single screw is inserted into the dens. There is no biomechanical advantage to using two screws (19, 34). However, if the first screw does not reduce the fracture gap satisfactorily, a second screw may be needed. A midline entry point is used for single screw fixation. An entry point 5 mm lateral to the midline is used for fixation of two screws. If two screws are to be inserted, the preoperative CT scan should be reviewed to determine whether the dens is wide enough to accommodate both screws.

A midline trough is cut into the anterosuperior edge of the C3 vertebral body and C2-C3 annulus with a rongeur to facilitate a flat trajectory into the tip of the dens. The cortical bone at the entry point for insertion of the drill is penetrated with a bone awl or high-speed drill to allow the K-wire to securely engage the bone as the drilling is initiated. If the fracture is subacute or chronic, curettes should be used to remove the soft tissue from the fracture site to facilitate fusion.

The K-wire enters the anterior portion of the C2 inferior endplate and is aimed rostrally until its tip engages the cortex of the tip of the

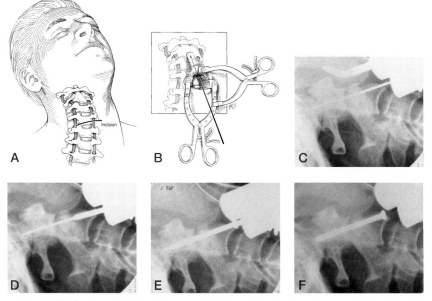

FIG. 11 Technique of odontoid screw fixation. Illustrations demonstrating the (**A**) transverse cervical incision and (**B**) placement of the Apfelbaum self-retaining retractor. Lateral fluoroscopic images showing (**C**) placement of the K-wire across the fracture line of a type II odontoid fracture and into the tip of the dens. (**D**) The hollow self-tapping screw is placed over the K-wire into C2. (**E**) Placement of the screw across the fracture site. (**F**) Final position of the screw after the K-wire was removed. [**A** and **B**, reproduced with permission from the Barrow Neurological Institute; **C–F**, reproduced with permission from (14).]

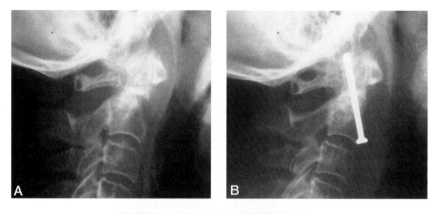

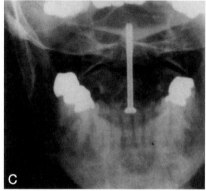

FIG. 12 (**A**) Preoperative and (**B**) postoperative lateral radiographs and (**C**) postoperative anteroposterior radiograph of a patient with a type II odontoid fracture treated with odontoid screw fixation.

dens (Fig. 11**C**). The trajectory of the K-wire is carefully monitored with fluoroscopic guidance and is adjusted as needed to avoid intradural penetration and neurologic injury. The trajectory should be as horizontal as possible to capture the tip of the dens and to prevent K-wire penetration through the posterior cortex of the dens into the spinal canal. A small amount of rostral penetration through the tip of the dens usually leaves the tip of the K-wire or screw adjacent to the alar and apical ligaments and does not endanger the spinal cord.

After the K-wire is in proper position, the screw length is measured. If the odontoid fragment is significantly distracted away from the C2 body, a screw that is shorter than the measured length is selected because the gap will be obliterated as the bone fragment is reduced. An appropriately sized, self-tapping, end-threaded cannulated screw is

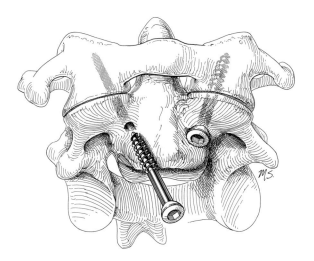

FIG. 13 Illustration of anterior atlantoaxial facet screw fixation. (Reproduced with permission from the Barrow Neurological Institute.)

inserted directly over the K-wire with a hollow screw driver (Fig. 11**D**). The tip of the screw should engage the tip of the dens, and the screw threads should not cross the fracture line in order to achieve a lag effect (Fig. 11**E**). Fluoroscopy should be used during screw placement to confirm the screw trajectory and to ensure that the K-wire is not advancing with the screw. The K-wire is removed after the screw is positioned satisfactorily in the dens (Fig. 11**F**). The screw head should sit flushly against the C2 body so that it does not protrude into the C2-C3 interspace. If the screw extends into the interspace, a lever effect can occur and cause the screw to loosen or to break loose from the bone. The patient usually wears a Philadelphia collar postoperatively until fusion is documented radiographically (Fig. 12**A–C**).

ANTERIOR C1-C2 TRANSARTICULAR SCREW FIXATION

The positioning and operative exposure for anterior C1-C2 transarticular screw fixation (17, 26, 36) is the same as that for odontoid screw fixation. Intraoperative open-mouth and lateral biplanar fluoroscopy is used to guide precise placement of the screw. The atlantoaxial joints are identified and decorticated bilaterally with curettes. The junctions of the C2 superior articular facets and the C2 body are identified, and the groove between these surfaces represents the drill entry points. The cortical bone is penetrated with a bone awl to prevent the drill bit from migrating as drilling is initiated. Pilot holes are drilled cephalad across each C2 superior facet into each C1 lateral mass. The trajectory of the pilot holes is monitored with biplanar fluoroscopy. A lateral trajectory is avoided to prevent injury to the vertebral arteries. A 3.5- or 4.0-mm diameter wide and 20- to 25-mm long lag screw is inserted into each pilot hole (Fig. 13). The screws should not penetrate beyond C1 into occipitoatlantal joints. Cannulated screws also may be used for this technique by applying the general principles previously described for anterior odontoid and posterior atlantoaxial facet screw fixation.

A Philadelphia collar or sternal occipital mandibular immobilizer brace is worn until fusion is documented radiographically. A halo brace is worn if this technique is being used as a salvage procedure to treat atlantoaxial instability after multiple failed posterior procedures or if the bone is very soft or osteoporotic.

REFERENCES

1. Aebi M, Etter C, Coscia M: Fractures of the odontoid process. Treatment with anterior screw fixation. **Spine** 14:1065–1070, 1989.

2. Apfelbaum R: Anterior screw fixation of odontoid fractures, in Rengachery SS, Wilkins RH (eds): *Neurosurgical Operative Atlas.* Baltimore, Williams & Wilkins, 1992, p 189.

3. Apfelbaum RI: Anterior screw fixation of odontoid fractures, in Apfelbaum RI (ed): *Scientific Information No. 24.* San Francisco, Aesculap, 1995, p 1.

4. Apostolides PJ, Dickman CA, Golfinos JG, et al.: Threaded Steinmann pin fusion of the craniovertebral junction. **Spine** 21:1630–1637, 1996.

5. Apostolides PJ, Zimmerman CG, Zerick WR, et al.: *Transoral Odontoidectomy Update: Report of 105 Cases.* Vancouver, BC, Congress of Neurological Surgeons Annual Meeting, 1993, p 55.

6. Apuzzo ML, Weiss MH, Heiden JS: Transoral exposure of the atlantoaxial region. **Neurosurgery** 3:201–207, 1978.

7. Böhler J: Screw-osteosynthesis of fractures of the dens axis. **Unfallheilkunde** 84:221–223, 1981.

8. Böhler J: Anterior stabilization for acute fractures and non-unions of the dens. **J Bone Joint Surg Am** 64:18–27, 1982.

9. Borne GM, Bedou GL, Pinaudeau M, et al.: Odontoid process fracture osteosynthesis with a direct screw fixation technique in nine consecutive cases. **J Neurosurg** 68:223–226, 1988.

10. Crockard HA: The transoral approach to the base of the brain and upper cervical cord. **Ann R Coll Surg Engl** 67:321–325, 1985.

11. Dickman CA, Crawford NR, Brantley AG, et al.: Biomechanical effects of transoral odontoidectomy. **Neurosurgery** 36:1146–1153, 1995.

12. Dickman CA, Crawford NR, Paramore CG: Biomechanical characteristics of C1-2 cable fixations. **J Neurosurg** 85:316–322, 1996.

13. Dickman CA, Douglas RA, Sonntag VKH: Occipitocervical fusion: Posterior stabilization of the craniovertebral junction and upper cervical spine. **BNI Q** 6:2–14, 1990.

14. Dickman CA, Foley KT, Sonntag VKH, et al.: Cannulated screws for odontoid screw fixation and atlantoaxial transarticular screw fixation. Technical note. **J Neurosurg** 83:1095–1100, 1995.

15. Dickman CA, Locantro J, Fessler RG: The influence of transoral odontoid resection on stability of the craniovertebral junction. **J Neurosurg** 77:525–530, 1992.

16. Dickman CA, Sonntag VKH: Wire fixation for the cervical spine: Biomechanical principles and surgical techniques. **BNI Q** 9:2–16, 1993.

17. Dickman CA, Sonntag VKH, Marcotte PJ: Techniques of screw fixation of the cervical spine. **BNI Q** 9:27–39, 1993.

18. Dickman CA, Sonntag VKH, Papadopoulos SM, et al.: The interspinous method of posterior atlantoaxial arthrodesis. **J Neurosurg** 74:190–198, 1991.

19. Doherty BJ, Heggeness MH, Esses SI: A biomechanical study of odontoid fractures and fracture fixation. **Spine** 18:178–184, 1993.

20. Etter C, Coscia M, Jaberg H, et al.: Direct anterior fixation of dens fractures with a cannulated screw system. **Spine** 16:S25–S32, 1991.

21. Geisler FH, Cheng C, Poka A, et al.: Anterior screw fixation of posteriorly displaced type II odontoid fractures. **Neurosurgery** 25:30–38, 1989.

22. Grob D, Crisco JJ 3d, Panjabi MM, et al.: Biomechanical evaluation of four different posterior atlantoaxial fixation techniques. **Spine** 17:480–490, 1992.

23. Grob D, Jeanneret B, Aebi M, et al.: Atlanto-axial fusion with transarticular screw fixation. **J Bone Joint Surg Br** 73:972–976, 1991.

24. Hadley MN, Martin NA, Spetzler RF, et al.: Comparative transoral dural closure techniques: A canine model. **Neurosurgery** 22:392–397, 1988.

25. Hadley MN, Spetzler RF, Sonntag VKH: The transoral approach to the superior cervical spine. A review of 53 cases of extradural cervicomedullary compression. **J Neurosurg** 71:16–23, 1989.

26. Lesoin F, Autricque A, Franz K, et al.: Transcervical approach and screw fixation for upper cervical spine pathology. **Surg Neurol** 27:459–465, 1987.

27. Magerl F, Seemann P-S: Stable posterior fusion of the atlas and axis by transarticular screw fixation, in Kehr P, Weidner A (eds): *Cervical Spine I*. Berlin, Springer-Verlag, 1987, p 322.

28. Marcotte P, Dickman CA, Sonntag VK, et al.: Posterior atlantoaxial facet screw fixation. **J Neurosurg** 79:234–237, 1993.

29. Masferrer R, Hadley MN, Bloomfield S, et al.: Transoral microsurgical resection of the odontoid process. **BNI Q** 1:34–40, 1985.

30. Menezes AH, VanGilder JC: Transoral-transpharyngeal approach to the anterior craniocervical junction. Ten-year experience with 72 patients. **J Neurosurg** 69:895–903, 1988.

31. Menezes AH, VanGilder JC, Graf CJ, et al.: Craniocervical abnormalities. A comprehensive surgical approach. **J Neurosurg** 53:444–455, 1980.

32. Montesano PX, Anderson PA, Schlehr F, et al.: Odontoid fractures treated by anterior odontoid screw fixation. **Spine** 16:33–37, 1991.

33. Paramore CG, Dickman CA, Sonntag VKH: The anatomical suitability of the C1-2 complex for transarticular screw fixation. **J Neurosurg** 85:221–224, 1996.

34. Sasso R, Doherty BJ, Crawford MJ, et al.: Biomechanics of odontoid fracture fixation. Comparison of the one- and two-screw technique. **Spine** 18:1950–1953, 1993.

35. Sonntag VKH: Occipitocervical and high cervical stabilization, in Rengachery SS, Wilkins RH (eds): *Neurosurgical Operative Atlas.* Baltimore, Williams & Wilkins, 1991, p 327.
36. Sonntag VKH, Dickman CA: Craniocervical stabilization. **Clin Neurosurg** 40:243–272, 1993.
37. Sonntag VKH, Kalfas I: Innovative cervical fusion and instrumentation techniques. **Clin Neurosurg** 37:636–660, 1991.
38. Spetzler RF, Dickman CA, Sonntag VKH: The transoral approach to the anterior cervical spine. **Contemp Neurosurg** 13:1–6, 1991.
39. Spetzler RF, Hadley MN, Sonntag VKH: The transoral approach to the anterior superior cervical spine. A review of 29 cases. **Acta Neurochir** 43:69–74, 1988.
40. Spetzler RF, Selman WR, Nash CL Jr, *et al.:* Transoral microsurgical odontoid resection and spinal cord monitoring. **Spine** 4:506–510, 1979.
41. Stillerman CB, Wilson JA: Atlanto-axial stabilization with posterior transarticular screw fixation: Technical description and report of 22 cases. **Neurosurgery** 32:948–954, 1993.
42. Van Gilder JC, Menezes AH: Craniovertebral abnormalities and their neurosurgical management, in Schmidek HH, Sweet WH (eds): *Operative Neurosurgical Techniques. Indications, Methods, and Results.* Philadelphia, W.B. Saunders, 1995, p 1719.

12

Surgery of Low-Grade Gliomas—Technical Aspects

MITCHEL S. BERGER, M.D.

When deciding how best to surgically approach a patient with a low-grade glioma involving the cerebral hemispheres, a number of critical issues must first be considered. The extent of resection ultimately determines both time-to-tumor progression and survival in the majority of these lesions. For instance, a complete tumor removal is curative for the cerebellar pilocytic astrocytoma or pleomorphic xanthoastrocytoma. However, for the diffusely infiltrative, subcortical astrocytic oligodendroglioma that involves midline structures, a biopsy-only approach may be all that is necessary to confirm the diagnosis and plan a therapeutic strategy. The other critical determinant that would affect the surgical approach is the proximity of the lesion to functional regions within the cerebral hemisphere, such as the rolandic cortex or language zones.

Low-grade gliomas have a propensity to be associated with small or large cysts that are the cause of the symptoms and signs that bring the patient to the attention of the physician. These cysts require an approach designed to empty their contents into the subarachnoid space, ventricle, or peritoneal cavity (*via* a shunt), depending on the amount of fluid produced. Another clinical problem frequently associated with low-grade gliomas of the cerebral hemispheres is occasional or medically refractory seizures. Controversy surrounds the need to address the seizure problem surgically by identifying and removing surrounding epileptic foci, or achieving seizure control by removing only the lesion. By necessity, all of these factors dictate the quality of the patient's life and must be factored into the surgical decision-making equation.

PREDICTING THE NATURAL HISTORY OF LOW-GRADE GLIOMAS

Figures 1 and 2 illustrate two problems that occur during the natural history of these particular lesions, namely, a change in the volume and biology of the tumor. In the first example, the size and infiltrative

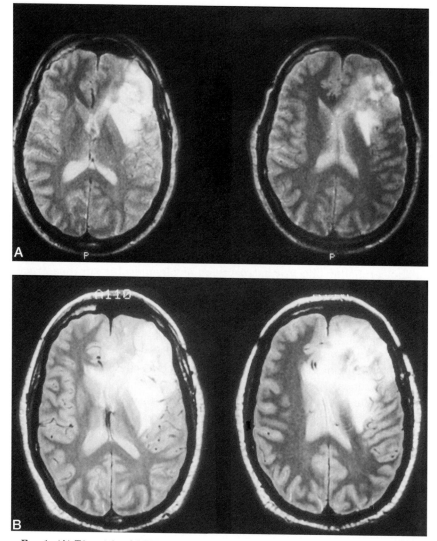

FIG. 1. (**A**) T2-weighted MRI scan of low-grade glioma involving left frontal lobe and anterior insula. (**B**) Progression of T2-weighted infiltrative tumor abnormality in a 24-month period.

dimensions of the low-grade glioma changed considerably over a 24-month period. At initial presentation, this tumor was readily resectable with functional mapping techniques, but at the time of progression demonstrated an anatomic substrate, *i.e.*, corpus callosum and internal capsule involvement, that prevented this from being resected

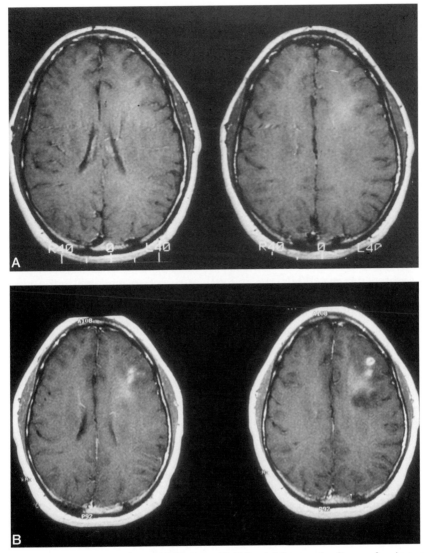

FIG. 2. (**A**) Contrast-enhanced MR scan of left frontal low-grade glioma, showing no contrast enhancement. (**B**) Contrast enhancement occurring within 18 months of the initial scan shown in Figure 2A.

aggressively. The second case depicted in Figure 2 shows that although the volume of the mass did not change, the tumor demonstrated contrast enhancement that coincided with a newly acquired anaplastic phenotype. This occurred within 18 months of the original scan, when the patient presented with a seizure and a noncontrast-appearing low-grade glioma. Thus, the role of surgery needs to be defined in the context of extent of resection and, ultimately, progression and survival. Tumors such as the pilocytic astrocytoma, ganglioglioma, subependymal giant cell astrocytoma, pleomorphic xanthoastrocytoma, desmoplastic astrocytoma, desmoplastic infantile ganglioglioma, dysembryoplastic neuroepithelial tumor, and ependymoma are all surgically curable lesions without the need for subsequent therapy.

On the contrary, if one considers the nonpilocytic astrocytic gliomas, oligodendrogliomas, and mixed gliomas, the role of surgery in affecting outcome is less clearly defined. This is primarily because of the lack of studies that consider the quantitative volume of tumor removed as well as the amount of tumor that remains after completing the resection. In a retrospective analysis performed on low-grade glioma patients at the University of Washington (1), not only the percent of resection but also the volume of residual disease was determined quantitatively based on the preoperative and postoperative T2-weighted images. When the percent of resection was evaluated with respect to tumor recurrence at a higher histologic grade, there was a higher likelihood, i.e., 37.5% versus 0%, that the tumor would recur with a malignant phenotype when less than 50% as opposed to 100% resection, respectively, was achieved. The mean time-to-tumor progression was also significantly prolonged, i.e., 24 months versus 63 months, when based on the percent of resection of less than 50% versus 100%, respectively. However, when the volume of residual disease was considered separately, the significance values became greater as the amount of remaining tumor following resection diminished. For example, when no tumor was visible on postoperative magnetic resonance (MR) imaging (0 cm^3), tumor recurrence was not seen in any patient during the median follow-up period of nearly 60 months following surgery. Yet, for those patients with over 10 cm^3 remaining following resection, a 30-month mean time-to-tumor progression was documented. In this latter group, 46.2% of patients developed a recurrence at a higher histologic grade, as opposed to none of the patients who underwent a complete resection (p = 0.0009). Thus, the extent of tumor removal defined in a quantitative fashion clearly affects the natural history of this type of brain tumor.

Notwithstanding, there are circumstances when a biopsy should be performed as opposed to considering a radical resection. A diffuse, infiltrative lesion extending throughout the subcortical white matter and involving midline structures is ideal for a diagnostic biopsy. Although the majority of these noncontrast-enhancing lesions are low-grade histologically, approximately 30% and 10% are anaplastic or glioblastomas, respectively (2). When a patient is unable to undergo a craniotomy or extensive anesthesia because of an accompanying medical illness, a biopsy is more appropriate. At times, the imaging studies confirm tumor progression, which must be confirmed histologically prior to instituting a therapeutic protocol. This might be particularly important when an enhancing focus of tumor develops in a region that previously did not enhance. In this circumstance, a metabolic imaging study may be misleading, indicating that the new focus is hypometabolic when the histologic sample obtained *via* a biopsy has become anaplastic or worse (Fig. 3). Even with the addition of ^{11}C thymidine to ^{18}fluorodeoxyglucose (^{18}FDG), position emission tomography (PET) may be unreliable in determining a change in the phenotype, thus empha-

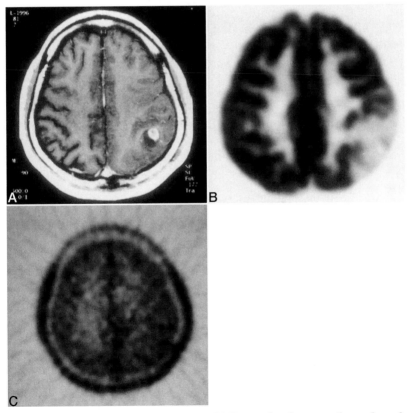

FIG. 3. (**A**) Contrast-enhancing T1-weighted MR scan showing a new focus of anaplastic degeneration within a low-grade glioma. (**B**) and (**C**) PET scanning with FDG and ^{11}C thymidine failing to demonstrate any evidence of hypermetabolism.

sizing the need to perform a biopsy prior to adding or switching treatment regimens.

Although the MR images provide exquisite detail with regard to anatomy, very little data, if any, are available to support the role of MR imaging in predicting the patient's clinical course. Contrast enhancement is perhaps the strongest predictor of outcome in that for the typical adult low-grade glioma, any evidence of contrast leaking into the tumor mass is indicative of at least an anaplastic glioma. However, any degree of contrast enhancement cannot be used to distinguish which type of glioma is present. This is certainly not true for pediatric cerebral hemispheric gliomas, which often enhance and may be associated with an accompanying cyst, indicative of an indolent, pilocytic histology. Table 1 describes several features associated with adult astrocytic gliomas. Based on findings such as a cyst, degree of mass effect, location, T2 *versus* T1 volume, cortical *versus* subcortical location, *etc.*, the histologic subtype of the tumor could not be predicted preoperatively when compared with the pathology specimen. Yet the intensity pattern as determined by T1-weighted MR scans may suggest tumor type, as depicted in Figure 4. Predominantly astrocytic gliomas have a strong propensity to be hypointense throughout the lesion, and are seldom isointense to normal brain. This is clearly not the case with oligodendrogliomas or the mixed oligoastrocytomas. Thus, the natural history of adult hemispheric gliomas may not be determined with any degree of certainty using MR imaging, except perhaps in predicting the histologic subtype (intensity pattern) or grade (contrast enhancement).

INTRAOPERATIVE LOCALIZATION STRATEGIES

Upon opening the dura, several observations should first be made. When the lesion involves the cortex, the gyral pattern is typically widened and the adjacent sulci are effaced. Because blood flow to the lesion is not significantly increased, there is absence of "red" veins, signifying a reduced oxygen extraction, as is seen in high-grade glio-

TABLE 1.
MRI Characteristics
Astrocytoma, Oligodendroglioma, Mixed Oligoastrocytoma

T1 INTENSITY*	Contrast enhancement
Cyst	T2 *vs.* T1 volume
Mass effect	Vascular flow voids
Hemorrhage	Diameter
Cortical *vs.* subcortical	Location

* MRI characteristic most closely associated with histology.

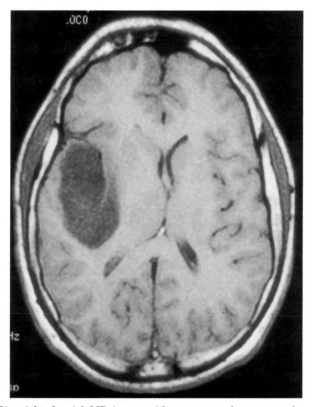

FIG. 4. T1-weighted axial MR image with contrast enhancement demonstrates a hypointense lesion consistent with an astrocytic glioma.

mas from rapid shunting of blood through the tumor capillary beds. The surface is often discolored and found to be pale or chalky white (Fig. 5). Large draining veins may be displaced or partially occluded. The consistency of a low-grade glioma is almost always predictable based on the MR imaging findings. The more hypointense (*i.e.*, darker gray) the lesion on the T1 weighted scan, the softer it is found to be during removal (Fig. 4). This is because of the finding microscopically of a loose, microcystic structure of the stroma with, at times, mucinous degeneration (Fig. 6). Isointense or hyperintense lesions tend to be significantly firmer than normal white matter. The color of infiltrated white matter ranges from light gray to off-white and should also be used to guide the resection under magnification. As the tumor removal proceeds toward the less infiltrated margin, the texture should be noted because it differs from the semi-firm consistency of normal white matter.

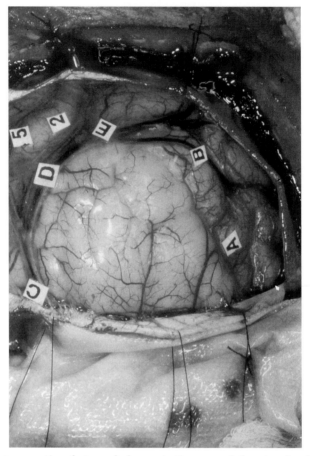

FIG. 5. Intraoperative photograph demonstrating expanded gyri and a chalky white appearance of a cortically based infiltrative low-grade glioma.

Several surgical methods are currently available, or will soon be possible, to help guide the tumor resection along with the general principles just described. Intraoperative ultrasound (IOUS) is invaluable for providing real time imaging of the lesion prior to and during the removal (Fig. 7). Low-grade gliomas are typically hyperechoic when imaged with ultrasound and demonstrate boundaries consistent with the T2-weighted MR images. Previous studies demonstrated a nearly precise correlation between ultrasound and MR imaging volumes of low-grade gliomas (3, 4). Thus, the boundaries of the lesion can be marked with surface letters, numbers of "fence-posted" with catheters that are passed under ultrasound guidance. This is quite differ-

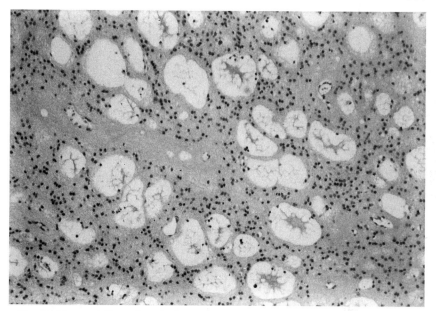

FIG. 6. Hematoxylin and eosin histology slide of mucinous degeneration within a low-grade glioma (×40).

ent from malignant or radiated gliomas because edema and gliosis, respectively, may result in false-positive echogenic regions that over-estimate the actual volume of the low-grade glioma. Notwithstanding, for a newly diagnosed case, IOUS is highly effective in demarcating tumor boundaries, as seen on preoperative MR imaging, and may help guide the resection by re-imaging during the procedure.

Surgical navigational systems have proven to be quite useful during both intra- and extra-axial tumor resections. Our experience at the University of Washington involves the use of temporarily implanted fiducial markers coupled with an infrared tracking system that relates the fiducial-based imaging study to the tip of the infrared mounted probe (Fig. 8). In this system, "real-time" images are produced in different reformatted images at the speed of up to 30 frames per second. This navigational system, i.e., ACUSTAR (Johnson & Johnson, Inc.) was developed at Vanderbilt University under the direction of Drs. George Allen and Robert Maciunas (5). This technology has an image-to-physical registration accuracy of less than 1 mm. The biggest problem with all of the systems currently available is the shift of intracranial contents that occurs during the course of the procedure as the tissue is removed and CSF is lost. However, when the patient is

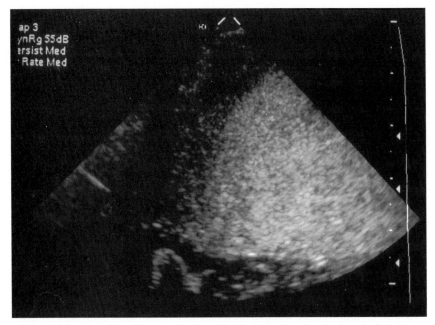

FIG. 7. Intraoperative ultrasound using a 5mH probe, showing the hyperechoic tumor mass and a relatively discreet margin adjacent to normal brain (hypoechoic).

positioned parallel or perpendicular to the floor, this shift may be readily calculated based on the beginning location of the cortical surface followed by intermittent determinations of the depth of the cortex compared with this initial demarcation. A method to compensate for the brain shift is to utilize an updating paradigm with IOUS, resulting in ongoing re-registration.

Efforts are underway to utilize the method of optical imaging to detect infiltrating tumor cells at the resection margin (6, 7). This is based on detecting the magnitude and time course of optical changes from the resection cavity after recording the patterns of reflecting red light back from the tissue with a microscope attached to a camera. This technique may be enhanced by using a dye compound, indocyanine green (ICG), which absorbs light in the far red spectrum. Figure 9 shows the typical pattern of optical changes in a low-grade glioma while an infusion of ICG is given to the patient during surgery. The peak response is greatest in the tumor-infiltrated brain and the clearance of the dye from the tumor is delayed when compared with non-tumor-infiltrated brain.

The ultimate ideal real time imaging feedback system to have during surgery to guide the extent of resection would be either an MR or

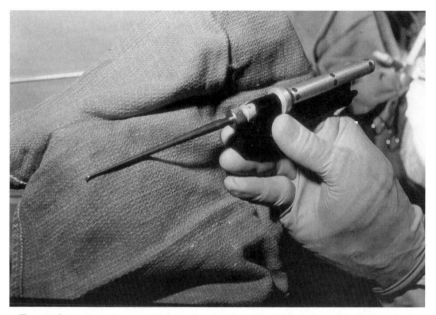

Fig. 8. Intraoperative surgical navigational probe with infrared emitting devices attached.

computed tomography (CT) scanner. The MR intraoperative system currently available is narrow in terms of operating in between the coils. In addition, it requires a specially built room with compatible instruments that are nonmagnetic. Alternatively, portable CT scan units are becoming available that are inexpensive and easy to move in and out of the operative field. Development and modification of both systems will occur during the future, and hopefully will be accessible and affordable. Preoperative imaging will identify an accompanying cyst in some low-grade hemispheric gliomas. When the cyst is encountered, it is essential to refer back to the appearance on the imaging studies to determine whether or not the cyst wall should be removed. When the cyst wall demonstrates contrast enhancement on MR or CT images, this indicates that the lining membrane is composed of tumor cells and must be removed. If no enhancement is seen, the cyst wall should remain in place and not be violated, to prevent injury to adjacent functional white matter (8). Diversion of the cyst contents into a natural cerebrospinal fluid (CSF) space will not be necessary following resection of all or most of the contrast-enhancing tumor tissue. However, in some circumstances where this is not possible and the cyst contents reaccumulate, a cyst-to-peritoneal shunt may be required. An

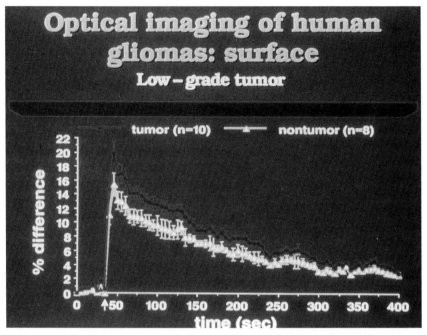

FIG. 9. Optical imaging enhanced with indocyanine green in patients with low-grade tumors. Note that the optical changes are different for the tumor *versus* the nontumor brain specimens. This is measured as clearance of the dye from the tumor in adjacent nontumor-infiltrated brain.

alternative approach would be to ablate the secretory component of the cyst lining with repetitive injections of ^{32}P isotope (9).

FUNCTIONAL STIMULATION MAPPING DURING THE RESECTION

The sine qua non during any resective procedure for a low-grade glioma is to maintain functional integrity of the adjacent cortex and subcortical white matter. At the same time, every possible attempt should be made to achieve a radical tumor removal that alleviates the symptoms and signs of mass effect. An additional goal of surgery is to eliminate or reduce the frequency of seizures in patients with medically refractory epilepsy. Several functional regions exist whereby the stimulation mapping techniques would serve as critical adjuncts to preserve their integrity. The primary motor and somatosensory areas collectively form the rolandic cortex and is bordered in front by the supplementary motor area. Posterior to the coronal suture, the premotor sulcus is nearly always found within 2.5 to 3.0 cm. The motor strip may be identified in the awake or asleep patient using currents be-

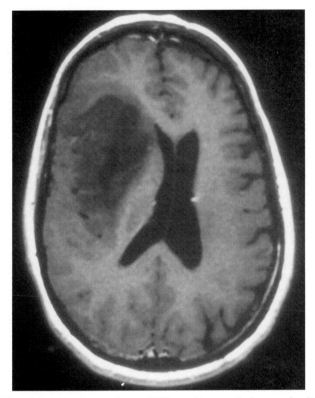

FIG. 10. T1-weighted contrast-enhanced MR axial image of a low-grade glioma involving the insula.

tween 2 mA and 16 mA, depending upon the anesthetic condition of the patient. This current is delivered *via* a bipolar stimulating electrode attached to a constant current generator, which yields biphasic square wave pulses (10). The same current that identifies the cortical site of neuronal orgin for both motor and sensory function is also able to depolarize axonal tracts in the subcortical white matter. Thus, when resecting tumor within or adjacent to the thalamus, insula, mesial temporal lobe, and spinal cord, stimulation of these descending white matter tracts is invaluable to avoid damage to these critical structures.

In the dominant hemisphere, the areas responsible for and subserving various language functions may also be identified with stimulation mapping. This includes Broca's area, which is located anterior to the inferior aspect of the face motor cortex, and reading and naming cortical sites, which may be located within regions of the temporal lobe including the anterior 3 to 4 cm, inferior parietal and posterior frontal

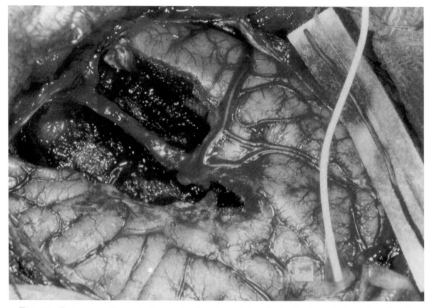

FIG. 11. Intraoperative photograph showing strip electrode inserted under the dura and identifying the motor strip. #1, face motor cortex. The resection involves the overlying superior temporal gyrus and the frontal operculum to achieve exposure to the underlying insula.

lobes (11, 12). Variability in all individuals makes it impossible to identify these functional sites with either anatomic imaging methods or surface landmarks identified during surgery. Nevertheless, functional localization methods with metabolic scans or specific MR sequences are better suited to identify motor and sensory cortical sites, as opposed to specific language tasks. Furthermore, functional imaging is not yet capable of subcortical localization for the descending motor, sensory, or language pathways. To better demonstrate the usefulness of the stimulation mapping methods, two illustrative cases are provided below.

Case of an Insular Low-Grade Glioma

The patient is a 43-year-old female who presented with intermittent complex partial seizures. MR imaging revealed a noncontrast-enhancing, hypointense lesion within the nondominant insula (Fig. 10). A frontotemporal craniotomy was performed with the patient asleep and the motor cortex was identified with 6 mA of stimulation-induced current. Temporarily implanted fiducials enabled the use of the surgical naviagation system for intraoperative localization prior to and

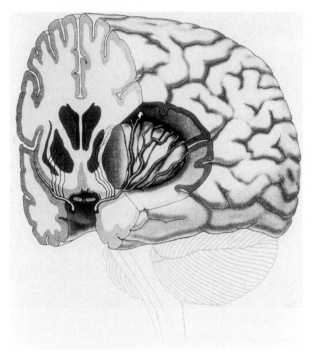

FIG. 12. Schematic drawing of insular tumor spreading apart the insular arteries and causing the lenticular striate vessels to be pushed mesially.

during the tumor removal. The first step in the procedure, following localization of the face and hand motor cortex *via* a stimulating strip electrode placed under the bone flap, is to remove the overlying non-functional superior temporal and frontal opercular gyri to achieve adequate exposure of the underlying insula (Fig. 11). It is imperative during this stage of the dissection to preserve the sylvian venous drainage system. Because of the large expansive tumor within the insula, the middle cerebral arteries are displaced and pushed apart, creating an excellent pathway into the tumor without having to sacrifice any of these insular triangle vessels (Fig. 12). The lateral lenticulostriate arteries are displaced mesially so that tumor removal should not result in injury to these critical vessels supplying portions of the internal capsule. The resection proceeds, using the navigational device to determine the depth of the removal and the proximity to the internal capsule, accounting for a shift of the intracranial contents during the course of the operation. Although the distance between the middle of the insula and the genu of the internal capsule averages 25 to 30 mm, the posterior portion of the insula is closest to the posterior limb of the

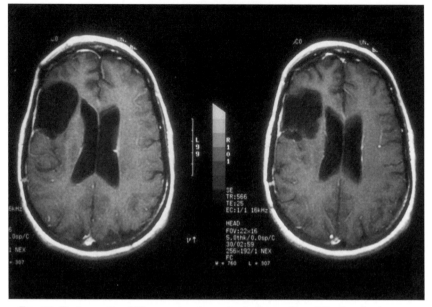

FIG. 13. Postoperative MR scan showing extent of resection of the insular tumor.

internal capsule at 7 to 10 mm. Because this is where the tumor mass is least bulky, it is critical to realize that potential injury to the motor pathways is greatest at this point. Thus, stimulation mapping should be repetitively done every 3 to 4 mm during the deepest part of the resection to avoid injury to this area. This is because current spread is usually no more than this aforementioned distance from the tips of the bipolar electrode. Postoperatively, the patient had an uneventful course without any motor deficits (Fig. 13).

Case of a Dominant Hemisphere Low-Grade Glioma

The three critical functions to be localized during tumor resections in this area include motor speech, naming, and reading. The patient in this case is a 32-year-old female who presented with facial motor seizures and speech arrest. These were intermittent in frequency. An MR imaging study demonstrated a noncontrast-enhancing, hypointense lesion involving the face motor area near the sylvian fissure (Fig. 14). Following a frontoparietal craniotomy under the influence of intravenous propofol, the patient was awakened and the dura was opened. The scalp is first anesthetized with a marcaine-lidocaine mixture that is also used to infiltrate around the middle meningeal artery to lessen headache from dural retraction. The first step in the language

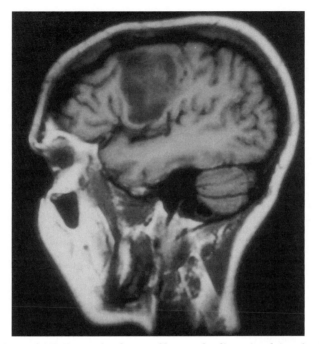

FIG. 14. Sagittal MR T1-weighted scan of low-grade glioma involving the face motor cortex of the dominant hemisphere.

mapping procedure is to identify the inferior aspect of the rolandic cortex with stimulation mapping at low, *i.e.*, 2 to 6 mA, currents. Using the same current, the patient is asked to count up to 50, during which each centimeter of cortex near the face motor area is stimulated to determine the site of speech arrest, *i.e.*, Broca's area. After this is accomplished, the cortical electrode array is placed on the brain surface and stimulation is induced with the bipolar electrode using increasing amperage to find the level of current that does not induce afterdischarge potentials. This is the current selected to map the exposed cortical surface during language mapping.

The patient is shown a series of pictures on slides depicting common objects with a leader phrase to read. Just prior to seeing the picture, the cortical site to be tested is stimulated with the current, as determined above, and documentation of dysnomia or anomia is accomplished. Each site is tested at least three times to determine if repetitive errors in naming and reading are significant (Fig. 15). Hesitation to name or read is not a contraindication to remove that cortical site. The essential as well as nonessential cortical sites are numbered with

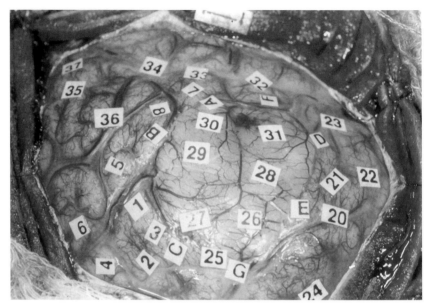

FIG. 15. Intraoperative map of face motor low-grade glioma showing the expanded tumor (underlying *26* through *30*), inferior rolandic cortex (*1* through *8*) and stimulation-induced site for anomia (*24*).

sterile paper tickets and remain in place until the resection is done and a photograph is taken to document the patient's brain map. In this case, the patient had a pronounced expressive dysphasia without any receptive dysfunction for nearly 8 weeks prior to returning to her baseline function. At that time she continued to have a very mild hesitation in motor speech, which was not a problem for the patient or her vocation.

Experience with tumor resections in the dominant hemisphere has resulted in the operative strategy of not removing any cortical or contiguous subcortical white matter within 10 mm of an essential site for language. This prevents any permanent damage from occuring with naming or reading (12). However, resections may come within millimeters of a motor cortical site, for speech or movement, without incurring a permanent deficit. Further work has shown that in approximately 8% of our functionally mapped patient population who harbor intrinsic glial neoplasms, functional tissue may be found within the tumor itself (13). Thus, it is not always safe to remove the tumor without first having the functional map in place to guide the resection. Finally, it should be noted that patients who have occasional seizure activity associated with a low-grade glioma are not candidates for simultaneous seizure mapping to identify epileptogenic foci adjacent to the mass, as these are usually not found. In this instance, tumor removal alone is usually all that is necessary to ensure a high likelihood of a seizure-free outcome. However, if the patient has intractable seizures refractory to antiepileptic drugs, electrocorticography is essential to use intraoperatively to identify seizure foci that typically reside adjacent to the tumor and not within its confines. Removing these separate seizure foci will yield the greatest possibility of achieving a seizure-free condition, or reducing the frequency or intensity of the seizures dramatically (14).

ACKNOWLEDGMENTS

This work was supported by NIH grant #1-UO1-CA62428-01, NIH #1-R21 CA70790-01, and The American Cancer Society Professor of Clinical Oncology Award (#071).

REFERENCES

1. Berger MS, Deliganis AV, Dobbins J, et al.: The effect of extent of resection on recurrence in patients with low grade cerebral hemisphere gliomas. **Cancer** 74: 1784–1791, 1994.
2. Chamberlain MC, Murovic JA, Levin VA: Absence of contrast enhancement on CT brain scans of patients with supratentorial malignant gliomas. **Neurology** 38:1371–1374, 1988.
3. LeRoux PD, Berger MS, Ojemann GA, et al.: Correlation of intraoperative ultrasound tumor volumes and margins with preoperative ultrasound tumor volumes and marings with preoperative computerized tomography scans: An intraoperative method to enhance tumor resection. **J Neurosurg** 71:691–698, 1989.
4. LeRoux P, Berger MS, Wang K, et al.: Low grade gliomas: Comparison of intraoperative ultrasound characteristics with preoperative imaging studies. **J Neurooncol** 13:189–198, 1992.
5. Maciunas RJ, Berger MS, Copeland B, et al.: A technique for interactive image-guided neurosurgical intervention in primary brain tumors, in (Maciunas RJ, guest ed) **Neurosurgery Clinics of North America** 1996, Vol 7, pp 245–266.
6. Haglund MM, Hochman DW, Spence AM, et al.: Enhanced optical imaging of rat gliomas and tumor margins. **Neurosurgery** 35:930–941, 1994.
7. Haglund MM, Berger MS, Hochman DW: Enhanced optical imaging of human gliomas and tumor margins. **Neurosurgery** 38(2):308–317, 1996.
8. Berger MS, Keles GE, Geyer JR: Cerebral hemispheric tumors of childhood. **Neurosurg Clin N Am** (Pediatric Neuro-Oncology) 34:839–852, 1992.
9. Lunsford LD: Stereotactic treatment of craniopharyngioma: Intracavitary irradiation and radiosurgery. **Contemp Neurosurg** 1:1–6, 1989.
10. Berger MS, Ojemann GA, Lettich E: Neurophysiological monitoring during astrocytoma surgery. **Neurosurg Clin N Am** 1:65–80, 1990.

11. Ojemann GA, Ojemann J, Lettich E, *et al.*: Cortical language localization in left, dominant hemisphere. **J Neurosurg** 71:316–326, 1989.

12. Haglund MM, Berger MS, Shamseldin M, *et al.*: Cortical localization of temporal lobe language sites in patients with gliomas. **Neurosurgery** 34:567–576, 1994.

13. Skirboll SL, Ojemann GA, Berger MS, *et al.*: Functional cortex and subcortical white matter located within gliomas. **Neurosurgery** 38:6478–685, 1996.

14. Berger MS, Ghatan S, Haglund MM, *et al.*: Low-grade gliomas associated with intractable epilepsy: Seizure outcome utilizing electrocorticography during tumor resection. **J Neurosurg** 79:62–69, 1993.

CHAPTER

13

Operative Techniques and Clinicopathologic Correlation in the Surgical Treatment of Cranial Rhizopathies (Honored Guest Lecture)

PETER J. JANNETTA, M.D., D.Sci.

Microvascular decompression procedures, like any procedure involving the cerebellopontine angle (CP angle), demand strict attention to technical detail. As the majority of these procedures are elective in nature, and as a substantial percentage of the patient population treated is elderly, complications related to faulty technique are poorly tolerated. Although the retromastoid craniectomy is a conceptually straightforward surgical approach, nuances of technique can make the difference between a successful outcome or catastrophe. For example, patient positioning, the size and shape of the craniectomy, the shape and size of the dural opening, and the angle of approach used after dural opening all vary, depending on the pathology being treated. Furthermore, without the proper approach, the relevant pathology for a particular cranial nerve syndrome may not be clearly visible.

As important as technique is to the successful execution of these procedures, an understanding of the likely neurovascular pathology responsible for a particular cranial rhizopathy will aid in both the recognition and manipulation of relevant pathologic relationships. The purpose of this presentation is to convey some of the lessons learned through the performance of more than 4000 microvascular decompression procedures over the last 30 years. The important technical concerns will be illustrated through a stepwise description of the retromastoid craniectomy as it is currently used for the treatment of cranial rhizopathies at the University of Pittsburgh. In addition, each technical description will be followed by a brief discussion of the types of pathology seen in the various compression syndromes.

I will begin this discussion with a description of the "Jannetta" retromastoid craniectomy in its generic form. I will then discuss the angles of approach and technical caveats for each of the individual cranial nerves and the lateral medulla. Finally, I will comment on the clinicopathologic correlations frequently encountered in the treatment of neurovascular compression syndromes.

THE JANNETTA RETROMASTOID CRANIECTOMY

The anatomic boundaries of the exposure afforded by the retromastoid approach are the tentorium superiorly, the petrous temporal bone laterally, the foramen magnum inferiorly, and the cerebellum and brainstem medially. As such, the retromastoid approach provides excellent exposure of cranial nerves V through XII, from their emergence from the brainstem to their entrance into the neural foramina. The blood vessels of the posterior fossa, including the vertebral arteries, basilar artery, posterior inferior cerebellar arteries (PICAs), anterior inferior cerebellar arteries (AICAs), and superior cerebellar arteries (SCAs) can also be visualized during all or part of their course (18). When performed properly, the majority of procedures can be performed with little to no cerebellar retraction.

POSITIONING

After the induction of general anesthesia and the placement of appropriate physiologic monitors and compression stockings, patients are placed in a three-point head holder. The patient is then gently lifted and rolled into the lateral decubitus (park bench) position with the affected side up. An axillary roll is placed just caudal to the dependent axilla, and a smaller roll is placed under the dependent knee to protect the peroneal nerve. The patient is securely fixed to the table with safety straps and 3-inch tape placed around the shoulders and hips. The shoulder is taped caudally and anteriorly, so as to provide an adequate working space in the retromastoid region. It is important to avoid excessive tension on the shoulder, as the brachial plexus may be injured. The trapezius muscle should be slightly stretched but easily deformable by light fingertip pressure. Final positioning of the patients head should result in a slightly (5°) vertex down position with the neck extended on the thorax and the head slightly flexed on the neck (similar to the military position of "attention"). The patient's face should be facing directly laterally or slightly (5°) down (6, 12). As will be discussed below, modifications may be made to facilitate exposure of particular cranial nerves. For example, in microvascular decompression procedures directed at the trigeminal nerve, it is most important to have the ipsilateral shoulder out of the way completely so as to allow a 45° caudal-to-rostral approach to the nerve. On the other hand, the vertex down position may be emphasized for cases involving the cranial nerve VII/VIII complex or lower cranial nerves, as this position allows for easier access to and manipulation of these structures.

INCISION

I currently limit my shave to a 2- to 3-cm strip extending from the top of the pinna to the upper neck. Prepping is done in the usual fashion; however, before draping, the mastoid process, the level of the external auditory meatus (EAM), and a line extending from the EAM to the inion, along the nuchal ridge are marked. The transverse sinus will lie just below the EAM-inion line, and the junction of the transverse and sigmoid sinus lies just at the intersection of this line, with a line extending rostrally along the posterior aspect of the mastoid process. The skin incision for a retromastoid approach should begin at the top of the pinna, 5–10 mm behind the hairline, and extend caudally along the hairline for a distance of 3–6 cm, depending on the operation being performed. For lower cranial nerve or lateral medullary compression syndromes, longer incisions are necessary to provide increased caudal exposure. In contrast, very small but well-placed incisions may provide adequate exposure for operations involving the trigeminal nerve. After the desired incision is marked, the patient is draped in a routine fashion, and a table-mounted self-retaining retractor (such as the Greenburg retractor system) is positioned so as to rest between the arms of the operating surgeon.

A good landmark for a well-placed incision is the insertion of the nuchal musculature, which will end approximately 1 cm below the rostral end of the incision. The musculature should be divided or split layer by layer to avoid inadvertent damage to the occipital vessels and nerves, which are located in the fascial planes between the muscle layers. As one approaches the foramen magnum, great care should be taken to avoid injury to the vertebral artery or one of its muscular branches, especially in older and atherosclerotic patients. Arterial pulsations may been seen or palpated through the musculature before visualization of the artery. Commonly, we avoid using the unipolar cautery in this region and perform the dissection with pickups and scissors. An adequate superficial dissection should expose the posterior aspect of the mastoid process, as well as the beginning of the digastric groove laterally and the floor of the posterior fossa caudally.

BONE FLAP

With the advent of the latest generation of high-speed pneumatic drills, it has become possible and, in the hands of some surgeons, almost routine to perform a suboccipital craniotomy in the retromastoid region. I still favor a craniectomy performed in the following manner, as I believe it to be a safe and straightforward technique. When used in conjunction with a methyl methacrylate cranioplasty, there is no palpable craniectomy defect; the incidence of postcraniectomy headaches is low; and the risk of injury to the dural sinuses is minimized. The occipital bone is perforated in the posterior and inferior quadrant of the bony exposure. The burr hole should be placed 5 cm behind the EAM in men and 4 cm behind the meatus in women along an extension of the line connecting the lateral canthus of the ipsilateral eye to the EAM (11). This places the burr hole away from the sinuses and the mastoid emissary vein. A second burr hole may be placed slightly laterally and superiorly if the bone is hard and thick. The dura is sharply dissected away from the bone, and rongeurs are used to remove bone to the edges of the dural sinuses, moving in a caudal-to-rostral and posterior-to-lateral direction. Frequently, air cells are encountered in the region of the mastoid root and, in a dolichocephalic patient, these air cells frequently extend posteriorly over the sigmoid sinus. Waxing of the air cells and other exposed bone edges aids in hemostasis and is essential for the prevention of cerebrospinal fluid rhinorrhea. It is essential to identify the edges of both the transverse and sigmoid sinuses, as well as their confluence. Once these landmarks are visualized, the craniectomy is tailored to the specific patient and pathology being treated. For example, the size of the craniectomy should be made larger in younger patients and in the early experience of the surgeon, and it should have a greater inferior extension for the treatment of lower cranial nerve rhizopathies and vascular compression of the lateral medulla (9).

At this point, I will discuss the dural openings and angles of approaches used for the treatment of the various cranial nerve syndromes.

TRIGEMINAL NEURALGIA

The dural opening for trigeminal neuralgia is a "T"-shaped opening, with the base of the T extending toward the confluence of the sinuses. Alternatively, a curvilinear incision based posteriorly may be used in older patients. The dural incision is taken right to the edge of the sinus, as a few extra millimeters of exposure may be gained by this maneuver. For the same reason, the dura is tacked up with sutures placed through the base of the dural flaps. The surgeon then moves inferiorly and faces in a anterosuperior direction, about 45° relative to the patient's axial plane. This position will allow the surgeon to perform a supralateral approach to the CP angle, angling over the supralateral surface of the cerebellum. The operating microscope is brought into play once the surgeon has established his/her position and is used for the remainder of the case. A rubber dam (made from an unused glove and cut slightly larger than a ½ × 1½-inch cottonoid) and cottonoid are folded and placed over the exposed cerebellum. A tapered (2 mm at the tip) microsurgical retractor blade is used to hold the rubber dam/cottonoid in place and bipolar forceps are used to unfold the distal 10–14 mm of the patty supralaterally, over the exposed cerebellum. The superficial arachnoid layers of the CP angle cistern usually bulge out toward the surgeon, especially with inspiration during mechanical ventilation. These arachnoid layers are sharply dissected, and any superficial bridging veins are coagulated and divided. As the arachnoid is divided, the petrosal venous system comes into view. The petrosal venous system usually consists of two or three veins coming together just before draining into the superior petrosal sinus, in an inverted "Y" type of configuration. I should note, however, that the veins may or may not be present, may be located more or less anteriorly or superiorly, and when present consist of a variable number of venous tributaries (4, 5). Some or all of the petrosal veins may require sacrifice to gain entrance to the CP angle cistern. These veins may be sacrificed with relative impunity and are best dealt with by doubly coagulating (coagulate, partially divide, recoagulate) and dividing away from the petrosal sinus.

Once the petrosal veins have been divided, the trigeminal nerve will come into view. The operating table may be rotated, and the microsurgical retractor may be manipulated so that the entire nerve, from brainstem to Meckel's cave can be well visualized. Adequate visualiza-

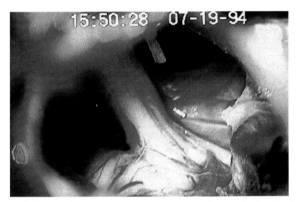

FIG. 1. Trigeminal neuralgia. This photograph was obtained during exploration of the CP angle in a 69-year-old woman with typical lower-division trigeminal neuralgia. Compression of the nerve, from an anterior and rostral direction, by the trifurcation of the SCA is clearly visible.

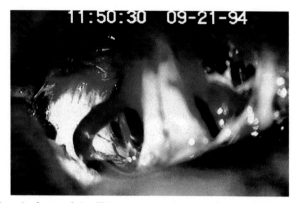

FIG. 2. Trigeminal neuralgia. This operative photograph was obtained at the time of reexploration of the CP angle in a 44-year-old man with lower facial pain. Although the AICA loop is clearly compressing the nerve from below, this is not responsible for the pain syndrome in this patient. Lower division pain is caused by rostral compression at the nerve root entry zone. Further exploration led to the discovery of a rostral cerebellar vein that was appropriately placed. Treatment of this vessel, along with the AICA, has resulted in a good outcome.

tion of the nerve is essential for the full appreciation of pathologic neurovascular relationships. For example, Figure 1 depicts a loop of the SCA compressing the nerve from an anterior and superior direction. This illustrates the most common finding seen in lower-division trigeminal neuralgia (4). Figure 2 demonstrates compression of the nerve from the caudal aspect by a loop of the AICA very well. This patient had lower-division trigeminal neuralgia, and, as I mentioned above, should have compression superiorly, at the nerve root entry zone. In fact, this patient illustrates an important point. He was referred to me after an unsuccessful exploration elsewhere. I surmise that the operating surgeon saw this large AICA loop, treated it, and went home. Further inspection of the nerve revealed a cerebellar vein running across the nerve root entry zone superiorly. This vein was treated, as was the AICA loop, and the patient is pain-free now, 18 months after his operation.

Compression of the nerve from an anterior and superior direction, usually by the SCA or one of its branches is the usual cause of lower facial trigeminal neuralgia. Of 1200 patients with trigeminal neuralgia treated with microvascular decompression, 69% had pain limited to the lower face (V2, V3, or V2 and V3), and 75% of all patients had compression of the nerve caused by the SCA. Isolated V2 pain, seen in 18% of the author's series, is seen most often in younger women. It is most often caused by compression along the side of the nerve. Although venous compression alone was found to be causal in only 12% of the entire series, it appears as though isolated V2 trigeminal neuralgia is more frequently caused by venous compression, frequently by a trigeminal vein (1, 4, 5).

Isolated first division trigeminal pain, is rare, occurring in only 3% of the author's series. When present, it is usually caused by a pontine surface vein, aberrant trigeminal vein, or loop of AICA compressing the nerve from below and laterally (portio major side of the nerve). V1 pain is encountered more frequently in combination with V2 pain (17% of author's series). The combination is again caused by compression from below and laterally (1, 4, 5).

HEMIFACIAL SPASM

A curvilinear dural incision, based laterally with the superior limb of the incision approaching the confluence of the sinuses, is used for microvascular decompression of the facial nerve. Stay sutures are placed, and the surgeon orients him/herself to face in an inferolateral direction. After introduction of the operating microscope, the rubber dam and cottonoid are placed in a caudal-lateral direction to expose the arachnoid overlying the glossopharyngeal and vagus nerves. This arachnoid and the arachnoid trabeculae in the region of cranial nerves IX and X are opened sharply, and the retractor is used to elevate the cerebellum off of the nerves until the choroid plexus, emerging through the foramen of Luschka, is visible. The retractor blade should now be adjusted so that it assumes a slightly caudal-to-rostral direction, with the tip of the retractor blade resting directly on or in front of the choroid plexus. This will allow visualization of the more medially placed facial nerve as it runs rostrally from the pontomedullary junction before joining the vestibulocochlear nerves. It may become necessary to rotate the operating table progressively toward the surgeon to achieve an adequate view of the facial nerve (6).

In classical hemifacial spasm, arteriolar crosscompression can be anticipated to occur from an anterior and caudal direction at the root entry zone. Figure 3 demonstrates the operative exposure of the nerve root entry zone of the facial nerve. Figure 3A–D is a step-by-step demonstration of our approach, centered on the choroid plexus just rostral to cranial nerves IX/X, inspection of a large PICA loop that was indenting the facial nerve as it left the pontomedullary junction, elevation of the offending vessel and, finally, padding the vessel with Teflon felt.

The PICA was found to be the offending vessel in 68% of patients in the most recent review of the authors series, with the AICA contributing to the pathology in 35% and the vertebral artery contributing in

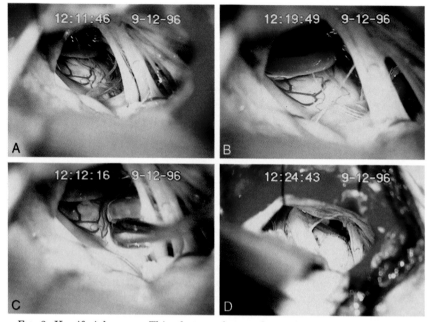

Fig. 3. Hemifacial spasm. This photograph was obtained during microvascular decompression of the facial nerve in a 57-year-old woman with a 10-year history of right-sided typical hemifacial spasm. The initial operative exposure, centered on the choroid plexus emerging from the foramen of Luschka, is depicted in **A**. **B** shows a higher-powered view of the PICA loop, which is deeply indenting the nerve in the region of the nerve root entry zone. **C** shows how the loop may be mobilized away from the nerve, and **D** demonstrates adequate padding with shredded Teflon.

24% (2). In atypical hemifacial spasm, which is characterized by a reversal of the usual rostral-to-caudal progression of spasm, pathologic vessels compress the nerve on its posterior (or rostral) aspect as it leaves the brainstem. Recognition and treatment of these pathologic vessels requires complete visualization of the facial nerve as it leaves the brainstem, as well as a learned anticipation of the causative pathology (6, 9, 12).

VERTIGO AND TINNITUS: "MENIERE'S DISEASE"

In the operative approach used for eighth nerve, the root entry zone of the eighth nerve must be dissected free from its caudal contact with the flocculus of the cerebellum more medially than in hemifacial spasm so that one can see veins at the brainstem, which may be causal. For decompression procedures aimed at the vestibular nerve, the pons above the nerve is exposed, and the flocculus of the cerebellum is elevated off of the nerve with the retractor, in a manner similar to opening the pages of a book, and the arachnoid trabeculae to the brainstem are sharply dissected (3).

The offending vessels responsible for both vertigo and tinnitus are commonly arteries in combination with one or more veins. The most frequently offending vessels are the labyrinthine artery, AICA, PICA, or some combination thereof. In nearly 20% of patients, however, the offending vessel will be a vein alone (3, 8, 13, 14). In patients with vertigo, the offending vessel will always be found at the brainstem, compressing the nerve root entry zone of the superior vestibular nerve. Figure 4 demonstrates the characteristic finding in patients with vertigo. This 66-year-old woman suffered from disabling vertigo for 18 months. Preoperative evaluation (brainstem-evoked responses) revealed her to have dysfunction of the left vestibular nerve. Operation revealed the characteristic compression of the superior vestibular nerve at the nerve root entry zone by both the AICA and a vein. Patients with dysequilibrium, but without true vertigo, will be found to have a compressive lesion just distal (about 1 mm) from the nerve root entry zone on the superior vestibular nerve. Patients with recalcitrant nausea have a compressing vessel located at the nerve root entry zone of the inferior vestibular nerve.

In patients with tinnitus, compression of the cochlear nerve may occur anywhere along the nerve, from the root entry zone to the internal auditory meatus. Figure 5A is an operative photograph obtained during a microvascular decompression procedure in a 53-year-old man with a 2-year history of left-sided tinnitus. A PICA loop can be

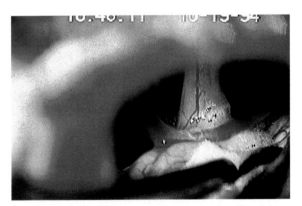

Fig. 4. Vertigo. This patient, a 66-year-old woman, had suffered from severe vertigo for 18 months at the time of operation. The AICA and a vein (which is covered by the AICA in this photo) were both compressing the nerve root entry zone of the superior vestibular nerve.

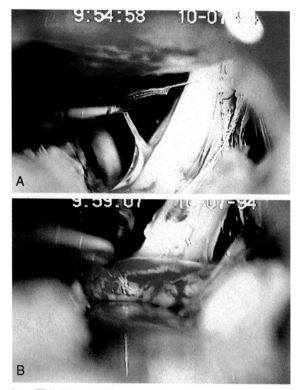

FIG. 5. Tinnitus. This 53-year-old man had a 2-year history of tinnitus on the left. A PICA loop can be seen running along the caudal side of the nerve in **A**. **B** demonstrates a medullary vein running along the nerve root entry zone of the cochlear nerve. Both of these vessels require treatment.

seen running along the caudal side of the cochlear nerve, as can a medullary vein at the nerve root entry zone (Fig. 5**B**). One type of compressive lesion that can be very difficult to treat is illustrated in Figure 6. This patient suffered from tinnitus, deep ear pain, and vertigo. Exploration revealed the AICA running between VII and VIII, compressing the nervous intermedius and the cochlear nerve. Furthermore, a small vein was found at the nerve root entry zone of the superior vestibular nerve. Thus, we were able to identify lesions responsible for each of his symptoms and treat him appropriately. Figure 6**B** shows the appearance of the nerve after division of the vein, division of nervus intermedius, and lateral mobilization of the AICA branch. This particular type of vascular compression (AICA running between fascicles and giving off a branch to the auditory canal and/or the pons) can be extremely difficult to treat effectively (3).

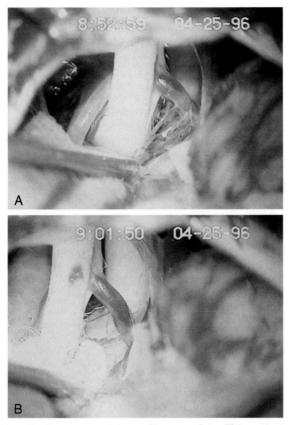

FIG. 6. Vertigo, tinnitus, nervus intermedius neuralgia. This patient with multiple complaints had multiple findings during exploration of the CP angle. An AICA loop is running between the facial and cochlear nerves and is compressing both the cochlear nerve and the nervus intermedius. There is also a vein running along the nerve root entry zone of the superior vestibular nerve. **B** demonstrates the final appearance of the nerve after decompression. The nervus intermedius has been divided, as has the vein compressing the superior vestibular nerve. The AICA loop has been padded away from the nerves as best as possible and has been moved laterally.

GLOSSOPHARYNGEAL NEURALGIA

To perform microvascular decompression of the glossopharyngeal nerve, the craniectomy should extend to the floor of the posterior fossa and follow the edge of the sigmoid sinus until it approaches the jugular bulb. The dura is opened in a fashion similar to that used in hemifacial spasm, except that the inferior extent of the dural opening will be greater. The surgeon moves slightly rostral relative to the patient and an inferolateral approach is used to expose the nerves. A significant number of patients will have a bridging cerebellar vein, which will require coagulation and division as the flocculus is gently elevated off of the IXth and Xth cranial nerves (17). Sharp arachnoidal dissection will allow the cerebellum to be elevated such that the entire cranial nerve IX/X complex is visible (Fig. 7).

Neurovascular compression will be caused by the PICA, vertebral artery, or a combination of one of these arteries and a vein in the great majority of patients (30/41 in the last series compiled from the author's data). If the offending vessel is a vein alone, as it was in 5 of the 41 patients reviewed, the vein may be moved away from the nerves, coagulated and divided. If the offending vessel is an artery and the compression is by a loop anteriorly, rostrally, or caudally (Fig. 7), then

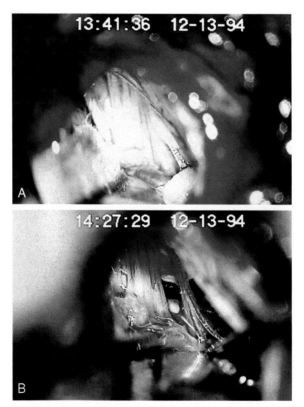

FIG. 7. Glossopharyngeal neuralgia. This photograph was taken during a microvascular decompression procedure in a 42-year-old man with right-sided throat pain. Cranial nerve IX can be seen compressed anteriorly by the vertebral artery (**A**), whereas cranial nerve X is compressed from its caudal aspect by PICA (**B**). Both of these vessels were treated, and the patient now remains pain-free.

the artery should be moved away and held off of the nerves with pieces of shredded Teflon felt. If the artery is running between the fascicles of the nerve, the artery should be moved distally along the nerve and held in place with small pieces of shredded Teflon felt. In performing these operations, it is important to remember that the perforating vessels in this region are physiologic end arteries without significant collateral supply. As such, they should be considered necessary for life and not interrupted. If bleeding from one of these small perforators does occur, gentle tamponade with a piece of Teflon, followed by patient irrigation with saline and hydrogen peroxide, will usually provide hemostasis (17).

ESSENTIAL HYPERTENSION

The approach taken for the treatment of essential hypertension is similar to that used for glossopharyngeal neuralgia on the left side. The compressing vessel responsible for hypertension is always an artery. The vertebral artery and/or the PICA are the most frequently involved vessels (7, 10, 15, 16). Preoperative magnetic resonance imaging will demonstrate the larger vessels responsible for the compression syndrome (16). These ectatic and frequently atherosclerotic vessels can be very difficult to mobilize (Fig. 8). Mobilization of these vessels requires the use of multiple, variable-sized pieces of Teflon felt placed initially away from the area of greatest compression. As the

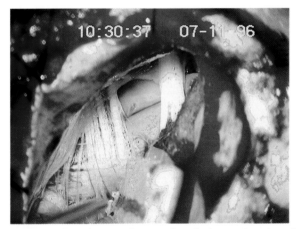

FIG. 8. Hypertension. This photograph was taken during exploration of the CP angle in an elderly woman with hemifacial spasm and essential hypertension. The large ectactic vertebral arteries deeply indent the lateral medulla in the region of the cranial nerve IX/X complex. Decompression of the lateral medulla in such cases can be extremely difficult.

artery is gradually elevated off the medulla, more pieces of felt are placed, moving toward the area of maximum compression. As mentioned previously, great care must be taken to preserve the perforating arteries in this region.

NOTES ON CLOSURE

After the appropriate cranial nerve(s) have been decompressed and absolute hemostasis has been achieved and verified with repeated Valsalva maneuvers, closure is begun. Every effort is made to achieve a watertight dural closure. A U stitch combined with a small piece of oxidized cellulose may be necessary for closing dura at the very edge of a sinus to ensure hemostasis. A combination of interrupted and running dural sutures, as well as the use of muscle patches may be necessary to achieve a truly watertight seal. Just before tying the final knot, the wound is filled with saline to reduce postoperative pneumocephalus. The bone edges should be rewaxed to prevent CSF rhinorrhea. A methylmethacrylate cranioplasty is performed to completely cover the bony deficit. Once formed, the cranioplasty is removed to allow for a final waxing of bone edges, as some of the wax may melt during the exothermic polymerization stage. Once the bone edges are waxed, the cranioplasty is replaced and the wound irrigated copiously. The deep muscles are then approximated with interrupted 2-0 suture. The wound is again irrigated, and the fascia is closed in a watertight fashion. Subcutaneous tissues and skin are then closed in layers, and a small dry dressing is applied.

ACKNOWLEDGMENTS

The author wishes to thank Daniel K. Resnick, M.D. for his assistance with preparation of the manuscript.

REFERENCES

1. Barker FG II, Jannetta PJ, Bissonnette DJ, et al.: Long term outcome of microvascular decompression for trigeminal neuralgia. **N Engl J Med** 334:1077–1083, 1996.
2. Barker FG II, Jannetta PJ, Bissonnette DJ, et al.: Microvascular decompression for hemifacial spasm. **J Neurosurg** 82:201–210, 1995.
3. Jannetta PJ: Neurovascular cross compression of the eighth nerve in patients with vertigo and tinnitus, in Samii M, Jannetta PJ (eds): *The Cranial Nerves.* Heidelberg, Germany, Springer-Verlag, 1981.
4. Jannetta PJ: Microvascular decompression of the trigeminal nerve root entry zone, in Rovit RL, Murali R, Jannetta PJ (eds): *Trigeminal Neuralgia.* Baltimore, Williams & Wilkins, 1990.
5. Jannetta PJ: Microvascular decompression of the trigeminal nerve for tic douloureux, in Youmans (ed): *Neurological Surgery.* Philadelphia, W.B. Saunders, 1996.

6. Jannetta PJ, Abbasy M, Maroon JC, et al.: Hemifacial spasm—Etiology and definitive microsurgical treatment: Operative techniques and results in 47 patients. **J Neurosurg** 47:321–328, 1977.

7. Jannetta PJ, Hamm IS, Jho HD, et al.: Essential hypertension caused by arterial compression of the left lateral medulla: A follow-up. **Perspect Neurol Surg** 3:107–125, 1992.

8. Jannetta PJ, Moller MB, Moller AR: Disabling positional vertigo. **N Engl J Med** 310:1700–1705, 1984.

9. Jannetta PJ, Resnick DK: Cranial rhizopathies, in Youmans (ed): *Neurological Surgery*. Philadelphia, W.B. Saunders, 1996, ed 4.

10. Jannetta PJ, Segal R, Wolfson SK: Neurogenic hypertension: Etiology and surgical treatment. **Ann Surg** 201:391–398, 1985.

11. Lang J Jr, Samii A: Retrosigmoid approach to the posterior cranial fossa: An anatomical study. **Acta Neurochir** 111:147–153, 1991.

12. Lovely TJ, Jannetta PJ: Technical aspects of microvascular decompression of the cranial nerves. **Contemp Neurosurg** 18(12):1–6, 1996.

13. Moller MB, Moller AR, Jannetta PJ: Diagnosis and surgical treatment of disabling positional vertigo. **J Neurosurg** 64:21–28, 1986.

14. Moller MB, Moller AR, Jannetta PJ, et al.: Vascular decompression surgery for severe tinnitus: Selection criteria and results. **Laryngoscope** 103:421–427, 1993.

15. Naraghi R, Gaab MR, Walter GF: Neurovascular compression as a cause of essential hypertension: A microanatomical study. **Adv Neurosurg** 17:182–187, 1989.

16. Naraghi R, Gaab MR, Walter GF, et al.: Arterial hypertension and neurovascular compression at the ventrolateral medulla. **J Neurosurg** 77:103–112, 1992.

17. Resnick DK, Jannetta PJ, Bissonnette DJ, et al.: Microvascular decompression for glossopharyngeal neuralgia. **Neurosurgery** 36:64–69, 1995.

18. Rhoton AL: Microsurgical anatomy of decompression operations on the trigeminal nerve, in Rovit RL, Murali R, Jannetta PJ (eds): *Trigeminal Neuralgia*. Baltimore, Williams & Wilkins, 1990.

14

Posterior Ventral Pallidotomy: Techniques and Theoretical Considerations

ROY A. E. BAKAY, M.D., PHILIP A. STARR, M.D., Ph.D.,
JERROLD L. VITEK, M.D., Ph.D., AND MAHLON R. DeLONG, M.D.

Pallidotomy was first utilized in the treatment of Parkinson's disease in the late 1940s and early 1950s. As is often true in functional neurosurgery, there have been a number of controversies surrounding this procedure, both in the past and the present. Our goal in this chapter is to discuss surgical techniques from our perspective and give the rationale for these techniques. We will point out, where appropriate, alternative methodologies. We will attempt to answer four very basic questions: Who is an appropriate surgical candidate? Where is the optimal target? How best to make the lesion? What are the anticipated results? The answer to each of these questions is critical and controversial.

THE APPROPRIATE CANDIDATE FOR PALLIDOTOMY

Historically, pallidotomy was used for many types of movement disorders. In the modern era, the only widely accepted indication is that of idiopathic Parkinson's disease. There is a small set of data that suggests that it may be helpful for segmental dystonia and possibly for hemiballismus. The focus here will be on Parkinson's disease (PD).

PD is a chronic, progressive, neurodegenerative disease that shows increasing incidence and prevalence with age (5, 8). PD was first described in the medical literature by James Parkinson in 1817. Cardinal symptoms of the disease are resting tremor, slowness of initiating (akinesia) and of executing movement (bradykinesia), rigidity, and postural instability. There may also be nonmotor symptoms and autonomic nervous system dysfunction (8). PD patients are frequently divided by symptoms into those who are tremor-dominant and those who are bradykinesia-rigidity dominant. Tremor-dominant patients tend to be younger at onset, slower in progression, and with better preserved cognitive function. These patients may benefit more from a thalamotomy. Those with predominant bradykinesia-rigidity, postural instability, and gait problems are usually older at onset, have more problems with dementia, and progress more rapidly. These patients may benefit more from a pallidotomy.

There is not a specific biological marker for PD, and the diagnosis is therefore clinical. Accurate diagnosis of PD requires ruling out other causes of Parkinson-like symptoms. These can be secondarily induced by various drugs, systemic diseases, or other neurodegenerative disorders. As many as 30 other disorders and diseases have features similar to PD. Autopsy findings have revealed that as many as 24% of patients diagnosed clinically as having idiopathic PD may not have the pathologic features of the disease, such as degeneration of neurons of the substantia nigra and the presence of Lewy bodies (3). There is a need for evaluation by a movement disorder specialist.

Patients with idiopathic PD who initially demonstrated a good response to levodopa but subsequently developed an unsatisfactory clinical response to maximum medical management are considered candidates for pallidotomy. Most patients, in addition to exhibiting the cardinal motor signs of PD (akinesia/bradykinesia, rigidity, tremor, and gait disorder/postural instability) also experience drug-induced dyskinesias, motor fluctuations, and freezing episodes. Many also experience dystonic posturing and pain. Our inclusion and exclusion criteria are as follows:

Inclusion criteria:

1. A clinical diagnosis of idiopathic PD. The diagnosis is based on the presence of at least two of the cardinal signs of this disorder (akinesia/bradykinesia, rest tremor, rigidity, or gait disorder/postural instability), with at least one of the signs being rest tremor or akinesia, as well as a history of a good response to levodopa therapy.
2. Hoehn and Yahr stage III or greater when "off."
3. Demonstrated response to levodopa.
4. Intractable disabling motor fluctuations (severe "on-off" periods, dyskinesias, or freezing episodes).
5. Unsatisfactory clinical response to maximum medical management.

Exclusion criteria:

1. Clinically significant medical disease that would increase the risk of developing pre- or postoperative complications (e.g., severe cardiac or pulmonary disease, diabetes mellitus, uncontrolled hypertension).

2. Evidence of secondary or atypical parkinsonism as suggested
   a. History of cerebral vascular accidents (CVAs), exposure to toxins, neuroleptics, or encephalitis.
   b. Neurologic signs of upper motor neuron or cerebellar involvement, supranuclear gaze palsy, or orthostatic hypotension.
   c. Magnetic resonance imaging (MRI) consistent with secondary parkinsonism (e.g., lacunar infarcts, pontine or cerebellar atrophy).
3. Significant dementia or depression.

These clinical criteria should serve only as a guide in determining whether or not a patient is a candidate for pallidotomy. There may be cases, for example, where patients do not meet all the inclusion criterion, yet are functionally disabled by their symptoms and would still benefit from pallidotomy. For example, consider patients with medically intractable predominantly unilateral parkinsonism who may not meet the Hoehn and Yahr criterion of stage III when "off." These patients may still be quite disabled by their symptoms and benefit substantially from pallidotomy. Pallidotomy is not indicated for patients with MRI evidence of severe cerebral, putaminal, or pallidal atrophy. Patients with "Parkinson's plus" syndromes, e.g., Shy-Drager syndrome, progressive supranuclear palsy, or olivopontocerebellar atrophy, generally do not benefit from surgery. Contraindications also include uncontrolled hypertension and severe swallowing difficulties. Patients who no longer respond to medications or whose response to medication does not fluctuate are not optimal candidates.

THE OPTIMAL TARGET

The basal ganglia are parts of larger, segregated circuits that involve the thalamus and cerebral cortex (10). A pathophysiological model has been elaborated and tested in which parkinsonian signs are viewed as resulting from increased activity of neurons in the "motor" portion of the internal pallidum, the major output nucleus of the basal ganglia, leading to increased inhibition of thalamocortical projection neurons and decreased activation of the precentral motor fields (Fig. 1). Increased internal pallidal activity is thought to result from striatal dopamine loss, leading to decreased inhibition of the internal pallidum via a monosynaptic ("direct") striatopallidal pathway and to excessive excitatory glutamatergic drive via a polysynaptic ("indirect") striatopallidal pathway. Current medical therapies for Parkinson's disease, aimed at systemically replacing dopamine, often lose their effectiveness after several years, with patients suffering from motor fluctuations and drug-induced dyskinesias. Therapeutic strategies have been

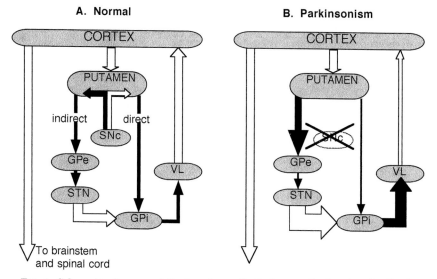

FIG. 1. Schematic diagram of the basal ganglia-thalamocortical motor circuit. *Open arrows*, excitatory connections; *filled arrows*, inhibitory connections. **(A)** Normal. The input (putamen) and output (GPi) nuclei of the basal ganglia are connected by indirect and direct pathways. Dopaminergic innervation of the putamen by substantia nigra, pars compacta (SNc) is inhibitory to striatopallidal fibers in the indirect pathway, but excitatory to striatopallidal fibers in the direct pathway. STN, subthalamic nucleus. **(B)** Parkinsonism. Changes in the widths of the *arrows* in comparison with **(A)** indicate changes in the relative influence of the pathway represented. When the putamen is deprived of dopaminergic innervation from SNc, the net result is that STN and GPi are overactive, thalamocortical projections are underactive, and the cortex is inhibited. **(C)** Parkinsonism, showing the compensatory effects of pallidotomy. Pallidotomy corrects for overactivity in the pallidothalamic projections, resulting in relative normalization of activity in the thalamocortical projection.

developed to reduce increased basal ganglia outflow directly by the placement of stereotactic lesions into the sensorimotor portion of the globus pallidus internis (GPi).

There is general agreement within contemporary neurosurgery that the lesion must be posterior and ventral in GPi to be effective. One school of thought is that a pure ansotomy is sufficient for clinical effect. An ansotomy should potentially eliminate the inhibitory output from GPi to the thalamus. However, a considerable amount of pallidothalamic output goes through the fascicularis lenticularis, which might not be affected with a small lesion. In addition, an isolated ansotomy should interrupt the output from globus pallidus externa (GPe) to the subthalamic nucleus, leading to further disinhibition of the subthalamic nucleus, and further excitation of the remaining GPi cells and of the remaining pallidothalamic fibers. Thus, a pure ansa lesion may well improve a number of parkinsonian signs but may not be the optimal area for lesioning. Another alternative is a more broad-based lesion encompassing the ansa, the motor elements of GPi, and the fascicularis lenticularis. This more extensive lesion is the basis of our surgical approach. Making a lesion too large in this area has the potential for increasing complications, and therefore careful shaping of the lesion is required. A final school of thought suggests that the optimal target is GPe. The theoretical basis of this is in eliminating the striatopallidal and pallidosubthalamic pathways so as to release the "normal function of the medial pallidum." The concept here is that both the direct and indirect pathways have been lesioned, and therefore stimulation and inhibition to GPi are somehow again balanced. The problems with such a concept are that the direct striatopallidal pathway is diffuse and therefore difficult to lesion completely, and because of the deficiency in striatal dopamine, it is already minimally functioning. The indirect pathway through the subthalamic nucleus is excitatory, and decreasing the pallidosubthalamic inhibition may produce the opposite effect of that which is desired. Although this type of lesion is described as a GPe lesion, all of the available information about lesions made in this area indicates that they incorporate the posterior elements of GPi and the ansa.

While the optimal target site remains to be definitively determined, we do know that the sensorimotor region in GPi is somatotopically arranged, with the leg more superior and medial and the arm more inferior and lateral. The boundaries between different somatotopic subdivisions of GPi are less well demarcated than in the thalamus or motor cortex. Nevertheless, the somatotopy of GPi is quite important inasmuch as we have observed that small single lesions based quite laterally tend to improve hand function more than leg, whereas those placed more medially tend to improve leg function more than hand. As a result, we have modified our approach to make both lateral and medial lesions to completely encompass both regions. We currently use a triangular pattern of lesioning that matches the shape of the posterior GPi. We believe this produces the maximum benefit from a posterior ventral pallidotomy.

MAKING THE LESION

Preparation of the Patient for Surgery

Since patients must be awake during the procedure, great care must be taken to fully inform them of the order of events and what to expect in the operating theater. Arrangements must be made to ensure that the anesthesia service does not write "routine" preoperative orders for these patients. No preoperative medicines should be given to the patient. No lines should be placed on the limb contralateral to the lesion. It is useful to instruct the patient to refuse placement of lines on the side of the body that needs to be evaluated intraoperatively. Prior to the start of surgery prophylactic antibiotics are given. The use of steroids is not necessary. Because patients must be awake and alert during the procedure, sedating medications should be used only if absolutely necessary and should be short-acting if possible. Monitoring equipment should be battery-powered to minimize potential interference with electrophysiologic recording. All antiparkinsonian medications are held after midnight in order to reduce drug-induced dyskinesias and allow the manifestation of parkinsonian motor signs. This is particularly important at the time of lesioning to enable immediate clinical assessment of the effect of lesioning. Patients with severe "off" periods who would experience significant difficulty being without medication overnight are allowed to take medication after midnight unless this is likely to result in dyskinesias in the morning during placement of the stereotactic frame. In these patients medication is stopped, based upon the patient's history, at a time that will allow them the most "on" time without the occurrence of drug-induced dyskinesias when the frame is being applied.

The initial target coordinates for stereotactic procedures historically are obtained by image-directed surgical methodology. The more information contained within the imaging technique, the more precise the initial probe placement. There has been an evolution from standard x-ray films which require correction for parallax, magnification, rotation, and tilt, to three-dimensional computed tomographic imaging techniques with three-dimensional reconstruction. Most of the current generation of computed tomography (CT) scanning units have software available for 3-D reformatting. Magnetic resonance imaging (MRI) permits multiplanar viewing and trajectory determination without the need for reformatting steps. The accuracy of MR techniques may not be as good as CT because the slices must be thicker (unless scan times are made very long). The fiducial markers are subject to multiple field distortions, and the error in identification of the fiducial markers is larger. Any MRI-compatible stereotactic frame can be used, but the Cosman-Roberts-Wells (CRW by Radionics, Cambridge, MA) and the Leksell frames (G frame by Electa, Atlanta, GA) seem best suited for functional stereotactic work. These are rectilinear systems with a semicircular arc fixed around the target, which allow easy translation of the arc in the X, Y, or Z direction, permit multiple targets to be reached without the need for additional calculations, and allow changes in the approach trajectory to a target without the need for manipulations of the frame coordinates.

We currently use the Leksell Series G stereotactic system and perform MRI only for target localization. MR images are acquired on a Phillips 1.5 T unit, using a fast-spin echo inversion recovery (FSE-IR) sequence, with TI = 200 msec, TR = 3000 msec, TE = 40 msec, acquisition mode = 2-D, matrix 256X512, NEX = 2. This protocol is modified from one in use at Oregon Health Sciences University (Bernard Coombs, Jerzy Szumoswski, and Kim Burchiel) and provides excellent visualization of the boundaries of GPi (Fig. 2).

With the Leksell system, determination of the target coordinates requires that MR images be parallel to one of the frame axes. The images should also be parallel or orthogonal to the patient's intercom-

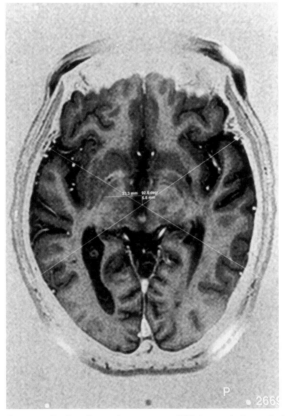

Fig. 2. This photograph of an inversion recovery MR image is 3 mm below the AC-PC plane. The lamina, GPe, and GPi are clearly visible for targeting.

missural (AC-PC) line, so that measurements based upon standard distances from the AC-PC line are accurate, and the morphology of anatomic landmarks in a particular plane remains consistent from case to case. Thus, the frame must be placed with its anteroposterior axis parallel to the patient's AC-PC line, without any rotation or lateral tilt. This is achieved by using the frame-mounted earplugs provided with the Leksell system, then adjusting the anteroposterior axis of the frame so that it is parallel to the orbitomeatal line. If the patient is seated with the head in a neutral position, the frame should be angled approximately 6° from the horizontal so that the anterior half of the ring is slightly higher than the posterior half. The frame is secured after infiltrating the scalp down to the periosteum with 1% lidocaine HCl with epinephrine. If a particularly long operation is anticipated, a mixture of 1% lidocaine HCl with 0.5% bupivacaine HCl in equal volumes can be used.

For the MRI, a cylindrical adapter is mounted to the frame and localizer so that the frame fits snugly into the headcoil. Imaging is performed in the axial and coronal planes with 2-mm slice thickness and 0 interslice distance. Using the MRI protocol described above, each set of images takes 10 minutes to acquire. On the axial cut best showing the AC and the PC, the length of the AC-PC line is measured. The tentative target is 2 mm anterior, 21 mm lateral, and 4 mm inferior to the mid-AC-PC point. These are the coordinates used by Leksell (9) and Laitinen et al. (6). Fine adjustments in the x and y coordinates are then made based upon direct visualization of the GPi and internal capsule, so that on the axial cut at the level of the AC-PC line, the target projects onto posterolateral GPi 2–3 mm from the GPi-GPe lamina and 0–1 mm from the internal capsule. Target coordinates are then independently determined on coronal imaging. We use the coronal cut passing through the point 2 mm ahead of the AC-PC midpoint. This can be found by first identifying the cut showing the AC in the midline, then moving posteriorly by the appropriate number of cuts (usually five cuts, or 10 mm) according to the patient's AC-PC length. The correct coronal plane should show the mammillary bodies inferior to the third ventricle. The tentative target is 21 mm lateral to the floor of the third ventricle. Fine adjustments in the x and z Leksell coordinates are then made, based upon direct visualization of the GPi and optic tract, so that the target is 2–3 mm medial to the GPi-GPe lamina, and 1 mm above the lateral edge of the optic tract.

In combining the two sets of coordinates from the two different imaging planes to derive one set of "consensus" coordinates, we tend to ignore the coordinate along the axis perpendicular to the plane of an image. Thus, the axial images are accurate for determining the x and

y coordinates, and the coronal images are accurate for determining the x and z coordinates.

In the Operating Room

Patients are positioned supine on the table during the opening of the cranium. This position helps to reduce the likelihood of an air embolus. After opening the cranium, the head is elevated 20–30° for the remainder of the procedure. A sterile field must be maintained over the scalp posterior to the eyebrows, but the patient's face and body are best left uncovered and a simple screen placed between the patient and the sterile field. It is very important to be able to see the affected side to observe spontaneous tremor as well as to test for strength and coordination. We prefer that the patient be able to see his/her body and the surrounding part of the room in order to provide orientation and reduce stress levels as much as possible. The anesthesia team should be on the side ipsilateral to the lesion. An arterial line for continuous blood pressure monitoring and intravenous line for administration of medications are essential. Short-acting narcotics are administered only if absolutely required for patient comfort. Individual small boluses are preferred so the surgeon knows how much medication is being given. The use of continuous drips is to be avoided because these are readily manipulated by the anesthesiologist without consultation with the surgeon. This is in contrast to any antihypertensive medication which needs continuous smooth delivery to ensure that the patient remains in a normotensive range. In the operating room setting, even the patient who is normally hypotensive may suddenly demonstrate remarkably increased systolic pressures; it is extremely important for the surgeon to be aware of the patient's blood pressure throughout the procedure and be assured that acute elevations have not occurred. Mean blood pressure should be kept at or below 90 mm Hg.

Head Stage and Electrophysiologic Equipment

Platinum-iridium glass-coated microelectrodes with a tip diameter of 2–4 μm and an impedance of 0.5–2.0 Mohms (at 1000 Hz) are used for recording. The electrode is placed in a stainless steel "carrier" tube (26 gauge) which is attached to a Kopf (David Kopf Instruments) water hydraulic microdrive that is attached to the stereotaxic frame. The microelectrode is advanced by both a coarse and a fine (micro) drive. Attached to the microdrive assembly is a high impedance preamplifier head stage to which the recording electrode and an indifferent lead in contact with the carrier tube are connected. The preamplifier is connected to standard electrophysiologic equipment for amplification, filtering, and discrimination of electrophysiologic signals. A Narashige

x-y stage has been adapted to fit on the stereotaxic head frame and acts as the base upon which the microdrive assembly is placed. The initial target coordinates are centered at 0-0 on the Narashige x-y stage, and subsequent adjustments in the medial-lateral and anterior-posterior plane are made by adjusting the coordinates of the x-y stage. This obviates the need for changing the coordinates of the stereotaxic frame and allows for more rapid and precise changes in coordinates.

Microelectrode Mapping Technique

Recording tracks are carried out in the parasagittal plane proceeding in the anterodorsal to posteroventral direction at an angle of approximately 30° anterior to the perpendicular from the AC-PC line. As the microelectrode is advanced, patterns of neural activity are noted throughout the track, and the depth from the starting position is recorded. The recorded single cell (unit) activity is displayed on an oscilloscope screen and connected to an audioamplifier for aural monitoring of the signal. Neural as well as electromyographic (emg) and other analog signals are stored on videotape for subsequent analysis. Based upon the characteristic neuronal discharge frequencies and patterns of striatal, GPe, GPi, and intralaminar border cells, the boundaries of the encountered nuclei are identified and fitted onto 2-D parasagittal maps drawn from the Schaltenbrand and Bailey Atlas (1). Within GPi, changes in neuronal discharge frequency in response to passive (sensory) or active (motor) movements of the patient's limbs, trunk, neck, and face are recorded. The location of responsive neurons are also mapped onto the Schaltenbrand and Bailey Atlas. After passing through the pallidum, the electrode may enter the optic tract or internal capsule. The optic tract is identified by listening for the evoked responses to light flashes (present in 87% of our cases) and/or by the patient's report of phosphenes evoked by stimulation (biphasic pulses, 300 Hz, 0.2 msec, 60 μA) through the microelectrode (present in 75% of our cases). Some patients (16%) were unable to identify the optic tract by microstimulation when present by light stimulation. The location of the corticospinal tract in the internal capsule is identified by characteristic motor responses to microstimulation. Multiple passes (3–9, mode = 4) of the microelectrode are made until sufficient data are collected to define the sensorimotor territory of GPi and the location of the optic and corticospinal tracts. We feel a minimum of two microelectrode passes are needed to define the anteroposterior and dorsoventral dimensions of GPi, and an additional pass is used to define the lateral edge of GPi. On occasion, due to unusual anatomy, 6–9 tracts have been needed. The initial trajectory is an average of 2.6 mm. from the center of the lesion determined physiologically.

Lesioning Procedure

Once the sensorimotor portion of the Gpi and its borders are defined and the target is selected, the recording microelectrode is replaced at exactly the same position with a 1.1-mm diameter lesioning electrode with a 3-mm exposed tip (Radionics, Cambridge, MA). The lesioning electrode is advanced to the upper border of the GPi based upon the physiologic map. Stimulation is carried out with cathodal pulses at 300 Hz and 0.2 msec pulse duration at current intensities varying from 0.2 to 2.0 mA. The effect upon mobility, tone, and tremor are observed. The presence of stimulation-induced movement or reports from the patient of speckles or flashes of light indicate activation of corticospinal or optic tract, respectively. The lesioning probe is advanced in 2-mm intervals until it approaches within 2 mm of the ventral border of GPi, based upon the physiologic recordings. At this point, the lesioning electrode is advanced in 0.5–1.0 mm increments until stimulation-induced tonic movements are induced at currents equal to or greater than 0.5 mA at 300 Hz or visual responses are reported at currents greater than or equal to 1.0 mA at 300 Hz. It is important to note that the majority (67%) of patients tested using varying current intensity or stimulation frequency do not report, nor have we been able to observe, any consistent change in mobility, tremor, or rigidity during stimulation in the portions of GPi which, when lesioned, result in significant improvement in these motor signs. Thus, stimulation-induced changes in parkinsonian motor signs cannot be relied upon to determine lesion placement.

At the lesion site, following determination of thresholds for the internal capsule and/or optic tract, the probe is warmed to 42°C. During this time the patient is examined for any change in strength, speech difficulty, or changes in visual fields. The patient is asked to read printed material and to report any change in vision such as blurring, distortion, or loss of text. If no adverse signs are observed, the persist for hours or days in some patients.

Our approach to lesioning by incremental increases in temperature is derived from observations of lesion size based upon experiments in egg white combined with MRI reconstructions of lesion size. We have made similar observations based upon reconstructions of lesion size from high-resolution MR images taken from patients in whom different temperatures were used to make the lesion. In our experience, lesioning at 75°C at a site where macrostimulation thresholds for developing phosphenes are >1.0 mA is safe for avoiding encroachment upon the optic tract, while macrostimulation thresholds >0.5 mA are safe for avoiding injury to the corticospinal tract.

In summary, we believe that by making multiple tracts rather than simply expanding a single track, one can more exactly shape the lesion against the adjacent structures to prevent collateral damage. Another technique to shape the lesion is to use a low temperature initially. By starting at 60° and increasing in increments of 5°–10°, one can optimize the lesion and minimize the potential complications. The patient is examined for optic tract or corticospinal tract injury throughout the lesioning process.

RESULTS

Complications in all contemporary series have been relatively low (1, 2, 4, 6, 7). The two major types of complications relate to the corticospinal tract and the optic tract. Previous reports have noted 14% (1) to 2% (6) with transient facial weakness and 4% with transient limb weakness (2, 6). Quadrantanopsia has been reported in from 0% (7) to 14% (6) of cases. Other complications, including the rare subdural hematoma or infection, have contributed to the overall morbidity. Evaluation of our first 128 patients demonstrates a morbidity of 3.9% with no perioperative mortality. We, however, have noted two patients who were worse following surgery and subsequently died several months later. Although these were debilitated patients, clearly the operation contributed to their demise. As with any surgical procedure, the complication rate in most studies has decreased with experience.

Contemporary studies demonstrate that pallidotomy can provide marked contralateral amelioration of the cardinal parkinsonian signs and drug-induced dyskinesias (1, 2, 4, 6, 7). Although none of these studies were randomized and only one (7) utilized blinded examiners, the results are clearly encouraging. In most studies 80% or better of the patients are reported improved. Much of this improvement is in terms of the drug-induced dyskinesias, but also in bradykinesia and rigidity. There is still controversy as to the degree to which tremor improves, but clearly it does improve. A number of studies with follow-up exceeding 1 year reported postsurgical decline in midline motor features, i.e., gait, postural stability, and freezing, but our preliminary results clearly demonstrate improvement that persists for at least 1 year. In most studies (1, 2, 6, 7) the improvement is predominantly in the "off" state. The "on-off" difference is frequently obliterated. Improvement has been suggested in the "on" stage by at least one investigator (4); however, the lack of an objective evaluator and the unconventional manner in which the data were obtained bring validity of these findings into question. All investigators indicate that less benefit is present on the ipsilateral side, although some improvement can be observed.

Our pilot study (1) clearly demonstrates that pallidotomy can ameliorate not only the cardinal signs of Parkinson's disease and drug-induced motor fluctuations and dyskinesias but can also improve quality of life. This improvement can be demonstrated quantitatively, with UPDRS scores improving 30% postoperatively. The Schwab and England scores improved from a mean of 49% preoperatively to 73% postoperatively. Physical and social functioning as well as vitality measures on Medical Outcome Scales also showed significant improvement postoperatively, reflecting the dramatic effect of pallidotomy on the patient's overall function and quality of life. Subsequent evaluation of these same patients demonstrates that those that were initially felt to have optimally placed lesions maintained this improvement for 2–3 years, whereas lesions placed more laterally, *i.e.*, including GPe or only partially including the sensorimotor area of GPi, demonstrate initial improvement that by 1–2 years is back to the preoperative baseline.

In summary, we believe that GPi sensorimotor pallidotomy is highly effective in treating nondemented patients with advanced Parkinson's disease improving akinesia/bradykinesia, tremor, rigidity, gait, and balance. Postoperatively most patients have reduced fluctuations with less severe "off" states and a greater percentage of "on" time. The "on" time is characterized by a lack of disability from drug-induced side effects. Pallidotomy also effectively relieves pain related to the parkinsonian state and improves physical and social functioning and vitality, without causing significant cognitive or psychiatric impairment. All of these findings, however, are based on relatively short follow-up and still await longitudinal evaluation to assess the true effectiveness of pallidotomy. Although a serious procedure with a definite morbidity rate, the pallidotomy's risk:benefit ratio clearly favors this procedure.

SUMMARY

1. Microelectrode mapping of the pallidum and adjacent structures allows for precise target identification and localization of critical structures, *i.e.*, optic tract, internal capsule, and external pallidum, which must be spared from lesioning.
2. Microelectrode mapping has provided physiologic-anatomic correlation for determining the optimal target location as related to clinical outcome and has helped to refine the role of stimulation as a tool for target localization.
3. The improved accuracy of this technique should result in more accurate lesion placement which should improve long-term outcome and decrease morbidity.

REFERENCES

1. Baron MS, *et al.:* Treatment of advanced Parkinson's disease by posterior GPi pallidotomy: 1-year results of a pilot study, in press, 1997.
2. Dogali M, *et al.:* Stereotactic ventral pallidotomy for Parkinson's disease. **Neurology** 45:753–761, 1995.
3. Hughes AJ, *et al.:* Accuracy of clinical diagnosis of idiopathic Parkinson's disease: A clinicopathological study of 100 cases. **J Neurol Neurosurg Psychiatry** 55:181–184, 1992.
4. Iacono RP, *et al.:* The results, indications, and physiology of posteroventral pallidotomy for patients with Parkinson's disease. **Neurosurgery** 36:1118–1125, 1995.
5. Kurland LT: Epidemiology: Incidence, geographic distribution and genetic considerations, in Fields WS (ed.) *Pathogenesis and Treatment of Parkinsonism.* Springfield, IL, Charles C Thomas, 1958, pp 5–43.
6. Laitinen LV, *et al.:* Leksell's posteroventral pallidotomy in the treatment of Parkinson's disease. **J Neurosurg** 76:53–61, 1992.
7. Lozano AM, *et al.:* Effect of GPi pallidotomy on motor function in Parkinson's disease. **Lancet** 346:1383–1387, 1995.
8. Rajput AH: Clinical features and natural history of Parkinson's disease (special consideration of aging), in Calne DB (ed): *Neurodegenerative Diseases.* Philadelphia, W.B. Saunders, 1994, pp 555–571.
9. Svennilson E, *et al.:* Treatment of parkinsonism by stereotactic thermolesions in the pallidal region: A clinical evaluation of 81 cases. **Acta Psychiatr Neurol Scand** 5:358–377, 1960.
10. Wichman T, *et al.:* Parkinson's disease and the basal ganglia: Lessons from the laboratory and from neurosurgery. **Neuroscientist** 1(4):236–244, 1995.

15

Surgical Techniques in Temporal Lobe Epilepsy

ANDRE OLIVIER, M.D., Ph.D.

The main purpose of this chapter is to provide an overview of various modalities of resection used in the treatment of temporal lobe epilepsy and to discuss their rationale, anatomic features, and technical aspects. This overview will be preceded by a brief review of the concept of mesial temporal lobe epilepsy and of the surgical anatomy of the temporal lobe. Although this chapter deals mainly with surgical techniques, reference will be made to results and complications obtained with these same techniques.

HISTORICAL PERSPECTIVE

Wilder Penfield was the first to discuss the modalities or extent of resections in relation to surgical outcome in patients treated for temporal lobe epilepsy (42,43). In 1954, he reported that additional resection of the hippocampus and uncus could transform a failed surgery into a successful one (44). The work of Scoville and Milner (60) and Penfield and Milner (45), which stressed the potential role of the hippocampus in memory function, had much to do in tailoring the temporal lobectomy. Indeed, from the mid-1950s until recently, the trend was to preserve as much as possible of the hippocampus. Thus, at the Montreal Neurological Institute (MNI), Rasmussen et al. (51–53, 55) performed an "anterior temporal lobectomy," in which the anterior temporal cortex, amygdala, and uncus were resected. If the postresection electrocorticogram showed active hippocampal spiking, they would then proceed with the resection of the anterior 1–1.5 cm of the hippocampus. Feindel, at the same institution, stressed the importance of resecting the amygdala in a radical fashion but routinely avoided the removal of the hippocampus for fear of memory impairment.

It is most interesting that Niemeyer (25, 26), in the mid-1950s, introduced the concept of selective removal of the hippocampus and amygdala at a time when classical "temporal lobectomy" was the standard. These structures by that time had already been shown experimentally and clinically to be important in the genesis of temporal lobe seizures (4, 10, 12, 15, 21, 68).

The refinement of the last decade in computer recording of epileptic activity and in brain imaging have forced the neurosurgeon to consider more and more specific, so-called "tailored resections" for each individual patient.

CONCEPT OF MESIAL TEMPORAL EPILEPSY

Insight into the role played by the mesiotemporal structures in human epilepsy is derived from various sources. Hughling Jackson (20) was the first to describe the autopsy findings showing a mesiotemporal lesion as the cause of psychomotor seizures. Echoing the original observations of Jackson, the many experimental studies of the 1950s, such as those of Kaada (22), Vigouroux et al. (68), Gastaut et al. (12), and Green and Shimamoto (15) as well as the observations in humans made by Feindel et al. (9, 10), Penfield and Jasper (44), and Morris (24), point to a very important role for the mesiobasal temporal structures in experimental and human epilepsies.

There is a large collection of data describing striking neuropathological changes in the mesiotemporal area in patients with temporal epilepsy. Hippocampal sclerosis and mesiotemporal sclerosis, including changes in the amygdala, have been reviewed in detail in a series of excellent studies (5, 7, 57). More recent work has shed light on some of the potential basic physiopathologic mechanisms responsible for mesiotemporal epilepsy (2, 11, 17, 58, 59, 61, 65). Further studies on mesiotemporal kindling have brought ample confirmation of the paramount importance of structures such as the uncus, amygdala, hippocampus, dentate gyrus, parahippocampus, entorhinal cortex, piriform, and perirhinal areas in the genesis of temporal seizures. Modern tracing techniques have revealed the bewildering functional complexity of these structures and the unsuspected richness of their connections with each other and with the basal ganglia and the neocortex (11, 18, 48, 61, 66). From the surgical point of view it is important to realize that all of these functional units are located in the mesiobasal part of the temporal lobe and represent in part or in toto the anatomic substratum of mesial temporal epilepsy.

From the electrodiagnostic standpoint, recordings with sphenoidal electrodes have shown a predominance of discharges in the mesiobasal structures in patients with temporal lobe epilepsy (54). The paramount importance of these mesial structures was also confirmed by recording and stimulation with intracranial depth and surface electrodes (14). In our series of patients studied with stereotactic electrodes for bitemporal epilepsy, an overwhelming percentage of the seizures was found to originate in the limbic structures (19, 31, 37, 38, 39, 49, 50, 62, 63). These seizure discharges started either in the hippocampus or amygdala but, more frequently, in the hippocampus with rapid spread from one structure to the other. Simultaneous "regional" limbic onset in both amygdala and hippocampus was also frequent. Seizures of strict neocortical onset were rare. However, quick spread of the discharges to and recruitment of the neocortex were the rule (49, 50).

Stimulation studies, with stereotactic electrodes placed in neocortical and limbic structures of the temporal lobe, have shown that many of the characteristic clinical features of temporal lobe epilepsy, such as the patient's habitual aura, can be reproduced by stimulation of the amygdala and hippocampus but rarely from the neocortical region (14). When electrical stimulation gave rise to seizures, these seizures were almost exclusively of limbic onset, slightly more often from the amygdala than from the hippocampus. These findings are in keeping with our intraoperative stimulation results under local anesthesia, in which the patient's habitual aura, psychic phenomena, automatisms, and after discharges were practically obtained only from stimulation through the deepest contacts of depth electrodes corresponding to the amygdala and hippocampus (A. Olivier, unpublished observations). They are also in keeping with the original work of Feindel et al. (9, 10) on the preoperative stimulation of the amygdala region in man and with the results of Halgren et al. (16) using strictly limbic stimulation.

Imaging studies of the past such as pneumoencephalography very often showed enlargement of one temporal horn in temporal lobe epilepsy (54). Magnetic resonance imaging (MRI) can now show in the living many of the characteristic changes described by the pathologists, particularly the mesial temporal sclerosis and the hippocampal atrophy (3). Furthermore, MRI can reveal a variety of additional lesions which can cause seizures such as gliomas, vascular malformations, and cortical dysplasias. Atrophic changes and volumetric assessments of these changes in specific structures can now be documented accurately with MRI (3).

The syndrome of mesiotemporal lobe epilepsy has been reviewed recently by Wieser et al. (70) The role of febrile convulsions in the pathogenesis of temporal epilepsy was stressed by Falconer et al. (8) and more recently by Abou-Kalil et al. (1) and Berkovic et al. (3). It is fair to say that the clinical manifestations of mesiotemporal epilepsy are in large part the same as those characteristic of "temporal lobe epilepsy," namely the presence of an aura (most often a hard-to-describe chest sensation), the alteration of consciousness, and the presence of oral and manual automatisms. Finally, the studies of

Wieser and Yasargil have shown that selective amygdalohippocampectomy can provide results comparable to those of more traditional temporal resections (19, 69, 71).

NEOCORTICAL EPILEPSY

That seizures can arise from neocortex is best shown by lesions that are confined to the surface of the temporal lobe such as vascular malformations, tumors, and dysplasias. The percentage of these types of seizures is low and probably in the vicinity of 15%.

SURGICAL ANATOMY OF THE TEMPORAL LOBE

Topographic Anatomy of the Temporal Lobe

In our approach to the topography of the temporal lobe we have been helped considerably by the work of Poirier and Charpy (46) and Duvernoy (6).

From the Sylvian fissure to the ambiens cisterna, one can envisage a series of seven temporal gyri disposed longitudinally and called, respectively, T1–T7. These are sequentially displayed on a coronal diagram (Fig. 1). Similarly, these gyri are separated and further identified by a series of seven longitudinal sulci which are designated by symbols: S1–S7 (Fig. 1). The first three gyri occupy the external surface of the lobe, while the fourth and fifth occupy its ventral surface.

The *first temporal gyrus* or T1 is very well demarcated dorsally and mesially by the Sylvian fissure and by a deep and long superior temporal sulcus below sometimes called the parallel sulcus or S1 (Fig. 2). T1 extends from the temporal pole backward into the posterior limb of the supramarginal gyrus according to a constant pattern (Fig. 2). Its depth, *i.e.*, its lateromesial extent is considerably larger posteriorly where it contains the transverse gyri of Heschl.

The *second temporal gyrus* (T2) is usually larger and more tortuous than the first one. Its dorsal aspect corresponds to the parallel or superior sulcus (S1). Posteriorly, its superior extent blends into the parietal lobe to form the posterior limb of the angular gyrus (Fig. 2). T2 is usually poorly separated from the third temporal gyrus (T3) by the second temporal sulcus (S2) which is rather inconsistent and often interrupted by bridges of tissue.

The *third temporal gyrus* (T3) occupies the inferolateral angle of the lobe. The *fourth temporal gyrus* (T4) or fusiform gyrus occupies its inferior surface. Narrow anteriorly where it emerges from the temporal pole, it becomes wider in the direction of the fourth occipital gyrus which has the same arrangement in the opposite direction (Fig. 3). The central portion of these two gyri fuse to form the fusiform lobule (Fig.

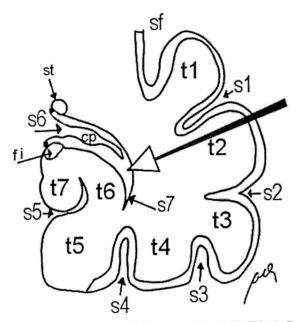

FIG. 1 Circumferential organization of the temporal gyri (T1–T7). t1, first superior or temporal gyrus; t2, second temporal gyrus; t3, third temporal gyrus; t4, fusiform gyrus; t5, parahippocampal gyrus; t6, hippocampus proper; t7, dentate gyrus; fl, fimbria; sf, sylvian fissure; s1, superior temporal sulcus; s2, s3, second and third temporal sulci; s4, collateral fissure; s5, hippocampal sulcus; s6, choroidal fissure; cp, choroid plexus; st, stria terminalis. The *large arrow* indicates the approach for transcortical, transventricular approach amygdalohippocampectomy

3). The fusiform gyrus is usually connected with the third temporal gyrus across the third sulcus (S3) by several anastomotic bridges. On its mesial side, however, it is very well demarcated from the fifth temporal gyrus (parahippocampal gyrus) by the collateral fissure (S4) remarkable by its depth and constancy. Originating in the occipital lobe, this fissure extends forward in the direction of the rhinal sulcus located just in front of the uncus (Figs. 3 and 4). Within the posterior extent of the temporal horn, the deepest part of the collateral fissure pushes the ventricular wall and forms the collateral eminence.

The *fifth temporal gyrus* (T5) is better known under the term of parahippocampal gyrus because of its close relation to the hippocampus proper with which it is continuous. It occupies the inner and inferior portion of the temporal lobe immediately below the hippocampus (Figs. 1 and 10). It is clearly demarcated laterally by the collateral fissure (S4) and mesially by the transverse fissure (ambiens cisterna).

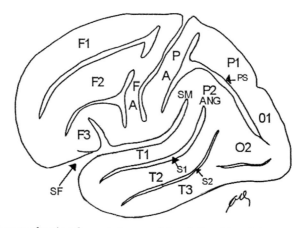

FIG. 2 Diagram showing the main topographic relationships of the temporal lobe with adjacent frontal, central, parietal, and occipital areas. Note the continuum of gyri, *i.e.*, how the first and second temporal gyri blend into the supramarginal and angular gyri and also how the supramarginal gyrus is continuous with the postcentral gyrus (see text). T1, T2, T3, first, second, and third temporal gyri; S1, S2, first and second temporal sulci; FA, precentral gyrus; PA, postcentral gyrus; F1, F2, F3, first, second, and third frontal gyri; 01, 02, first and second occipital gyri; PS, intraparietal sulcus; P1, superior parietal lobule; P2, inferior parietal lobule; SM, supramarginal gyrus; ANG, angular gyrus; SF, sylvian fissure. [Reproduced with permission from Poirier and Charpy (46).]

It is important to realize that its anterior extent does not reach the temporal pole but terminates about 2 cm behind and mesial to it by bending on itself from below upward to form an abrupt elbow, the two limbs of which become in contact to form the uncal sulcus (Figs. 3–5). This bend or genu gives rise to the hippocampal lobule which is demarcated from the temporal pole by the rhinal sulcus. The uncal sulcus contains the hippocampal artery and is continuous posteriorly with the hippocampal sulcus (S5) (Figs. 1, 10, and 12). Thus, the parahippocampal gyrus is separated externally and mesially from the anterior extent of the fourth temporal gyrus and from the temporal pole by the rhinal sulcus which forms a notch at approximately 2 cm behind the temporal pole. This sulcus which runs mainly in the vertical plane extends into the inferior surface of the temporal lobe in the direction of the collateral sulcus without reaching it (Figs. 3 and 4). Posteriorly the parahippocampal gyrus is divided into two parts by the anterior extent of the calcarine sulcus, a superior one which becomes the isthmus of the cingulate gyrus and an inferior one which is continuous with the lingual gyrus of the occipital lobe (Figs. 3 and 4). To

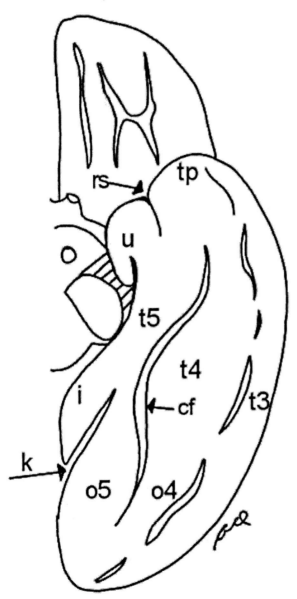

FIG. 3 Ventral aspect of temporal lobe. tp, temporal pole; t3, third temporal gyrus; t4, fourth temporal gyrus (fusiform); t5, fifth temporal gyrus (parahippocampus); o5, fifth occipital gyrus (lingual gyrus); o4, fourth occipital gyrus (fusiform gyrus); i, isthmus; k, proximal segment of calcarine fissure; cf, collateral fissure; u, uncus; tp, temporal pole; rs, rhinal sulcus. Note that the parahippocampal (T5) gyrus does not reach the pole but bends on itself to form the uncus. Posteriorly T5 is divided by the proximal portion of the calcarine fissure (K) to form the isthmus of the cingulate gyrus and the lingual gyrus (o5) of the occipital lobe. Note the course and importance of the collateral fissure (CF). [Reproduced with permission from Poirier and Charpy (46).]

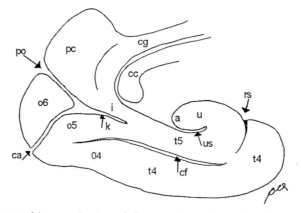

FIG. 4 Topographic organization of the mesial surface of the temporal lobe. The fusiform gyrus (T4) runs from the occipital pole to the temporal pole. The parahippocampal gyrus (T5) does not reach the pole but bends on itself to form the hippocampal lobule (uncus). Posteriorly it is subdivided by the proximal segment of the calcarine sulcus (K) into the isthmus of the cingulate gyrus and the lingual gyrus (o5). u, uncus; a, apex of uncus; us, uncal sulcus; rs, rhinal sulcus; cf, collateral fissure; cg, cingulate gyrus; k, anterior segment of calcarine sulcus; ca, calcarine sulcus; i, isthmus; po, parietooccipital fissure; pc, precuneus; o6, cuneus (sixth occipital gyrus); o5, lingual gyrus (fifth occipital gyrus); o4, fourth occipital gyrus. [Reproduced with permission from (46).]

the parahippocampal gyrus (T5) are annexed specific structures such as the uncus, the hippocampus, the fimbria, and the dentate gyrus.

The uncus is a conical shaped lobule formed by the bending of T5 on itself and corresponds roughly to the hippocampal lobule described above (Figs. 4 and 5). Its dorsomedioventral convex surface can be subdivided into several small gyri including the semilunar gyrus superiorly, the uncinate gyrus inferiorly, and the intralimbic gyrus posteriorly (6). Its apex made by the intralimbic gyrus is continuous with the fimbria, a relationship well seen by retracting the choroid plexus. The hippocampal sulcus (S5) is very deep and pushes inward the ventricular wall giving rise to the hippocampus proper (Figs. 1 and 10). Its two pial walls are usually intimately adherent one to the other and contain numerous small vessels. These pial layers may be separated in cases of hippocampal atrophy. The internal wall of the sulcus is formed by the external surface of the dentate gyrus, while its external wall is formed by cortex of the hippocampus and of the parahippocampal gyrus (subicular area) (Figs. 1 and 10). Its lateral ventricular border corresponds to the ventricular sulcus, a crucial landmark (Figs. 1 and 10). When the ventricle is opened the hippocampus appears as a white bulging structure with a crescent shape and an external convexity. The

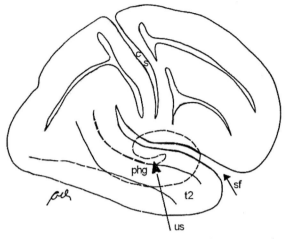

FIG. 5 Projection of parahippocampus gyrus (PHG) and uncus over lateral surface of temporal lobe. sf, sylvian fissure; us, uncal sulcus; t2, second temporal gyrus; cs, central sulcus; phg, parahippocampal gyrus.

hippocampal formation (hippocampus and parahippocampus) surrounds the cerebral peduncle over a distance of about 5 cm.

The *hippocampus* is virtually sitting over the *parahippocampal gyrus* forming a separate convolution (T6) (Figs. 1 and 10). Its anterior portion or head is short and wide with a width of 15–18 mm. It occupies the rostral extent of the temporal horn and blends mesially into the posterior part of the uncus. Over its ventricular surface can be found several small indentations and digitations which are due to the meandering course of the hippocampal artery within the hippocampal sulcus. Its midportion or "body" normally measures 8–10 mm in width and blends posteriorly into a narrower portion called the "tail" which extends backward and upward into the trigone of the ventricle. The fimbria is a narrow flat white band which runs horizontally along the internal border of the hippocampus just above the dentate gyrus. Its dorsal aspect represents the inferior edge of the choroidal fissure (Fig. 10). It terminates anteriorly at the apex of the uncus in relation with the intralimbic gyrus. Posteriorly it is continuous with the fornix.

The *dentate gyrus* (T7) is a C-shaped gray ribbon running parallel and underneath the fimbria and is located between it and the parahippocampal gyrus, from which it is separated by the hippocampal sulcus (Figs. 1 and 10). The term hippocampal formation refers to both the parahippocampal gyrus and hippocampus proper.

Vascular Anatomy of the Temporal Lobe

VENOUS ANATOMY

Prior to carrying out any temporal resection it is important to have a clear idea of the venous pattern of the temporal area which can vary considerably from one patient to another. The superficial sylvian vein is constant and is located over the sylvian fissure. Not infrequently it may run over the first temporal gyrus. Sometimes two veins may run parallel and may empty anteriorly into a single trunk. It receives branches from the suprasylvian (frontocentroparietal) and from the infrasylvian (temporal) areas. It usually drains forward and empties into a sinus at the pole of the middle fossa. Exceptionally this vein will continue to run under the ventral surface of the temporal lobe and empties in the transverse sinus. At times the venous drainage goes backward and downward to the transverse sinus, forming the so-called "vein of L'Abbé." More rarely the predominant drainage is upward toward the superior longitudinal sinus through a vein of Trolard which drains over the central area. The venous drainage over the ventral surface is more difficult to evaluate. One must keep in mind that large veins may be running forward and also emptying at the pole of the temporal lobe. They should be visualized as the resection proceeds and the consequence of their occlusion evaluated. At times it is preferable to simply "skeletonize" a vein and leave it intact. The venous drainage of the mesiobasal areas forms a different entity. The region of the hippocampal formation drains through the vein of Rosenthal which runs in the superior part of the ambiens cisterna. This vein as well as the deep sylvian veins are not in the surgical field, and only their tributaries need to be visualized. These are the sulcal veins in the region of the collateral fissure, hippocampal fissure, and endorhinal sulcus.

ARTERIAL ANATOMY AS IT APPLIES TO TEMPORAL RESECTIONS

The *M1 segment* or horizontal segment of the middle cerebral artery corresponds to the anterosuperior limit of the amygdala region (Fig. 6). It is important to keep in mind the position and orientation of its lenticulostriate branches in the resection of the most dorsal part of the amygdala.

The *M2 segments* (usually two in number) run within the sylvian fissure over the insula and should be visualized subpially in the removal of the first temporal gyrus.

The *M3 segment* run from the edges of the insula (circular sulcus) to the superior temporal sulcus. These can be seen subpially as the T1 gyrus is resected. They should be clearly visualized in the subarachnoidal space as they run over and around the first temporal gyrus, passing underneath the sylvian veins.

The *M4 segments* correspond to the intrasulcal branches within the superior temporal sulcus (S1) and their continuation over the second gyrus (T2).

The anterior *choroidal artery* takes its origin from the internal carotid just before it branches into middle and anterior cerebral arter-

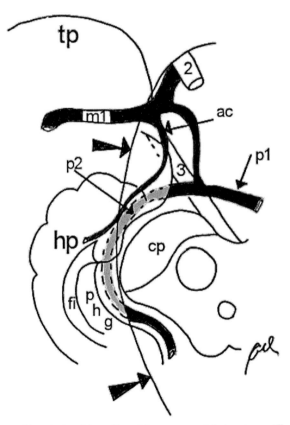

FIG. 6 Topographic relationships of basal temporomesial structures. The m1 segment of the middle cerebral artery (m1) (within the sylvian fissure) corresponds to the anterosuperior border of the amygdala region. The posterior cerebral artery runs along the posterior and inferior border of the uncus and within the ambiens cisterna along the mesial border of the parahippocampus gyrus. The anterior choroidal artery runs over the dorsomedial part of the amygdalouncal complex. The ventromedial part of the uncus is sitting over the third nerve. Note the relative position of the free edge of tentorium indicated by the *large arrows*. tp, temporal pole; 2, optic nerve; 3, oculomotor nerve; ac, anterior choroidal artery; hp, hippocampus; fi, fimbria; phg, parahippocampal gyrus.

ies. It runs over the dorsomedial surface of the amygdala within the endorhinal sulcus before entering the temporal horn just behind the dorsal and posterior aspect of the amygdala where it forms the "choroidal point" by giving rise to numerous branches that form the choroid plexus (Fig. 6).

The choroidal point is an important surgical landmark. It is located at the anterior limit of the choroidal fissure where the fimbria and stria terminalis join to form the velum terminale (6). The choroid plexus in itself is also a crucial landmark. By retracting it mesially (upward), the fimbria and choroidal fissure can be visualized, and by retracting it laterally over the hippocampus the stria terminalis can be seen (Fig. 7). By pulling backward its anterior extent, the entrance of the anterior choroidal artery in the ventricle can be visualized as well as the region of the velum terminale. One should also be familiar with the anatomy of the posterior communicating artery and its relationship with the ventral portion as well as the course of both P1 and P2 segments of the posterior cerebral artery as they course within the crural and ambiens cisterna along the cerebral peduncle (Fig. 6). Usually, the hippocampal artery arises from the P1 segment close to the free edge of the tentorium.

DIFFERENT MODALITIES OF TEMPORAL RESECTION

Several modalities of cortical resections have evolved in the surgical treatment of temporal lobe epilepsy from the standard lobectomy to the selective amygdalohippocampectomy. We will review the main modalities of cortical resection with emphasis on the rationale, anatomic features, and technical aspects.

In reviewing the series of patients on whom we operated for temporal lobe epilepsy, it was found appropriate to subdivide these patients into specific categories according to the surgical modality used. This also includes cases where an obvious lesion, static or tumoral, was encountered.

"Temporal lobectomy" as the word implies is the removal of the entirety of the temporal lobe. Thus, this term should be reserved to designate a total removal of the temporal lobe, including all gyri and limbic structures. This is a rare occurrence nowadays. The term "anterior temporal lobectomy" is also a misnomer from the anatomic standpoint. It is preferable to use the term "temporal resection" indicating more specifically the extent of cortex and limbic structures that has been removed.

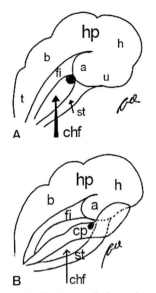

FIG. 7 (**A**) To illustrate how the fimbria and the stria terminalis correspond to the edges of the choroidal fissure (CHF) and how they merge at the apex of the uncus. chf, choroidal fissure; st, stria terminalis; h,b,t, head, body, and tail of hippocampus; a, apex of uncus; fi, fimbria; hp, hippocampus; u, uncus. The *black dot* represents entrance of the anterior choroidal artery in the fissure. (**B**) Relationship of the choroid plexus (cp) with the choroidal fissure (chf). When the plexus is displaced mesially the fimbria (fi) is visualized. When displayed laterally the region of the stria terminalis (st) is seen. When its anterior extent is displaced posteriorly, the anterior edge of the fissure and the region of the apex of the uncus (a) is seen. hp, hippocampus; h, head of hippocampus; b, body of hippocampus; a, apex of uncus; chf, choroidal fissure.

Corticoamygdalohippocampectomy (CAH)

CAH corresponds to the standard temporal procedure carried out at the Montreal Neurological Institute over the years (Figs 8 and 9). Essentially it is a temporal neocortical resection which extends habitually 4.5 cm along the sylvian fissure on the dominant side and 5 cm on the nondominant hemisphere (27–30, 32, 42, 43). The resection is performed typically by the technique of gyral emptying with subpial aspiration of cortex (56). The procedure is accomplished by bipolar coagulation and perforation of both the arachnoid and pia along the first temporal gyrus. With an ultrasound dissector (CUSA, Valleylab, Richmond Hill, Ontario) the gyral content is removed along a series of small transarachnoidpial holes (Fig. 8). Once the cortex has been fragmented and resected with ultrasound, one proceeds with the division of the small opercular branches of the middle cerebral artery corresponding to segment M3 and running from the sylvian fissure to the superior temporal sulcus underneath the sylvian vein. In dividing these arterial branches it is important to leave a sufficient arterial stump in case bleeding occurs during their division in order not to damage the sylvian vein. At this stage of the procedure, it is also important to study the pattern of bypassing arteries and veins in order to avoid subsequent ischemic changes behind the line of resection. The posterior line of resection is extended downward across the superior temporal sulcus and the lateral gyri to the collateral fissure. At this point both upper and lower surfaces of the superior sulcus are exposed, coagulated, and divided. The line of incision is brought forward through the fusiform gyrus. The first temporal gyrus is further emptied exposing the M2 branches of the middle cerebral artery. This dissection is carried out subpially leaving intact these vascular trunks. The temporal white matter peduncle is easily identified under the lower M2 trunk and is transected in the direction of the temporal horn. The neocortex is then resected "en bloc."

Opening of the temporal horn is usually facilitated by following the collateral fissure. The ventricle is usually just dorsal to the bottom of the exposed fissure. (Fig. 10). The surgical landmarks of the limbic structures become clear by elevating the roof of the temporal horn and

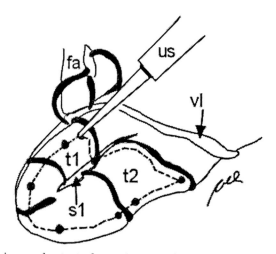

FIG. 8 Technique and extent of resection over the temporal cortex. A series of pial perforations is made and joined with the ultrasound dissector (us). Sulci and gyri are defined by the perigyral and intrasulcal course of the temporal arteries. Recognition of their course provides anatomic landmarks and ensures complete hemostasis during the resection. fa, precentral gyrus; t1, first (superior) temporal gyrus; t2, second temporal gyrus; s1, superior temporal sulcus; us, ultrasound dissector (cusa); vl, vein of L'Abbé. *Dotted line,* line of cortical excision.

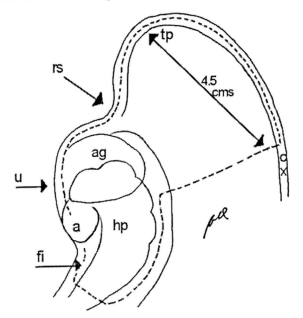

FIG. 9 Transverse diagram showing the habitual extent of cortical and limbic resections in corticoamygdalohippocampectomy in dominant hemispheres. The extent of resection along the sylvian fissure is based on recognition of the precentral sulcus rather than preresection measurements which can be misleading. cx, temporal cortex; hp, hippocampus; fi, fimbria; u, uncus; ag, amygdala; a, apex of uncus (intralimbic gyrus); rs, rhinal sulcus.

displacing upward the choroid plexus to expose the fimbria (Figs. 7A and B, 10). The space lateral to the hippocampus is called the lateral ventricular cleft and is limited ventrally by the ventricular sulcus which is a crucial surgical landmark (Fig. 10). The space anterior to the hippocampus is the anterior cleft. The posteroinferior edge of the amygdala corresponds to the anterior border of the temporal horn where it usually forms a mild bulge. The first step in the removal of the hippocampal formation consists in dissecting just lateral to the ventricular sulcus over the collateral eminence. Using the ultrasonic dissector an endopial resection of the parahippocampal gyrus is then performed from backward to forward mesial to the collateral fissure (Fig. 10, 12). In this manner the tentorium edge and the ambiens cisterna are exposed subpially. Care is taken not to damage the posterior cerebral artery located at the mesial border of the parahippocampal gyrus. The hippocampus proper is then tilted laterally into the parahippocampal cavity which provides better visualization of the fimbria. The line of transection is extended mesially through the

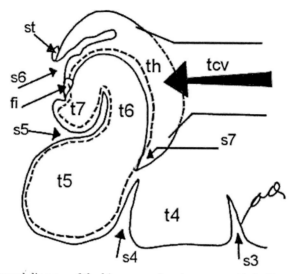

Fɪɢ. 10 Coronal diagram of the hippocampal region proper. t4, fusiform gyrus (fourth temporal gyrus); t5, parahippocampal gyrus; t6, hippocampus proper; t7, dentate gyrus; fi, fimbria; s3, third temporal sulcus; s4, collateral fissure (fourth temporal sulcus); s5, hippocampal fissure; s6, choroidal fissure; s7, ventricular sulcus; th, temporal horn. The *large arrow* indicates the transcortical transventricular approach for selective amygdalohippocampectomy (TCV). The *dotted line* shows the extent of resection of the hippocampal formation.

fimbria and dentate gyrus exposing the entrance of the hippocampal sulcus. The hippocampus body or tail is transected and then lifted upward and forward, bringing in sight the hippocampal sulcus which becomes a most important landmark. Posteriorly the hippocampal sulcus is a virtual space which opens anteriorly into the large uncal sulcus which contains the hippocampal arteries and veins. By lifting up the hippocampus, the small arteries and veins entering and leaving the core of the hippocampus are clearly visualized, coagulated, or simply teased off the hippocampus. By extending the dissection anterior to the sulcus, the uncus is then entered. A radical resection of the uncus is carried out again by endopial aspiration with the ultrasound instrument (Fig. 12). This maneuver is simplified by identifying the anterior extent of the fimbria which leads into the conical posterior aspect of the uncus called the apex (Fig. 7**A** and **B**). The free edge of the tentorium is also and important landmark. The uncus can be carefully emptied with the ultrasonic dissector set at very low parameters, *i.e.*, vibration and suction set at 10–15% of the full strength. Meticulous care should be taken to recognize the cerebral peduncle which is visualized through the pia of the ambiens or crural cisternae. More anteriorly the apex of the uncus merges into the ambiens gyrus which is mesial to the free edge of the tentorium, anterior to the cerebral peduncle and dorsal to the oculomotor nerve (Fig. 6). By leaving the pia intact and resecting only the cortex, the basal cisterna can be clearly identified first along the free edge of the tentorium seen through the pia. The oculomotor nerve is visualized and follows back to the first segment of the posterior cerebral artery (P1) (Fig. 6). The resection of the uncus takes care of the removal of most of the amygdala since the anterior portion of the uncus is in part the mesial extension of the amygdala. Surgically the anterior border of the amygdala area corresponds to the sylvian vallecula which contains the M1 segment of the middle cerebral artery. Dorsally, its limits can only be defined by identifying the endorhinal sulcus located over the dorsomesial extent of the uncus proper. To properly assess and carry out the resection of the dorsal extent of the amygdala, the entrance of the anterior choroidal artery in the ventricle must be visualized and if possible its courses followed within the endorhinal (supraamygdalar) sulcus.

Corticoamygdalectomy (CA)

The corticoamygdalectomy as the name implies consists in an anterior temporal cortical resection combined to a removal of the amygdala with sparing of the hippocampal formation proper. Usually the neocortical resection itself has been rather limited to the anterior 4–4.5 cm of cortex. We have used this modality of resection mainly in patients with severe memory impairment and more specifically in those who have failed the ipsilateral amytal test for memory. Work from our institution (23) has shown that this modality when used in patients with fragile memory has been of some help in controlling the seizure tendency while avoiding memory disturbance. Overall, however, the results on seizure tendency have not been satisfactory. In this procedure the cortical resection is carried out along the sylvian fissure but is limited to the anterior 4–4.5 cm of the three temporal gyri. The temporal horn is opened for purpose of identifying the hippocampus proper which is left undisturbed as well as the corresponding extent of the parahippocampal gyrus. As complete as possible a resection of the amygdala and of the uncus is carried out. It is practically impossible to avoid encroachment of the anterior part of the hippocampus within the uncus itself.

Selective Amygdalohippocampectomy (SeAH)

As mentioned earlier this procedure was introduced by P. Niemeyer in the mid-1950s and represented a significant departure from the standard lobectomy which was in vogue at that time (Figs. 11 and 12). Niemeyer and Niemeyer and Bello (25, 26) suggested a transcortical approach through the second temporal gyrus approaching the hippocampus and the amygdala transventricularly.

Yasargil has developed a different approach to perform the amygdalo-hippocampectomy by using the transsylvian route (72). By dividing the arachnoid over the sylvian fissure the bottom of the circular sulcus is exposed. An incision is then made in between two opercular temporal arteries, the temporal peduncle is transected and the ventricular horn exposed. The hippocampal formation is then resected by an extrapial approach as far laterally as the collateral fissure. The amygdala is removed by subpial aspiration.

For the performance of selective amygdalohippocampectomy we have adopted an approach similar to that suggested by Niemeyer (33, 35). A key-hole incision measuring 2–3 cm is made either within the depth of the first temporal sulcus (S1) or preferably along the upper border of the second temporal gyrus (T2) just below the sulcus and in front of the central sulcus. (Figs. 1 and 12) By using the ultrasonic dissector, a corridor of approximately 4–5 mm in height is fashioned down to the ependymal lining which is also opened with the same instrument (Figs. 10 and 12). Retractors are then inserted which

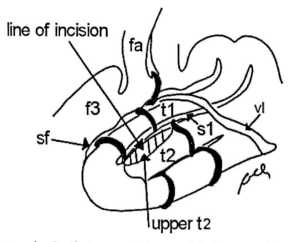

FIG. 11 Diagram showing the transcortical approach to the temporal horn for selective amygdalohippocampectomy. The incision is made in the superior part of t2, along the superior temporal sulcus (s1) anterior to the central sulcus. t1, t2, first and second temporal gyri; fa, precentral gyrus; f3, third frontal gyrus; vl, vein of L'Abbé; s1, first superior temporal sulcus; p2, inferior parietal lobule; t1, superior temporal gyrus; t2, second temporal gyrus; sf, sylvian fissure.

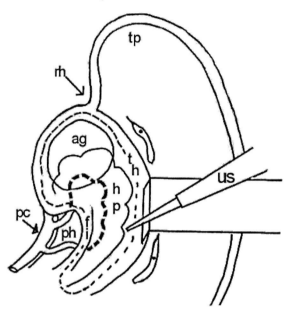

FIG. 12 Diagram in the transverse plane to illustrate the transventricular approach for amygdalohippocampectomy using a strictly subpial approach with ultrasonic dissector. rh, rhinal sulcus; ag, amygdala; tp, temporal pole; us, ultrasound (cusa); ph, parahippocampal gyrus; fi, fimbria; pc, posterior cerebral artery; hp, hippocampus.

provide unobstructed view of the hippocampus proper (Fig. 12). The serial anatomic landmarks for the hippocampal removal are then established in a stepwise fashion. First the lateral ventricular sulcus located between the hippocampus proper and the lateral wall of the horn is identified (Fig. 10). Then the fimbria and the apex of the uncus are visualized on the inner side by lifting up the choroid plexus (Fig. 7**A** and **B**). The ependymal lining must be opened sufficiently to see the bulge of the amygdala and the tip of the horn anteriorly and also the beginning of the hippocampal tail posteriorly. The resection proper is done as described previously by transecting just lateral to the ventricular sulcus and carrying out an endopial intragyral removal of the parahippocampal gyrus along its anteroposterior extent (Figs. 10 and 12). In dissecting the cortex mesially within the parahippocampal gyrus care is taken not to injure the posterior cerebral artery which runs over its mesial border (Fig. 6). It can be visualized through the pia. Dissection is then carried out forward into the parahippocampal gyrus, and the anterior portion of the uncus is entered. The hippocampus proper is then tilted laterally into the empty cavity of the parahippocampal gyrus revealing the fimbria which is transected along its length exposing the medial part of the dentate gyrus. It is transected at the junction of the body and the tail and then lifted up exposing the perforating vessels arising from the hippocampal artery. These are coagulated and divided or simply teased out, and the sulcus is followed forward inside the uncus. At this point, the content of the anterior portion of the uncus is also resected by a subpial aspiration care being taken not to endanger the cerebral peduncle. The entire content of the uncus is emptied, including the segment which fills the basal cisterna. Extreme care should be taken to identify the dorsomesial extent of the amygdala which corresponds to the endorhinal sulcus in order to perform a radical removal of the amygdala itself. A reliable landmark in this area is the entrance of the anterior choroidal artery into the ventricular cavity, where it fans out to form the choroidal plexus (choroidal point). If further resection of the posterior extent of the hippocampus and parahippocampal gyrus is desired, it is achieved by subependymal and endopial aspiration backward in the direction of the tectal cisterna, along the cerebral peduncle and the P2 segment of the posterior cerebral artery. The posterior extent of the hippocampal formation resection corresponds to the lateral mesencephalic sulcus which runs vertically between the cerebral peduncle and the tectum.

Secondary Amygdalohippocampectomy (SecAH)

REOPERATIONS IN TEMPORAL LOBE EPILEPSY

Further insight into the role of the hippocampal formation and uncus in temporal lobe epilepsy has been gained on the basis of reoperations when only or predominantly the hippocampus and uncus were resected (13, 40, 41, 67).

This procedure can be performed safely through a small dural opening over the previous surgical cavity. Only the temporal extent of the craniotomy needs to be opened. In doing these procedures it is most important to carry out the dural opening as anterior and inferior as possible to avoid damage to the middle artery branches which may have sagged downward in the cavity and which may be adherent to the dura. For any reoperation if no previous operative photographs are available it is recommended to perform an angiogram in order to assess the presence of a vein of L'Abbé and the configuration of the sylvian vein. Once the intracavity membranous formations have been dissected and the ventricular horn reopened, the same technique described above for the removal of limbic structures is followed.

Tailored Resection Associated with a Lesion in the Temporal Lobe

The advent of MRI has forced neurosurgeons to consider various tailored resections most appropriate for a visualized lesion. Within the confines of the temporal lobe, two broad types of removal associated with a lesion can be recognized depending on the proximity of this lesion to the limbic structures. If the lesion is superficial and involves the neocortex only or if it is located at the posterior extent of the temporal lobe it appears preferable to remove only the lesion and the gliotic tissue surrounding it, especially if this lesion is well demarcated such as is often the case with cavernous hemangiomas or hamartomas. On the other hand, if the lesion is also of small volume but located within the limbic structures or in their immediate vicinity it is preferable to remove both the lesion and the amygdala and the hippocampal formation. Further studies are needed to determine which is the optimal approach. It may very well be that each case will need to be considered on an individual basis. Whatever the nature and extent of these lesions, the same endopial approach described above should be used.

USE OF IMAGE-GUIDED SURGERY IN TEMPORAL LOBE EPILEPSY

We have published elsewhere the use of a frameless stereotaxic technique in the surgical treatment of epilepsy (34, 36). This modality of image-guided surgery (ISG (Allegro Viewing Wand), Mississauga, Ontario) has been particularly useful for procedures on the temporal lobe. This approach has been useful for centering the craniotomy in relation to the underlying temporal and central gyri (Fig. 13). It has been particularly useful to reduce the size of the craniotomy in selective amygdalohippocampectomy and to center the cortical incision along the anteroposterior extent of the upper T2 gyrus and in front of the central sulcus, particularly in the dominant hemisphere. The use of a stereotaxic pointer has facilitated the entrance to the ventricle and has helped to verify the position of surgical instruments during the procedure and to determine with precision both the anterior and posterior extent of the resection along the brainstem (Fig. 14). This technique has also been useful to determine and measure precisely the extent of neocortical resection along the floor and along the sylvian fissure. Finally, it can be used to place acute depth electrodes with a greater precision within the amygdala and hippocampus and to archive data generated by recording and stimulation during electrocorticography (34, 36).

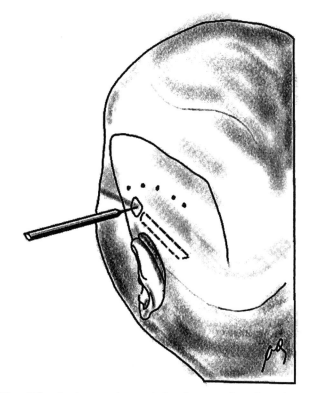

Fig. 13 Use of the viewing wand to optimize the centering of craniotomy and assess location of cerebral structures including sulci and gyri. For example, the relative position of the amygdala, hippocampus, and sylvian fissure can be displayed over the scalp.

COMPLICATIONS

In a personal series of 811 craniotomies and resective procedures for epilepsy on the temporal lobe, the number of complications that can be devised in a surgical and neurologic group has been very low. Of significance, there have been a series of 11 scalp infections, 5 cases of osteomyelitis, 3 cases of subdural empyemas, and 6 cases of epidural hematomas.

Fortunately, there has been no instance of mortality nor significant permanent neurologic morbidity. We estimate that the number of cases of transient postoperative dysphasia in procedures done on the dominant lobe has been well below 10%. No patient has had a persistent incapacitating dysphasia. Similarly with the approach used, there is no instance of clinically significant visual field deficits.

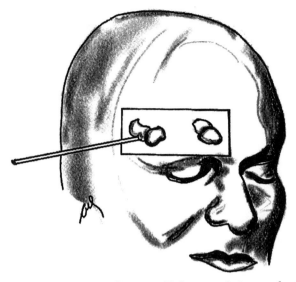

FIG. 14 To illustrate the concept of image-guided surgery in temporal epilepsy. Structures of interest (here the hippocampus and the amygdala) can be reconstructed, color-coded, and targeted with a pointer. This technique is of considerable help in ingraining three-dimensional surgical anatomy and in defining surgical approaches.

In our series of now over 130 cases of selective amygdalohippocampectomy there has been no visual field deficit, one case of transient third nerve paresis associated with the removal of a ganglioglioma of the uncus, and three instances of transient dysphasia including one case of severe anomia which lasted for 2 weeks.

RESULTS ON SEIZURE TENDENCY

In presenting the results on seizure tendency we have used the following classification:

Class 1: seizure free

Class 2: rare seizures (maximum 3/year)

Class 3: >90% seizure reduction (without monthly seizure)

Class 4: 60–90% or more seizure reduction (with monthly seizures)

Class 5: <60% seizure reduction (without significant improvement in quality of life)

The presence of an aura was documented preoperatively in 88% of all categories of temporal resections. After a radical resection of the amygdala (4/5) associated with hippocampal resection the aura disappeared in 84% of these cases (Tables 1, 2).

TABLE 1

Results of Temporal Resection (703 Patients Followed Up for a Minimum of 1 yr)

Type of Surgery	No. Patients	CL 1 (%)	CL 2 (%)	CL 3 (%)	CL 4 (%)	CL 5 (%)
CA	114	40	3	5	18	34
CAH	391	77	8	5	7	3
Seeah	109	85	5	3	3	4
SecAH (reop)	89	62	14	10	9	5

TABLE 2

Postoperative Medication (591 Patients Followed up for a Minimum, of 1 yr)

Medication	%	%
None	36	
Being tapered	20	
Less	25	
Arrested or reduced		81
Same	11	
More	3	
Different	5	

Of the 602 patients to whom a questionnaire was sent, 540 (89.7%) replied. To the question *"Do you feel that, on the overall, you have benefitted from the operation? If yes, in what sense?"* 510 patients or 94.4% answered yes and 30 or 5.6% replied no. Memory was felt to be subjectively the same or better in 83.7%, and it was felt to be worse in 16.3%.

DISCUSSION

In 1954 Penfield (28) indicated on the basis of a second operation that further hippocampal removal could transform a failed operation into a successful one. In the ensuing years, instead of extending the idea of removing the hippocampus in a more radical fashion, the trend was to do a "temporal lobectomy" with sparing of the hippocampus. This approach stemmed from the work of Scoville and Milner (60) and Penfield and Milner (45) which stressed the risk for memory after bilateral hippocampal damage. Nevertheless, by 1958, Niemeyer and Bello (25, 26) had suggested a selective removal of the amygdala and hippocampus on the basis of available clinical and experimental evidence for the crucial role of the amygdala and hippocampus in seizures of temporal lobe origin. Feindel studying Penfield's material had also demonstrated the paramount role played by the amygdala in the temporal lobe automatisms and seizures (9, 10).

The standard procedure for temporal resection used in most centers had been that of "en bloc" resection preconized among others by M. Falconer (8) and later by Polkey in England and Price *et al.* (47, 48) and Crandall (12) in the United States. At the Montreal Neurological Institute, the standard technique has been that of an anterior temporal resection including the amygdala and the anterior hippocampus. This approach departed from the "en bloc" resection due to the fact that it was carried out mainly as a subpial aspiration of the mesiobasal structures. At MNI, until the mid-1970s, the extent of hippocampal resection was based mainly on the degree of epileptiform activity detected during electrocorticography following initial removal and could vary from an anterior to a total removal of the hippocampus (Rasmussen).

Also at the MNI, this author in a series of 200 consecutive cases between 1971 and 1981 a standard approach to temporal resection was used where a maximum of 4.5 cm of cortex was removed on the dominant side with usually a resection of 1.5–2 cm of the hippocampus and sometimes more (27).

In the author's present updated series of 739 patients, 10% have had a removal of the amygdala only, and of those who had a removal of the hippocampus, 69% had a minimum of 2.5 cm removed.

In 1984, Spencer in a series of 36 patients also suggested that the resection of lateral cortex could be limited to 4.5 cm over the lateral cortex and recommended a radical removal of the hippocampus through this limited anterior cortical resection (64).

Our work with chronic depth electrode recording has indeed confirmed the overwhelming predominance of temporal seizure onset from limbic structures (37, 39, 62). In patients with bitemporal epilepsy it has been shown that the seizures arise predominantly from one temporal lobe and within that temporal lobe from the amygdala or hippocampus in more than 80% of the time (62). Seizures of neocortical onset have been relatively rare but well documented. We have used extensively the technique of preoperative sphenoidal recording electrocorticography with surface and depth electrodes to define the level of onset of seizures. Combining these approaches and relying more and more heavily on the morphologic changes seen in the limbic structures on MRI we have carried out more and more frequently the transcortical selective amygdalohippocampectomy which has become the procedure of choice in cases of mesiotemporal limbic epilepsy, *i.e.*, when the seizure pattern, the EEG findings, and the morphologic stigmata are congruent. The final outcome of these different approaches needs to be further studied.

The problem of lesionectomy or removal of a lesion and its surrounding tissue is being studied at different centers at the present time. In many instances the mere removal of the lesion can arrest or control the seizure, but it has not been demonstrated yet in a large series to what extent the results obtained are superior when the lesion and the entire epileptic area are resected. When a superficial lesion appears to be the source of seizures and if the same lesion has a potential for bleeding or is suspected of being a tumor, the approach of choice is to perform a radical removal of that lesion and await for the result on the seizure tendency. Should seizures persist a second operation would be justified. For lesions located in the immediate vicinity of the amygdala and hippocampus it would appear preferable to remove both the lesion and the amygdala and hippocampus especially if these structures are reduced in volume. However, it appears preferable to leave the hippocampus alone if it is not encroached or reduced in size when the dominant temporal lobe is involved. Again further studies are needed to confirm or invalidate this approach. Whatever the nature, location, and extent of a temporal lesion causing seizures, the same endopial approach should be followed with strict adherence to the sequence of landmarks described above.

CONCLUSION

Temporal resections are no longer considered as a single standard type of resective procedure. The temporal "en bloc" lobectomy may still have its place in specific instances. However, the advances in intracranial recording and in brain imaging and consideration of patients with impaired memory has imposed upon the surgeon to consider various types of resections individualized for each specific patient. Thus, procedures such as corticoamygdalectomy or corticoamygdalohippocampectomy have been implemented. Over the last decade there has been a definite trend in reducing the extent of neocortical resection and increasing the amount of limbic structure removal. This has led surgeons in many centers to use more and more frequently selective limbic removal by a variety of approaches. We have found that the transcortical T2 or transsulcal S1 approach was entirely satisfactory from the technical standpoint and could be performed with the use of an ultrasound dissector. This technique differs from that developed by Yasargil in that it is a transventricular subependymal and entirely subpial procedure minimizing the manipulations of the sylvian and brainstem vessels. In both approaches, a transcortical incision has to be done. The amount of white matter fibers disruption may in fact be less with the direct transcortical approach as compared with the transsylvian one which involves the transection of the temporal white matter peduncle.

Finally, the display of small epileptogenic lesions potentially tumoral or vascular in nature has been a definite incentive to carry out more restricted resections limited to the lesion and the immediate surrounding gliotic tissue. This may be entirely satisfactory as a first-stage approach which could be followed by a second operation at a later date if the need arises. When such a small lesion is located within or in the immediate vicinity of the limbic structures it appears preferable to remove both the lesions and the low threshold limbic structures.

Reoperation and further removal of limbic structures can be done safely if a meticulous technique is used to avoid damage to both venous and arterial vessels. Assuming that the proper indications have been followed in the patient selection, the use of the technique described in this chapter will lead to a high degree of success on seizure tendency with minimal morbidity.

The understanding and proper use of the ultrasonic endopial technique are intimately related to a practical knowledge of arterial and venous anatomy of the brain. The same approach is used for removal of glial tumors that occupy the gyri and the vascular malformations that basically occupy sulci. The endopial technique is the basis of the microsurgical approach to the brain itself.

REFERENCES

1. Abou-Kalil B, Andermann E, Andermann F, *et al.:* Temporal lobe epilepsy after prolonged febrile convulsions: Excellent outcome following surgical treatment. **Epilepsia** 34(5):878–883, 1993.

2. Babb TL: Research on the anatomy and pathology of epileptic tissue, In Lüders H (ed): *Epilepsy Surgery.* New York, Raven Press, 1991, 719–727.

3. Berkovic SF, Andermann F, Olivier A, *et al.:* Hippocampal sclerosis in temporal lobe epilepsy demonstrated by magnetic resonance imaging. **Ann Neurol** 29:175–182, 1991.

4. Cadilhac J: Hippocampe et épilepsie. Montpellier, France, Imprimerie Paul Dehan, 1955, p 205.

5. Corsellis JAN: The incidence of Ammon's horn sclerosis. **Brain** 80:193–208, 1957.

6. Duvernoy H: The human hippocampus. Munich, Germany, J. F. Bergman Verlag, 1988, pp 166.

7. Earle KM, Baldwin M, Penfield W: Incisural sclerosis and temporal lobe seizures produced by hippocampal herniation at birth. **Arch Neurol Psychiatry** 69:27–42, 1953.

8. Falconer MA, Hill D, Meyer A, *et al.:* Treatment of temporal lobe epilepsy by temporal lobectomy: Survey of findings and results. **Lancet** 1:827–835, 1955.

9. Feindel W, Penfield W: Localization of discharge in temporal lobe automatism. **Arch Neurol Psychiatry** 72:605–630, 1954.

10. Feindel W, Penfield W, Jasper H: Localization of epileptic discharge in temporal lobe automatism. *Transactions of the American Neurological Association*, 1952, pp 14–17.
11. Gale K: Subcortical structures and pathways involved in convulsive seizure generation. **J Clin Neurophysiol** 9(2):264–277, 1992.
12. Gastaut HR, Vigouroux R, Naquet R: Lésions épileptogènes amygdalo-hippocampiques provoquées chez le chat par l'injection de "créme d'albumine". **Rev Neurol** 87:607–609, 1952.
13. Germano I, Poulin N, Olivier A: Reoperation for recurrent temporal lobe epilepsy. **J Neurosurg** 81:31–36, 1994.
14. Gloor P, Olivier A, Quesney LF, *et al.*: The role of the limbic system in experimental phenomena of temporal lobe epilepsy. **Ann Neurol** 12(2):129–144, 1982.
15. Green JD, Shimamoto T: Hippocampal seizures and their propagation. **Arch Neurol Psychiatry** 7:687–702, 1953.
16. Halgren E, Walter RD, Cherlow DG, *et al.*: Mental phenomena evoked by electrical stimulation of the human hippocampal formation and amygdala. **Brain** 101:83–117, 1978.
17. Houser CR, Miyashiro JE, Swartz BE, *et al.*:Altered patterns of dynorphin immunoreactivity suggest mossy fiber reorganization in human hippocampal epilepsy. **J Neurosci** 10:267–282, 1990.
18. Insausti R: Comparative anatomy of the entorhinal cortex and hippocampus in mammals (Review). **Hippocampus** 3(Spec No):19–26, 1993.
19. Ives JR, Thompson CJ, Gloor P, *et al.*: The on-line computer detection and recording of spontaneous temporal lobe epileptic seizures from patients with implanted depth electrodes via a radiotelemetry link. **EEG J** 37:199–213, 1974.
20. Jackson JH, Colman WS: Case of epilepsy with tasting movements and "dreamy state" with very small patch of softening in the left uncinate gyrus. **Brain** 21:580–590, 1898.
21. Jasper HH, Kershmann J: Electroencephalographic classification of the epilepsies. **Arch Neurol Psychiatry** 45:903–943, 1941.
22. Kaada BR: Somatomotor, autonomic and electrographic responses to electrical stimulation of "rhinencephalic" and other structures in primates, cat and dog: A study of responses from limbic, subcallosal, orbito-insular, pyriform and temporal cortex, hippocampus, fornix and amygdala. **Acta Physiol Scand Suppl** 83:1–285, 1951.
23. Kim H-I, Olivier A, Jones-Gotman M, *et al.*: Corticoamygdalectomy in memory-impaired patients. **Stereotact Funct Neurosurg** 58:162–167, 1992.
24. Morris AA: Temporal lobectomy with removal of uncus, hippocampus and amygdala. **Arch Neurol Psychiatry** 76:479–496, 1956.
25. Niemeyer P: The transventricular amygdalo-hippocampectomy in temporal lobe epilepsy, In Baldwin M, Bailey P (eds): *Temporal Lobe Epilepsy*. Springfield, IL, Charles C Thomas, 1958, 461–482.
26. Niemeyer P, Bello H: Amygdalo-hippocampectomy in temporal lobe epilepsy. Microsurgical technique. **Excerpta Medica** 293:20(abst 48), 1973.
27. Olivier A: Surgical management of complex partial seizures, In A. R. Nistico G, Di Perri R, Meinardi H (eds): *Epilepsy: An Update on Research and Therapy*. New York, Liss, 1983, pp 315–323.

28. Olivier A: Commentary: Cortical resections, In Engel J Jr (ed): *Surgical Techniques in the Epilepsies.* New York, Raven Press, 1986, pp 405–416.

29. Olivier A: Risk and benefit in the surgery of epilepsy: Complications and positive results on seizures tendency and intellectual function. **Acta Neurol Scand** 78(suppl 117):114–121, 1988.

30. Olivier A: Surgery of epilepsy: Methods. **Acta Neurol Scand** 78(suppl 117):103–113, 1988.

31. Olivier A: Relevance of removal of limbic structures in surgery for temporal lobe epilepsy. **Can J Neurol Sci** 18:628–635, 1991.

32. Olivier A: Surgery of the mesial temporal epilepsy, In Shorvon S, Dreifuss F, Fish D, *et al.* (eds): *The Treatment of Epilepsy.* London, 1996, vol 53, pp 689–698.

33. Olivier A: Standardized versus focus resection in the surgery of temporal lobe epilepsy, In Pawlik G, Stefan H (eds): *Focus Localization: Multimethodological Assessment of Localization-Related Epilepsy.* Berlin, Germany, 1996, 383–402.

34. Olivier A, Alonso-Vanegas M, Comeau R, *et al.*: Image-guided surgery of epilepsy. **Neurosurg Clin North Am** 7(2):229–243, 1996.

35. Olivier A, Cukiert A, Palomino-Torres X, *et al.*: Transcortical selective amygdalo-hippocampectomy: Microsurgical technique and results (abstr.). *Proceedings of the American Epilepsy Association.* Seattle, December 1992.

36. Olivier A, Germano I, Cukiert A, *et al.*: Frameless stereotaxy for surgery of the epilepsies: Preliminary experience. Technical note. **J Neurosurg** 81:629–633, 1994.

37. Olivier A, Gloor P, Ives J: Investigation et traitement chirurgical de l'épilepsie bitemporale. **Union Med** 109:1–4, 1980.

38. Olivier A, Gloor P, Ives JP: Stereotaxic seizure monitoring in patients with "bitemporal epilepsy." Indications, techniques and results. **Proc Am Assoc Neurol Surg,** no 14, Toronto, 1977.

39. Olivier A, Gloor P, Quesney LF, *et al.*: The indications for and the role of depth electrode recording in epilepsy. **Appl Neurophysiol** 46:33–36, 1983.

40. Olivier A, Tanaka T, Andermann F: Reoperations in temporal lobe epilepsy (abstr.). **Epilepsia** 29:678, 1988.

41. Olivier A, Tanaka T, Andermann F: The significance of limbic structure removal in the surgery of temporal lobe epilepsy, based on reoperations. *Proceedings of the Xth Meeting of the World Society for Stereotactic and Functional Neurosurgery.* Maebashi, Japan, October, 1989, p 171.

42. Penfield W, Baldwin M: Temporal lobe seizures and the technique of subtemporal lobectomy. **Ann Surg** 134:625–634, 1952.

43. Penfield W, Flanagin H: Surgical therapy of temporal lobe seizures. **Arch Neurol Psychiatry** 64:491–500, 1950.

44. Penfield W, Jasper H: *Epilepsy and the Functional Anatomy of the Human Brain.* Boston, Little Brown, 1954, pp 815–816.

45. Penfield W, Milner B: Memory deficit produced by bilateral lesions in the hippocampal zone. **Arch Neurol Psychiatry** 79:475–497, 1958.

46. Poirier P, Charpy A: *Traité d'Anatomie Humaine.* Paris, Masson, 1921, p 796.

47. Polkey CE: Anterior temporal lobectomy at the Maudsley Hospital, London. In Engel J Jr (ed): *Surgical Treatment of the Epilepsies.* New York, Raven Press, 1989, pp 641–645.

48. Price JL, Russchen F, Amaral DG: The amygdaloid complex, In Bjorklund A, Hokfelt T, Swanson LW (eds): *Handbook of Chemical Neuroanatomy.* Amsterdam, Elsevier, 1987, vol 5, pp 279–388.

49. Quesney LF: Clinical and EEG features of complex partial seizures of temporal lobe origin. **Epilepsia** 27(suppl 2):S27–S45, 1986.

50. Quesney LF, Olivier A, Andermann F, et al.: EEG and clinical manifestations of frontal and temporal lobe seizures. **Can J Neurol Sci** 14:252–253, 1987.

51. Rasmussen T: Surgical treatment of patients with complex partial seizures. **Adv Neurol** 11:415–449, 1975.

52. Rasmussen T: Surgical aspects of temporal lobe epilepsy, results and problems. Acta Neurochirurgica, Suppl. 30: *Advances in Stereotactic and Functional Neurosurgery* 4. F.J. Gillingham, J. Gybels, ER Hitchcock & G. Szikla (eds). Springer-Verlag, Vienna 13–24, 1980.

53. Rasmussen T: Surgical treatment of complex partial seizures: Results, lessons and problems. **Epilepsia** 24(suppl 1):65–76, 1983.

54. Rasmussen T, Branch C: Temporal lobe epilepsy. Indications for and results of surgical therapy. **Postgrad Med J** 31:9–14, 1962.

55. Rasmussen T, Jasper H: Temporal lobe epilepsy: Indication for operation and surgical technique In Baldwin M, Bailey P (eds): *Temporal Lobe Epilepsy.* Springfield, IL, Charles C Thomas, 1958, 440–460.

56. Sachs E: The subpial resection of the cortex in the treatment of Jacksonian epilepsy (Horsley operation) with observations on area 4 and 6. **Brain** 58:492–523, 1935.

57. Sano K, Malamud N: Clinical significance of sclerosis of the cornu ammonis. **Arch Neurol Psychiatry** 70:40–53, 1953.

58. Sato M, Racine RJ, McIntyre DC: Kindling: Basic mechanisms and clinical validity. **Electroencephologr Clin Neurophysiol** 76:459–472, 1990.

59. Scheibel ME, Scheibel AB: Hippocampal pathology in the temporal lobe epilepsy: A Golgi study. In Brazier MAB (ed): *Epilepsy, Its Phenomena in Man.* UCLA Forums in Medical Sciences. New York, Academic Press, 1973, p 17.

60. Scoville W, Milner B: Loss of recent memory after bilateral hippocampal lesions. **J Neurol Neurosurg Psychiatry** 20:11–21, 1957.

61. Sloviter RS: The functional organization of the hippocampal dentate gyrus and its relevance to the pathogenesis of temporal lobe epilepsy. **Ann Neurol** 35:640–654, 1994.

62. So N, Gloor P, Quesney LF, *et al.*: Depth electrode investigations in patients with bitemporal epileptiform abnormalities. **Ann Neurol** 25:423–431, 1989.

63. So N, Olivier A, Andermann F, et al.: Results of surgical treatment in patients with bitemporal epileptiform abnormalities. **Ann Neurol** 25:432–439, 1989.

64. Spencer DD, Spencer SS, Mattson RH, *et al.*: Access to the posterior medial structures in the surgical treatment of temporal lobe epilepsy. **Neurosurgery** 15:667–671, 1984.

65. Sutula T, Cascino G, Gavazos J, *et al.*: Mossy fiber synaptic reorganization in the epileptic human temporal lobe. **Ann Neurol** 26:321–330, 1989.

66. Swanson LW, Kohler C, Bjorklund A: The limbic region. In Bjorklund A, Hokfelt T, Swanson LW (eds): *The Septohippocampal System: Handbook of Chemical Neuro-*

anatomy. Vol. 5: *Integrated Systems of the CNS,* Part 1. Amsterdam, Elsevier 1987, pp 125–277.

67. Tanaka T, Yonemasu Y, Olivier A, *et al.:* Clinical analysis of reoperation in cases of complex partial seizures. **Neurol Surg (Jpn)** 17:933–937, 1989.

68. Vigouroux R, Gastaut HR, Badier M: Provocation des principales manifestations cliniques de l'épilepsie dite temporale par stimulation des structures rhinencéphaliques chez le chat non-anaesthésié. **Rev Neurol** 85:505–508, 1951.

69. Wieser HG: Selective amygdalohippocampectomy: Indications, investigative techniques and results. In *Advances and Technical Standards in Neurosurgery.* Symon L, *et al.* (eds): Wien, Austria, Springer, 1986, vol 13, pp 40–133.

70. Wieser HG, Engel J Jr, Williamson PD, *et al.:* Surgically remediable temporal lobe syndromes, In Engel EJ Jr (ed): *Surgical Treatment of the Epilepsies.* New York, Raven Press, 1993, ed 2, pp 49–63.

71. Wieser HG, Yasargil MG: Die "Selective amygdohipokampektomie" Als chirurgische behandlungsmethode du mediobasal-limbischen epilepsie. **Neurochirurgia (Stuttg)** 25:39–50, 1982.

72. Yasargil MG, Teddy PJ, Roth P: Selective amygdalo-hippocampectomy: Operative anatomy and surgical technique. In Symon L, *et al.* (eds): *Advances and Technical Standards in Neurosurgery.* Wien, Austria, Springer, 1985, vol 12.

CHAPTER

16

Carotid Endarterectomy: How the Operation Is Done

CHRISTOPHER M. LOFTUS, M.D., F.A.C.S.

OVERVIEW

Carotid surgery changes every year. We now have proven efficacy for carotid endarterectomy in symptomatic patients with of ≥70% of linear stenosis (16, 17) and, according to those whose believe in ACAS (myself included) (6, 13), in asymptomatic patients with ≥60% stenosis as well. In this chapter I hope to describe what I consider to be basic, careful, and safe techniques for carotid reconstruction, as well as outline the scientific foundation for the various operative decisions facing the cerebrovascular surgeon. There is more than one way to perform any given operation, and all variations cannot be demonstrated here. A more complete discussion of indications, special considerations, and nuances of surgical technique can be found in more detailed technical writings (12, 14, 15).

I have personally tried both conventional loupe-magnified and formal microscopic repair of the internal carotid artery (ICA) at various stages of my career. At this time I use the 3.5× loupe-magnified technique, with placement of a Hemashield patch graft in every case. Whereas microscopic endarterectomy is certainly elegant, yielding a repair that is nearly invisible to the naked eye, it did not seem to impact my incidence of restenosis or acute occlusion. Primary patch graft placement, however, has essentially eliminated these problems in the 1½ years that I have used it.

TECHNIQUE CHOICES

Anesthetic Technique

Proponents of local anesthesia stress the advantages of patient response to questioning as a superior monitoring technique in assessing the need for shunt placement and in reducing postoperative morbidity and shortening length of stay. Monitoring under local anesthesia consists of direct patient questioning and performance of a simple task with the opposite hand during crossclamping. The risk of patient

243

disorientation from ischemia with subsequent movement and contamination of the operative field can be minimized by careful monitoring and sedation by the anesthetist. We have recently analyzed our own institutional data, comparing the incidence of electroencephalogram (EEG) changes and the need for shunting between two surgeons, a vascular surgeon who uses only local anesthesia with EEG, and myself, using general anesthesia with EEG (22). The incidence of EEG changes and shunt placement was less in this series with local anesthesia. There was no difference, however, in stroke rate, complications, outcome, or length of stay. A complete description the technique and its advantages can be found in Harbaugh's recent article (10).

To my understanding, general anesthesia remains the technique of choice for carotid artery surgery in most centers, and is my preference in almost all cases. The acceptance of local anesthesia is increasing, however, particularly with new emphasis on reducing length of stay. Some have suggested that carotid surgery be performed essentially as an outpatient procedure (4) although I have strong reservations about this, particularly in patients with associated risk factors. I have on several occasions performed successful carotid endarterectomies under local anesthesia when the patients had pulmonary problems so severe that postoperative ventilator dependence was a risk.

Monitoring Techniques

Monitoring techniques fall into two broad categories: (a) tests of vascular integrity, such as stump pressure measurements, xenon rCBF studies, transcranial Doppler and, to a lesser extent, intraoperative OPG, Doppler/duplex scanning, and angiography, and (b) tests of cerebral function, such as EEG, EEG derivatives, and/or somatosensory-evoked potential (SSEP) monitoring. The suitability of near-infrared spectroscopy (NIRS) for carotid surgery monitoring is unclear at present (20). The choice of technique will depend on the surgeon's preference and the resources available at the institution. In my practice I use full-channel EEG interpreted by a neurologist on-line. I also perform audible Doppler examination of the carotid tree after the arterial repair.

Intraoperative Shunting

The necessity for indwelling arterial shunt during carotid endarterectomy is one of the most widely debated and long-standing controversies in neurovascular surgery. Carotid surgeons generally align themselves into three groups: those who use shunts in every case; those who use shunting when indicated by some form of intraoperative monitoring (see above); and those who never shunt, no matter what the clinical or monitoring situation. Although I was trained in universal shunting, I believe this is excessive, and I perform monitoring-dependent shunting based on EEG criteria. In my experience I shunt about 15% of carotid endarterectomies; this increases to about 25% if the contralateral carotid is occluded. When a shunt is placed and flow is reestablished, the monitoring should return to baseline, and if this does not occur, the shunt must be evaluated for possible thrombosis or misplacement. I auscultate the shunt with a Doppler probe that works well to confirm patency and shunt flow. I have had only one case in which a demonstrably patent shunt did not restore the EEG; the shunt was removed and replaced twice in an unsuccessful attempt to improve the EEG; the patient awakened clinically normal from the procedure, despite my obvious concerns.

Arteriotomy Techniques

Some areas of controversy exist concerning technical performance of the carotid arterial repair. Objective data on these subjects are scarce, no doubt owing to the difficulty in documenting the individual contribution of such minor factors to success or failure in large series of patients. A few topics, however, are worthy of mention.

PATCH GRAFTING

Most surgeons favor patch grafting of the internal carotid repair in cases of recurrent stenosis, and many use patch grafts selectively in a primary repair in which the internal carotid lumen has been sufficiently narrowed to raise questions about postoperative stenosis and possible thrombosis. As already mentioned, I have gone to 100% patching with Hemashield graft material, as described by Ojemann and Ogilvy (18). The use of autologous vein does incur the risk of central patch rupture, with possible disastrous consequences, and a high femoral donor site, rather than the ankle, is preferable. The recent article of Yamamoto *et al.* citing the extensive Mayo Clinic patching experience is very instructive (23).

TACKING SUTURES

The use of tandem sutures to secure the distal intima in the ICA has been deemed unnecessary by some, yet has been cited by others as one of the major technical improvements in reducing carotid surgical morbidity. Although such sutures have the potential to narrow the internal carotid lumen, this risk seems low in comparison to the possibility of intimal dissection if a loose flap is left behind. Both Patterson (19) and Ferguson (7, 8), among others, point out that tacking sutures become unnecessary if the internal carotid arteriotomy is carried far enough to visualize normal intima distal to the plaque. These arguments are reasonable, and certainly I am a strong proponent of an arteriotomy that extends well above the zone of diseased internal carotid, however, I have not been entirely satisfied with the clean feathering of intima distally in some cases and have become accustomed to placing distal tacking sutures in approximately 25% of my arterial repairs without ill effects.

HEPARINIZATION

Intravenous heparin is routinely administered at some point before arterial crossclamping and repair. The dose, which may vary from 2500–10,000 units, appears to be of little consequence and is a matter of individual preference. I give 5000 units when the artery is first being dissected, and I do not reverse the anticoagulation. There is no evidence that this single dose of anticoagulant contributes to intraoperative or postoperative bleeding any more than the preoperative antiplatelet or anticoagulant agents most carotid patients have received. In my patients who are heparinized because of crescendo transient ischemic attacks (TIAs) or an intraluminal thrombus, I routinely operate with full anticoagulation on board, and I have occasionally maintained full heparinization postoperatively in patients with prosthetic heart valves or a contralateral symptomatic lesion requiring a second surgery. If meticulous attention is paid to technique, this is not a problem.

SURGICAL TECHNIQUE

There are several cardinal principles of carotid reconstruction:

• Complete knowledge of the patient's vascular anatomy.

• Complete vascular control at all times.

• Anatomic knowledge to prevent harm to adjacent structures.

• Assurance of a widely patent repair free of technical errors.

It is my feeling that the meticulous anatomic dissection and identification of vital cervical structures needed to minimize postoperative complications can be achieved only with a bloodless field. Accordingly, I do not consider elapsed time to be a factor in the performance of carotid surgery. In my institution, carotid endarterectomy requires from 2–2½ hours of operating time, and the average crossclamp time is between 30 and 40 minutes. No untoward effects from the length of the procedure have been observed in any patient, and I am convinced that the risk of cervical nerve injury or postoperative complications related to hurried closure of the suture line is significantly reduced by meticulous attention to detail.

Two surgeons trained in the procedure are always present during carotid surgery. Both surgeons stand on the operative side, with the primary surgeon facing cephalad and the assistant facing the patient's feet. The operative nurse may stand either behind or across the table from the primary surgeon. The patient is positioned supine on the operating room table, with head extended and turned away from the side of operation (Fig. 1). Several folded pillow cases are placed between the shoulder blades to facilitate extension of the neck, and the degree of rotation of the head is determined by the relationship of the external carotid artery (ECA) and ICA on preoperative angiography. The carotid vessels are customarily superimposed in the anteroposterior plane, and moderate rotation of the head will swing the internal carotid laterally into a more surgically accessible position. In those patients in whom the internal carotid can be seen angiographically to be laterally placed, the head rotation need not be as great. On the other hand, occasional patients will demonstrate an internal carotid that is rotated medially under the external carotid, and in such cases no degree of head rotation will yield a satisfactory exposure (Fig. 2). In these cases the surgeon must be prepared to mobilize the external carotid more extensively and swing it medially to expose the underlying internal carotid (even tacking it up to medial soft tissues, if necessary).

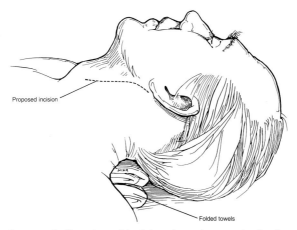

FIG. 1 I prefer a vertically oriented incision along the anterior border of the sternocleidomastoid muscle, which tails off toward the mastoid process. [Reproduced with permission from (12).]

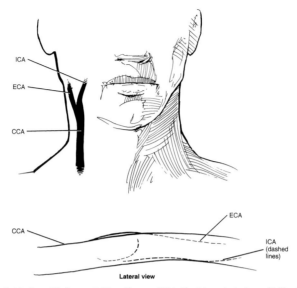

FIG. 2 The "side-by-side" carotid implies an ICA that is rotated medially to the ECA on the AP arteriogram. This will significantly complicate exposure of the carotid system and needs to be determined preoperatively for best results. [Reproduced with permission from (12).]

The position of the ICA bifurcation likewise has been determined before surgery from the angiogram, and the skin incision is planned accordingly. A linear incision along the anterior portion of the sterno-mastoid muscles is always used. This may go as low as the suprasternal notch and as high as the retroaural region, depending on the level of the bifurcation. The skin and subcutaneous tissues are divided sharply to the level of the platysma, which is always identified and divided sharply as well. Self-retaining retractors are then placed, and the underlying fat is dissected to identify the anterior edge of the sternocleidomastoid muscle (Fig. 3). Retractors are left superficial at all times on the medial side to prevent retraction injury to the laryngeal nerves but laterally may be more deeply placed. Dissection proceeds in the midportion of the wound down the sternomastoid muscle until the jugular vein is identified. It is to be emphasized that the jugular vein is the key landmark in this exposure. In some corpulent individuals the vein is not readily apparent, and a layer of fat between it and the sternocleidomastoid must be entered to locate the jugular itself. If this is not done, it is possible to fall into an incorrect plane lateral and deep to the jugular vein. As soon as the jugular is identified, dissection is shifted to go along the medial jugular border, and the

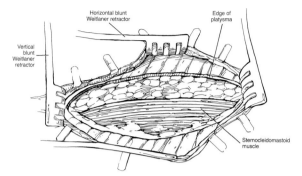

FIG. 3 The anterior border of the sternocleidomastoid muscle lies deep to the platysma and is the key landmark in a carotid exposure. [Reproduced with permission from (12).]

vein is held back with blunt retractors. The importance of the blunt retractor in preventing vascular injury at this point cannot be over-emphasized. In this process, several small veins and one large common facial vein are customarily crossing the field and need to be doubly ligated and divided (Fig. 4). The underlying carotid artery is soon identified once the jugular has been retracted. Most often, I come upon the common carotid artery first, and at the point of first visualization, the anesthesiologist is instructed to administer 5000 units of intravenous heparin which, as mentioned earlier, is never reversed. Dissection of the carotid complex is then straightforward, and the common

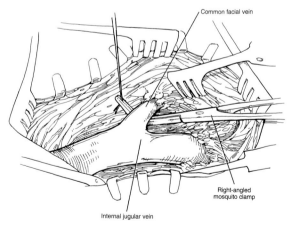

FIG. 4 The common facial vein will need to be double-ligated and divided in every case. After this retraction of the jugular vein gives the first exposure of the common carotid artery. [Reproduced with permission from (12).]

carotid artery (CCA), ECA, and ICA are isolated with the gentlest possible dissection and encircled with 00 silk ties (or vessel loops, if preferred) passed with a right angle clamp. Rarely, in unusually high ICA exposures, a ligature carrier has proven useful to pass the tie about the distal ICA. Injection of the carotid sinus is not routinely done; however, the anesthesiologist is notified when the bifurcation is being dissected, and if any changes in vital signs ensue, the sinus is injected with 2–3 ml of 1% plain xylocaine through a short 25-g needle. Although the carotid complex is completely exposed, the common and external carotids are not dissected free from their underlying beds in order to prevent postoperative kinking and coiling of these vessels. These arteries are dissected circumferentially only in those areas where silk ties or clamps are placed around them. Posterior dissection is more extensive in the region of the ICA, where posterior tacking sutures may later be placed and tied.

The common carotid silk is passed through a wire loop, which is then pulled through a rubber sleeve, thereby facilitating constriction of the vessel around an intraluminal shunt if this becomes necessary. The external and internal carotid ties are merely secured with mosquito clamps. Particular attention is paid to the superior thyroid artery, which is dissected free and secured with a double-loop 00 silk ligature. A hanging mosquito clamp keeps tension on this occlusive Pott's tie. Occasionally, multiple branches of this artery are identified on the preoperative angiogram, and these must be individually dealt with so that no troublesome backbleeding will ensue during the procedure through ignorance of these vessels. It is also essential that the external carotid silk tie (and subsequent crossclamp) be placed proximal to any major external branches, lest unacceptable backbleeding occur during the arteriotomy and repair.

Proper placement of the retractors facilitates the control of the carotid system. The hanging mosquitoes and silk ties are draped over these retractor handles to keep the field uncluttered. Of particular note is a blunt hinged retractor that is invaluable in exposing the ICA when a far distal exposure is necessary (Fig. 5). Dissection of the ICA must be complete and clearly beyond the distal extent of the plaque before crossclamping is performed. A clear plane can be developed if the jugular vein is followed distally and dissection follows the plane between the lateral carotid wall and the medial jugular border. By following this plane, the hypoglossal nerve is readily identified as it swings down medial to the jugular and crosses toward the midline over the internal carotid. We prefer to mobilize the nerve along its lateral wall adjacent to the jugular vein, after which it can be isolated with a vessel loop and gently retracted from the field. This has seldom yielded

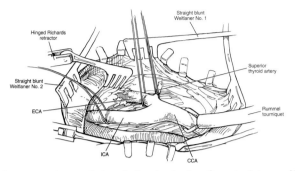

FIG. 5 Total exposure is mandatory before beginning the arteriotomy. All vessels are encircled with silk ties. The blunt hinged modified Richards retractor is placed so as to open up the high exposure over the distal ICA. [Reproduced with permission from (12).]

transient hypoglossal paresis, which seems to result instead in cases in which the nerve is not visualized and is blindly retracted. Inadvertent transection of the hypoglossal nerve has never been seen.

It is vital to have adequate exposure of the internal carotid and control distal to the plaque before opening the vessel. The extent of the plaque can be readily palpated with some experience by a moistened finger. There is also a visual cue in which the vessel becomes pinker and more normal-appearing distal to the extent of the plaque. If high exposure is needed, the digastric muscle can be cut with impunity, although this is necessary only in a small percentage of cases. When complete exposure is achieved, the final step in preparation for cross-clamping is to ensure that a small Javid clamp can be fitted in the region of the ICA and rotated 180° so that it lies underneath the vessel (Fig. 6). In most cases this requires additional adventitial dissection

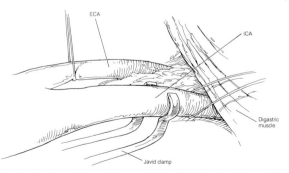

FIG. 6 A small Javid clamp is sized around the distal internal carotid in case shunt placement is required. This clamp will snug the vessel around the shun tubing, eliminating backbleeding. [Reproduced with permission from (12).]

behind the vessel to create a "window" in which the clamp head can be freely turned. This important step is necessary to facilitate rapid insertion of an intraluminal shunt if required. I also use a sterile marking pen to draw the proposed arteriotomy line along the vessel, which is helpful in preventing a jagged or curving suture line.

The monitoring system is then rechecked, and the encephalographer is notified of impending crossclamping. Once a suitable period of baseline EEG has been recorded, the common carotid is occluded with a large DeBakey vascular clamp, and small, straight bulldog clamps are used to occlude the ICAs and ECAs. A no. 11 blade is then used to begin the arteriotomy in the common carotid, and when the lumen is identified, a Pott's scissors is used to cut straight up along the marked line into the region of the bifurcation and then up into the internal until normal internal carotid is entered (Fig. 7). The incision should be up the midline of the vessel; lateral deviation will increase the difficulty of hemostatic arterial repair. In severely stenotic vessels with friable plaques the lumen is not always easily discerned, and false planes within the lesion are often encountered; great care must be taken to ensure that the back wall of the carotid is not lacerated and that the true lumen is identified before attempted shunt insertion. A quick release of the ICA bulldog clamp can demonstrate the lumen by backflow if necessary.

Changes in the EEG mandate a rapid trial of induced hypertension. If there is no immediate reversal of these changes, an intraluminal shunt is used. I use a 15-cm straight shunt fashioned from a no. 8 pediatric feeding tube, which is cut by the scrub nurse so that a black marker dot is directly in the center of the shunt. The shunt is first

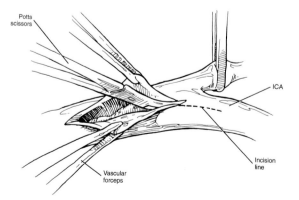

Fig. 7 The Pott's angled scissors are used to cut directly up the center of the vessel wall, following the line previously drawn. [Reproduced with permission from (12).]

inserted into the CCA and secured by pulling up on the silk ties; a mosquito clamp then holds the rubber sleeve in place to snug the silk around both the vessel and the intraluminal shunt. The shunt tubing is held closed at its midportion with a heavy vascular forceps, then briefly opened to confirm blood flow and evacuate any debris in the shunt tubing (Fig. 8). Suction is then used by the assistant to elucidate the lumen of the internal carotid and the distal end of the shunt tubing is placed therein. After the shunt is again bled, flushing any debris from the internal carotid, the bulldog clamp is removed, and the shunt is advanced up the internal carotid until the black dot lies in the center of the arteriotomy. The shunt, if properly placed, should slide easily up the internal carotid, and no undue force should be used to prevent intimal damage and possible dissection. The small Javid clamp is then used to secure the shunt distally in the internal carotid. Visualization of the dot in the center of the arteriotomy confirms constant correct positioning of the shunt. A hand-held Doppler probe can be applied to the shunt tubing to audibly confirm flow.

With or without the shunt, the plaque is next dissected from the arterial wall with a Freer elevator. A vascular pickup is used to hold the wall, and the Freer elevator is moved from side to side, developing a plane first in the lateral wall of the arteriotomy (Fig. 9). The plaque is usually readily separated in a primary case, and I go approximately halfway around the wall before proceeding to the other side. The plaque is then dissected on the medial side of the common carotid and transected proximally with a Pott's or Church scissors. A clean feathering away of the plaque is almost never possible in the common

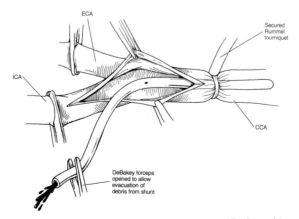

FIG. 8 After placing the shunt down the common carotid, the tubing is flushed to eliminate air and debris. [Reproduced with permission from (12).]

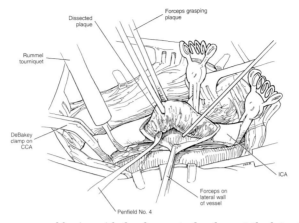

FIG. 9 Plaque removal begins with development of a plane at the lateral edge of the arteriotomy. Either the Freer dissector or a Penfield no. 4 dissector work well. [Reproduced with permission from (12).]

carotid, and the goal here is to transect the plaque sharply, leaving a smooth transition zone. Attention is then directed to the ICA, where likewise the plaque is dissected, first laterally and then medially, and then an attempt is made to feather the plaque down smoothly from the ICA. However, I find in some cases no matter how far up the ICA I go that a shelf of normal intima remains and that tacking sutures are required (Fig. 10). Attention is finally directed to the final point of plaque attachment at the orifice of the external carotid. The vascular pickup is used to grip across the entire plaque at the external carotid opening, and with some traction on the plaque, the external carotid can

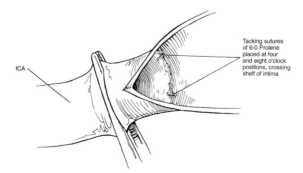

FIG. 10 When tacking sutures are required, they are placed from the inside out with a double-armed 6-0 Prolene suture. The knot is thus left outside the vessel, and the intimal edge is held down by the stitches. [Reproduced with permission from (12).]

be marsupialized such that the plaque can be dissected quite far up into that vessel. I like to free the external plaque by sweeping around it with a Penfield no. 4 dissector and/or a curved mosquito clamp so that it is well freed up before eversion/avulsion is attempted. The plaque usually stops at the first major external branch. Plaque is often tethered in the external carotid by the bulldog clamp, and as long as the plaque lumen is held closed with the heavy forceps, this clamp can be removed without untoward bleeding, allowing avulsion of the distal plaque. The bulldog must be quickly reapplied to stem copious back-bleeding that occurs when the plaque is removed from the external. It should be stressed that if plaque removal is inadequate in the external carotid thrombosis may ensue that can occlude the entire carotid tree with disastrous results. If there is any question as to incomplete removal of external plaque, I do not hesitate to extend the arteriotomy up the external carotid itself and close it via a separate suture line.

After gross plaque removal, a careful search is made for remaining fragments adherent to the arterial wall. Suspect areas are gently stroked with a peanut sponge, and every attempt is made to remove all loose fragments in a circumferential fashion, elevating them the complete width of the vessel until they break free at the arteriotomy edge. Although it is important to remove all loose fragments, no attempt is made to elevate firmly attached fragments that pose no danger of elevating or breaking off.

Several special aspects of plaque removal need to be considered. The simplest to remove are the soft, friable plaques with intraplaque hemorrhage and thrombus that dissect quite readily and from which fragments are easily removed. The more difficult are the severely stenotic, stony hard plaques, in which a plane of dissection at the lateral border of the carotid may not be readily apparent. This situation is analogous to the gross appearance in a case of recurrent carotid stenosis. In several of my cases of this type, plaque removal, even in the gentlest fashion, resulted in areas of thinning in which only an adventitial layer is left in the posterior wall of the carotid. These cases have been treated by primary plication with one or two double-armed interrupted stitches of 6-0 Prolene placed in the same fashion as the tacking sutures, and no untoward consequences have ensued. Likewise, I have occasionally encountered an intraluminal thrombus emanating from a congenital web or shelf in the lumen of the vessel, and this has been successfully plicated with a posteriorly placed stitch of double-armed 6-0 Prolene. In all cases, the goal is to leave as smooth an arteriotomy bed as is possible, with minimal areas of denudation or roughness available as sites for thrombus formation.

Attention is then directed to the arterial repair. If desired, the operating microscope can be brought into the field at this point or, in some cases, a bit sooner to allow for removal of the small fragments under high magnification (1, 9, 21). My personal preference is to continue with 3.5× loupe magnification. As previously mentioned, tacking sutures are used in the distal internal carotid in some of our cases. Double-armed sutures of 6-0 Prolene are placed vertically from the inside of the vessel out, such that they traverse the intimal edge and are tied outside the adventitial layer (Fig. 10). Most often, two such sutures are used, placed at the four and eight o'clock positions. I then proceed to fashion the Hemashield patch.

The patch material is placed over the arteriotomy and cut to the exact length of the opening. After removal from the field, the ends are trimmed and tapered to a point with Church scissors. Each end of the patch is then anchored to the arteriotomy with double-armed 6-0 Prolene sutures, and the needles are left on and secured with rubber shod clamps (Fig. 11). The medial wall suture line is closed first, and a running nonlocking stitch is brought from the ICA anchor to the CCA anchor, where it is tied to a free end of the CCA anchor Prolene (Fig. 12). The lateral wall is then closed (with the remaining limb of the ICA

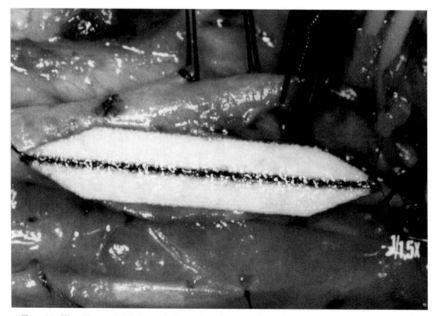

FIG. 11 The Hemashield patch is secured at each end with an anchor stitch of 6-0 Prolene, and the needles are left attached for later use.

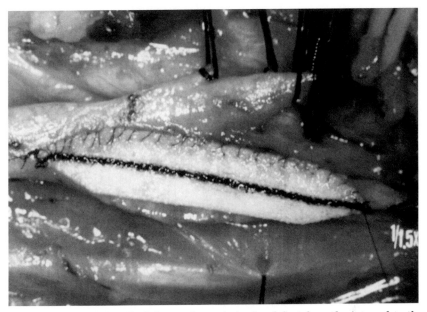

FIG. 12 The medial wall of the patch repair is closed first from the internal to the common carotid, and the two stitch ends are tied together.

anchor stitch) from the ICA to just below the level of the carotid bulb (Fig. 13). At this point the second arm of the CCA anchor stitch is used to run up the CCA lateral wall to meet the ICA limb. Small bites are taken just at the arterial edge throughout (being certain, however, that all layers are included), and sutures are placed relatively close together to prevent leaks. Care is also taken that no stray adventitial tags or suture ends are sewn into the lumen, where they might induce thrombosis. Several millimeters of unsewn vessel are left on the lateral wall, ensuring room to remove the shunt, if one has been used. After the electroencephalographer is again notified, the shunt is double-clamped with two parallel straight mosquitoes, then cut between them and removed in two sections, one from each end. A common error at this point is to mistakenly entangle the suture material in the shunt clamps and, thereby, hamper smooth shunt removal. With or without shunt, the arteriotomy is completely closed as follows: All three vessels are first opened and closed sequentially to ensure that backbleeding is present from the ICA, ECA, and CCA. The two stitches are then held taut by the surgeon while the assistant introduces a heparinized saline syringe with blunt needle into the arterial lumen. The vessel is filled with heparinized saline, and in this process all air is evacuated from

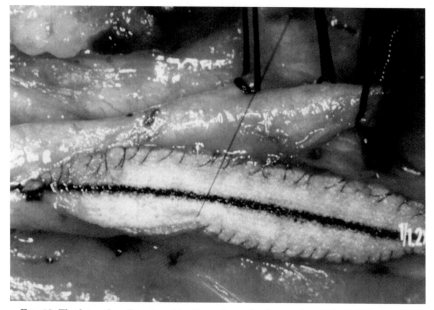

FIG. 13 The lateral wall is closed halfway down the internal and then with the second stitch halfway up the common. This photograph shows the internal closed, in preparation for the common repair.

the intraluminal space (Fig. 14). As the stitches are drawn up and a surgeon's knot is thrown, the blunt needle is withdrawn, allowing no air to enter. Seven or eight further knots are then placed in this most crucial stitch. The clamps are removed first from the external carotid, then from the common carotid and finally, some 10 seconds later, from the ICA (Fig. 15). In this fashion, all loose debris and remaining microbubbles of air are flushed into the external carotid circulation. Meticulous attention is paid to evacuation of all debris and air before opening the internal carotid in every case. However, in the rare case in which there is a known external carotid occlusion (although most of these can be reopened at surgery with an ECA endarterectomy), this technique is extremely crucial, as there is no external carotid safety valve, and all intraluminal contents will be shunted directly into the intracranial circulation.

When the clamps have been removed, the suture lines are inspected for leaks, which are customarily controlled with pressure, patience, and Surgicel gauze. In occasional cases, a single throw of 6-0 Prolene is necessary to close a persistent arterial hemorrhage. Suture repairs of bleeding points are more likely if a patch graft has been placed. It is

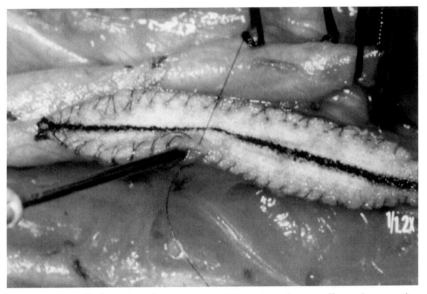

FIG. 14 After the lateral wall common carotid repair, only a small opening remains, through which the shunt can be removed and backbleeding checked. A blunt needle is then inserted, and heparinized saline fills the vessel while the knots are secured.

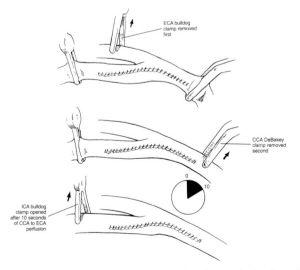

FIG. 15 Sequence of clamp removal. [Reproduced with permission from (12).]

almost never necessary to reapply clamps to the artery if the repair has been properly performed. The repair is then lined with Surgicel, and the three vessels are tested with a hand-held Doppler to ensure patency. Retractors are removed, and hemostasis is confirmed both along the jugular vein and from the surrounding soft tissues. Persistent oozing is often encountered in these patients who have often received large doses of antiplatelet agents in addition to their intraoperative heparin. A final Doppler check is made, and the wound is closed in layers. The carotid sheath is first closed to provide a barrier against infection, and the platysma is then closed as a separate layer to ensure a good cosmetic result. Either running or interrupted subcuticular stitches may be used to close the skin edges, which are then apposed with Steristrips. A Hemovac drain is routinely used and left inside the carotid sheath. It is removed on the first postoperative day. Patients are restarted on aspirin the day after surgery and are discharged in 2–3 days.

I manage any postoperative neurologic deficit, including TIA alone, with immediate angiography. In my experience lesser measures, such as duplex scanning, are inadequate to facilitate definitive surgical decision making in these patients, in whom quick judgments and emergent surgery may be required. Any occluded carotid postop is reexplored and repatched immediately, although since adopting the primary Hemashield patch repair my incidence of postop occlusion has been zero.

Special Surgical Considerations

BILATERAL CAROTID ENDARTERECTOMY

Bilateral carotid endarterectomy runs the risk not only of extreme swings of blood pressure from concurrent denervation of both carotid sinuses but also the risk of bilateral cranial nerve injury. For this reason, when bilateral carotid endarterectomy is required in my patients, I stage these procedures 6 weeks apart and have the patient examined by an otolaryngologist to ensure that no occult cranial nerve or vocal cord dysfunction is present before the second procedure. Unilateral nerve dysfunction in the cervical region is troublesome, but a bilateral dysfunction can be disabling. I have, on several occasions, deferred second side surgery and maintained the patient on medical therapy when an occult vocal cord paralysis was diagnosed.

INTRALUMINAL THROMBUS

The problem of surgical timing in patients with angiographically demonstrated propagating intraluminal thrombus remains an open question among cerebrovascular experts (2, 11). In patients who present with TIAs (which, in my experience, have always resolved with anticoagulation) and an intraluminal thrombus I have opted for delayed surgery (at 6 weeks after repeat angiography) in every case, and have never seen a negative outcome from intercurrent embolization once heparin is instituted. Likewise there is a small subset of patients with postoperative neurological events (most often, TIA) after carotid endarterectomy who are found to have a fresh thrombus adherent to the suture line, partially occluding the artery, and which is presumably the source of embolic phenomena. If there is no other angiographic evidence of technical inadequacy I have chosen to manage these patients conservatively as well, with full anticoagulation and 6-week follow-up arteriography. In every case the thrombus has resolved, and there have been no negative neurological outcomes in our series with this plan of management. Despite the surgeon's natural inclination to fix a problem with bold action, I have found that a measured conservative approach yields good results in cases of fresh or propagating thrombus and in our experience is superior to undertaking a high-risk surgical procedure.

TANDEM LESIONS OF THE CAROTID SIPHON

In the NASCET trial symptomatic patients were excluded if the degree of siphon stenosis exceeded that at the carotid bifurcation (17). The presence of stenotic disease at the carotid siphon has been proposed as a contraindication to carotid endarterectomy because of both inability to pinpoint the symptomatic source and the reputed increased possibilities of postoperative occlusion from decreased carotid flow velocity. This has not been my experience, and I do not hesitate to operate on patients with tandem lesions if I am convinced that an active plaque at the carotid bifurcation is the source of their embolic phenomena.

RECURRENT CAROTID STENOSIS

There is a small but finite incidence of recurrent carotid stenosis after primary carotid endarterectomy. Aside from technical inadequacies, it has been difficult to identify risk factors associated with recurrent carotid stenosis, although continuation of smoking habits after endarterectomy has proved to be a significant risk factor in several studies (3, 5), whereas hypertension, diabetes mellitus, family history, lipid studies, aspirin use, and coronary disease may not be as important.

Reoperation for carotid stenosis is a technically difficult procedure. It is associated with significantly higher risks than primary endarterectomy. In our institution, the possibility of reoperation for carotid stenosis is entertained in patients who present with angiographically proven disease and classical neurological symptoms referable to the appropriate artery or with documented progression to severe stenosis while being followed with annual serial duplex examinations.

CONCURRENT CORONARY/CAROTID DISEASE

It is well-established that patients with ECA disease have a higher than normal incidence of coronary disease, as well as other peripheral vascular problems. Indeed, the risk of perioperative myocardial infarction exceeds the risk of perioperative stroke in many clinical series' of carotid endarterectomy. Several major questions arise when planning treatment for concurrent coronary/carotid disease. These include the following questions: What is the risk of coronary revascularization in a patient with a high-grade asymptomatic stenosis or bruit? In patients with symptomatic carotid disease, what is the appropriate workup of the coronary circulation? If surgical degrees of both carotid artery and coronary artery disease are identified in the same patient, what is the appropriate surgical management—staged carotid followed by coronary revascularization, combined procedure, or "reverse staged" coronary revascularization followed by delayed carotid endarterectomy?

The first question regarding asymptomatic bruit in symptomatic coronary patients is straightforward. ACAS has now shown a surgical benefit for lesions ≥60%, and I recommend that these be staged before coronary revascularization whenever possible.

The second question, regarding appropriate workup of coronary disease in symptomatic carotid artery patients, is a more difficult one. In this situation, workup is customarily guided by the patient's history and symptomatology. It has been my practice to obtain cardiology consultation in any patient with a history of angina, known heart disease, or abnormal resting ECG. The workup proceeds with a thallium stress test with exercise or dipyridamole, and if there is any evidence of myocardial ischemia, coronary angiography is performed.

When the results of cardiac evaluation indicate the need for coronary revascularization, the question becomes one of timing of the surgical procedures. My preference is to do staged procedures whenever possible. With careful hemodynamic monitoring and good anesthetic technique, we are routinely able to perform safe unilateral carotid endarterectomies before coronary revascularization. An occasional patient with severe unstable angina may require a combined procedure, but this entails a significantly higher surgical risk, so I attempt staged procedures whenever possible. Most series' dealing with "reverse-staged" coronary carotid procedures (*i.e.*, the coronary artery revascularization first with delayed carotid endarterectomy) discuss them in the context of asymptomatic carotid disease. Whereas I previously felt that "reverse-staged" procedures in asymptomatic patients were unindicated, I now feel that for unstable coronary disease with an unacceptable cardiac anesthetic risk, a "reverse-staged" procedure may be appropriate, because the ACAS data has validated surgery on silent carotid lesions.

In conclusion then, it is my preference to aggressively work up any patient with cardiac symptoms before carotid endarterectomy. If procedures in both circulations are indicated, staged procedures are preferable unless the coronary circulation disease makes anesthesia for carotid endarterectomy an untenable proposition. In such cases a combined procedure may be acceptable. I see no indication for "reverse-staged" procedures in symptomatic patients and would *prefer* to reconstruct asymptomatic carotid stenosis of ≥60% first, whenever possible.

CONCLUSIONS

Now that cooperative study data is available to support the clear superiority of surgery in the management of both asymptomatic (≥60%) and symptomatic carotid stenosis (≥70%), carotid artery reconstruction will undergo continued technical refinements. There will be additional data forthcoming from NASCET for the "moderate" stenosis group of patients with linear stenosis of 30–69%, and patients continue to be entered into that trial at present. The cerebrovascular surgical community will also face challenges from cardiologists and radiologists who seek to treat carotid patients with angioplasty and stenting. At present there is *no* level one evidence to support the efficacy of endovascular treatment, whereas such evidence clearly exists for surgical treatment.

Many of the basic neurovascular principles are standard, but I have seen relaxation of some old "taboos" (such as contralateral occlusion, tandem stenosis, and fresh stroke). In my opinion this expanded acceptance of carotid surgery arises from more rigorous training and credentialing of surgeons, improved monitoring and anesthetic techniques, and the scientific application of cooperative trial methodology to the carotid problem.

The surgical methods presented here have been successful in producing acceptable postoperative results in a broad spectrum of carotid patients. Minor technical details that may vary among surgeons are probably of little significance. On the other hand, subtleties of technique that may add operative time to the "routine" carotid assume greater importance when difficult lesions or high exposures are encountered, or when the patient is unstable. The importance of a good outcome under these more difficult circumstances leads me to approach all carotid surgery, no matter how simple it may seem, with the same technical approach. Perhaps the most important factor in ensuring technically acceptable carotid surgery is the availability of a skilled cerebrovascular surgeon with a demonstrable morbidity and mortality below 3% and a proper understanding of both vascular principles and cerebral physiology.

REFERENCES

1. Bailes J, Spetzler RF: *Mirosurgical Carotid Endarterectomy.* Philadelphia, Lippincott-Raven, 1996.
2. Biller J, Adams HP, Boarini D, *et al.:* Intraluminal clot of the carotid artery. **Surg Neurol** 25:467–477, 1986.
3. Clagett G, Rich N, McDonald P, *et al.:* Etiologic factors for recurrent carotid artery stenosis. **Surgery** 2:313–318, 1983.
4. Collier PE, Friend SZ, Gentile C, *et al.:* Carotid endarterectomy clinical pathway: An innovative approach. **Am J Med Qual** 10:38–47, 1995.
5. Dempsey RJ, Moore R, Cordero S: Factors leading to early reoccurrence of carotid plaque after carotid endarterectomy. **Surg Neurol** 43:278–283, 1995.
6. Executive Committee for the Asymptomatic Carotid Atherosclerosis Study: Endarterectomy for asymptomatic carotid stenosis. **JAMA** 273:1421–1428, 1995.
7. Ferguson GG: Extracranial carotid artery surgery. **Clin Neurosurg** 29:543–574, 1982.
8. Ferguson GG: Carotid endarterectomy: Indications and surgical technique. **Int Anesthesiol Clin** 22:113–121, 1984.
9. Findlay JM: Carotid microendarterectomy. **Neurosurgery** 32:792–798, 1993.
10. Harbaugh R: Carotid surgery under local anesthesia. **Techn Neurosurg** 3, in press, 1997.
11. Heros RC: Carotid endarterectomy in patients with intraluminal thrombus. **Stroke** 19:667–668, 1990.
12. Loftus CM: *Carotid Endarterectomy: Principles and Technique.* St. Louis, Quality Medical Publishing, 1995.
13. Loftus CM, Hopkins LN: Paradoxical indications for carotid endarterectomy. **Neurosurgery** 36:99–100, 1995.
14. Loftus CM, Quest DO: Technical controversies in carotid artery surgery. **Neurosurgery** 20:490–495, 1987.
15. Loftus CM, Quest DO: Technical issues in carotid surgery 1995. **Neurosurgery** 36:629–647, 1995.
16. MECS European Carotid Surgery Trial: Interim results for symptomatic patients with severe (70–99%) or with mild (0–29%) carotid stenosis. **Lancet** 337:1235–1243, 1991.
17. North American Symptomatic Carotid Endarterectomy Trial Collaborators: Beneficial effect of carotid endarterectomy in symptomatic patients with high grade stenosis. **N Engl J Med** 325:445–453, 1991.
18. Ojemann RG, Ogilvy CS: Patch angioplasty. **Techn Neurosurg** 3, in press, 1997.

19. Patterson RH: Technique of carotid endarterectomy, in Smith RR (ed): *Stroke and the Extracranial Vessels*. New York, Raven Press, 1984, pp 177–185.
20. Samra SK, Dorje P, Zelenock GB, *et al.:* Cerebral oximetry in patients undergoing carotid endarterectomy under regional anesthesia. **Stroke** 27:49–55, 1996.
21. Spetzler RF, Martin N, Hadley MN, *et al.:* Microsurgical endarterectomy under barbiturate protection: A prospective study. **J Neurosurg** 51:147–150, 1986.
22. Wellman BJ, Loftus CM, Kresowik T, *et al.:* The differences in electroencephalographic changes in awake versus anesthetized carotid endarterectomy patients, in *Joint Section on Cerebrovascular Surgery, 2nd Annual Meeting*. Anaheim, CA, 1997.
23. Yamamoto Y, Piepgras DG, Marsh WR, *et al.:* Complications resulting from saphenous vein patch graft after carotid endarterectomy. **Neurosurgery** 39:670–676, 1996.

CHAPTER

17

Monitoring in Traumatic Brain Injury

PAUL G. MATZ, M.D., AND LAWRENCE PITTS, M.D.

OVERVIEW

Although outcome after traumatic brain injury (TBI) appears to be improving, head injury still represents a major public health problem, and many patients with severe TBI die or do poorly. Thus, continuing improvements in treatment are needed. Despite extensive publications regarding management of TBI in the United States, treatment varies considerably among and possibly even within institutions. In a survey of centers treating TBI, only 28% reported that they frequently used intracranial pressure (ICP) monitoring, because these centers were predominantly level I centers in which severe TBI is treated frequently. Seven percent of centers surveyed, however, never used ICP monitoring (17).

To better guide management of TBI and other brain disorders, in the past several years, technological improvements have expanded the scope of physiologic and biochemical monitoring. Although still largely used in clinical experimental settings, such monitoring now more routinely includes determination of cerebral blood flow (CBF), jugular venous saturation ($SjvO_2$), and cerebral metabolic rate of oxygen consumption ($CMRO_2$). It is likely that multimodality monitoring (23) will be much more common and that ICP monitoring will be routine. Therefore, an understanding of monitoring after TBI is paramount.

Physiology

Trauma resuscitation, surgical intervention, and intensive care management after TBI serve to optimize flow of well-oxygenated blood to the brain (3). The rationale for aggressive management in these settings is to avoid ischemia, which occurs when $CMRO_2$ exceeds the brain's supply of oxygen [CBF × arteriovenous oxygen difference ($AVDO_2$)]. $CMRO_2$ is sometimes reduced after trauma because of decreased brain oxygen requirements (50). However, CBF and $CMRO_2$, which are usually tightly matched, may also become uncoupled (39), and despite low oxygen requirements, ischemia may follow TBI (50).

Therefore, adequate CBF depends less on an absolute value and more on a CBF needed to sustain the patient's $CMRO_2$ at any given time (39; Fig. 1).

CBF is equal to the cerebral perfusion pressure (CPP) divided by the cerebrovascular resistance (CVR). CPP is defined as the mean arterial pressure (MAP) minus ICP. When cerebral autoregulation is intact, CVR changes with CPP to keep CBF relatively constant over a wide range of CPP values (roughly, 50–150 mm Hg). Because of unknown changes of CVR with altered CPP, estimations of CBF using CPP are often erroneous. After TBI, at least two events can occur. First, pressure autoregulation may be disrupted or only partially preserved (10, 23, 32, 33). TBI may shift the pressure autoregulatory curve to the right, and a previously "normal" CPP may become inadequate and precipitate plateau waves (53). Secondly, regional and global CBF in the first 6 hours after TBI may not be coupled to CPP (10). If CVR is increased as a result of vasospasm or microcirculatory changes, CBF will fall for a given CPP, and ischemia may result (39). If CVR is decreased because of traumatic vasoparalysis, CPP may underestimate CBF, and hyperemia may ensue (39).

Indications

Disrupted autoregulatory mechanisms and biochemical cascades initiated by trauma are exacerbated by further ischemia and render the injured brain extremely sensitive to alterations in perfusion that are

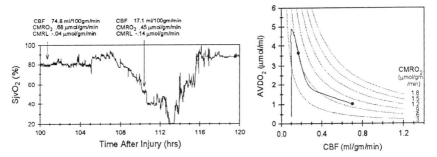

FIG. 1 After TBI, ischemic episodes occur despite an overall reduction in $CMRO_2$. Panel **A** demonstrates an episode of jugular venous desaturation and the concurrent changes in $CMRO_2$, CBF, and cerebral metabolic rate of lactate production (CMRL). In this instance, $CMRO_2$ and CBF are diminished; however, CBF is reduced to a greater degree, and ischemic results are evidenced by a fall in $SjvO_2$ and an increase in CMRL. In panel **B**, these data are plotted relative to CBF and O_2 extraction. As CBF falls for a given $CMRO_2$, $AVDO_2$ rises until infarction develops. Then, O_2 requirements no longer exist, and $AVDO_2$ falls precipitously. [Reproduced with permission from (50).]

well-tolerated by the normal brain (3, 10). Secondary brain insults such as hypoxia and hypotension may occur after TBI and are powerful determinants of outcome (10, 17). Hypotension significantly increases mortality; mortality after severe TBI triples if systolic blood pressure remains below 90 mm Hg for 30 minutes or longer in the ICU (6). Although hypotension often happens during transport, it also can commonly occur in the intensive care unit (ICU) (10, 18, 62). Decreased CPP, *i.e.*, brain hypotension, may be caused by impaired autoregulation, systemic hypotension, intracranial hypertension, hydrocephalus, hematoma, cerebral edema, vasospasm, or herniation (39). Consequently, more severely injured patients tend to require more support to maintain adequate CPP (53). Reduced CPP after TBI correlates with poor outcome (53). Some degree of intracranial hypertension occurs in 50–75% of patients after TBI, and its duration also correlates with increased morbidity and mortality (17, 33). However, no clinical signs are associated with low CBF until it has fallen to a level close to the threshold for permanent neuronal damage (39). Therefore, a strong argument can be made for aggressive monitoring in the setting of TBI. Monitoring may help determine whether the CBF is rising or falling, if the brain is hyperemic or ischemic, if autoregulation is preserved, and if a therapy is achieving its endpoint (39).

There are several ideal goals for a monitoring system in the setting of TBI. Monitoring systems should allow the physician to make an estimation of CBF and, if possible, $CMRO_2$ to avoid brain ischemia. They should be portable for use at the bedside to minimize patient transport and noninvasive to minimize the risk of infection and hemorrhage. Optimally, the monitor would directly measure the required parameter, continuously whenever possible, and yield quantitative rather than relative values. Because the degree and nature of focal injuries vary widely after TBI, a monitor ideally would yield global and regional determination of parameters. To increase the ease and acceptability of monitoring, artifacts should be minimized. Because no one system begins to reach all of these goals for monitoring the TBI patient, we can understand the current need for multimodality monitoring (9).

ICP MONITORING

ICP monitoring is the oldest and most common form of cerebral monitoring in the setting of TBI or indeed any other brain pathology. ICP monitoring provides at least two important perspectives to the clinician. First, it quantifies the influence that mass effect from TBI has on the brain and indicates the tendency toward herniation (33). Secondly it permits direct determination of CPP. In addition to allowing optimization of CPP, it allows the clinician to limit the risks of administration of agents commonly used to treat intracranial hypertension by applying them only when needed (33, 53). After TBI in one series, 81% of adults had interventions based on ICP monitoring (15). In the pediatric population, 88% of children had therapy based on ICP measurements (49). Generally, ICP monitors are recommended in patients who have a Glasgow Coma Score (GCS) less than or equal to 8 or a GCS motor score less than 5. One study has identified a subset of patients with GCS less than 8 and with normal CT scans who were not at risk for intracranial hypertension and did not necessarily require ICP monitoring unless two of the following three characteristics were present: age above 40, evidence of posturing, or previous episodes of hypoxia or hypotension (45).

ICP monitors consist of four basic types: the fiberoptic parenchymal monitor, the ventricular catheter, the subdural catheter, and the sub- or epidural bolt (42, 46). Pressure transduction from the subdural catheter and epidural bolt is exerted through a fluid-filled external transducer (42). The ventricular catheter can be transduced through a fiberoptic or a fluid-filled transducer; both of these methods yield similar results in the ventricular catheter (7). Each type of monitor has particular advantages and disadvantages. The fiberoptic parenchymal monitor is accurate and can be placed rapidly at the bedside. However, it cannot be "zeroed" each day and, subsequently, may drift (46). In addition, CSF cannot be removed. Because the catheter enters the parenchyma, the ICP value does not necessarily represent global ICP and should be placed on the side of the pathology (32). The ventricular catheter has advantages similar to those of the parenchymal monitor but, in addition, CSF can be withdrawn to lower ICP. Unfortunately, the risk of hemorrhage and infection are higher in a ventricular catheter, and insertion can be difficult in the setting of TBI if the ventricles are small (45, 47). Both the sub- or epidural bolt and subdural catheter are inexpensive, simple monitoring systems with few complications. Unfortunately, neither of them permits removal of CSF, and both can become occluded with debris (42). They, like the parenchymal monitor, may not represent global ICP and should be placed on the side of greatest pathology (32, 42). Epidural catheters or bolts are generally the least accurate systems and generally are not used now (42, 46).

Similar complications have been observed in all ICP monitoring systems. Infection is the most common complication but varies slightly in location, depending on the type of system. Infection can occur in any anatomic space, resulting in scalp abscess, osteomyelitis, subdural empyema, brain abscess, meningitis, or ventriculitis. Ventriculitis and meningitis are far more common with ventricular catheters, and an overall infection rate (or, at least, contamination rate) of 0–12% has been previously described (45, 47). With fiberoptic parenchymal monitors, CSF space infections are far less likely, and an infection rate of 0–1.7% has been reported (15, 46). In children, an infection rate of 0.3% has been observed for all monitoring (49).

Hemorrhage is another possible complication in ICP monitoring. Like infection, hemorrhage can occur in any anatomic space, producing intraventricular, intracerebral, subdural, and epidural hematomas. Parenchymal hematomas are more common with ventricular catheters because they penetrate the brain to a greater degree (32). The hemorrhage rate is 0–5% for fiberoptic intraparenchymal monitors (15, 46) and 1–6% for ventricular catheters (45, 47). In the pediatric population, the hemorrhage rate has been observed to be 0.3% (49). Other pitfalls include technical malfunction of the monitors, especially fracture of the fiberoptic transducer. Technical malfunction occurred at a rate of 6% in adults and 3.6% in children (15, 49). Because hemorrhage and infection are two main complications, coagulopathy and immunosuppression are relative contraindications to ICP monitoring (32).

When systolic blood pressures are transmitted to the brain, a characteristic ICP wave form is generated with three successively smaller peaks representing the peak of systole, the tidal wave, and the dicrotic notch. As intracranial hypertension develops, the wave form morphology is altered as a result of decreased brain compliance. The peaks no longer become successively smaller, and the ICP wave form becomes more pyramidal in shape (23, 32, 59). Therefore, careful ICP monitoring with wave form analysis can demonstrate intracranial hypertension that alters brain compliance (59). Pressure-volume dynamics of the brain also can be followed with ICP monitoring (4). After TBI, if pressure autoregulation is preserved, increases in CPP produce an increase in brain compliance while increases in CPP without pressure autoregulation produce decreased compliance because of to hyperemia (4).

Because ICP monitoring is continuous, quantitative, and global, it is well-suited not only to guide the intensive care management of TBI patients but also to diagnose the delayed intracranial hypertension that develops in as many as 31% of patients (Fig. 2). This process can occur as a result of a delayed hematoma, hypoxia, vasospasm, or hyponatremia 3–10 days after TBI and correlates with a worsened outcome (60).

TRANSCRANIAL DOPPLER ULTRASONOGRAPHY

Transcranial Doppler ultrasonography (TCD) permits observation of flow velocity (FV) in the proximal vessels of the circle of Willis through

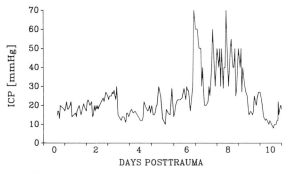

FIG. 2 Intracranial hypertension can occur in delayed fashion after severe TBI. In this case, the patient's ICP was slightly abnormal until the 6th day after injury. At that time, severe intracranial hypertension ensued, and a poor outcome resulted. ICP monitoring easily detects delayed intracranial hypertension. [Reproduced with permission from (60).]

transcranial insonation. Insonation sites can be transtemporal, transforaminal, transorbital, or submandibular, depending on the vessel insonated (23). Through observation of FV, a qualitative estimate of CBF can be obtained. In addition, the difference between systolic and diastolic FV yields a pulsatility index (PI), which is useful in estimating brain compliance (20). Comparison of the intracranial middle cerebral artery (MCA) FV to the extracranial internal carotid artery (ICA) FV produces a Lindegaard ratio (37), which is a marker for vasospasm. In patients with TBI, TCD can be used to demonstrate vasospasm (Fig. 3) and predict cerebral compliance changes using a system that is portable and noninvasive. However, TCD only permits qualitative estimates of regional CBF and generally is not a continuous monitoring system.

TCD can be a useful tool in diagnosing and preventing secondary ischemia in the ICU. In one study after severe TBI, 34% of patients had elevation of FV (Fig. 3). A subset of these patients had unilateral regional elevation of FV and went on to develop infarction in the territory supplied by the vessel insonated (8). In patients with traumatic hematomas, FV was also decreased on the side of the compressive lesion, and FV reduction correlated with reductions in CPP (55). In a different group of patients with TBI, intracranial hypertension and reduction in CPP produced increases in $AVDO_2$ and PI (Fig. 4) and a decrease in FV. Adequate treatment of the cerebral hypoperfusion resulted in reductions in $AVDO_2$ and PI and an increase in FV (Fig. 4). Maneuvers that lead to a reduction in ICP without improvement in CPP did not produce these changes (9). Relative changes in the FV and

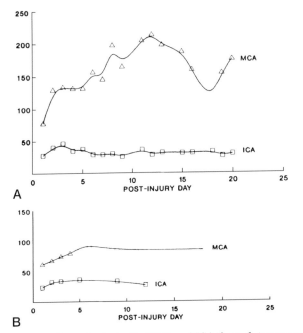

FIG. 3 By monitoring flow velocity in the MCA and ICA through transcranial Doppler, posttraumatic vasospasm can be detected. In this series of patients FV were measured in centimeters per second on consecutive days after TBI. Posttraumatic vasospasm, as evidenced by increasing MCA FV above 120 cm/sec without change in ICA FV, was observed in a subset of patients 5–15 days after TBI (A). The remainder of the patients (B) had no evidence of vasospasm on TCD ultrasonography. [Reproduced with permission from (40).]

PI obtained by TCD ultimately may assist the clinician in treating ICP and CPP after TBI.

By correlating ^{133}Xe CBF and TCD, Martin et al. observed that 27% of patients developed elevated MCA FV in a pattern consistent with that of vasospasm. In these patients, the region of highest MCA FV correlated to the region of lowest CBF consistent with a picture of reduced CBF resulting from vasospasm (Fig. 3). In 17% of patients, both elevated MCA FV and traumatic subarachnoid hemorrhage (SAH) were observed (40). In a similar study, Romner et al. observed that 41% of patients with traumatic SAH had significantly elevated MCA FV (52). The combination of traumatic SAH and vasospasm on TCD correlates with a poor outcome (40, 58). After TBI, FV is often reduced in the first few days. FV then increases and may peak from 5–13 days after TBI in a pattern consistent with the vasospasm observed after spontaneous SAH (40, 58; Fig. 3). In the absence of

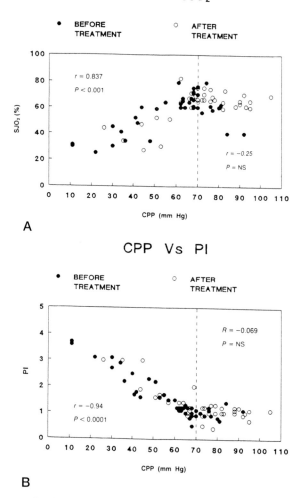

FIG. 4 The use of multimodality monitoring for patients with TBI demonstrates the consequences of cerebral hypoperfusion. In this group of patients, CPP, before and after treatment, was monitored simultaneously with PI and SjvO$_2$ saturation. Correlation coefficients (r values) and their statistical significance (P values) were obtained between CPP and PI or SjvO$_2$ before and after treatment. Cerebral hypoperfusion resulted in jugular venous desaturation and increased O$_2$ extraction before treatment (A). CPP and SjvO$_2$ changes had a linear correlation with a statistically significant correlation coefficient before treatment. (A). Reductions in CPP may result in or may be the product of reductions in cerebral compliance. Reduced cerebral compliance with diminished CPP in this group of patients resulted in an increase in the pulsatility index (B). CPP and PI changes had a negative correlation to each other before treatment that yielded a statistically significant correlation coefficient (B). In both of these examples, treatment to increase brain perfusion improved the jugular venous oxygen saturation and decreased the pulsatility index. [Reproduced with permission from (9).]

traumatic SAH, vasospasm, manifested by increased FV and an elevated Lindegaard ratio, was found to have a far shorter duration than that observed in the setting of traumatic SAH (40). Increasing FV after TBI may also be associated with cerebral hyperemia, depending on vascular resistance at the time (52, 58). Both hyperemia and vasospasm have been associated with diminished pressure autoregulation after TBI (58).

TCD may also provide information about brain compliance after TBI. After TBI, PI was observed to increase in regions ipsilateral to the traumatic lesion. Furthermore, these increases in PI correlated with the onset of intracranial hypertension and reduced brain compliance (20). Ten days after a minor TBI in one patient, PI was observed to increase during surgical hypotension. This result suggested either loss of autoregulation or an unexpectedly reduced brain compliance (30).

JUGULAR VENOUS SATURATION MONITORING

$SjvO_2$ monitoring permits continuous observation of oxygen saturation of blood leaving the cranium through a fiberoptic catheter inserted into the internal jugular vein (IJ) and threaded retrograde into the jugular bulb (1). Measurement of $SjvO_2$ permits calculation of the $AVDO_2$ [$AVDO_2$ = 1.39 × hemoglobin concentration × (SaO_2 − $SjvO_2$)]. Using CPP as an estimate for CBF, a rough estimation can be made of $CMRO_2$ when $SjvO_2$ is used in conjunction with CPP monitoring (39, 50). $SjvO_2$ monitoring is portable, provides continuous monitoring of venous saturation, and yields a direct, quantitative, global value of $SjvO_2$.

From a technical standpoint, the catheter is inserted retrograde into the IJ over a guide-wire, using sterile technique (1, 23, 50). Venous puncture of the IJ usually requires rotation of the head. Therefore, suspected cervical spine injury, in addition to coagulopathy, is a relative contraindication (1). Successful insertion of an IJ catheter without head rotation has been described and uses a point directly above the lateral border of the sternocleidomastoid at the level of the cricoid cartilage (63). A skull film is used to ensure that the catheter is at the jugular bulb. Controversy exists as to which IJ to use to reduce sampling error. A 5–15% difference in $SjvO_2$ between the IJs has been described (50). Often, the IJ that yields the higher ICP when compressed will be chosen (36). If ICP changes are similar after compression, the IJ ipsilateral to the lesion will be selected. If the lesion is diffuse, then the right IJ has been used, because it is often the dominant one (1, 36). Complications include carotid puncture (3–4%) and line sepsis (0–5%) (36, 50). Unfortunately, artifacts are common with $SjvO_2$ monitoring (5–55%) (12, 18, 36) and usually occur when the fiberoptic catheter is obstructed by the vessel wall. Other causes of artifact are breakage of the optical fiber, obstruction of the catheter lumen with blood, looping of the catheter in the IJ, and poor correlation between fiberoptic and laboratory oximeters (1, 13, 36, 54).

Continuous monitoring of $SjvO_2$ has demonstrated multiple episodes of early (less than 3 days) and late venous desaturation ($SjvO_2$ <50% for 10 minutes) in the period after TBI (12, 18, 36). Episodes of early venous desaturation were observed in 39.6% of TBI patients, usually within 24 hours of injury (18). Desaturations often lasted less than 1 hour and, therefore, were likely to go undetected by intermittent monitoring (18; Fig. 5). They were more likely to occur in patients with reduced CBF (18, 54). An increase in $AVDO_2$ in the face of decreasing CBF suggested that CBF was barely adequate for a given $CMRO_2$ and that ischemia was imminent (Fig. 1). Understandably, venous desaturations after TBI correlated with poor outcome and increased mortality

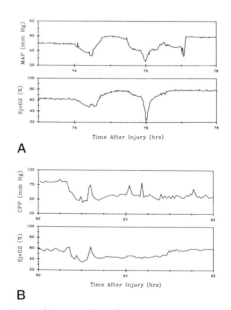

FIG. 5 $SjvO_2$ reduction and increased cerebral extraction of oxygen occurs for a variety of reasons. Often, systemic hypotension will reduce the supply of oxygen to the brain, causing increased extraction and reduced $SjvO_2$ **(A)**. These episodes can be of short duration and may be missed by monitoring modalities that are not continuous. In addition to systemic hypotension, brain hypotension resulting from reduced CPP from intracranial hypertension or hypocarbia reduces the available oxygen supply to the brain and results in increase oxygen extraction and reduced $SjvO_2$ **(B)**. Often, these changes are brief and cannot be detected without continuous monitoring. [Reproduced with permission (54).]

(18, 54; Fig. 6). Late venous desaturations (greater than 3 days) accounted for 26% of desaturations (12) and tended to be prolonged. The global hypoxia treatment that precipitated these desaturations (it was unresponsive to treatment) proved deleterious and correlated with poor outcome independent of ICP (12).

Venous desaturations resulted from various pathophysiologic processes, all of which reduced the flow of oxygen to the brain. Desaturations occurred with reduced arterial oxygen as a result of hypoxia or hypotension, or with increased cerebrovascular resistance from hypocapnia or vasospasm (36, 54; Fig. 5). Finally, cerebral hypoperfusion attributable to intracranial hypertension also precipitated venous desaturation (36; Figs. 4 and 5). Interestingly, venous desaturations caused by cerebral hypoperfusion from systemic hypotension were immediate; yet, venous desaturations from cerebral hypoperfusion from elevated ICP were delayed (54). In certain cases, the degree of venous desaturation may have been underestimated because of extracerebral mixing of venous blood (54).

$SjvO_2$ monitoring also may provide information regarding changes in brain compliance similar to those seen with pulsatility indices and

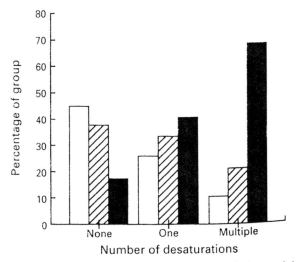

FIG. 6 After TBI, subsequent episodes of brain hypoperfusion and hypoxia were deleterious. Episodes of decreased O_2 supply to the brain, as evidenced by jugular venous desaturations, strongly correlated with outcome. With successive desaturations, mortality (*shaded bars*) increased significantly. Severe disability (*lined bars*) tended to be stable, whereas good recovery (*open bars*) fell precipitously. With multiple jugular venous desaturations, poor outcome as defined by mortality plus severe disability was almost 90%. [Reproduced with permission from (19).]

TCD. Cerebral hemodynamic reserve represents the ability of the brain to tolerate reduction in CPP without an increase in oxygen extraction (13). Cerebral reserve can be determined if ICP and $SjvO_2$ are monitored. After severe TBI, patients with initial severe brain swelling had a compromised cerebral reserve with significant oxygen extraction for a given fall in CPP. This observation suggested that a given CPP provided just enough CBF to prevent ischemia and that reduction in the CPP resulted in increased oxygen extraction. This scenario improved over the course of one day. Conversely, those patients with moderate brain swelling had a normal cerebral reserve and did not extract more oxygen with a fall in CPP. This cerebral reserve status became compromised if cerebral swelling was exacerbated over the course of a day (13).

CEREBRAL BLOOD FLOW—CLEARANCE TECHNIQUES

Without a direct measurement of CVR, measurement of CPP provides only an estimation of CBF (41). TCD ultrasonography itself only suggests relative CBF based on patterns of FV. Because of errors inherent in the indirect techniques, an argument can be made for direct measurement of CBF in the setting of TBI (3, 39, 44). The classic method for direct measurement of CBF is using the uptake and clearance of an inert, diffusible gas that is proportional to blood flow (3, 39). Nitrous oxide was the first gas used (26), but this technique only yielded a measurement of global CBF and was invasive (3, 39). Currently, radioisotopes of inert gases such as ^{133}Xe can be used to determine regional CBF. In this technique, the radioactive gas is inhaled until the brain levels are stable; radiation dosage is minimized because only trace doses are required (3, 39). [133]Xe washout is measured noninvasively by multiple portable detectors that allow determination of regional CBF (3). ^{133}Xe-CBF often has poor resolution, though, with areas of high CBF concealing areas of low CBF. In addition, the technique does not provide continuous determination of CBF (3). Since Xe has high radiographic density, CBF can be determined after inhalation of a high concentration of Xe and then measuring its washout regionally by using rapid serial computerized tomography (CT) scans (3, 39). Xe-CT provides better resolution and quantification of CBF than does the ^{133}Xe-CBF technique. However, the technique is not portable, and large concentrations of Xe that may produce somnolence are often required (3).

CBF determination can rapidly detect ischemia after TBI. In patients with severe TBI, ischemic flows were detected in 28% of cases (3, 51). Many of these ischemic flows were detected within 6 hours of TBI, and CBF determination detected within the first 6 hours after TBI was often lower than during any other period after TBI (3; Fig. 7). Mean CBF after TBI correlated with outcome, and patients with early ischemic flows usually died within 48 hours of injury (3, 51; Fig. 7). When CBF was correlated with the results of CT scanning, ischemia was observed in 40–50% of cases with subdural hematoma or diffuse brain swelling. In patients with epidural hematomas or focal contusions, ischemia was present in only 0–6% of cases (3, 44). Because ischemia often occurs early after TBI, immediate determination of ischemia by direct CBF measurement can prove difficult and impractical (44). Because ischemia is so often associated with subdural hematoma or diffuse brain swelling in the early period after TBI, an argument can be made to assume that ischemia is present and to treat it accordingly before initial CBF determination (44).

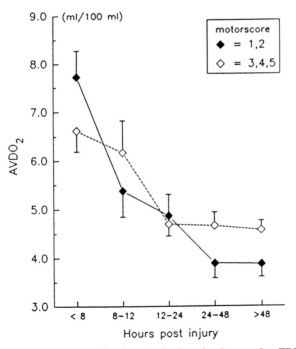

FIG. 7 Cerebral ischemia often develops in the first few hours after TBI. In patients with severe TBI and reduced motor score on the Glasgow Coma Scale, AVDO$_2$ is greatest in the first few hours after injury and is higher in patients with a lower motor score (*black diamonds*). The large values of AVDO$_2$ are consistent with increased oxygen extraction resulting from cerebral ischemia (Reproduced with permission from Bouma GJ, Muizelaar JP, Choi SC, *et al.*: Cerebral circulation and metabolism after severe traumatic brain injury: The elusive role of ischemia. **J Neurosurg** 75:690, 1991.)

In a series of patients, mean CBF was determined for 10 days after severe TBI. Ischemia was present in 25% of these patients. In this subset of patients, hypocapnia and hypotension did not appear to contribute to the low CBF. Hyperemia was observed in 30% of overall group (51). CBF in excess of metabolic demand produces hyperemia. Hyperemia after TBI results from impaired metabolic coupling and may produce vascular engorgement and cerebral swelling (3). Direct CBF measurement may diagnose hyperemia and alterations of vascular reactivity in the early stages and allow for targeted therapy of CBF.

CBF—MICROCIRCULATORY MONITORING

In addition to CBF techniques that detect the washout of a given marker in large regions of brain tissue, CBF in the cerebral microcirculation can be monitored more locally by means of a probe placed on the brain or the skull. Currently, three techniques have been used clinically: laser Doppler flow (LDF), thermal diffusion flow (TDF), and near-infrared spectrometry (NIRS). Unlike TCD, which measures flow velocity in large conductance vessels, these techniques measure CBF continuously in the microcirculation and tissue (28, 41, 56). However, each has specific advantages and disadvantages related to technique and equipment (14, 19, 27, 28, 41, 56).

In the LDF technique, CBF is measured by means of a flexible, optical-light conducting probe that guides monochromatic laser light to biologic tissues and records Doppler-shifted, back-scattered light (28, 41; Fig. 8). Moving structures such as red blood cells will produce a Doppler frequency shift in relation to stationary structures, and the signal generated is a result of red cell flux (28). Probes can be placed at

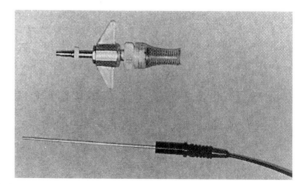

FIG. 8 The laser Doppler flowmetry probe can be inserted intraoperatively or at the bedside though a bolt. The LDF probe is small and monitors microcirculatory flow in a small area of cortex beneath the probe. [Reproduced with permission from (28).]

the bedside through a stationary bolt (28; Fig. 8) or in the operating room tunneled through a separate incision (41). LDF provides a continuous measure of relative microcirculatory flow using a portable detector (28). However, LDF does not produce quantitative data, records flow of only a small tissue volume, and does not provide information on flow direction (28, 41). Furthermore, artifact has been observed from local tissue pressure, large vessels, laceration of the cortex, or movement (28, 41).

In a group of patients with severe TBI, LDF was used to monitor alterations in CBF without complication. In 27% of these patients, LDF artifact precluded CBF monitoring (28). In the remainder of the group, LDF demonstrated a clear correlation between mean red blood cell flux and CPP. Furthermore, LDF was able to detect an autoregulatory breakpoint in these patients below which CPP was inadequate (28). Often, TCD and LDF results were tightly coupled; however, in certain instances, hyperemia was detected by LDF in the microcirculation while TCD measurements did not change (28). One hypothesis for this observation was that LDF could sense some local flow perturbations that TCD could not. In a different, smaller group of patients with severe TBI, LDF monitoring demonstrated that mean local CBF increased as the clinical condition improved. The pattern of CBF also changed over time as clinical improvement occurred. Patients who were severely comatose had low, fluctuating CBF inversely related to ICP. As neurologic function improved, CBF increased; but fluctuations in CBF were observed that were unrelated to respiration or ICP waves. When complete recovery occurred, no variations were observed in CBF. In these patients, Meyerson et al. hypothesized that the pattern of LDF flow changes correlated with various stages in the recovery of the microcirculation. In addition, they thought that LDF monitoring could reveal the effects of certain drugs on the microcirculation (41).

The TDF measures CBF using a flexible Silastic sheath with two gold plates on the undersurface (Fig. 9). The gold plates are positioned on the cortical surface, and each plate contains a thermistor that can be heated. Often, the distal plate is heated, and the proximal plate is kept normothermic. CBF is then inversely proportional to the temperature gradient between plates, and a quantitative measurement for CBF can be obtained (14, 56). TDF sheaths are normally placed intraoperatively and tunneled through a separate small incision; however, they can be placed at the bedside (14; Fig. 9). TDF provides continuous, quantitative, real-time measurements of CBF on a portable system. However, the technique is invasive and, like the LDF, records only a small tissue volume (14, 56). The sheath cannot be placed over a sulcus

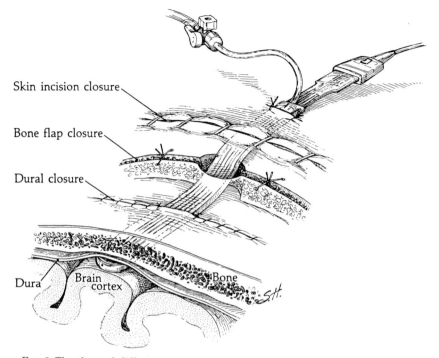

Skin incision closure

Bone flap closure

Dural closure

Dura   Brain   Bone
        cortex

FIG. 9 The thermal diffusion probe measures CBF in the microcirculation by monitoring the temperature gradient between two plates placed on the cortical surface. The
probe is placed intraoperatively and tunneled through the craniotomy and out a separate
incision. [Reproduced with permission from (14).]

or a major vessel and is best suited for homogeneous states of flow and
perfusion, such as those observed after diffuse cerebral swelling (14).

TDF was used for continuous monitoring of CBF in a small group of
patients with severe TBI. In one-half of the patients, ischemic levels of
CBF were observed at some interval after TBI. In the other half of the
group, hyperemic levels of CBF were recorded. Sustained low CBF
measurements in these patients were associated with vasospasm and,
often, brain death. Hyperemic CBF levels were often associated with
poor outcome and intracranial hypertension (14). In a larger group of
patients with TBI, TDF was used to monitor CBF for 7 days. Thirty-
three percent of the comatose patients had ischemic levels of CBF in
the first 8 hours after injury. An improving CBF in these patients
correlated with good outcome (56). Unfortunately, artifact prevented
use of TDF in 35% of patients. In both studies, the threshold CBF for
survival of cortical function obtained using TDF correlated well with
measurements obtained using Xenon, N_2O, and H_2 clearance (14, 56).

The three major light-absorbing molecules in the brain are oxyhemoglobin (HbO_2), deoxyhemoglobin (Hb), and cytochrome aa_3 (19). NIRS allows noninvasive monitoring of relative changes in the chromophore levels of HbO_2 and Hb through detectors placed on the scalp (27; Fig. 10). Absorption of light by HbO_2 and reduced HB is detected by using light at a wavelength near 760 nm (near infrared). The NIRS unit is a portable unit with a probe that consists of two tungsten filament lamps placed 3.5 cm on either side of a 760-nm light detector (19; Fig. 10). NIRS offers the advantage of portable, continuous, noninvasive, regional monitoring of hemoglobin oxygenation. NIRS monitoring can be performed only over a small region, and it is prone to artifact from stray light sources, scalp blood flow, and arrest of NIRS signal as a result of stray light. The NIRS can also be distorted by drift and temperature changes (27).

Using multimodality monitoring, including TCD, LDF, ICP, and $SjvO_2$, 38 ischemic or hyperemic events were monitored in nine patients with TBI who demonstrated large decreases or increases in CPP. In these patients, NIRS detected 37 (97%) of the changes, whereas $SjvO_2$ monitoring detected only 20 (53%) of the changes (Fig. 11). Hypoxia, intracranial hypertension, and reduced cerebral perfusion caused decreased levels of oxyhemoglobin (Fig. 11). Hyperemia was associated with increased CBF and increased levels of oxyhemoglobin (27). In 46 patients with TBI, NIRS was performed to assess for changes in optical density consistent with hematoma formation (19). In this group of patients, hematomas resulted in significantly higher changes in optical density between hemispheres than did diffuse injury (Fig. 10). Furthermore, epidural and subdural hematomas had significantly higher changes in optical density than intracerebral hematomas (19). In those patients with extraaxial hematomas, the change in optical density correlated with hematoma thickness (19). Hence, NIRS proved to be a continuous, inexpensive way to monitor for development of an intracranial hematoma. Unfortunately, localization of the hematoma and detection of bilateral and chronic hematomas proved to be a technical problem (19).

METABOLIC MONITORING WITH EMISSION TOMOGRAPHY

Measurement of CBF and $CMRO_2$ can be performed simultaneously and directly by monitoring the metabolic rate of some substrates themselves, using radionuclide tracers (2, 16, 22, 35, 39). Positron emission tomography (PET) uses emission CT to measure the *in vivo* distribution of positron-emitting radionuclides; regional CBF and regional $CMRO_2$ can be determined by measuring ^{15}O in brain slices, whole blood, and plasma during inhalation of $C^{15}O_2$ and $^{15}O_2$ (16). Use

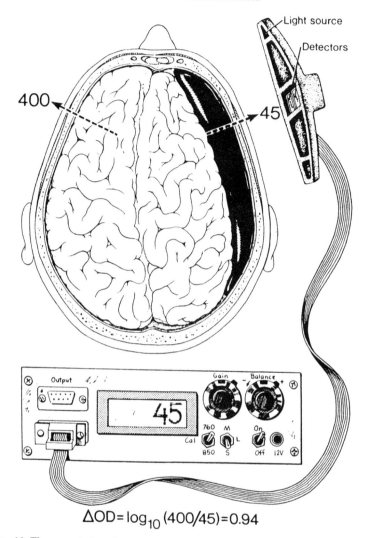

$$\Delta OD = \log_{10} (400/45) = 0.94$$

FIG. 10 The near-infrared spectroscopy probe consists of two tungsten filaments placed on either side of a near-infrared (760-nm) light detector. The probe measures changes in Hb oxygenation by monitoring changes in near infrared light absorbency or optical density. The apparatus is portable and noninvasive. [Reproduced with permission from (19).]

of the tracer [^{18}F]fluorodeoxyglucose permits measurement of the cerebral metabolic rate of glucose consumption [CMRG1] (2). PET provides a method to obtain direct, quantitative measurements of CMRO$_2$

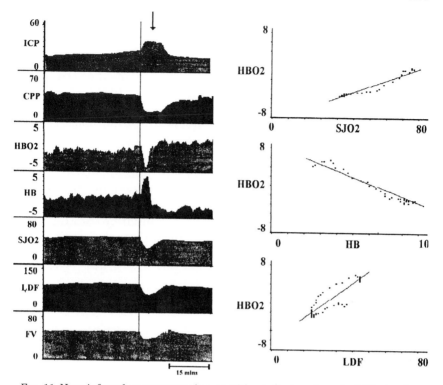

FIG. 11 Near-infrared spectroscopy is a sensitive indicator of cerebral Hb desaturation. In this patient with TBI, near-infrared spectroscopy detected a reduction in the level of HbO₂ and an increase in the level of deoxyhemoglobin. Simultaneous multimodality monitoring demonstrated intracranial hypertension, cerebral hypoperfusion, jugular venous desaturation, and reduction of laser Doppler and transcranial Doppler flow velocities (**A**). All of these changes were consistent with cerebral ischemia. Reduction of the Hb level correlated with jugular venous desaturation and reduction in cortical cerebral blood flow (**B**). [Reproduced with permission from (27).]

in any region of the brain with good resolution. Reproducibility is often within 5% (16).

PET affords the opportunity to study regional O_2 supply and use simultaneously, as well as regional glucose use. In doing so, uncoupling of CBF and $CMRO_2$ and CMRG1 can be quantified (2, 16). After acute and chronic ischemia, uncoupling was observed between glucose supply and use in ischemic tissue. Furthermore, uncoupling was also observed between $CMRO_2$ and CMRG1, with glucose metabolism much greater than oxygen metabolism. These results suggested a high rate of anerobic metabolism of glucose in ischemic tissue (2).

PET has not been used often in TBI patients for several reasons. First, PET is costly and requires specialized instrumentation not widely available (22). It is somewhat invasive, is not portable, does not provide for continuous monitoring, and has decreased sensitivity at high flow rates. Resolution of the tomograph can be diminished as a result of partial volume effect. Inaccurate head positioning makes reproducibility and serial measurements difficult (16). Because of these problems, a different technique, single-photon emission computed tomography (SPECT), has become more popular.

SPECT is performed with radiolabeled amines that are highly lipophilic, have high brain extraction, and are flow-limited (22). One popular tracer is N-isopropyl I-123 p-iodoamphetamine. The tracers and equipment used to perform SPECT scanning are cheaper and more widely available than those for PET. Unfortunately, SPECT yields qualitative data. Also, the resolution obtained through SPECT is inferior to that obtained by PET (39). Quantitative data has been obtained using SPECT following a stroke. Quantitation of a SPECT scan requires a normal hemisphere in the same patient and involves comparison of emissions from the abnormal hemisphere to the normal hemisphere (22).

A group of patients with acute focal ischemia were studied, using SPECT scanning to measure CBF and CT scanning to determine regions of infarction. In half the patients, the initial SPECT abnormality delineated the exact area of infarct eventually observed on CT. In the other half of the group, the SPECT abnormality was larger than that observed on CT (22). A second group of stroke patients showed similar findings (35). In these patients, the SPECT image correlated well with the severity of the initial symptoms but not with outcome (35). In many of these cases, SPECT was obtained in the first few hours after symptoms; it was hypothesized that SPECT scanning at this point demonstrated both reversibly and irreversibly injured neurons (22, 35). In the setting of TBI, SPECT has not been studied significantly because of difficulties with its resolution, as well as with quantitation of its measurements. SPECT has also not gained in use because of the popularity of other methods for measuring CBF.

ELECTROPHYSIOLOGIC MONITORING

To complement the measurement of metabolic parameters in the injured brain, electrophysiologic monitoring in TBI can provide a functional assessment of the neural structures involved in the tested pathway (23, 57). Functional monitoring can be performed through electroencephalography (EEG)- or sensory-evoked potentials (SEP). SEP can be subdivided into somatosensory-evoked potentials (SSEP), visual-evoked potentials (VEP), and auditory brainstem responses (ABR). Electrophysiologic monitoring augments the neurologic examination and provides useful information when other measures of neural function are limited by coma or medication (21, 45, 57).

EEG measures spontaneous electrical activity in the superficial cortex through scalp electrodes. When compared with SEP, the signal amplitudes of EEG are large and represent activity in the underlying cortex. EEG can be performed on a portable apparatus, is noninvasive, and can record global and regional function. However, EEG does not give quantitative results and can be performed continuously only with difficulty. After TBI, EEG results were more abnormal when measured closer to the time of injury or after alterations in consciousness. Global EEG abnormalities resolved faster than focal ones (57). Although debatable, EEG results predicted bad outcome but were unable to predicate good outcome; furthermore, no specific pattern of EEG abnormality was representative of TBI (57). When used in the setting of TBI, certain problems have arisen with EEG. EEG changes have lagged behind the clinical course. EEG results vary with time, and the optimal period for obtaining EEG after TBI has not been determined. EEG results also vary with region, and the optimal region for EEG after TBI has not been determined (57). Also EEG interpretations can be done by relatively few physicians in the intensive care setting.

SEPs represent minute electrical responses generated in sensory pathways in response to stimulation of that sensory modality (21). SEPs are quantified according to amplitude, latency, and conduction. The SEP technique can be performed using a portable machine and can yield quantitative information regarding regional SEPs. Unfortunately, determination of SEP generally does not provide continuous monitoring. Unlike EEG, SEP monitoring is relatively resistant to artifact from sedation and can be used to assess the function of subcortical structures (21, 38, 57). After TBI, SEP has been used as an adjunct to the neurologic examination in monitoring the clinical condition (21, 45). SSEP, VEP, and ABR have all been used together in multimodality monitoring, and simultaneous usage of these modes of SEP yields a powerful predictor of outcome after TBI (51, 52). SEP can also be used in determination of brain death (38, 57). Injury to peripheral structures such as nerves, eyes, and ears may preclude usage of SSEP, VEP, and ABR, respectively. Because of inherently small amplitude, SEP may be difficult to detect above electrical noise generated in the ICU (21, 57).

After TBI, SSEP has been reported to have a higher correlation with outcome than other modes of SEP (29). After severe TBI, SSEP was compared in patients with diffuse brain injury, those with focal contusions greater than 2.5 cm, and those with normal CT scans. No significant difference was observed on initial SSEP in these patients. However, in those patients with diffuse brain injury and focal contusions, SSEP recordings deteriorated 22.6% and 41.2%, respectively. In those patients with normal CT scans, SSEP recordings improved 51.1% (29). In another group of patients with severe TBI, bilaterally preserved SSEP recordings 70 msec after a stimulus correlated with good outcome. Poor outcome was correlated with absent SSEP recordings 50 msec after a stimulus (43). In those patients whose SSEPs deteriorated, an increase in $AVDO_2$ was observed, suggesting an impairment in oxygen delivery or use (43).

Although often studied in severe TBI, electrophysiological abnormalities have been observed following lesser insults. After minor TBI, Varney *et al.* followed a group of patients with theta bursts on EEG (61). Interestingly, 78% of these patients complained of symptoms similar to those described in the setting of complex partial seizures. When treated with antiepileptic drugs, 67% of these patients experienced improvement in their symptoms.

Although various electrophysiologic techniques have been applied to TBI patients, there has been great variability in the findings in almost all groups. Certainly EEGs are critical if seizures are suspected in acute or chronic injury phases, and some clinicians use EEG burst-suppression to determine the dosage of barbiturates for induced coma (25). However, because of common discrepancies between electrophysiologic studies and clinical status or outcome, these modalities have not been used as routinely in TBI patients as the clinical examination, CT scanning, or other cerebral monitoring methods.

BRAIN MICRODIALYSIS

Investigators have been able to sample neurochemicals directly *in vivo* by infusing small amounts of fluid through one lumen of a microcatheter into the brain and analyzing tiny amounts of extracellular neurochemicals in the effluent retrieved through a second lumen. This technique is referred to as microdialysis. Experimental animal studies of microdialysis after brain ischemia and traumatic injury have been reported over the past several years, and initial reports are appearing on the use of microdialysis in humans with these insults.

Microdialysis of multiple neurochemicals including lactate, pyruvate, aspartate, and glutamate was performed in 10 patients with spontaneous SAH for as long as 11 days. The lactate:pyruvate ratio and glutamate levels were successively elevated and correlated with outcome (48). Kanthan and Shuaib observed very high concentrations of glutamate, glycine, and γ-aminobutyrate in a patient with severe

TBI (24). Langemann *et al.* monitored brain glucose, lactate, and pH in the dialysate (phD) of four patients with TBI and found that glucose and the glucose:lactate ratio correlated to a certain degree with the clinical courses of these patients (34). In two patients with TBI and one with subarachnoid hemorrhage, these investigators also measured glucose, lactate, and phD, as well as several antioxidants, including ascorbic acid, uric acid, glutathione, and cysteine. Again the researchers observed a relationship between changes in neurochemical levels and clinical phenomena such as hypoxia or intracranial hypertension (31). Bullock *et al.* observed glutamate and aspartate concentrations 600-fold greater than baseline in a patient with vascular cerebral infarction. Interestingly, the duration of excitatory amino acid elevation in this patient was longer than that observed in animal studies (6). Bullock *et al.* also recently presented preliminary data in 60 TBI patients in whom they measured brain O_2, CO_2, pH, temperature, glutamate, aspartate, potassium, lactate, and glucose, along with ICP and CPP. Excitatory amino acid elevation correlated most closely with elevated potassium or intracranial hypertension. Elevated lactate concentration correlated neither with cerebral hypoperfusion nor poor outcome. Of the parameters examined in their study, brain oxygen monitoring appeared to be the most practical and useful in guiding therapy and influencing outcome (5; R. Bullock, presentation at ICRAN5, Riccione, Italy, September 1996).

Microdialysis appears to be a most promising tool for monitoring brain chemistry and response to treatment. At present, it is an expensive and laborious technique and has been approved only for experimental use. If the monitoring system costs can be lowered and sufficient data collected to ensure its reliability and usefulness such that it can be approved for routine clinical use, microdialysis and brain gas determinations may become essential features of future monitoring in TBI.

SUMMARY

In the past several years, improvements in technology have advanced the monitoring capabilities for patients with TBI. The primary goal of monitoring the patient with TBI is to prevent secondary insults to the brain, primarily cerebral ischemia. Cerebral ischemia may occur early and without clinical correlation and portends a poor outcome. Measurement of ICP is the cornerstone of monitoring in the patient with TBI. Monitoring of ICP provides a measurement of CPP and a rough estimation of CBF. However, with alterations in pressure autoregulation, measurement of CPP does not always allow for determination of CBF. To circumvent this problem, direct measurements of CBF can be performed using clearance techniques (^{133}Xe, N_2O, Xe-CT) or invasive monitoring techniques (LDF, TDF, NIRS). Although direct and quantitative, clearance techniques do not allow for continuous monitoring. Invasive CBF monitoring techniques are new, and artifactual results can be problematic.

The techniques of jugular venous saturation monitoring and TCD are well-established and are powerful adjuncts to ICP monitoring. They allow the clinician to monitor cerebral oxygen extraction and blood flow velocity, respectively, for any given CPP. Use of TCD may predict posttraumatic vasospasm before clinical sequelae. Jugular venous saturation monitoring may detect clinically occult episodes of cerebral ischemia and increased oxygen extraction. Jugular venous saturation monitoring optimizes the use of hyperventilation in the treatment of intracranial hypertension.

Although PET and SPECT scanning allow direct measurement of $CMRO_2$, these techniques have limited application currently. Similarly, microdialysis is in its infancy but has demonstrated great promise for metabolic monitoring. EEG and SEP are excellent adjuncts to the monitoring arsenal and provide immediate information on current brain function. With improvements in electronic telemetry, functional monitoring by EEG or SEP may become an important part of routine monitoring in TBI.

REFERENCES

1. Andrews PJ, Dearden NM, Miller JD: Jugular bulb cannulation: Description of a cannulation technique and validation of a new continuous monitor. **Br J Anaesth** 67:553–558, 1991.
2. Baron JC, Rougemont D, Soussaline F, *et al.*: Local interrelationships of cerebral oxygen consumption and glucose utilization in normal subjects and in ischemic stroke patients: A positron tomography study. **J Cereb Blood Flow Metab** 4:140–149, 1984.
3. Bouma GJ, Muizelaar JP: Cerebral blood flow in severe clinical head injury. **New Horiz** 3:384–394, 1995.
4. Bouma GJ, Muizelaar JP, Bandoh K, *et al.*: Blood pressure and intracranial pressure-volume dynamics in severe head injury: Relationship with cerebral blood flow. **J Neurosurg** 77:15–19, 1992.
5. Bullock R, Zauner A, Myseros JS, *et al.*: Evidence for prolonged release of excitatory amino acids in severe human head trauma: Relationship to clinical events. **Ann N Y Acad Sci** 765:290–297, 1995.
6. Bullock R, Zauner A, Woodward J, *et al.*: Massive persistent release of excitatory amino acids following human occlusive stroke. **Stroke** 26:2187–2189, 1995.
7. Chambers KR, Kane PJ, Choksey MS, *et al.*: An evaluation of the camino ventricular bolt system in clinical practice. **Neurosurgery** 33:866–868, 1993.

8. Chan KH, Dearden NM, Miller JD: The significance of posttraumatic increase in cerebral blood flow velocity: A transcranial Doppler ultrasound study. **Neurosurgery** 30:697–700, 1992.

9. Chan KH, Dearden NM, Miller JD, et al.: Multimodality monitoring as a guide to treatment of intracranial hypertension after severe brain injury. **Neurosurgery** 32:547–553, 1993.

10. Chesnut RM: Secondary brain insults after head injury: Clinical perspectives. **New Horiz** 3:366–375, 1995.

11. Chestnut RM, Marshall SB, Piek J, et al.: Early and late systemic hypotension as a frequent and fundamental source of cerebral ischemia following severe brain injury in the Traumatic Coma Data Bank. **Acta Neurochir Suppl (Wien)** 59:121–125, 1993.

12. Cruz J: On-line monitoring of global cerebral hypoxia in acute brain injury: Relationship to intracranial hypertension. **J Neurosurg** 79:228–233, 1993.

13. Cruz J, Gennarelli TA, Alves WM: Continuous monitoring of cerebral hemodynamic reserve in acute brain injury: Relationship to changes in brain swelling. **J Trauma** 32:629–634; discussion 634–635, 1992.

14. Dickman CA, Carter LP, Baldwin HZ, et al.: Continuous regional cerebral blood flow monitoring in acute craniocerebral trauma. **Neurosurgery** 28:467–472, 1991.

15. Eddy VA, Vitsky JL, Rutherford EJ, et al.: Aggressive use of ICP monitoring is safe and alters patient care. **Am Surg** 61:24–29, 1995.

16. Frackowiak RS, Lenzi GL, Jones T, et al.: Quantitative measurement of regional cerebral blood flow and oxygen metabolism in man using ^{15}O and positron emission tomography: Theory, procedure, and normal values. **J Comput Assisted Tomogr** 4:727–736, 1980.

17. Ghajar J, Hariri RJ, Narayan RK, et al.: Survey of critical care management of comatose, head-injured patients in the United States. **Crit Care Med** 23:560–567, 1995.

18. Gopinath SP, Robertson CS, Contant CF, et al.: Jugular venous desaturation and outcome after head injury. **J Neurol Neurosurg Psychiatry** 57:717–723, 1994.

19. Gopinath SP, Robertson CS, Grossman RG, et al.: Near-infrared spectroscopic localization of intracranial hematomas. **J Neurosurg** 79:43–47, 1993.

20. Goraj B, Rifkinson-Mann S, Leslie DR, et al.: Correlation of intracranial pressure and transcranial Doppler resistive index after head trauma. **Am J Neuroradiol** 15:1333–1339, 1994.

21. Greenberg RP, Mayer DJ, Becker DP, et al.: Evaluation of brain function in severe human head trauma with multimodality evoked potentials. Part 2. Localization of brain dysfunction and correlation with posttraumatic neurological conditions. **J Neurosurg** 47:163–177, 1977.

22. Hill TC, Magistretti PL, Holman BL, et al.: Assessment of regional cerebral blood flow (rCBF) in stroke using SPECT and N-isopropyl-(I-123)-p-iodoamphetamine (IMP). **Stroke** 15:40–45, 1984.

23. Jordan KG: Neurophysiologic monitoring in the neuroscience intensive care unit. **Neurol Clin** 13:579–626, 1995.

24. Kanthan R, Shuaib A: Clinical evaluation of extracellular amino acids in severe head

trauma by intracerebral in vivo microdialysis. **J Neurol Neurosurg Psychiatry** 59:326–327, 1995.

25. Kassell NF, Hitchon PW, Gerk MK, *et al.*: Alterations in cerebral blood flow, oxygen metabolism, and electrical activity produced by high dose sodium thiopental. **Neurosurgery** 7:598–603, 1980.

26. Kety SS, Schmidt CF: The determination of cerebral blood flow in man by the use of nitrous oxide in low concentrations. **Am J Physiol** 143:53–66, 1945.

27. Kirkpatrick PJ, Smielewski P, Czosnyka M, *et al.*: Near-infrared spectroscopy use in patients with head injury. **J Neurosurg** 83:963–970.

28. Kirkpatrick PJ, Smielewski P, Czosnyka M, *et al.*: Continuous monitoring of cortical perfusion by laser Doppler flowmetry in ventilated patients with head injury. **J Neurol Neurosurg Psychiatry** 57:1382–1388, 1994.

29. Konasiewicz SJ, Moulton RJ: Electrophysiologic assessment of intracerebral contusions in closed head injury. **J Trauma** 37:370–374.

30. Lam AM: Change in cerebral blood flow velocity pattern during induced hypotension: A non-invasive indicator of increased intracranial pressure? **Br J Anaesth** 68:424–428, 1992.

31. Landolt H, Langemann H, Mendelowitsch A, *et al.*: Neurochemical monitoring and on-line pH measurements using brain microdialysis in patients in intensive care. **Acta Neurochir Suppl (Wien)** 60:475–478, 1994.

32. Lang EW, Chesnut RM: Intracranial pressure: Monitoring and management. **Neurosurg Clin N Am** 5:573–605, 1994.

33. Lang EW, Chesnut RM: Intracranial pressure and cerebral perfusion pressure in severe head injury. **New Horiz** 3:400–409, 1993.

34. Langemann H, Mendelowitsch A, Landolt H, *et al.*: Experimental and clinical monitoring of glucose by microdialysis. **Clin Neurol Neurosurg** 97:149–155, 1995.

35. Lee RG, Hill TC, Holman BL, *et al.*: Predictive value of perfusion defect size using N-isopropyl-(I-123)-p-iodoamphetamine emission tomography in acute stroke. **J Neurosurg** 61:449–452, 1984.

36. Lewis SB, Myburgh JA, Reilly PL: Detection of cerebral venous desaturation by continuous jugular bulb oximetry following acute neurotrauma. **Anaesth Intensive Care** 23:307–314, 1995.

37. Lindegaard KF, Nornes H, Bakke SJ, *et al.*: Cerebral vasospasm diagnosis by means of angiography and blood velocity measurements. **Acta Neurochir (Wien)** 100:12–24, 1989.

38. Litscher G, Schwarz G, Kleinert R: Brain-stem auditory evoked potential monitoring: Variations of stimulus artifact in brain death. **Electroencephalogr Clin Neurophysiol** 96:413–419, 1995.

39. Martin NA, Doberstein C: Cerebral blood flow measurement in neurosurgical intensive care. **Neurosurg Clin N Am** 5:607–618, 1994.

40. Martin NA, Doberstein C, Zane C, *et al.*: Posttraumatic cerebral arterial spasm: Transcranial Doppler ultrasound, cerebral blood flow, and angiographic findings. **J Neurosurg** 77:575–583, 1992.

41. Meyerson BA, Gunasekera L, Linderoth B, *et al.*: Bedside monitoring of regional cortical blood flow in comatose patients using laser Doppler flowmetry. **Neurosurgery** 29:750–755, 1991.

42. Mollman HD, Rockswold GL, Ford SE: A clinical comparison of subarachnoid catheters to ventriculostomy and subarachnoid bolts: A prospective study. **J Neurosurg** 68:737–741, 1988.
43. Moulton RJ, Shedden PM, Tucker WS, *et al.*: Somatosensory evoked potential monitoring following severe closed head injury. **Clin Invest Med** 17:187–195, 1994.
44. Muizelaar JP, Schroder ML: Overview of monitoring of cerebral blood flow and metabolism after severe head injury. **Can J Neurol Sci** 21:S6–11, 1994.
45. Narayan RK, Kishore PR, Becker DP, *et al.*: Intracranial pressure: To monitor or not to monitor? A review of our experience with severe head injury. **J Neurosurg** 56:650–659, 1982.
46. Ostrup RC, Luerssen TG, Marshall LF, *et al.*: Continuous monitoring of intracranial pressure with a miniaturized fiberoptic device. **J Neurosurg** 67:206–209, 1987.
47. Paramore CG, Turner DA: Relative risks of ventriculostomy infection and morbidity. **Acta Neurochir (Wien)** 127:79–84, 1994.
48. Persson L, Valtysson J, Enblad P, *et al.*: Neurochemical monitoring using intracerebral microdialysis in patients with subarachnoid hemorrhage. **J Neurosurg** 84:606–616, 1996.
49. Pople IK, Muhlbauer MS, Sanford RA, *et al.*: Results and complications of intracranial pressure monitoring in 303 children. **Pediatr Neurosurg** 23:64–67, 1995.
50. Ritter AM, Robertson CS: Cerebral metabolism. **Neurosurg Clin N Am** 5:633–645, 1994.
51. Robertson CS, Contant CF, Gokaslan ZL, *et al.*: Cerebral blood flow, arteriovenous oxygen difference, and outcome in head injured patients. **J Neurol Neurosurg Psychiatry** 55:594–603, 1992.
52. Romner B, Bellner J, Kongstad P, *et al.*: Elevated transcranial Doppler flow velocities after severe head injury: Cerebral vasospasm or hyperemia? **J Neurosurg** 85:90–97, 1996.
53. Rosner MJ, Rosner SD, Johnson AH: Cerebral perfusion pressure: Management protocol and clinical results. **J Neurosurg** 83:949–962, 1995.
54. Sheinberg M, Kanter MJ, Robertson CS, *et al.*: Continuous monitoring of jugular venous oxygen saturation in head-injured patients. **J Neurosurg** 76:212–217, 1992.
55. Shigemori M, Kikuchi N, Tokutomi T, *et al.*: Monitoring of severe head-injured patients with transcranial Doppler (TCD) ultrasonography. **Acta Neurochir Suppl (Wien)** 55:6–7, 1992.
56. Sioutos PJ, Orozco JA, Carter LP, *et al.*: Continuous regional cerebral cortical blood flow monitoring in head-injured patients. **Neurosurgery** 36:943–949, 1995.
57. Sloan TB: Electrophysiologic monitoring in head injury. **New Horiz** 3:431–438, 1995.
58. Steiger HJ, Aaslid R, Stooss R, *et al.*: Transcranial Doppler monitoring in head injury: Relations between type of injury, flow velocities, vasoreactivity, and outcome. **Neurosurgery** 34:79–85, 1994.
59. Takizawa H, Gabra-Sanders T, Miller JD: Changes in the cerebrospinal fluid pulse wave spectrum associated with raised intracranial pressure. **Neurosurgery** 20:355–361, 1987.
60. Unterberg A, Kiening K, Schmiedek P, *et al.*: Long-term observations of intracranial

pressure after severe head injury: The phenomenon of secondary rise of intracranial pressure. **Neurosurgery** 32:17–23, 1993.

61. Varney NR, Hines ME, Bailey C, *et al.*: Neuropsychiatric correlates of theta bursts in patients with closed head injury. **Brain Inj** 6:499–508, 1992.

62. Vernon DD, Woodward GA, Skjonsberg AK: Management of the patient with head injury during transport. **Crit Care Clin** 8:619–631, 1992.

63. Willeford KL, Reitan JA: Neutral head position for placement of internal jugular vein catheters. **Anaesthesia** 49:202–204, 1994.

III

General Scientific Session III
Analysis Of Outcome

18

Outcome Analysis in Lumbar Spine: Instabilities/Degenerative Disease

RICHARD G. FESSLER, M.D., Ph.D.

As the cost of medical care has become increasingly more expensive, the demand for analysis of patient outcome has likewise become greater. At the same time, however, the specific information requested in "outcome analysis" has changed. Whereas until recently outcome analysis specifically referred to "medical" outcome, it now is also interpreted to mean "quality of life," "patient satisfaction," and, most specifically "cost-effectiveness."

To prepare ourselves to provide this information on outcome analysis, we need to examine several key questions:

1. Why do we need outcome analysis?
2. What is outcome data?
3. How do you get outcome data?
4. What outcome data currently exists?
5. What tools to collect data currently exist?
6. How do we know which tools to use?
7. How do we evaluate agencies selling outcome analysis services?

This chapter will review each of these questions.

WHY DO WE NEED OUTCOME ANALYSIS?

"Idealistically," the best reason to pursue accurate analysis of our outcomes is to document for each of us the true results of our surgical and nonsurgical interventions. These data could be used for self-improvement of surgical and nonsurgical care, as well as for comparison to the "average outcome" on a local, regional, or national scale. Furthermore, these results could be used to give patients accurate statistics regarding the probability of specific results for specific surgeons, as well as for predicting the outcomes of specific patients. Less idealistically, but probably more importantly, we are rapidly approaching the point at which managed care organizations and payers will demand this information for contract negotiations and for referral of patients.

WHAT IS OUTCOME DATA?

Current definitions of outcome data include a variety of related measures. These include not only medical outcome but also functional outcome, return to work, quality of life, patient satisfaction, and cost-effectiveness.

Medical Result

Outcome analysis of the medical result in degenerative disease of the lumbar spine includes evaluation of a variety of parameters. First, was there a return of motor or sensory function that was lost before surgery? Second, what is the amount of residual pain that the patient is experiencing in either his/her back or leg? Third, if a discectomy was performed, was there a recurrent disc herniation? Fourth, if a fusion was performed, was the fusion successful, or did a pseudarthrosis occur? Fifth, has the patient continued on narcotic or nonnarcotic medication at the same dose and frequency as was used preoperatively? Finally, did the patient suffer any neurologic or vascular complications, or did a CSF leak, an infection, or spondylolisthesis occur as a result of the surgery?

Functional Outcome

Analysis of functional outcome falls into two categories. Absolute range of motion can be objectively tested by physical therapists for each range of motion of the lumbar spine and lower extremities. The second area of functional outcome is assessed by the patient in activities of daily living. Is the patient able to engage in strenuous activities that require running or lifting? Can the patient move heavy objects, use a vacuum cleaner, or engage in moderate sports activities, such as bowling or playing golf? Can the patient carry groceries or lift relatively light objects? Is the patient proficient at climbing multiple sets of stairs or even one set of stairs? How well does the patient do in activities that require bending, kneeling, or stooping? Is the patient able to walk several blocks or one block? Finally, is the patient capable of personal hygiene activities, such as self-bathing or self-dressing?

Return to Work

A relatively new area of assessment is the time period after surgery before the patient can return to work. Furthermore, the type of work to which the patient is to return is also assessed. Can the patient return to the same job he or she did before surgery? Can the patient return to work but to a job requiring less strenuous activity? Are the patient's overall physical abilities at work altered or are they the same? Did the patient require rehabilitation before being able to work? Finally, if the patient was not able to return to his/her previous type of employment, was a retraining program necessary to return the patient to some type of work?

Quality of Life

Quality of life can be analyzed through a variety of patient self-assessment questionnaires that address how illness has impacted the patient's life. These questionnaires can vary from simple "visual analog scales," through which the patient's assessment of his/her pain is assessed, to a variety of more detailed questionnaires that assess pain, depression, or quality of life in general. They include the Beck Depression Inventory, McGill-Melzack Pain Questionnaire, Sickness Inventory Profile, Coping Strategies Questionnaire, Symptom Checklist 90, Sickness Inventory, and the Oswestry Scale. Each of these questionnaires assesses the patient's perception of his/her quality of life, either through reported level of depression or reported level of impact of sickness on daily activities.

Patient Satisfaction

Patient satisfaction is frequently assessed through exit questionnaires administered by hospital personnel regarding the patient's perception of his/her hospital stay and his/her satisfaction with the care received in the hospital. Although these data may have implications for the patient's immediate postoperative period, they provide minimal predictability for the patient's long-term satisfaction with the surgical outcome; this has been assessed more effectively through a more recent tool known as SF-36.

Cost-Effectiveness

Finally, one of the most important outcome measures recently requested is cost-effectiveness. This measure includes the cost of the preoperative treatment, including evaluation, medications, physical therapy, injection therapy, and counseling. It also includes the cost of the procedure itself, including the surgeon's fee, the anesthesiologist's fee, the fee of critical care physicians (if included), consultations, and pharmacy. Furthermore, it includes the cost of ancillary services, including radiology, laboratory, physical therapy, room charge, and implantable devices. Finally, cost-effectiveness is reflected in the length of stay, length of rehabilitation, length of stay in the intensive care unit, and reliability and rapidity of filling out the multiple forms requested by insurance carriers, rehabilitation services, and attorneys.

HOW DO YOU GET OUTCOME DATA?

Outcome data can be collected through any of several means. First, each individual surgeon can collect his/her own outcome data, or a group of surgeons can collect their data together. This requires that each individual or group either device or buy scales to assess the above measures. Also, office personnel will be needed to administer the scales, as well as to collect and analyze the data.

A second option, which is currently being exercised by several hospitals, is that outcome evaluations are conducted by each hospital. They generally take the format of patient satisfaction surveys or cost data. Most frequently, these outcome evaluations do not include sufficient information on medical outcome to be used for this type of assessment. Finally, numerous outside agencies are currently available to perform these services for individuals, groups, or hospitals. These services are frequently available on a cost-per-patient basis, a cost-per-physician basis, or they can be contracted on a yearly basis.

WHAT OUTCOME DATA CURRENTLY EXIST?

Currently, there are no outcome data that address all of the above issues. Most medical literature addresses only medical and functional outcome. Specifically regarding degenerative disease of the lumbar spine, the majority of the medical literature has been criticized for using retrospective data collection, using analysis by surgeons involved with the patient's surgery, and having relatively small numbers of patients in each report. One recent publication that is not subject to these criticisms is that of Zdeblick et al. (12). In this prospective randomized evaluation, patients undergoing lumbar fusion were divided into three groups. Group One patients received no posterior instrumentation. Group Two patients received a semirigid posterior construct. Group Three patients received a fully rigid posterior instrumentation construct. Each patient was evaluated on the basis of fusion rate, pain level, and return to work. This study found a higher fusion rate, less pain, and a greater rate of return to work with increasing rigidity of the construct.

An alternative study evaluated the risk for undergoing second surgical procedures in patients undergoing lumbar fusion after worker-compensable injuries in the state of Washington (6). This retrospective data analysis concluded that instrumentation doubled the risk of a second surgery and that "outcome of lumbar fusion performed in injured workers was worse than reported in published case series." Other groups have retrospectively evaluated the data of the Social Security Administration and likewise questioned the effectiveness of surgery for low back disease (2–5, 9, 11). It is interesting to note that the criticisms of "retrospective data review and analysis by surgeons" does not seem to apply to these apparently "antisurgery" publications, which are retrospective data reviews by nonsurgeons. It would seem reasonable to propose that the criteria to which one group is expected to conform would be equally valid for all other groups.

Several authors have closely evaluated return-to-work rates after lumbar spine surgery (1, 7, 8, 10). Based on these evaluations, the best predictors for return to work after lumbar spine surgery would appear to be (*a*) preinjury job satisfaction, (*b*) Minnesota Multiphasic Personality Inventory scales I and II, and (*c*) the presence of a personality disorder. It is very interesting to note that a physician's assessment of the morbidity of an injury is not predictive of a patient's return to work (10).

WHAT TOOLS TO COLLECT DATA EXIST?

Some of the accepted tools used to measure outcome have previously been mentioned. These include:

1. Coping Strategies Questionnaire
2. McGill-Melzack Pain Questionnaire
3. SF-36 Health Questionnaire
4. Multi-dimensional Pain Inventory
5. Sickness Inventory Profile
6. Beck Depression Inventory
7. Symptom Check-List 90
8. Prolo Scale

Given the above tools and others are similar to them, how do we know which tools to use? Scientifically, the best tools are those that will have demonstrable validity, reliability, and predictability. Validity will have been determined through peer-reviewed publications that demonstrate that the attributes proposed for assessment are, in fact, assessed when compared to accepted measures. Reliability is demonstrated through repeated analysis of the same group demonstrating equivalent results. Predictability is ascertained through demonstrating that given a specific manipulation (such as surgery), an identifiable group of patients will reliably have a predictable result.

Economically, measurement tools must be relatively inexpensive to use, and they must be easy for patients to complete. Despite these desirable scientific and economic factors, however, it is difficult to predict what "payers" will use their own assessment of outcome. Ideally, one would hope that the most scientifically sound measures are chosen for general use. Ethically, we must absolutely reject the use of a tool chosen solely because it justifies the least amount of treatment.

HOW DO WE EVALUATE AGENCIES SPELLING OUTCOME ANALYSIS SERVICES?

When one decides to either collect one's own outcome data or use an agency for that service, there are numerous factors to consider in one's decision. First, at this time the most reasonable measures available, which appear to be well-founded in the literature and supported by the National Institute of Health are: (a) the MMPI, (b) the SF 36, (c) the Beck Depression Inventory, and (d) the McGill-Melzak Pain Questionnaire. Based on their widespread use and demonstrated reliability, all of these would appear to be excellent measures for inclusion in one's outcome analysis package.

The services offered must include an easy mechanism for data input. This could be performed by filling in dots on a card and sending the cards to the data analysis agency, or via direct computer entry, after which discs are mailed or data is downloaded to the data analysis organization. Definite data collection timepoints must be identifiable, and a definite schedule of reports with data interpretation must be offered. In addition, there must be a mechanism for handling missing data points. Absolute data security must be insured.

A definite mechanism of data input must be made available. This can be done on the basis of a descriptor, such as herniated disc disease, lumbar stenosis, or spondlyolisthesis, or it can be done on the basis of an ICD-9 code. Each has its benefits and disadvantages, but whichever is chosen, it must be adhered to uniformly. In addition, if one intends to use data analysis for competitive marketing, one must know what comparison groups are available with which one's data would be contrasted.

Finally, in evaluating an outside agency for their service, it must be determined whether the hardware will be supplied by the agency, or whether it will be bought independently by the physician or physician's group. The software maintenance and upgrades must be clearly defined and penalties put in place for failure so as to provide appropriate maintenance in a timely fashion. Reporting periods must be clearly defined. The reports must be readable, and interpretation of the results must be clear.

SUMMARY

In summary, expectations for outcome analysis have changed over the last several years. It is no longer the case that outcome analysis is expected to be done by academic institutions alone. Surgeons in private practice are rapidly approaching the time when outcome analysis of personal results will be necessary for competitive marketing purposes. In addition, the definition of outcome analysis has been considerably expanded from medical outcome to include functional outcome, return to work, quality of life, patient satisfaction, and cost-effectiveness. The above discussion has considered several aspects of data outcome analysis for degenerative disease of the lumbar spine. It is the intent of this review to help surgeons prepare themselves for changing expectations in their new medical environment.

REFERENCES

1. Bernard TN: Repeat lumbar spine surgery: Factors influencing outcome. **Spine** 15:2196–2206, 1993.
2. Cherkin DC, Deyo RA, Loeser JD, *et al.:* An international comparison of back surgery rates. **Spine** 19:1201–1206, 1994.
3. Ciol MA, Deyo RA, Kreuter W, *et al.:* Characteristics in Medicare beneficiaries associated with reoperation after lumbar spine surgery. **Spine** 19:1329–1334, 1994.
4. Deyo RA, Cherkin D, Conrad D: The back-pain outcome assessment team. **Health Serv Res** 25:733–737, 1990.
5. Deyo RA, Cial MA, Cherkin DC, *et al.:* Lumbar spinal fusion: A cohort study of complications, reoperations, and resource use in the Medicare population. **Spine** 18:1463–1470, 1993.
6. Franklin GW, Haug J, Heyer NJ, *et al.:* Outcome of lumbar fusion in Washington State workers' compensation. **Spine** 19:1897–1904, 1994.
7. Gallagher RM, Rauh V, Haugh LD, *et al.:* Determinants of return to work among low back pain patients. **Pain** 39:55–67, 1989.
8. Grubb SA, Lipscomb HJ: Results of lumbosacral fusion for degenerative disc disease with and without instrumentation. **Spine** 17:349–355, 1992.
9. Kent DL, Haynor DR, Larson EB, *et al.:* Diagnosis of lumbar spinal stenosis in adults: A metaanalysis of the accuracy of CT, MR, and myelography. **Am J Roentgeno** 158:1135–1144, 1992.
10. LaCroix J, Powell J, Lloyd G, *et al.:* Low back pain: Factors of value in predicting outcome. **Spine** 15:495–499, 1990.
11. Turner JA, Herron L, Deyo RA: Metaanalysis of the results of lumbar spine fusion. **Acta Orthop Scand Suppl** 251:120–122, 1993.
12. Zdeblick TA: A prospective, randomized study of lumbar fusion. **Spine** 18:983–991, 1993.

19

Upper Cervical Spine Trauma: Outcome Assessment

JOSEPH T. ALEXANDER, M.D., AND REGIS W. HAID, JR., M.D.

Trauma to the cervical spine remains an important problem for modern society, despite efforts at prevention, such as *Think First,* ongoing improvements in automotive and workplace safety, and campaigns against drunken driving. A disproportionate number of the victims of cervical trauma are young males, and the leading causes remain motor vehicle accidents and sports/leisure injuries. Improvements in the initial stabilization and management of these patients have improved the long-term survival rate as fewer patients succumb to the acute complications of cervical injuries. This has led to increased focus on the issues of rehabilitation, long-term outcome, and return to work and/or the activities of daily living, which can be summed up as "quality of life." The cost of treatment for cervical trauma can be significant, both in terms of acute care and long-term rehabilitation. Payers, both private insurers and governmental agencies, are beginning to demand data on the outcome of treatments rendered, and this will certainly be the case for cervical trauma as well.

"Cervical trauma" is an extremely broad topic, including a diverse group of injuries with radically different treatments and outcomes. One can consider cervical trauma from the standpoint of injury to the spinal cord, nerve roots, bones, intervertebral disc, ligaments, or myofascial components. Even within the category of bony injury, there is considerable heterogeneity among groups such as atlantal, axial, and subaxial injuries. To be meaningful, analysis of outcome must focus on a very specific group, so that one can compare "apples to apples" (21). For the purposes of this discussion, we will limit our review to acute, type II fractures of the odontoid process, because this is a common cervical injury that most practicing neurosurgeons would feel comfortable in managing.

Outcome has generally been considered from the standpoint of the fracture type, mechanism of injury, characteristics of the patient, and neurological status. Traditional outcome studies have focused on "hard data," which could also be called "physician-derived," such as radiographic studies, fusion rate, biomechanical features of surgical constructs, and the morbidity/mortality rates for a procedure (30, 37). Recently, some observers have suggested that outcome should be evaluated in a different way, from the standpoint of the patient (15). Meaningful data can be collected on "patient-centered" factors such as pain, satisfaction, ability to participate in work and leisure activities, and "quality of life" (30). Payers and other overseers of medical care are also beginning to demand data on patient satisfaction, return to work, and even cost-effectiveness (9, 31, 36). If physicians are to maintain a leading role in the management of medical problems, it will be increasingly necessary to have comprehensive outcome data organized in such a way that our treatment decisions can be justified (3, 21, 31, 33). In this review, we will examine the data available in regard to outcome for treatment of acute, type II odontoid fractures, both in terms of the traditional measures of outcome, as well as the emerging, patient-oriented outcome paradigm.

TREATMENT OF ODONTOID FRACTURES

Fractures of the axis are most commonly across the base of the odontoid process (5, 18). Nonoperative treatment options include immobilization with various cervical and cervicothoracic braces or the halo device. Operative treatment options include direct fracture fixation with an anterior odontoid screw procedure or posterior atlantoaxial fusion with wire, clamps, or transarticular screw technique. Operative intervention has been advocated as a primary treatment modality or may be reserved for patients who fail nonoperative management strategies. On beginning this project, we harbored the notion that a general consensus existed as to the best treatment option for this common cervical injury, and that we would be able to derive a meaningful conclusion from a meta-analysis of the available literature. However, following an extensive literature search and critical review of the data, we concluded that no *demonstrable* consensus exists, and that a meta-analysis could not be done (21). In the following section, selected papers will be discussed to illustrate the limits of our current understanding of this problem.

Ekong *et al.,* were early advocates of the use of halo immobilization for odontoid fractures. Although they reported a 41% nonunion in a series of 22 patients in 1981, they noted the improvement in early mobilization and shortened hospital stay that the halo provided (13). Dunn and Seljeskog reported the results of 80 patients treated with immobilization in 1986 (12). About 70% were treated in a halo device, the remainder with skeletal traction, bed rest, or a hard collar. They reported an overall 26% radiographic nonunion rate but did not break this down by the type of immobilization used. They recommended halo management for acute, nondisplaced fractures in younger patients and suggested consideration of operative treatment for the older patient, the displaced fracture, or a case of delayed diagnosis. In a prescient comment, they concluded that ". . . in today's cost-conscious medical environment, one cannot help but reflect on the economics of various forms of treatment (12)."

Hadley et al., in 1989, gave an interim report on the experience at the Barrow Neurological Institute in the treatment of odontoid fractures (19). At that time, there were 68 patients with acute fractures treated with either a halo device, Philadelphia collar, or SOMI. At 12 weeks, 19 patients had failed to fuse, for a failure rate of 28%. Of these 19 patients, 5 healed after further halo treatment, whereas 14 required operative stabilization. In this study, the single most important prognostic feature was the degree of displacement of the fragment. For patients with less than 6 mm of displacement, halo management was recommended, whereas operative treatment was reserved for those with a greater degree of displacement or failure of halo therapy. Bucholz and Cheung, in 1989, reported a failure rate of 13% in a small group of 15 patients treated with a halo device for at least 3 months, followed by a Philadelphia collar for 1 month (4). Mandabach et al. found a similar success rate for halo treatment of odontoid fractures in the pediatric population, with a 20% rate of failure of halo immobilization (23).

Fairholm et al. demonstrated the potential harmful outcome for patients with untreated odontoid fractures, in reporting a series of 51 generally younger patients with neurological deterioration resulting from nonunion (17). However, Ryan and Taylor questioned the importance of achieving a radiographic union in their analysis of 35 cases of odontoid fractures in elderly patients, and recommended SOMI or collar treatment in this patient population (29). Harrigan et al. found a high fatality rate after odontoid fracture in a series of 19 elderly patients but also concluded that elderly patients with minimally displaced fractures could be treated with a SOMI or collar (20).

Polin et al. recently added to the controversy brewing over immobilization. The premise of their study was that "the need for rigid fixation, demonstrated by the use of the halo vest in many institutions, has never been rigorously substantiated" (25). They reviewed 37 patients with type II odontoid fractures treated at one institution over a long period. Patients were nonrandomly assigned to treatment with either a Philadelphia collar (18 patients) or a halo (19 patients.) They had no cases of neurological deterioration during treatment. Seven patients were unstable by flexion-extension radiographs, for a failure rate of 19%. However, there were an additional five patients that had an unhealed fracture line but were stable on flexion-extension radiographs that were considered "successes" by the authors. Based on this small, nonrandomized series, they concluded that "the lack of a significant difference in the rates of instability and the need for late fusion between the groups argues that the treatments can be used equivalently" (25). Conversely, Duncan and Esses recently concluded that "because of the unacceptable rate of nonunion and because of their documented lack of immobilization of the upper cervical spine, collars or braces should probably not be used as a primary treatment in most instances (11)."

Clark and White compared immobilization with operative management in 1985 (5). In their series of 96 patients with type II odontoid fractures, 18 patients were untreated, and 3 had an orthosis. These 21 patients had a 100% nonunion rate. Thirty-eight patients were treated with a halo device with a 34% nonunion rate. Thirty-four patients underwent operative stabilization (26 posterior, 8 anterior) with a nonunion rate of 6%. Based on this experience, they recommended operative intervention as the primary treatment modality (5).

Among the options for surgical intervention, there are numerous small case series advocating various surgical approaches. Dickman *et al.* reported a 100% fusion rate in a group of 8 patients treated with posterior atlantoaxial wiring with autologous bone graft (10). Aldrich *et al.* reported a 100% fusion rate in 10 patients treated with a posterior atlantoaxial fusion with a Halifax clamp and autologous bone (1). Marcotte *et al.* reported a 100% fusion rate in six patients treated with posterior C1-C2 transarticular screws, posterior interspinous wiring, and autologous bone graft (24). Geisler *et al.* reported a 100% fusion rate in a series of 9 patients treated with an anterior odontoid screw procedure, although there were 2 unrelated perioperative deaths in this series (16). Rainov *et al.* reported a fusion rate of 100% in a larger series of 30 patients, using a somewhat different anterior odontoid screw technique but noted a 12% rate of complications, such as decreased neck motion or persistent neck pain (26).

The brief summary listed above is in no way an exhaustive review of the literature on the treatment of type II odontoid fractures, nor is it meant to advocate any one treatment method over another. Rather, it is meant to illustrate the shortcomings of the current literature regarding this problem. All of the studies are nonrandomized and typically use historical controls (if any). Most include only a small number of patients and have heterogenous entry and outcome criteria. In many cases, we had to reevaluate the presented data to cull out only acute, type II fractures, so the numbers we present may not tally with the overall numbers in any given paper. Outcome data was presented almost entirely from the standpoint of radiographic healing rates, with little attention to patient-derived outcome measures, such as pain, function, satisfaction, or return to work. For these reasons, we were unable to make any rigorous conclusions or present any modern outcome data from the existing literature.

OUTCOME ANALYSIS AND SPINE SURGERY

One can ask: Why are outcome studies important in cervical spine trauma at all? We as neurosurgeons are the experts in this area. Isn't our professional judgment enough? Until recently, the opinion of an individual physician was sufficient "proof" of the necessity for a particular treatment. Whether we like it or not, this era is coming to a close. There are a number of different factors that together are forcing a change in the delivery of medical care in the United States. We will briefly review some of these influences, and then outline our suggestions for a study of the outcome of the management of odontoid fractures, which could serve as a model for the analysis of other management problems in spine surgery.

Efficacy research can be defined as that done to determine whether a procedure works at all. Effectiveness research is that undertaken to determine whether a procedure works well when applied to the general population and what the patient-oriented outcomes of the procedure are (21). As Keller noted, "Frequently, procedures and technologies are widely disseminated and used solely on the basis of their efficacy even though effectiveness studies have never been conducted" (21). Raskob et al. go on to say that, "Frequently, the so called evidence for effectiveness and safety of an experimental therapy has been based on selected case reports, uncontrolled series of cases, clinical experience, or even published 'expert' opinion (27)." Gartland noted that, "Authors, journals, program committees and professional societies must share the blame for the publication of flawed studies that are designed using inappropriate strategies" (15). These criticisms are certainly relevant in considering the literature on the treatment of type II odontoid fractures.

More sophisticated databases collected by medical researchers, the insurance industry, and governmental agencies have shown considerable differences in the manner in which particular medical problems may be treated in different regions of the country (35), often with no discernible difference in outcome but with potentially large cost differences. Keller noted that "it does appear that variations in practice patterns are more clearly related to uncertainty about the best way to treat clinical problems than to financial incentives for physicians to do more" (21). Traditionally, physicians have only been held to the standard of care within their community. Now through improvements in communication and travel, the "community" is being expanded to include ever larger geographic divisions, and we may eventually be held to a national standard of care. This once again highlights the need for accurate outcome data.

New surgical treatments have rarely been evaluated by rigorous testing programs before widespread adoption by the surgical community (17, 27). For practical and ethical reasons, double-blinded, randomized, placebo-controlled studies of surgical procedures are not possible. For many of the same reasons, it can be difficult to evaluate a surgical *versus* a nonsurgical treatment for a particular disease (28). Raskob *et al.* pointed out that new therapies have "often been assumed to be of clinical benefit based on pathophysiologic knowledge, which is then uncritically accepted as hard evidence of clinical efficacy" (27). Perhaps the single greatest obstacle is our own attitudes toward randomized studies. As Gross noted in a critique of orthopaedic outcome trials,

> It is difficult for surgeons to accept a clinical trial if they harbor a preconceived belief that one of the treatments to be used may be inferior to the other. At present, they prefer to analyze their results retrospectively and to accept the fact that subsequent findings may demonstrate that the treatment they chose was inferior. If surgeons are to participate in randomized, controlled trials, they must accept the concept that not only are they responsible for the ultimate clinical outcome after the patient has been operated on, but also that they have a responsibility to establish, as expeditiously as possible, the relative values of available options of treatment. [(Reprinted with permission from (17).]

These concerns are by no means limited to neurosurgical practice. Across the board, physicians are being asked to prove the effectiveness of a wide range of interventions, with the threat of financial or regulatory control if we do not comply. A recent example is the use of right heart (Swan-Ganz or PA) catheterization for critically ill patients. Previous attempts at randomized studies had failed because of the strongly held feelings of physicians that the procedure was beneficial (8). Connors *et al.* performed a rigorous observational study that found both an increase in mortality and an increase in resource use associated with the procedure (7). Dalen and Bone noted, in an accompanying editorial that "If such a randomized controlled trial is not undertaken, then it is time to pull the PA catheter, and we would recommend that the FDA issue a moratorium on the use of flow-directed PA catheters (8)."

Despite these problems, meaningful research can be done, given sufficient incentive. To date, the best known examples of this type of work relevant to neurosurgery are the outcome studies of the external-internal carotid artery bypass procedure (28) and the carotid endarterectomy trials. Our feelings toward this type of research are irrelevant. It will be undertaken by other participants in the medical arena without our participation, and we must become involved if we want to maintain our leadership in this field (31, 33).

Raskob *et al.* have identified the key features of an acceptable clinical study (27):

1. The trial must be prospective, with a concurrent control group.
2. The patients must be randomly allocated between groups.
3. The groups must be comparable.
4. Well-defined, objective endpoints must be used. Because surgical trials cannot be double-blinded, the outcome assessment should be performed by an independent observer.
5. All clinically relevant outcomes should be reported.
6. A sufficient number of patients must be studied to allow valid conclusions, and appropriate statistical methods should be used to analyze the data.

Objective endpoints are not merely the traditional, physician-derived data such as fusion rates or mortality. Patient-derived outcome measures can also be reliably assessed (22, 30) and will in fact be required in the future. Cost-effectiveness will likewise be increasingly important (6, 9, 32, 34).

We have demonstrated that no consensus exists as far as the treatment of acute, type II odontoid fractures is concerned. Furthermore, the available literature regarding this condition is deficient, particularly in regard to modern, patient-derived outcome parameters. For this reason, we suggest that a new study of this condition should be undertaken. To achieve significance in terms of adequate numbers of patients in a reasonable amount of time, a multicenter trial would be necessary. Uniform entry and outcome criteria would be needed, including "patient-derived" measures. Difficult choices will be needed to limit the number of experimental groups, because there are so many options currently available. Perhaps most importantly, the participants will need an open mind, because opinions on the "best" treatment of this condition are strongly held. In a recent editorial, Benzel pointed out that "We all should remain critical of our current management techniques and continuously look for better ways to manage

complex problems, particularly those with relatively high treatment
failure rates (2)."

REFERENCES

1. Aldrich EF, Weber PB, Crow WN: Halifax interlaminar clamp for posterior cervical fusion: A long-term follow-up review. **J Neurosurg** 78:702–708, 1993.
2. Benzel EC: Nonoperative management of types II and III odontoid fractures: The Philadelphia collar versus the halo vest. **Neurosurgery** 38(3):457, 1996.
3. Bourne RB, Keller RB: Controversy: Outcomes research. **Spine** 20(3):384–387, 1995.
4. Bucholz RD, Cheung KC: Halo vest versus spinal fusion for cervical injury: Evidence from an outcome study. **J Neurosurg** 70:884–892, 1989.
5. Clark CR, White AA: Fractures of the dens. **J Bone Joint Surg Am** 67(9):1340–1348, 1985.
6. Clark RE: Understanding cost-effectiveness. **Spine** 21(5):646–650, 1996.
7. Connors AF, Speroff T, Dawson NV, et al.: The effectiveness of right heart catheterization in the initial care of critically ill patients. **JAMA** 276(11):889–897, 1996.
8. Dalen JE, Bone RC: Is it time to pull the pulmonary artery catheter? **JAMA** 276(11):916–918, 1996.
9. Detsky AS, Naglie IG: A clinician's guide to cost-effectiveness analysis. **Ann Intern Med** 113(2):147–154, 1990.
10. Dickman CA, Sonntag VKH, Papadopoulis SM, et al.: The interspinous method of posterior atlantoaxial arthrodesis. **J Neurosurg** 74:190–198, 1991.
11. Duncan RW, Esses SI: Dens fractures: Specifications and management. **Semin Spine Surg** 8(1):19–26, 1996.
12. Dunn ME, Seljeskog EL: Experience in the management of odontoid process injuries: An analysis of 128 cases. **Neurosurgery** 18(3):306–310, 1986.
13. Ekong CEU, Schwartz ML, Tator CH, et al.: Odontoid fracture: Management with early mobilization using the halo device. **Neurosurgery** 9(6):631–637, 1981.
14. Fairholm D, Lee ST, Lui TN: Fractured odontoid: The management of delayed neurological symptoms. **Neurosurgery** 38(1):38–43, 1996.
15. Gartland JJ: Orthopaedic clinical research: Deficiencies in experimental design and determinations of outcome. **J Bone Joint Surg Am** 70(9):1357–1364, 1988.
16. Geisler FH, Cheng C, Poka A, et al.: Anterior screw fixation of posteriorly displaced type II odontoid fractures. **Neurosurgery** 25(11):30–37, 1989.
17. Gross M: A critique of the methodologies used in clinical studies of hip-joint arthroplasty published in the English-language orthopaedic literature. **J Bone Joint Surg Am** 70(9):1364–1371, 1988.
18. Hadley MN, Browner C, Sonntag VKH: Axis fractures: A comprehensive review of management and treatment in 107 cases. **Neurosurgery** 17(2):281–289, 1985.
19. Hadley MN, Dickman CA, Browner CM, et al.: Acute axis fractures: A review of 229 cases. **J Neurosurg** 71:642–647, 1989.
20. Harrigan WC, Powell FC, Elwood PW, et al.: Odontoid fractures in elderly patients. **J Neurosurg** 78:32–35, 1993.
21. Keller RB: Outcomes research in orthopaedics. **J Bone Joint Surg Am** 75(10):1562–1574, 1993.

22. Laupacis A, Rorabeck CH, Bourne RB, et al.: Randomized trials in orthopaedics: Why, how and when? **J Bone Joint Surg Am** 71(4):535–543, 1989.
23. Mandabach M, Ruge JR, Hahn YS, et al.: Pediatric axis fractures: Early halo immobilization, management and outcome. **Pediatr Neurosurg** 19:225–232, 1993.
24. Marcotte P, Dickman CA, Sonntag VKH, et al.: Posterior atlantoaxial screw fixation. **J Neurosurg** 79:234–237, 1993.
25. Polin RS, Szabo T, Bogaev CA, et al.: Nonoperative management of types II and III odontoid fractures: The Philadelphia collar versus the halo vest. **Neurosurgery** 38(3):450–456, 1996.
26. Rainov NG: Direct anterior fixation of odontoid fractures with a hollow spreading screw system. **Acta Neurochir (Wien)** 138:146–153, 1996.
27. Raskob GE, Lofthouse RN, Hull RD: Methodological guidelines for clinical trials evaluating new therapeutic approaches in bone and joint surgery. **J Bone Joint Surg Am** 67(8):1294–1297, 1985.
28. Relman AS: The Extracranial-Intracranial Arterial Bypass Study: What have we learned? **N Engl J Med** 316(13):809–810, 1987.
29. Ryan MD, Taylor TKF: Odontoid fractures in the elderly. **J Spinal Disord** 6(3): 397–401, 1993.
30. Spratt KF, Weinstein JN: Measuring clinical outcomes, in Wiesel SW, Weinstein JN, Herkowitz HN, et al. (eds): *The Lumbar Spine*. Philadelphia, W.B. Saunders, 1995, ed 2, pp 1313–1338.
31. Tarlov EC: Patient-based health status measurement: A tool for assessing the effectiveness of spinal surgery. **Perspect Neurol Surg** 5(2):149–153, 1994.
32. Task Force on Principles for Economic Analysis of Health Care Technology: Economic analysis of health care technology. **Ann Intern Med** 123(1):61–70, 1995.
33. Travis RL: The quest for quality. **Perspect Neurol Surg** 6(2):149–160, 1995.
34. Udvarhelyi IS, Colditz GA, Rai A, et al.: Cost-effectiveness and cost-benefit analyses in the medical literature. **Ann Intern Med** 116(3):238–244, 1992.
35. Wennberg JE: Practice variations and the challenge to leadership. **Spine** 21(12): 1472–1478, 1996.
36. Wiesel SW: A new Era in spine surgery? FDA panel approves fusion cages—After sharply criticizing new studies. **The BackLetter** 11(7):73–84, 1996.
37. Wiesel SW: Provocative new study on spinal fusion: Do patients assess the outcome of spine surgery accurately? **The BackLetter** 11(9):97–105, 1996.

20

Low-Grade Gliomas: In Search of Evidence-based Treatment

MARK BERNSTEIN, M.D., F.R.C.S.C.

BACKGROUND TO THE PROBLEM

Malignant glial neoplasms are usually fatal in adults, but the value of aggressive treatment as soon as imaging shows the lesion both to prolong life and ameliorate neurologic symptoms is clear in most cases. Although radiation has been shown in randomized trials to prolong life for patients with anaplastic astrocytoma and glioblastoma (43), no randomized study has demonstrated unequivocally the value of aggressive surgery for these patients, but the rapid growth of these tumors and their common production of symptoms and signs of focal deficit and/or increased intracranial pressure because of their mass makes aggressive surgical decompression a matter of common sense for many cases. In others that are diffuse and/or deep, stereotactic biopsy followed by radiation is the appropriate approach. Despite aggressive therapy these tumors are invariably fatal, with median survival of approximately 15 months for glioblastoma and 3 years for anaplastic astrocytoma; however, the value of early and aggressive treatment is relatively clear.

Low-grade gliomas (LGG), including the histologic subtypes of fibrillary astrocytoma, oligodendroglioma, and mixed oligoastrocytoma occurring in the supratentorial compartment of adults have a more variable biological behavior for which the value of treatment and the timing of treatment are of less clear-cut value than for their malignant counterparts. A series of retrospective reviews provides conflicting and inconclusive results about the role of observation, stereotactic biopsy, aggressive surgery, and radiation for treating these tumors, and there exists significant variability in the therapeutic approach on the part of clinicians and in the clinical course of the disease in individual patients (32).

There are approximately 1500 new cases of LGG in North America each year (9). Most patients present with their initial symptoms approximately 1–2 decades younger than patients presenting with malignant gliomas. More than one-half of the patients present with a seizure and are neurologically intact. Imaging typically demonstrates a low-density, nonenhancing lesion on computed tomography (CT) and magnetic resonance imaging (MRI) which may be lobar and relatively discreet (Fig. 1), superficial but indiscreet (Fig. 2), deep and diffuse (Fig. 3) or somewhere inbetween (Fig. 4). Most are not associated with mass effect on imaging, but a number demonstrate considerable mass effect sometimes in a neurologically intact patient (Fig. 5) or sometimes in a patient with signs of increased intracranial pressure (Fig. 6).

The median survival time in adults with LGG is approximately 4–7 years, ranging up to 10 years in some series (11, 16, 20–24, 26–30, 35–37, 39, 41, 44), and the 10-year survival rate ranges from approximately 15 to 45% (13, 16, 24, 28, 35–37). Tumor recurrence is defined

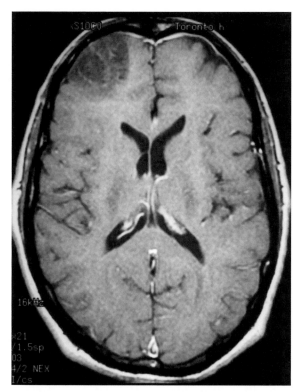

Fig. 1 Axial gadolinium-enhanced T1-weighted MRI of a 49-year-old engineer presenting with a 2-year history of nocturnal grand mal seizures and neurologically intact on examination. The patient was treated with radical resection and remains clinically well with no disease on MRI 30 months after surgery. The histology was mixed oligodendroglioma-astrocytoma. No radiation was given.

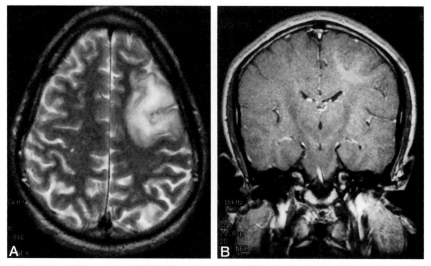

FIG. 2 Axial T2-weighted MRI (**A**) and coronal gadolinium-enhanced T1-weighted MRI (**B**) showing presumed left frontal LGG in a 17-year-old student presenting with one focal motor seizure and neurologically intact. The patient is being followed without biopsy or any treatment and remains clinically well with stable MRI 8 years after initial imaging.

by worsening of neurologic symptoms and signs, progression of lesion on imaging, and transformation to a more anaplastic histology. Management issues that remain controversial in the adult include: whether or not to observe (with or without tissue diagnosis), the role of stereotactic biopsy, the role of aggressive resection, and the role of radiation. In general, neurologic deficit above and beyond seizure activity and evidence of enhancement (30) and/or mass effect (37) on imaging is interpreted as suggestive of a more aggressive lesion with a worse prognosis, and most clinicians recommend treatment when confronted with a patient with any of these clinical/imaging features although, even in this scenario, there is no good evidence that aggressive treatment from the beginning is necessary or beneficial in terms of survival. When treatment is elected, aggressive surgery is usually done for lobar lesions and stereotactic biopsy for deep or diffuse lesions; conventional fractionated radiation via regional fields to a dose of at least 50 Gy would usually follow. Older age is suggestive of a poorer prognosis, and patients over 40 generally warrant treatment from the beginning (21, 30). Behavior is also a function of histologic subtype, with diffuse fibrillary astrocytoma having the worst prognosis and oligodendroglioma the best (35). The clinical scenario that is devoid of putative

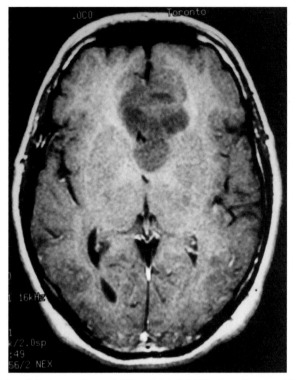

FIG. 3 Axial gadolinium-enhanced T1-weighted MRI of a 42-year-old immunology research scientist presenting with several month history of brief episodes of forgetfulness and neurologically intact on examination. Stereotactic biopsy revealed astrocytoma. No radiation was given, and the patient remains stable clinically and on imaging 3 years after biopsy.

negative prognostic factors and the subject of most controversy is the scenario of a young adult (*i.e.*, under 40 years) who presents with a seizure and no hard interictal neurologic deficit and who has a low-density intraaxial lesion on MRI without enhancement and without mass effect. A number of authors have examined the predictive value regarding survival of molecular and cellular markers and proliferation indices found within LGGs (8, 15, 25).

In this report we will examine available information regarding the role of observation, biopsy, surgery, and radiation for presumed or confirmed adult supratentorial LGG, and the ongoing process to develop evidence-based practice parameters for this challenging neurooncologic conundrum. Excluded from this discussion are pilocytic astrocytoma, brainstem tumors, and optic pathway gliomas, all of

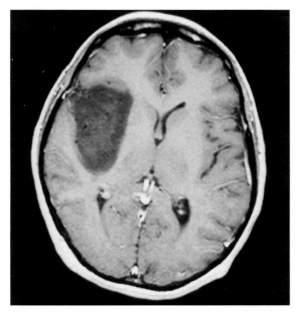

FIG. 4 Axial gadolinium-enhanced T1-weighted MRI showing presumed right fronto-temporal subcortical LGG in a 41-year-old woman with a 1-year history of focal sensory seizures involving the left arm and neurologically intact on examination. The patient had been treated for Hodgkin's disease 10 years earlier. The patient preferred observation only, and she remains stable clinically and on imaging 2 years after initial imaging without tissue diagnosis or treatment.

which present their own particular set of questions regarding diagnosis and treatment.

PROBLEMS WITH PUBLISHED OUTCOME REPORTS

The literature on survival of patients with LGG consists predominantly of class II and class III evidence, poorly controlled retrospective reviews for the most part (6, 45). There are numerous problems intrinsic to these studies that render their recommendations inconclusive and nondefinitive: (*a*) The numbers of patients in each treatment arm being compared are generally small. (*b*) The criteria for selection of patients for various treatment regimens (*e.g.*, radiation *versus* no radiation) are not specified. (*c*) The series often consist of patients from various imaging eras (*i.e.*, pre-CT, CT pre-MRI, MRI). (*d*) The minimum follow-up is often shorter than the usually accepted median survival of 5 years. (*e*) The degree of surgical resection is often based on surgeons' descriptions, as opposed to being based on postoperative imaging. (*f*) There is a lack of multivariate analysis in some series; and

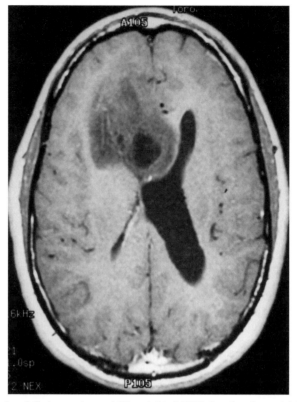

FIG. 5 Axial gadolinium-enhanced T1-weighted MRI showing deep right frontal presumed LGG with mass effect in a 28-year-physical education teacher who experienced one grand mal seizure and was normal on neurological examination. The patient chose the nontreatment option and remains well and seizure-free on carbamazepine, with stable MRI 4 years after initial imaging.

numerous others. Although the use of sophisticated statistical analysis may glean useful information from these studies, conclusions about outcome are not reliable and not definitive. These concerns apply to all full-length papers on survival in LGG patients, with the exception of one small randomized study carried out by the Southwest Oncology Group that concluded that postradiation chemotherapy with lomustine (CCNU) added no survival benefit for patients with LGG (11). Although this paper is of interest, as it is at least a randomized study and qualifies as class I data, it is of relatively little help in solving the usual LGG dilemma, as the more fundamental questions relate to the value of the role of surgery and of radiation for this disease that have not been conclusively resolved.

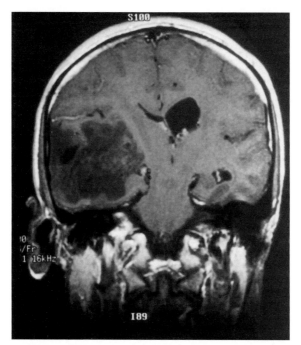

FIG. 6 Coronal gadolinium-enhanced T1-weighted MRI showing right temporal presumed LGG with mass effect in a 22-year-old man with a 1-year history of mild right-sided headaches. He had early papilledema on examination. Aggressive subtotal resection revealed histology of low-grade astrocytoma with prominent microcystic change. The patient was treated with adjuvant conventional fractionated radiation and remains stable 3.5 years after surgery.

OBSERVATION

The concept of discovering a suspected LGG on imaging of a patient and then deferring treatment and choosing a course of observation may seem unthinkable to some clinicians, especially for a disease with a median survival much worse than that of breast cancer, and for a disease that almost always turns into an anaplastic astrocytoma or glioblastoma in adults. However, a number of clinicians exercise this option, and this approach has been critically examined in the literature and found to be safe (5, 33). There are many weaknesses in the latter study, but certainly there is at least circumstantial evidence that deferring treatment until clinical/imaging/histologic progression occurs is not detrimental to selected patients. In other words, all patients with LGG will eventually be treated, but the question is when: Should treatment begin at initial discovery of the lesion or at time of progression? One other study of observation alone involved a group of patients with deep-seated lesions undergoing stereotactic biopsy only; median survival for the 70 patients was 3 years (12).

The advantages of a simple course of observation include: deferring the risk of treatment, deferring the cost of treatment, and honoring some patients' wishes to remain a "nonpatient" for as long as possible. Advantages of not waiting but treating from the beginning include: satisfying some patients' (and doctors') needs to treat a serious condition as early and as aggressively as possible and making the assumption that treatment given for a new tumor might be more effective than giving it when the tumor is demonstrating more biologically aggressive and, therefore, possibly more treatment-resistant behavior.

STEREOTACTIC BIOPSY

Stereotactic biopsy is an effective and relatively safe means of obtaining a specific tissue diagnosis of a glioma, although it is well-known that sampling error can lead to misleading results when derived from a small sample (7, 38). Furthermore, many feel that if a course of observation is selected for a particular patient with a suspected supratentorial LGG, why put him/her through the risk of a biopsy, which for all intraaxial lesions may be as high as 6% but is likely less for low-grade, as opposed to anaplastic, gliomas (3, 4). In the author's personal series of almost 500 stereotactic biopsies, 70 have disclosed LGG, and three were complicated for a morbidity rate of 4.3%. Of these three patients, one incurred a major neurological deficit secondary to intracerebral hemorrhage (1.4%), whereas the other two incurred minor morbidity from an intracerebral hematoma and a subarachnoid hemorrhage (2.9%).

It is well-known that an imaging diagnosis of LGG may be inaccurate in up to one-third of patients (3, 18), but if the lesion indeed is a more anaplastic lesion, it will be demonstrated as such on subsequent close clinical and imaging monitoring, and appropriate action will be taken. This potential delay in therapy is unlikely to have detrimental effects for the patient, unless the patient progresses too far and incurs a known poor prognostic factor for outcome of therapy—a lower functional (i.e., Karnofsky) status. Therefore, if observation only is deemed an acceptable option for selected patients with a suspected LGG, it appears that the neurosurgeon can defer the risk of biopsy until intervention is needed, based on imaging and/or clinical progression of the lesion.

Regarding the role of biopsy, as opposed to aggressive resection vis-á-vis the impact on patient survival, there are no randomized studies examining this question, but as presented below, there are a number of papers that, using retrospective review, suggest that biopsy is as good as aggressive resection regarding survival (30, 35, 37, 44). There are also one-armed, noncomparative studies that provide strong circumstantial evidence that some patients having stereotactic biopsy followed by radiation perform as well as or better than historical controls receiving aggressive resection followed by radiation (22).

RESECTION

There have been a number of retrospective reviews examining the value of aggressive surgical resection of malignant gliomas and LGGs (1, 2, 16, 29, 30, 35, 37, 39). None are randomized studies, and it is doubtful that a randomized study could ever be executed to solve definitively the question of whether aggressive surgery confers improved survival in the subset of patients who do not require surgery for obvious immediate resolution of increased intracranial pressure and/or significant focal neurological deficit. The major problem with papers dealing with this subject is that in nonrandomized studies patients are likely to be selected for either gross total resection, subtotal resection, or biopsy based on preoperative clinical and imaging features and intraoperative findings. These parameters might well represent the true determining prognostic factor(s) in outcome, irrespective of the actual extent of surgery and, therefore, the extent of resection may simply be an associated factor or epiphenomenon (19).

Using the tool of retrospective review with the known pitfalls outlined above, a number of authors have examined the role of aggressive surgery in determining the outcome of patients with LGG and have found statistically significant survival benefit favoring more aggressive surgical resection (16, 28, 29), but a similar number have not (30, 35, 37, 44). All of these studies have a number of the problems outlined above pertaining to comparisons of survival results in groups of patients treated in different ways and assessed retrospectively. One recent article reported outcome as a function of imaging findings and found that the incidence of recurrence and the probability of anaplastic transformation were dependent on the preoperative and postoperative tumor volumes whereas the time to recurrence was inversely related to tumor volume (2).

RADIATION

The same type of information as is available regarding extent of resection exists regarding the role of radiation therapy with all the same inherent weaknesses in the methods and the conclusions reached. A number of papers conclude that there is a statistically significant survival advantage with the use of radiation after surgery

(35, 37). Furthermore, the study of Shaw et al. suggests a dose-response relationship, with patients receiving more than 53 Gy having superior 5- and 10-year survival rates, as opposed to those of patients receiving less than 53 Gy (35). A similar number of articles report no survival benefit for patients receiving postoperative radiation (16, 29, 30, 44), although one of these did find a significant benefit in the subset of patients over 40 years old who underwent biopsy or subtotal resection (29). Another report observed an increase in the time to anaplastic transformation from 3.7 to 5.4 years when postoperative radiation was used, as opposed to the use of surgery alone (41). It cannot be emphasized often enough that all of these articles suffer from one or more of the problems outlined above, which renders the conclusions nondefinitive.

One other type of outcome study compared neuropsychological function in 3 groups of 20 patients—two groups of adult LGG patients, one receiving radiation and the other not, and a third group of controls who did not harbor brain tumors (40). Test scores were worse for the LGG patients, as opposed to the controls, with no significant difference between irradiated patients and those not receiving radiation.

RANDOMIZED STUDIES ON RADIATION

The European Organization for the Research and Treatment of Cancer (EORTC) trial 22844 demonstrated no survival difference between groups of adult LGG patients treated with two doses of radiation (45 Gy in 25 fractions *versus* 59.4 Gy in 33 fractions to regional fields) after biopsy or resection (17). This study accrued 379 patients between 1985 and 1991. Another randomized study examining two doses of radiation after surgery was conducted by NCCTG/RTOG/ECOG (NC-CTG 86-72-51) in the United States and closed accrual in November 1994 with 100 evaluable patients having been randomized to each arm (50.4 Gy in 28 fractions *versus* 64.8 Gy in 36 fractions). This paper will not be published for another several years.

Regarding randomized studies for the "nonbelievers" in radiation, one trial is almost complete, and two others are about to begin. EORTC study 22845 randomized patients to observation *versus* radiation (54 Gy in 30 fractions) after resection or biopsy; patients were stratified for histology (astrocytoma *versus* oligodendroglioma or mixed oligoastrocytoma) and for degree of resection (biopsy *versus* partial, subtotal, or gross total resection). Closure of accrual is anticipated in late 1996 after 300 patients have been entered, and data analysis will be forthcoming a few years after that. A number of American cooperative groups with RTOG as the coordinating center are about to initiate a study with the two following arms: observation/delayed radiation for low-risk patients (under age 40, gross total resection, flow cytometrically determined % S-phase < 6%) *versus* radiation ± PCV chemotherapy for high-risk patients (age over 40 and/or stereotactic biopsy or subtotal resection, and/or % S-phase >/= 6%). Patients will be stratified for grade (St. Anne-Mayo grade 1 *versus* grade 2), histology (astrocytoma *versus* oligodengroglioma *versus* oligoastrocytoma), and Karnofsky Performance Status (70 and 80 *versus* 90 and 100). The University of Toronto has just started a randomized study comparing observation-delayed radiation *versus* radiation up front (50 Gy in 25 fractions to regional fields) in adults with supratentorial low-grade astrocytoma after stereotactic biopsy or resection. Patients will be stratified for age (18–39 *versus* 40 years old and over), presentation (seizures only *versus* focal deficit), extent of surgery (biopsy *versus* resection), and location (lobar *versus* deep). In addition to time to recurrence and survival, other endpoints will include MR cerebral blood volume measurement and spectroscopy, detailed neuropsychological testing, and assessment of molecular markers of tumor progression, including p53, EGF receptor, and *ras* activation. Other Canadian and possibly American centers are being recruited in this study.

DEVELOPMENT OF LGG PRACTICE PARAMETERS

Definitions

Development of practice parameters is an initiative that is becoming widespread and was initiated primarily to aid in health-care cost containment and also to help provide clinicians with evidence-based algorithms to help them give the best care to their patients, based on available evidence (10, 14, 34, 42, 45). Also implicit in the development of practice parameters were medicolegal implications in that it was assumed that the individual risk of litigation in a medical case might be less if a physician is treating the patient according to locally/nationally/internationally accepted practice parameters (10, 34, 42, 45).

Possible conclusions of the process of development of practice parameters include three levels of recommendation: standards (accepted principles of patient management that reflect a high degree of clinical certainty); guidelines (recommendations for patient management that reflect a particular strategy or range of management strategies that reflect a moderate clinical certainty); and options (other strategies for patient management for which there is unclear clinical certainty because of inconclusive or conflicting evidence or opinion). Standards are intended to be applied rigidly in virtually all cases; exceptions will be rare and difficult to justify (10). A neurooncologic example of a standard would be the administration of conventional fractionated radiation to a young patient with a reasonable Karnofsky performance status after resection of a glioblastoma. Guidelines are intended to be more flexible. They should be followed in most cases but depending on the patient, guidelines can and should be tailored to fit individual needs. An example might refer to the resection of a presumed lobar glioblastoma producing mild symptoms and signs in a young patient. Deviations from guidelines will be fairly common and are justifiable in individual circumstances (10). Options are neutral with respect to recommending an intervention; they merely note that different interventions are available, none of which has compelling evidence in its favor (10). An example might be the scenario of a 75-year-old patient presenting with one seizure and harboring a small dominant frontal presumed glioblastoma on MRI; treatment options would include resection or stereotactic biopsy.

The types of evidence available from the literature upon which the process of parameter development depends heavily are classified into: class I (evidence provided by one or more well-designed randomized controlled clinical trials); class II (evidence provided by one or more well-designed clinical studies such as case control or cohort studies); and class III (evidence provided by expert opinions, nonrandomized historical controls, and case reports) (6).

Relating practice parameters to levels of clinical evidence, standards are usually based on class I evidence or overwhelming evidence from class II studies that directly addresses the question at hand or from decision analysis that directly addresses the issues. Guidelines are based on class II evidence that directly addresses the issue, decision analysis that directly addresses the issue, or strong consensus of class III evidence. Options are based on inconclusive or conflicting evidence from retrospective reviews and/or expert opinion.

The Process for LGG

The process followed for LGG was that described in general for the development of practice parameters (45). In 1994 a LGG Practice Parameters Team was assembled in a cooperative effort of the American Association of Neurological Surgeons and Congress of Neurological Surgeons via the Joint Section on Tumors, the American Academy of Neurology, and the American Society of Therapeutic Radiology and Oncology. A Chair (Dr. E. Shaw, a radiation oncologist) and two co-chairs were selected (Dr. L. Recht, a medical concologist, and Dr. M. Bernstein, a neurosurgeon). Other members of the team included neurosurgeons (Dr. M. Camel, Dr. S. Haines, Dr. J. Rock, Dr. M. Rosenblum), medical oncologists (Dr. T. Byrne, Dr. B. O'Neill), and a radiation oncologist (Dr. M. Shea). Other members included advisors on practice parameters from neurosurgery (Dr. R. Florin, Dr. B. Walters) and from neurology (Dr. J. Rosenberg).

A Medline search was performed using the following key words: adult, supratentorial, low-grade glioma, astrocytoma, oligodendroglioma, oligoastrocytoma, computed tomography, magnetic resonance imaging, surgery, radiation therapy, and chemotherapy. Also a citation search was performed, using three papers from the peer-reviewed medical literature that the team members considered oft-cited "classic" papers on the subject (20, 33, 35). Each abstract of all citations was reviewed by all team members, and 60 were chosen for further in-depth review, based on the following criteria: English language, after 1975, peer-reviewed original work, and addressing natural history, recurrence, survival, or quality of life in patients managed with observation (with or without biopsy), biopsy, resection, or radiation. Each paper was evaluated by at least three team members according to a standardized assessment protocol developed by the team. The quality of evidence from each citation was classified into class I, II, and III evidence. As a result of this process which as of October 1996 was not complete, 15 papers were selected from the published literature for the development of practice parameters.

Preliminary Results for LGG

The process is not final but will be shortly and the practice parameters will be published in due course. For the scenario of a young (*i.e.*, < approximately 40 years of age) adult with a supratentorial LGG with no neurologic deficit, and no enhancement or mass effect on MRI, the author's personal recommendations are as follows:

1. Observation without a biopsy is an option.
2. Observation after a biopsy showing LGG is an option.
3. Aggressive surgical resection is an option.
4. Aggressive conventional fractionated radiation is an option.

For the scenario of a patient approximately more than 40 years of age and/or with neurological deficit and/or evidence of enhancement and/or mass effect on imaging, treatment from the beginning is an option. If treatment is elected, for lobar tumors, aggressive surgical resection, followed by radiation, is advised. For deep or diffuse tumors, stereotactic biopsy, followed by radiation, is advised.

CONCLUSIONS

LGGs are generally slow-growing lesions in young, otherwise healthy adults about which there is immense controversy and both uncertainty and strength of conviction on the part of clinicians as to how these patients should best be treated. Rigorous scrutiny of the literature does not provide compelling evidence for treatment, as opposed to observation; for aggressive removal, as opposed to biopsy; or for radiation, as opposed to no radiation, for the common scenario of a young adult with seizure(s) only, a normal interictal neurological examination, and a suspected LGG on MRI without enhancement or mass effect. Randomized studies that are completed and awaiting data analysis or are about to begin will provide important class I evidence that will provide clearer practice parameters on the most optimal, cost-effective treatment. Until the results of such studies are available, clinicians must continue to manage disease in these patients on a case-by-case basis.

REFERENCES

1. Albert FK, Forsting M, Sartor K, et al.: Early postoperative magnetic resonance imaging after resection of malignant glioma: Objective evaluation of residual tumor and its influence on regrowth and prognosis. **Neurosurgery** 34:45–61, 1994.
2. Berger MS, Deliganis AV, Dobbins J, et al.: The effect of extent of resection on recurrence in patients with low grade cerebral hemisphere gliomas. **Cancer** 74: 1784–1791, 1994.
3. Bernstein M, Guha A: Biopsy of low-grade astrocytomas. **J Neurosurg** 80:776–777, 1994.
4. Bernstein M, Parrent AG: Complications of CT-guided stereotactic biopsy of intra-axial lesions. **J Neurosurg** 81:165–168, 1994.
5. Cairncross JG, Laperriere NJ: Low-grade glioma: To treat or not to treat? **Arch Neurol** 46:1238–1239, 1989.
6. Canadian Task Force on the Periodic Health Examination: The periodic health examination. **Can Med Assoc** 121:1193–1254, 1979.
7. Chandrasoma PT, Smith MM, Apuzzo MLJ: Stereotactic biopsy in the diagnosis of brain masses: Comparison of results of biopsy and resected surgical specimen. **Neurosurgery** 24:160–165, 1989.
8. Coons SW, Johnson PC, Pearl DK, et al.: Prognostic significance of flow cytometry deoxyribonucleic acid analysis of human oligodendrogliomas. **Neurosurgery** 34: 680–687, 1994.
9. Davis FG, Malinski N, Haenszel W, et al.: Primary brain tumor incidence rates in four United States regions, 1985–1989: A pilot study. **Neuroepidemiology** 15:103–112, 1996.
10. Eddy DM: Designing a practice policy: Standards, guidelines, and options. **JAMA** 263:3077–3084, 1990.
11. Eyre HJ, Crowley JJ, Townsend JJ, et al.: A randomized trial of radiotherapy versus radiotherapy plus CCNU for incompletely resected low-grade gliomas: A Southwest Oncology Group study. **J Neurosurg** 78:909–914, 1993.
12. Franzini A, Leocata F, Cajola L, et al.: Low-grade glial tumors in basal ganglia and

thalamus: Natural history and biological reappraisal. **Neurosurgery** 35:817–821, 1994.

13. Gannett DE, Wisbeck WM, Silbergeld DL, *et al.*: The role of postoperative irradiation in the treatment of oligodendroglioma. **Int J Radiat Oncol Biol Phys** 30:567–573, 1994.

14. Guyatt GH, Sackett DL, Cook DJ, *et al.*: Users' guide to the medical literature. II How to use an article about therapy or prevention. A. Are the results of the study valid? **JAMA** 270:2598–2601, 1993.

15. Ito S, Chandler KL, Prados MD, *et al.*: Proliferative potential and prognostic evaluation of low-grade astrocytoma. **J Neurooncol** 19:1–9, 1994.

16. Janny P, Cure H, Mohr M, *et al.*: Low grade supratentorial astrocytoma: Management and prognostic factors. **Cancer** 73:1937–1945, 1994.

17. Karim ABM, Maat B, Hatlevoll R, et al: A randomized trial on dose-response in radiation therapy of low-grade cerebral glioma: European Organization for Research and Treatment of Cancer (EORTC) Study 22844. **Int J Radiat Oncol Biol Phys** 36:549–556, 1996.

18. Kondziolka D, Lunsford LD, Martinez AJ: Unreliability of contemporary neurodiagnostic imaging in evaluating suspected adult supratentorial (low-grade) astrocytoma. **J Neurosurg** 79:533–536, 1993.

19. Laperriere NJ, Bernstein M: Removal of malignant astrocytomas (letter). **Neurosurgery** 22:440, 1988.

20. Laws ER, Taylor WF, Clifton MB, *et al.*: Neurosurgical management of low-grade astrocytoma of the cerebral hemispheres. **J Neurosurg** 61:665–673, 1984.

21. Loiseau H, Bousquet P, Rivel J, *et al.*: Astrocytomes des bas grade sus-tentoriels de l'adulte: Facteurs pronostics et indications therapeutiques a propos d'une serie de 141 patients. **Neurochirurgie** 41:38–50, 1995.

22. Lunsford LD, Somaza S, Kondziolka D, *et al.*: Survival after steretoactic biopsy and irradiation of cerebral nonanaplastic, nonpilocytic astrocytoma. **J Neurosurg** 82:523–529, 1995.

23. McCormack BM, Miller DC, Budzilovich GN, *et al.*: Treatment and survival of low-grade astrocytoma in adults—1977–1988. **Neurosurgery** 31:636–642, 1992.

24. Medbery CA, Straus KL, Steinberg SM, *et al.*: Low-grade astrocytomas: Treatment results and prognostic variables. **Int J Radiat Oncol Biol Phys** 15:837–841, 1988.

25. Montine TJ, Vandersteenhoven JJ, Aguzzi A, *et al.*: Prognostic significance of Ki-67 proliferation index in supratentorial fibrillary astrocytic neoplasms. **Neurosurgery** 34:674–679, 1994.

26. Nijjar TS, Simpson WJ, Cadalla T, *et al.*: Oligodendroglioma: The Princess Margaret Hospital Experience (1958–1984). **Cancer** 71:4002–4006, 1993.

27. Nitta T, Sato K: Prognostic implications of the extent of surgical resection in patients with intracranial malignant gliomas. **Cancer** 75:2727–2731, 1995.

28. North CA, North RB, Epstein JA, *et al.*: Low-grade cerebral astrocytomas: Survival and quality of life after radiation therapy. **Cancer** 66:6–14, 1990.

29. Philippon JH, Clemenceau SH, Fauchon FH, *et al.*: Supratentorial low-grade astrocytomas in adults. **Neurosurgery** 32:554–559, 1993.

30. Piepmeier JM: Observations on the current treatment of low-grade astrocytic tumors of the cerebral hemispheres. **J Neurosurg** 67:177–181, 1987.

31. Pu AT, Sandler HM, Radany EH, *et al.*: Low grade gliomas: Preliminary analysis of failure patterns among patients treated using 3D conformal external beam irradiation. **Int J Radiat Oncol Biol Phys** 31:461–466, 1995.

32. Recht LD, Bernstein M: Low-grade gliomas. **Neurol Clin** 13:847–859, 1995.

33. Recht LD, Lew R, Smith TW: Suspected low-grade glioma: Is deferring therapy safe? **Ann Neurol** 31:431–436, 1992.

34. Rosenberg J, Greenberg MK: Practice parameters: Strategies for survival into the nineties. **Neurology** 42:1110–1115, 1992.

35. Shaw EG, Scheithauer BW, Gilbertson DT, *et al.*: Postoperative radiotherapy of supratentorial low-grade gliomas. **Int J Radiat Oncol Biol Phys** 16:663–668, 1989.

36. Shaw EG, Scheithauer BW, O'Fallon JR, *et al.*: Mixed oligoastrocytomas: A survival and prognostic factor analysis. **Neurosurgery** 34:577–582, 1994.

37. Shibamato Y, Kitakabu Y, Takahashi M, *et al.*: Supratentorial low-grade astrocytoma: Correlation of computed tomography findings with effect of radiation therapy and prognostic variables. **Cancer** 72:190–195, 1993.

38. Soo TM, Bernstein M, Provias J, *et al.*: Failed stereotactic biopsy in a series of 518 cases. **Stereotact Funct Neurosurg** 64:183–196, 1996.

39. Steiger HJ, Markwalder RV, Seiler RW, *et al.*: Early prognosis of supratentorial grade 2 astrocytomas in adult patients after resection or stereotactic biopsy: An analysis of 50 cases operated on between 1984 and 1988. **Acta Neurochir (Wien)** 106:99–105, 1990.

40. Taphoorn MJB, Schiphorst AK, Snoek FJ, *et al.*: Cognitive functions and quality of life in patients with low-grade gliomas: The impact of radiotherapy. **Ann Neurol** 36:48–54, 1994.

41. Vertosick FT, Selker RG, Arena VC: Survival of patients with well-differentiated astrocytomas diagnosed in the era of computed tomography. **Neurosurgery** 28:496–501, 1991.

42. Vibbert S: *What Works?* Grand Rounds Press, Whittle Direct Books, 1993.

43. Walker MD, Green SB, Byar DP, *et al.*: Randomized comparisons of radiotherapy and nitrosoureas for the treatment of malignant glioma after surgery. **N Engl J Med** 303:1323–1329, 1980.

44. Westergaard L, Gjerris F, Klinken L: Prognostic parameters in benign astrocytomas. **Acta Neurochir (Wien)** 123:1–7, 1993.

45. Woolf SH: Practice guidelines: a new reality in medicine. II. Methods of developing guidelines. **Arch Intern Med** 152:946–952, 1992.

21

Outcome After Microvascular Decompression for Typical Trigeminal Neuralgia, Hemifacial Spasm, Tinnitus, Disabling Positional Vertigo, and Glossopharyngeal Neuralgia (Honored Guest Lecture)

PETER J. JANNETTA, M.D., D.Sci.

Microvascular decompression (MVD) has become increasingly popular as a treatment for many cranial nerve disorders since its introduction as a treatment for trigeminal neuralgia. In this chapter, we discuss the results of outcome studies performed at the University of Pittsburgh on patients who underwent MVD for the following disorders: typical trigeminal neuralgia (1, 2), hemifacial spasm (3), tinnitus (4), disabling positional vertigo (5), and glossopharyngeal neuralgia (6). The accrued experience in our unit with MVD for these five syndromes now totals over 4000 patients. Although the majority of these operations were performed by the sole author, patients operated by other surgeons were also included in the outcome studies. I am grateful to these surgeons for allowing us to include their results in this report.

MICROVASCULAR DECOMPRESSION FOR TYPICAL TRIGEMINAL NEURALGIA (TN)

Methods

PATIENTS

All 1185 patients who underwent MVD for typical TN at the Presbyterian-University Hospital (PUH), Pittsburgh, Pennsylvania, between January 1, 1972 and December 31, 1991 were included in this study, which was reported in 1996 (1). Criteria for typical TN included lancinating, shock-like pain located within the distribution of one or more trigeminal nerve branches. Most patients could consistently provoke pain attacks by touching trigger points, talking, chewing, or brushing their teeth. Some patients, particularly those with long histories of TN, noted aching pain between paroxysms. However, if major pain characteristically lasted seconds to minutes, atypical TN was diagnosed. These 369 patients were excluded from this series. Patients with typical TN posterior fossa tumor have been the subject of a separate report from our group (7). Eleven patients had concomitant ipsilateral glossopharyngeal neuralgia (GPN), 10 had ipsilateral hemifacial spasm (HFS; painful tic convulsif, and one had contralateral HFS. Overall, 1336 operations were performed in 1185 patients (1204 sides). Operative technique was described in this author's previous work (8).

DATA COLLECTION AND OUTCOME CRITERIA

Operative findings, complications, and presence or absence of individual symptoms of TN were prospectively recorded and maintained in a computerized database. Operative results were first assessed at clinic follow-up or by telephone. All patients were then sent an annual questionnaire beginning in 1980, which addressed presence or absence of facial pain, quality of the pain (if present), and persistence of any operative complications. A description of any follow-up treatment required for facial pain was also requested (whether with medications, or another operative procedure). For the purposes of this report, follow-up was terminated in January 1993; postoperative facial numbness was assessed with a special questionnaire in January 1994. This questionnaire requested reporting of facial numbness on a five-point scale: no postoperative numbness at any time, transient postoperative numbness (entirely resolved by the time of the questionnaire), and mild, moderate, and severe persistent numbness.

An outcome of "excellent" was assigned if the patient was free of lancinating facial pain, or at least 98% pain-free, without medication for TN. (Some patients reported taking medication for contralateral TN. If the operated side was pain-free under these circumstances, a grade of "excellent" was assigned.) A grade of "partial" relief or "good" outcome was assigned if TN symptoms were relieved by 75% or greater. Intermittent treatment with low doses of medication for TN was considered compatible with partial success. If more than 25% of preoperative symptoms were present without medication, or if chronic medication was resumed at any dose, a grade of "failure" was assigned. Facial pain that was constant, aching, or burning in character was not considered a criterion for failure, because such symptoms were commonly present prior to MVD in patients who had previously undergone ablative procedures. Burning and aching facial pain are discussed separately below. Relief of these symptoms, when they existed preoperatively as a result of prior ablative treatments for TN, was not expected from MVD. The performance of any subsequent operative procedure (percutaneous or open) was considered a failure of the initial

MVD. If the patient was graded as a failure or partial success at the time of first postdischarge evaluation, failure was considered to have taken place 1 month postoperatively.

Outcome assessment, whether in clinic or by questionnaire, was performed by personnel other than the operating surgeon. Statistical methods were described previously (1).

Results

DEMOGRAPHICS, PREOPERATIVE SYMPTOMS AND PRIOR TREATMENT

A total of 1204 first MVDs for typical TN were performed in 1185 patients during the study period. Patients with less than 1 year follow-up (49 of 1204 sides; 4.1%) were included in calculation of demographic statistics, operative findings, and complications, and excluded from outcome analysis. Immediate postoperative results for these patients were not different from patients with more extended follow-up (Mann-Whitney U test; $P > 0.5$). Patients who underwent bilateral MVDs were counted as two separate patients. (Bilateral MVDs were performed in 19 patients; TN contralateral to the operated side occurred either pre- or post-MVD in 76 patients; 6.5%. Bilateral TN was the subject of a prior report from our group (9).

Median patient age at operation was 57 years (range, 5 to 87). At time of operation, patients' mean life expectancy based on age- and sex-specific tables for the 1987 United States population (10) was 25 years (median, 23 years). Male-to-female ratio was 40:60. Symptoms were right-sided in 62% of patients. Median age at onset of symptoms was 49 years (range, 2 to 82 years). Median preoperative duration of symptoms was 6 years (range, less than 1 year to 44 years). There was no significant change in preoperative duration of symptoms during the 20-year study period.

TABLE 1.
Distribution of symptoms in patients with typical TN
(1204 previously unoperated sides)

Divisions involved	No. of patients	Percent (%)
V_1 only	33	2.8
V_2 only	213	17.7
V_3 only	176	14.6
V_{1+2}	207	17.2
V_{2+3}	427	35.4
V_{1+3}	0	0.0
V_{1+2+3}	148	12.3

The distribution of pain between the three branches of the trigeminal nerve is shown in Table 1. Patients with longer preoperative duration of symptoms had pain in more divisions of the trigeminal distribution (mean duration of symptoms: 6.8, 7.2, 8.7 years for patients with pain in one, two, or three divisions respectively; P < 0.005).

Previous treatment with medication was nearly universal: 93% of patients had been treated with carbamazepine, 52% with phenytoin, and 14% with baclofen. Two medications had been used by 47% of patients, and all three in 7%. In general, patients reported significant relief of TN from these medications (particularly carbamazepine), but developed intolerable side effects or had recurrent tics despite medication. Some patients had pain refractory to medication at presentation.

Prior operative treatments for TN are shown in Table 2. Peripheral nerve injections, avulsions, or sections had been performed in 17%, radiofrequency gasserian lesions (RFLs) in 8%, and glycerol rhizolyses in 4%. Spiller-Frazier procedures or other destructive procedures directed toward the trigeminal ganglion or root (posterior fossa rhizotomies, injections of alcohol, phenol, or hot water) had been performed in 3% of patients. In all, 27% had undergone one or more ablative trigeminal procedures prior to MVD.

Duration of symptoms before MVD was highly correlated with the prior performance of an ablative procedure. Patients without such procedures had a shorter mean preoperative duration of symptoms: 6.4

TABLE 2.

Relative risks of facial hypalgesia, hypesthesia, and decreased corneal reflex in patients with prior operative procedures for TN[a]

	Prior RFL (N = 110)	Prior RAL (N = 42)	Prior PNS (N = 216)	Prior glyc (N = 58)	Prior MVD (N = 56)
Hypalgesia	4.0[b]	5.8[b]	5.2[b]	1.0	1.2
	(2.2–7.2)	(2.1–16.2)	(3.4–8.0)	(0.4–2.1)	(0.6–2.8)
Hypesthesia	6.7[b]	5.3[b]	5.2[b]	0.8	2.3
	(3.4–12.9)	(1.9–15.0)	(3.4–8.1)	(0.3–1.8)	(1.0–5.2)
Decreased corneal reflex	4.4[b]	4.6[b]	2.5[b]	0.6	2.2
	(2.3–8.4)	(1.8–11.7)	(1.4–4.4)	(0.1–2.6)	(1.8–5.7)

[a] Preoperative findings in 1204 sides without prior MVD; findings in a separate group of 56 patients who underwent prior MVD elsewhere also shown. Values shown are the odds ratios for the type of sensory deficit specified at left, for patients with prior treatments specified in column head compared to patients without any prior ablative procedure. In parentheses: 99% confidence intervals. *RFL*, radiofrequency lesion; *RAL*, other retrogasserian ablative lesion (see text); *PNS*, peripheral nerve section or avulsion; *glyc*, glycerol rhizolysis.
[b] P < 0.0001.

years (25th to 75th percentile, 3 to 8 years), compared with 9.4 years (25th to 75th percentile, 5 to 16 years) for those who had undergone one or more such procedures (t test $P < 0.001$). Apart from subtle decreases in sensation in the trigeminal distribution in some patients, there were no characteristic physical findings. Many patients had slight degrees of facial hypesthesia (36%) or hypalgesia (36%). The corneal reflex was decreased or absent in 8.5% of patients. Preoperative duration of symptoms and number of involved divisions were not significantly related to the presence of hypesthesia, hypalgesia, or a decreased corneal reflex.

The probability of a preoperative sensory deficit was highly related to prior operative treatment for TN (Table 2). Both prior RFLs and prior retrogasserian ablative procedures conveyed relative risks of 4.0 to 6.7 of hypalgesia, hypesthesia and decreased corneal reflex; prior peripheral nerve destructions (PNDs) had similar relative risks of facial hypalgesia and hypesthesia, and a slight excess risk of decreased corneal reflex. Prior glycerol rhizolysis carried no excess risk of facial hypalgesia, hypesthesia, or decreased corneal reflex. Prior MVD at another institution (a separate group of 56 patients) carried a minor but statistically significant risk of hypesthesia and decreased corneal reflex, but no additional risk of hypalgesia.

OPERATIVE FINDINGS

Operative findings are summarized in Table 3. The most frequent operative finding (76% of patients) was trigeminal compression by the

TABLE 3.

Vessels found to compress the trigeminal nerve in 1204 consecutive previously unoperated sides with typical TN

Vessel	First operation N (total 1204)	Percent (%)	Reoperation N (total 132)	Percent (%)
SCA	909	75.5	27	20.5
AICA	116	9.6	4	3.0
PICA	8	0.7	0	0
Vertebral	19	1.6	0	0
Basilar	9	0.7	0	0
Labyrinthine	3	0.2	1	1.0
Unnamed small artery	186	15.4	47	35.6
Vein	822	68.2	95	72.0
Vein only	151	12.5	49	37.1
Vein and artery	671	55.7	46	34.8
Unnamed small artery or vein only	223	18.5	102	77.3

Abbreviations: SCA, superior cerebellar artery; AICA, anterior inferior cerebellar artery; PICA, posterior inferior cerebellar artery.

superior cerebellar artery (SCA). A vein was thought to contribute to compression in 68% of patients and to be the sole compressing vessel in 13%.

Compression of the trigeminal nerve by an ectatic vertebral or basilar artery was more frequently found in older patients (odds ratio [OR] 1.06/year, 95% confidence interval [CI] 1.01 to 1.1, P = 0.01), in males (OR 3.6, 95% CI 1.6 to 8.4, P < 0.005), and in patients with hypertension (OR 8.2, 95% CI 3.6 to 19, P < 0.001). MVD in patients with vertebrobasilar compression was the subject of a prior report from our group (11). A small unnamed artery or vein as sole compressing vessel was more frequent in female patients (OR 1.6, 95% CI 1.2 to 2.1, P < 0.005).

OPERATIVE COMPLICATIONS

Operative complications are shown in Table 4. There were two operative deaths. The first occurred in a 79-year-old woman who suffered a postoperative hemispheric stroke. The second occurred in a 69-year-old woman who suffered a brainstem and cerebellar infarction,

TABLE 4.
Operative complications in 1336 MVDs for typical TN

Complication	First operatins (N = 1204)	Reoperations (N = 132)	Total (N = 1336)
Operative death	2	0	2
Brainstem infarct	0	1	1
Cerebellar hematoma	2	0	2
Supratentorial hematoma	2	0	2
Cerebellar edema	4	0	4
Hydrocephalus	2	0	2
Facial paresis			
transient	5	4	9
permanent, mild	0	1	1
permanent, severe	0	1	1
Hearing loss, ipsilateral			
permanent, mild	1	0	1
permanent, severe	14	1	15
Extraocular muscle palsies			
trochlear, transient	11	0	11
trochlear, permanent	2	0	2
abducens, transient	2	0	2
Facial numbness, severe	11	11	22
CSF leak	17	3	20
Pseudomeningocele	4	0	4
Bacterial meningitis	4	1	5
"Chemical meningitis"	198	27	225

Other complications: pneumonia (2), septicemia (1), subendocardial myocardial infarction (1), transverse sinus thrombosis (1), pulmonary embolus (1), contralateral moderate permanent hearing loss (1).

apparently due to occlusion of the SCA by the implant. Both deaths occurred before the introduction of intraoperative brainstem-evoked response (BSER) monitoring. Since 1980, when monitoring of BSERs was introduced at PUH, there have been no deaths in 773 consecutive first MVDs for typical TN.

Six patients had infarction, edema, or hemorrhage of the ipsilateral cerebellar hemisphere, of whom five required cerebellar resection. There was one postoperative supratentorial subdural hematoma and one supratentorial intracerebral hematoma, both requiring evacuation. All patients recovered without permanent sequelae.

Severe facial numbness occurred after 11 (0.9%) first MVDs for typical TN and after 11 reoperations (8%). Numbness as a sequela of MVD is discussed in further detail below. There were no cases of postoperative anesthesia dolorosa (facial anesthesia with severe paresthesia). Burning and aching facial pain were reported by 3% and 4% of patients, respectively, after a single MVD and no ablative procedures. Of the 878 patients with no prior ablative procedures, three reported postoperative treatment with a tricyclic antidepressant drug or related medication for burning or aching pain. Of the 326 patients with prior ablative procedures, four reported postoperative treatment with tricyclic antidepressant or related drugs for burning or aching pain that was not clearly attributed to the ablative procedure. Burning and aching facial pain were more commonly reported by the 96 patients with radiofrequency lesions of the trigeminal ganglion before MVD (burning pain, $P < 0.001$; aching pain, $P = 0.002$), but not by those who had had other ablative procedures.

Fifteen patients (1.2%) suffered loss of hearing in the ipsilateral ear, of whom 14 had severe loss. In addition, a single patient lost hearing to a moderate degree in the contralateral ear. Hearing loss was not significantly correlated with patient age, sex, decompression of the facial as well as the trigeminal nerve, or repositioning of any specific artery.

Intraoperative monitoring of BSERs was first used at PUH in 1980, although several years passed before it became routine. Before the introduction of BSERs, ipsilateral hearing was lost in 11 of 431 operations (2.6%); after 1979 the rate fell to five of 773 operations (0.6%). The difference between the complication rate for the two time periods was statistically and clinically significant (OR 4.0, 1972 to 1979 higher than 1980 to 1991; 95% CI 1.4 to 12, $P < 0.01$).

Five patients (0.4%) suffered transient facial weakness. No permanent facial weakness resulted from a first MVD for typical TN.

Fifteen patients suffered postoperative extraocular movement abnormalities. Eleven of 13 trochlear palsies resolved completely; two persisted for more than 1 year. Two abducens palsies occurred (one ipsilateral and one contralateral); both resolved completely.

Wound complications were all satisfactorily managed without lasting sequelae. Two patients developed hydrocephalus after MVD and required a lumbo- or ventriculoperitoneal shunt.

OUTCOME AFTER MVD

For 1204 patients who underwent first MVD for typical TN at PUH during the study period, the follow-up rate 5 years post-MVD was 91%, and 87% 10 years post-MVD. Median follow-up for the 1155 patients followed 1 year or more was 6.2 years. A total of 8714 patient-years of follow-up information was accrued.

Actuarial survival for the group as a whole (Kaplan-Meier estimator) was 93% 10 years post-MVD and 70% 20 years post-MVD. A total of 121 patients (10%) were lost to follow-up for reasons other than death. These patients had the same outcome distribution immediately prior to loss as the remainder of the group (Mann-Whitney U test, P = 0.14). A proportional hazards model found higher rates of loss for younger patients (P < 0.001) and for patients who lost hearing as an operative complication (P = 0.005). Immediate postoperative relief of TN, postoperative facial weakness, and numbness were not significantly related to chance of loss to follow-up.

During the first postoperative week full relief of TN was achieved in 82% of patients; 16% had partial relief, and 2% had no relief. Disregarding results of reoperations, 1 year after MVD, 75.2% of patients had excellent results and 8.9% had partial relief (total 84.1%). Ten years after MVD 63.5% had excellent results and 3.5% had partial relief (total 67.0%; Fig. 1A).

A total of 132 patients (11%) were submitted to reoperation for recurrent or refractory symptoms prior to January 1, 1992. Results and complications of reoperations are reported below.

Including results of all operations per patient, 1 year after MVD, 79.7% of patients had excellent results and 7.6% partial relief (total 87.3%); 10 years after MVD, 69.6% had excellent results and 4.2% partial relief (total 73.8%; Fig. 1B).

Life-table analysis was used to estimate the annual chance of tic recurrence after a first MVD for typical TN (Fig. 2). Because all failures that occurred prior to the first outpatient follow-up or questionnaire response were assumed to have occurred 1 month postoperatively, the values for postoperative years 1 and 2 are distorted (some failures actually occurring in year 2 having been assigned to year 1). The risk of TN recurrence (transition from the "excellent" group to either the "good" or "poor" groups) fell below 2% per year by 5 years

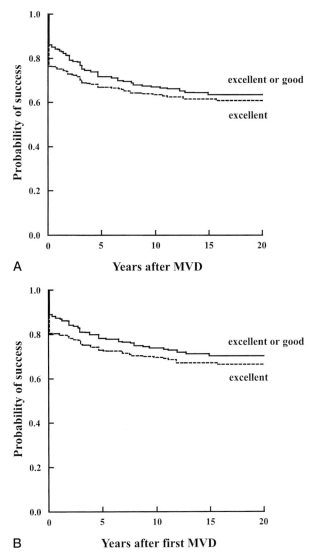

FIG. 1. (A) Kaplan-Meier plot showing long-term outcome for all previously unoperated patients (1204 sides; results of first MVD only). The *dashed line* represents chances of excellent relief of TN after first MVD; the *solid line* represents chances of a good or excellent result. (B) Kaplan-Meier plot showing long-term outcome for all previously unoperated patients (1204 sides). Final results after one or two operations per patient are shown. *Dashed line*, chance of excellent results; *solid line*, chance of good or excellent results. See text for grading of success.

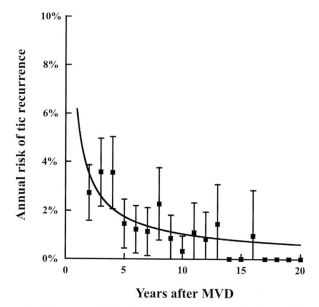

Years after MVD

Fig. 2. Plot showing annual risk of recurrence of trigeminal neuralgia after MVD. Recurrence is defined as the transition from the "excellent" to either the "good" or "poor" result groups. For each postoperative year (starting with year 2), the life-table recurrence rate is shown, with error bars representing 95% confidence intervals. A fitted power function curve is also shown. The recurrence rate falls below 2% per year by postoperative year 5, and below 1% per year by postoperative year 10.

after MVD and below 1% by 10 years after MVD. The annual recurrence rate during the second postoperative decade was 0.7% (9 recurrences in 1251 patient-years).

Of 282 patients in whom MVD was considered to have failed, 34% resumed chronic medication for TN, 20% underwent ablative procedures on the trigeminal nerve, and 22% reported both types of therapy. No further treatment for TN was reported to be necessary by 24% of patients in whom MVD was considered to have failed by our criteria.

OUTCOME BY SUBGROUP

Four Cox proportional hazards models were constructed to identify variables predicting operative success. In two models, excellent or good/excellent results after first MVD only were considered success; in the other two models, the same criteria were used, but results of all operations were included. Variables examined included patient age and sex, side and duration of symptoms, number of trigeminal divisions involved by pain, history of prior ablative procedures on the trigeminal nerve, presence of trigger points, preoperative hypesthesia or hypalgesia, coincident symptoms of contralateral TN, ipsilateral HFS or GPN, anatomic findings at operation, performance of partial trigeminal rhizotomy (21 patients; 1.7%), and degree of immediate postoperative relief. Variables were considered significant if they entered at least two models at the P < 0.05 level.

The most significant variable in all four models was immediate postoperative relief of TN. Patient sex was the second most significant variable in three of four models, with less frequent recurrence in male patients. Three of four models contained venous compression of the trigeminal root entry zone as a significant predictor of long-term failure. Duration of preoperative symptoms (greater or less than 8 years) entered two models, with longer duration of preoperative pain predicting failure in both models that considered "partial success" as failure. Bilateral TN or ipsilateral HFS were not related to failure in any of the models. The performance of an ablative procedure or partial rhizotomy before MVD did not increase chances of tic recurrence in any model. Characteristics of the four models are summarized in Table 5; the univariate effects of the four significant covariates are shown in Figure 3.

TABLE 5.

Characteristics of four Cox proportional hazards models of postoperative pain relief after MVD for typical TN. The hazard ratio and P value for each covariate are shown. Models: 1, excellent results, first MVD only; 2, excellent or good results, first MVD only; 3, excellent results, final results after one or two operations per patient; 4, excellent or good results, final results after one or two operations per patient.

	Model			
	1	2	3	4
Sex (male)				
hazard ratio	0.74	0.76	0.70	0.71
P value	0.006	0.02	0.003	0.01
Duration of symptoms greater than 8 years				
hazard ratio	1.25	1.12	1.32	1.18
P value	0.03	0.3	0.01	0.2
Vein at operation				
hazard ratio	1.20	1.27	1.40	1.46
P value	0.1	0.05	0.008	0.006
Immediate postoperative relief of pain				
hazard ratio	0.35	0.30	0.39	0.35
P value	<0.0001	<0.0001	<0.0001	<0.001

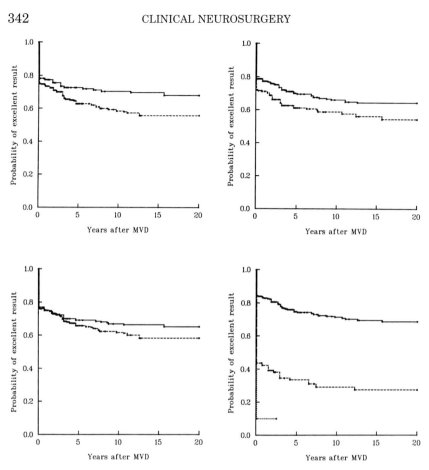

FIG. 3. Kaplan-Meier plots showing the effect of univariate stratification of outcome by the four prognostic factors found to be significant in a Cox proportional hazards model. (A) Effect of patient sex (*solid line*, male patients; *dashed line*, female patients). (B) Effect of preoperative duration of symptoms (*solid line*, less than 8 years; *dashed line*, more than 8 years). (C) Effect of venous compression of the trigeminal root entry zone (*solid line*, no venous compression; *dashed line*, venous compression). (D) Effect of immediate postoperative relief (*solid line*, complete relief; *dashed line*, partial relief; *dotted line*, no relief).

FACIAL NUMBNESS AND TIC RELIEF AFTER MVD

Of 1204 patients who underwent MVD for typical trigeminal neuralgia during the study period, 522 had a single MVD on a single side only, had not undergone ablative procedures before or after MVD, and were still being followed in 1994. Of these, 494 returned questionnaires in 1994 that included a question about facial numbness (95% response rate); 480 questionnaires contained an answer to the specific question addressing facial numbness (92% specific response rate). These questionnaire responses were the basis of our recently reported investigation of the relationship between postoperative facial numbness (an index of intraoperative trauma to the trigeminal nerve) and the success of MVD for typical tic (2).

Of these 480 patients, 59% were female; median age was 56 years; the mean number of trigeminal divisions affected by tic was 1.8. Patients in the study group differed from other patients operated during the same 20-year period with respect to the following variables: preoperative duration of symptoms (shorter by 1 year in the numbness study group), frequency with which an SCA or vein was considered to be compressing the trigeminal root entry zone (both slightly more likely in the study group), and year of surgery (surgery more recent in the study group). Median follow-up time for this group of patients was 7.9 years (range, 2.1 to 21.5 years).

POSTOPERATIVE FACIAL NUMBNESS: INCIDENCE AND RISK FACTORS

After a single MVD, 67.9% of patients reported that they had never had facial numbness and 14.8% recalled transient postoperative numbness (total, 82.7% without persistent numbness). The remaining 17.3% of patients reported some degree of persistent facial numbness (11.9% mild, 4.4% moderate, and 1.0% severe). There was no significant univariate association between postoperative numbness and the following variables: patient age, sex, side and duration of symptoms, number of involved trigeminal divisions, and preoperative presence of subtle trigeminal hypesthesia or hypalgesia on preoperative physical examination.

Two operative findings were significantly related to postoperative numbness in univariate analysis. When trigeminal compression by the SCA was found at operation, postoperative numbness was less likely (Mann-Whitney $P = 0.009$). When a vein was found, postoperative numbness was more likely (Mann-Whitney $P < 0.001$). When numbness was stratified as persistent *versus* transient or none, a multivariate logistic regression model that included a variable equal to time between MVD and questionnaire (to adjust for regression of numbness over time and for bias introduced by the statistical methodology (12)) showed that both operative findings (SCA and vein) were independently significant in predicting persistent postoperative facial numbness (SCA: OR 0.51, 95% CI 0.29 to 0.87, $P = 0.01$; vein: OR 2.5, 95% CI 1.2 to 5.2, $P = 0.01$).

POSTOPERATIVE FACIAL DYSESTHESIA: INCIDENCE AND RISK FACTORS

Burning and aching facial pain were reported by 3.3% and 4.8% of patients, respectively, after a single MVD and no ablative procedures. Burning and aching facial pain were reported more frequently by patients who also reported postoperative facial numbness (Table 6). Of 83 patients with persistent facial numbness, 9.6% reported burning and 14.5% reported aching facial pain. Of 397 patients without persistent facial numbness, 2.0% reported burning and 2.8% reported aching facial pain. In univariate logistic regression analysis, burning and aching facial pain were both more common if facial numbness was present after MVD (OR 1.8 [burning; P = 0.005] and 1.9 [aching; P < 0.001] for each point on the numbness rating scale). When numbness was stratified as persistent *versus* transient or none, odds ratios for persistent numbness were 5.2 for burning pain (P = 0.001) and 5.9 for aching pain (P < 0.001). There was no relationship between reported postoperative burning or aching facial pain and patient age, sex, side or duration of symptoms, number of involved trigeminal divisions, or operative findings of compression by the SCA or a vein.

TEMPORAL TRENDS

Temporal trends in self-reported facial numbness, burning and aching facial pain, and risk factors for numbness were tested using logistic regression analysis with the year of surgery as the independent variable. Significant temporal trends were found for persistent facial numbness (more likely in patients with more recent surgery, P = 0.008; Fig. 4) and for the finding of a compressing vein at surgery (more likely in patients with more recent surgery, P < 0.001). There were no significant temporal trends in the presence of a compressing SCA at

TABLE 6.
Relationship between facial numbness after microvascular decompression and facial dysesthesias *

	Burning pain			Aching pain		
	OR	95% CI	P value	OR	95% CI	P value
Numbness (per point, 5-point scale)	1.8	(1.2–2.7)	0.005	1.9	(1.3–2.7)	<0.001
Persistent numbness (yes/no)	5.2	(1.9–14)	0.001	5.9	(2.5–14)	<0.001

* OR, odds ratio; CI, confidence interval. P values shown reflect univariate logistic regression analysis.

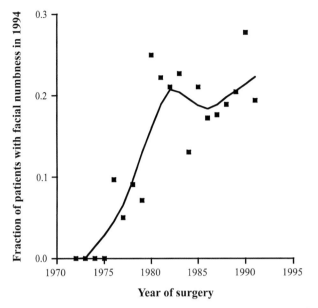

FIG. 4. Scatterplot showing the chance of persistent facial numbness after MVD for typical tic, by year of operation. *Squares* indicate the proportion of patients undergoing MVD in the indicated years who reported persistent facial numbness by questionnaire in 1994. A LOWESS-smoothed trend line (119) is also shown (tension parameter = 0.4). The trend toward less frequent persistent facial numbness in patients who underwent MVD earlier in the study period was statistically significant (logistic regression, P = 0.007). In a subgroup of 372 patients undergoing MVD in 1980 or later, there was no significant temporal trend in persistent facial numbness (P = 0.95).

surgery or in the incidence of postoperative burning or aching facial pain.

LONG-TERM PAIN RELIEF AND POSTOPERATIVE NUMBNESS

Because a temporal trend was observed in the incidence of reported persistent facial numbness during the study period, all outcome analyses were stratified by a variable equal to years between MVD and questionnaire response (12).

In univariate analysis, slightly better long-term tic relief was observed in patients without persistent facial numbness, but the trend was not statistically significant (P = 0.3; Fig. 5). A Cox multivariate proportional hazards model was used to adjust for the four variables found to be prognostic in this patient population (1): sex, duration of symptoms longer than 8 years, operative finding of a compressing vein, and degree of immediate postoperative relief. After adjustment for the

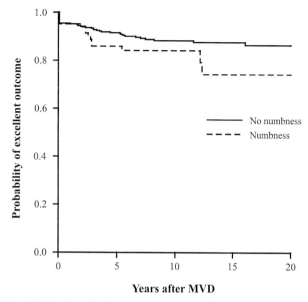

FIG. 5. Kaplan-Meier plot showing univariate stratification of outcome after MVD for trigeminal neuralgia by presence or absence of postoperative persistent facial numbness. Results are for 480 patients who underwent a single MVD on a single side with no prior or subsequent ablative procedures. *Solid line*, no persistent facial numbness; *dashed line*, persistent facial numbness. Less frequent tic recurrence was seen in patients without persistent facial numbness, but the trend was not statistically significant (P = 0.26).

other prognostic factors, persistent facial numbness was still not significantly related to tic relief (P = 0.4).

Subgroup analyses were performed on three patient groups: 381 patients in whom trigeminal compression by the SCA was found at operation (with or without additional venous compression), 120 patients in whom the SCA was the only compressing vessel found, and 372 patients operated since 1980. In the patient subgroup with SCA trigeminal compression found at operation, persistent facial numbness was not a significant prognostic factor in univariate analysis (P = 0.7) or after adjustment for the other four prognostic factors (P = 0.8). In the group with the SCA as sole compressing vessel, lack of persistent facial numbness significantly predicted successful long-term tic relief both in univariate analysis (P = 0.02) and after adjustment for the other three prognostic factors (P = 0.03).

Patients who underwent MVD in 1980 or later constituted a subgroup in whom there was no temporal trend in persistent facial numbness (logistic regression P = 0.95; Fig. 4). As discussed below, analysis of this subgroup was performed to minimize the bias introduced in an analysis of survival (*i.e.*, tic relief) by a treatment outcome variable (*i.e.*, facial numbness). In this patient subgroup, better long-term tic relief was observed in patients without persistent facial numbness in univariate analysis, but the trend was not statistically significant, either in univariate analysis (P = 0.19) or after adjustment for the other prognostic factors (P = 0.3).

REOPERATIONS

Eleven percent of the patients in this series (132 of 1204) underwent reoperation for persistent or recurrent tic symptoms. Ten percent were performed within 30 days of the initial MVD and 58% were less than 2 years after initial MVD. The vessels most frequently found to compress the trigeminal nerve at reoperation were veins or unnamed small arteries (Table 3).

Complications after reoperation are summarized in Table 4. There was no operative mortality. One patient had transient dysarthria and right arm ataxia. We classified this event as a brainstem infarction, although there was no brainstem abnormality seen by magnetic resonance (MR) imaging; all symptoms cleared completely. Cranial nerve complications were more frequent after reoperations. Four patients had transient facial weakness and an additional two patients had facial weakness that persisted more than 1 year.

Performance of a second MVD was a risk factor for postoperative facial numbness. Fifty patients who had undergone two MVDs and no ablative procedures on a single side were sent questionnaires requesting information on facial numbness; 45 responded (90% response rate). After their second MVD, 18% of patients reported that they never had numbness and 11% recalled transient postoperative numbness (total 29%). The remaining 71% reported some degree of persistent numbness (29% mild, 33% moderate, and 9% severe). Self-reported facial numbness was significantly more likely after a second MVD than after a single MVD, both in univariate analysis (Mann-Whitney P < 0.001) and in a multivariate logistic regression model that adjusted for the finding of an SCA or a vein at first operation (P < 0.001). Reoperations were not followed by higher rates of postoperative burning or aching facial pain in a logistic model that included the effects of prior RFL and facial numbness post-MVD (P > 0.1).

Reoperations were not as successful as first MVDs (Fig. 6). Five years after reoperation, 45% of patients had excellent results, and 51% had good or excellent results. Ten years after reoperation results were 42% excellent and 47% good or excellent. As after first MVDs, the majority of failures after reoperation occurred within the first 2 years,

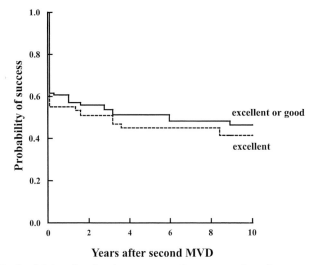

FIG. 6. Kaplan-Meier plot showing outcome after reoperations for recurrent trigeminal neuralgia after a first MVD (132 sides). *Dashed line*, chance of excellent results; *solid line*, chance of good or excellent results.

with few failures occurring after 5 years postreoperation. A Cox model found only one variable that significantly predicted long-term postoperative pain relief after reoperation: immediate postoperative relief of tic pain (P < 0.01).

PATIENT ASSESSMENT OF OUTCOME

Of 875 patients whose most recently returned questionnaire was available for review, 99.7% of those assigned outcomes of "excellent" and 93% of those assigned outcomes of "partial relief" considered their results to have been successful. Interestingly, nearly half (48%) of those whom we assigned an outcome of "failure" considered their own results to have been successful. Extrapolating these percentages to the entire series would predict an 87% "success" rate of MVD for typical TN.

Discussion

Microvascular decompression for typical trigeminal neuralgia is a safe and effective technique for the relief of tic symptoms. The operation, as presently performed at our center, has low rates of morbidity and near-zero mortality. The following discussion briefly compares our experience with MVD for tic to reported experiences with other medical, surgical, and radiosurgical treatments for trigeminal neuralgia.

More extensive reviews of the various treatments available for tic are also available (13, 14).

MEDICAL TREATMENT FOR TRIGEMINAL NEURALGIA

Numerous medications have been used to treat TN, and many remain in current use (15, 16). The present gold standard for tic treatment is carbamazepine (Tegretol). About 70 to 80% of patients with typical TN will have excellent relief from this drug. Over 90% of those who respond well have pain relief within 48 hours of starting the drug. Dosage should be guided by the patient's symptoms. There is no need to achieve a minimum "therapeutic" level by laboratory measurement. Some patients require very small chronic doses, or can take the drug intermittently as needed. Others have tic that is refractory to carbamazepine even at high doses, causing intolerable side effects.

The long-term success rate of carbamazepine has not been well established. In one retrospective study (17), of the 69% of patients with initially satisfactory tic relief from carbamazepine, only 56% still had satisfactory tic relief 10 years later. There are many reasons for failure of carbamazepine. Some patients develop breakthrough pain, while others have side effects that require the drug to be stopped: hyponatremia, leukopenia, or rash. Breakthrough pain in a patient on carbamazepine can be treated by adding a second drug or by tapering the carbamazepine and substituting another drug. If carbamazepine is stopped abruptly in a TN patient who has had significant relief from the drug, a severe paroxysm of TN may follow.

Second-line drugs for TN include phenytoin, baclofen, valproic acid, and clonazepam. The choice between these agents is not guided by firm published evidence (18), although phenytoin is often tried first. Although GABA pentin is frequently prescribed for TN, there is insufficient published evidence for its efficacy. In general, all of these agents are significantly less effective than carbamazepine. Given the variety of safe and effective surgical treatments available for TN, prolonged periods of time spent on trials of partially effective drugs are probably too often pursued.

SURGICAL TREATMENTS FOR TRIGEMINAL NEURALGIA (OTHER THAN MICROVASCULAR DECOMPRESSION)

Operative tic treatments in current use include peripheral neurectomies, percutaneous radiofrequency heat lesions of the gasserian ganglion (RFL) (19), retrogasserian glycerol rhizolysis (glycerol injection into the trigeminal cistern) (20), and trigeminal ganglion balloon microcompression (21). These procedures all cause controlled injury to the trigeminal nerve, ganglion, or root.

The least invasive surgical treatment for TN is peripheral neurectomy (22, 23). The supraorbital nerve can be avulsed at its exit from the skull through the supraorbital foramen. The infraorbital nerve is usually approached through an intraoral Caldwell-Luc incision, although extraoral approaches have also been described. The inferior alveolar and lingual nerves can be exposed through incisions on the posterior mandibular mucosa. The procedures can be repeated if tic recurs (22). Peripheral neurectomies have been in use for many years and have high initial success rates and few complications, although the short duration of tic relief makes them a less attractive option, except for the patient with a limited life expectancy.

Radiofrequency gasserian lesions (RFL) are created using a needle passed percutaneously into the gasserian ganglion. The technique has been reported in detail (19, 24–26). Electrical stimulation can be used during the procedure to ensure that the lesion created is within the desired portion of the ganglion. Hypalgesia is an expected result of the procedure. Because the success rate of the procedure is correlated with the likelihood of postoperative numbness (27–32), some surgeons create a denser lesion that includes analgesia and/or hypesthesia for light touch as well. Most surgeons report initial success rates in excess of 90%. The reported long-term success rate varies widely between different series: some groups reported 10-year pain-free rates as high as 78% (27), while others found that only 20% of patients remained pain-free 6 to 7 years after radiofrequency gasserian lesions (33, 34). Most authors have not used actuarial reporting methods, rendering comparison between series difficult.

The principal complication of the RFL procedure is facial dysesthesia. In a compilation of about 9,000 RFL cases reported by various authors, Sweet (35) found that 10% had dysesthesias that were controlled by drugs and 4% had anesthesia, analgesia, or hypalgesia dolorosa (presumably not controlled by drugs). Relatively higher dysesthesia rates are reported by authors who create denser RFL lesions, with higher rates of facial numbness. In the series reported by Taha et al. (27), 7% of patients with mild hypalgesia after RFL reported facial dysesthesia, compared with 15% of those with dense hypalgesia, and 36% in those with analgesia.

After RFL, successful tic relief is correlated with the degree of facial numbness produced. Latchaw et al. (28) reported that patients with substantial, moderate, or no sensory deficit had 5-year tic recurrence rates of 0%, 46%, and 74%, respectively. Broggi et al. (29) found that patients with analgesia after RFL had a 7.5% tic recurrence rate, whereas those with hypalgesia had a 41% recurrence rate. In our series (1, 2), a prior RFL was a significant predictor of pre-MVD facial numbness (Table 2), showing that patients who do not achieve successful tic relief are also frequently left with numb faces. Facial dysesthesias were also reported significantly more frequently by patients who had undergone RFL before MVD. Other complications of RFL procedures, such as intracranial hemorrhage, palsies of other cranial nerves, or death are rare (35).

A percutaneous technique that causes numbness less frequently than RFL is the retrogasserian glycerol rhizolysis, in which glycerol is injected into the trigeminal cistern. The technical details of the procedure have been reported (20, 36, 37). Initial success rates of the procedure are high, usually 80 to 90% (25). The median time to tic recurrence, based on reports using actuarial methods (37–43) is between 16 and 36 months. The procedure can be repeated, but immediate success rates are lower and recurrence is faster (median time to recurrence, about 1 year (39, 40, 43)). General anesthesia is used, which is an advantage over RFL for patients who cannot tolerate discomfort during the procedure.

Compared with RFL lesions, the glycerol rhizolysis has a lower rate of postoperative facial numbness (44). The rate of mild loss of light touch sensation has been reported to be less than 30% (37) to 70% (45). Bergenheim et al. (46) reported that deficits in light touch and pinprick sensation improved during the first year after glycerol rhizolysis, and Arias (47) noted that the majority of sensory deficits after glycerol rhizolysis had resolved by 3 months postoperatively. In our MVD series, a glycerol rhizolysis pre-MVD was not associated with increased rates of facial hypalgesia or hypesthesia on pre-MVD physical examination (Table 2). Most investigators agree that the chance of tic recurrence is lower in patients with sensory loss after glycerol rhizolysis (38, 44, 46, 48). Some authors disagree (49). In one report that suggested that patients with sensory loss after glycerol rhizolysis had a higher rate of tic recurrence, facial sensation at last follow-up was used as the stratifying variable, an analytical technique that introduces a strong bias in favor of apparently longer pain relief in patients without numbness (12). The rate of sensory loss increases after more than one glycerol rhizolysis: Lunsford (36, 37) reported a rate of less than 30% after one rhizolysis, compared with 50% after two, and 70% after three rhizolyses. Significant loss of corneal sensation is uncommon after glycerol rhizolysis, and anesthesia dolorosa is rare.

A newer percutaneous treatment for tic is balloon microcompression, in which a small balloon is introduced into Meckel's cave and used to physically compress the trigeminal ganglion (21). The technique has been described in detail (50, 51). Reported initial success rates have ranged between 78 and 100% (25, 52). A median time-to-tic recurrence of about 3.5 years has been reported (53). Most patients have some degree of sensory loss initially, and minor dysesthesias are reported in as many as 20% of patients (53). Successful tic relief is probably correlated with the presence of sensory loss (51), as has been noted for each of the other percutaneous procedures. Significant loss of corneal sensation and anesthesia dolorosa both appear to be very uncommon sequelae. Temporary masseter weakness is seen in the majority of patients but tends to resolve in less than a year (52).

An even less "invasive" treatment for tic is stereotactic radiosurgery using the Gamma Knife (54). The nerve root entry zone is the target for a single dose of between 60 and 90 Gy. Sixty-seven percent of patients who were treated with doses above 65 Gy achieved complete pain relief, which began between 1 and 8 weeks after radiosurgery in most responders. Six percent of patients had facial paresthesias. Long-term results with this technique are not yet known. Although perhaps less invasive than percutaneous methods, this technique appears to have the lowest initial success rate of the procedures described in this chapter, and the durability of response in patients who do achieve good pain relief is unknown.

MICROVASCULAR DECOMPRESSION FOR TRIGEMINAL NEURALGIA

MVD for typical tic has been shown to be safe and effective in reports from our group (1, 8, 55–59) and from other centers around the world (60). As presently practiced at our institution, the operation is routinely performed through an 8-cm skin incision, with a 5-cm craniectomy, no use of intraoperative retraction, operating time between 50 and 90 minutes, and postoperative hospital time between 2 and 4 days for most patients. Including first MVD procedures for both atypical and typical TN, there have been only two postoperative deaths from MVD of the trigeminal nerve at PUH.

Although direct comparisons between series are hindered by differing definitions of operative success, our results are similar to those in other studies of tic recurrence after MVD using actuarial methods (34, 42, 61–66). The annual tic recurrence rate in our patients fell below 2% by 5 years postoperatively and below 1% by 10 years postoperatively. The large size and extended follow-up in our cohort (288 patients pain-free 10 years after MVD) provide a more precise estimate of the annual recurrence rate after MVD than those previously available (2 to 3.5% (61, 62)). During the second postoperative decade, the annual recurrence rate in our patients was 0.7%.

Other groups have studied the relationship between various prognostic factors and the success of MVD in relieving tic. The large size of our patient cohort allowed us to use multivariate Cox analysis to identify four factors that were correlated with long-term tic recurrence. The factors that predicted higher tic recurrence rates after MVD in our patients were female sex, preoperative symptoms for longer than 8 years, decompression of a vein at operation, and lack of immediate postoperative tic relief.

Women have been noted to have a higher rate of tic recurrence in some previous studies (61, 67, 68), although other groups have disagreed with this conclusion (42, 69–71). We found a similar trend toward more frequent recurrence of symptoms in women after MVD for HFS (see below).

Longer preoperative history of tic was reported as a risk factor for tic recurrence after MVD by some groups (61, 67, 72–74) but not by others (42, 65, 70, 71). This was the least important of the four factors we identified. It has been suggested that patients with shorter preoperative histories of tic might have higher success rates because of spontaneous remissions that are part of the natural history of the disease, but such remissions are unlikely to occur in patients with preoperative histories as long as 8 years. More severe changes in the trigeminal nerve from longstanding vascular compression are another possible explanation for this observation.

The number of trigeminal divisions affected by tic was not a prognostic factor in our series or in other reports (61). Preoperative sensory deficit or history of a trigeminal ablative procedure, previously reported as unfavorable prognostic factors (42, 62, 68, 73–75), were not significant in our analysis.

Operative findings at MVD have been correlated with outcome by a number of previous investigators (62, 65, 66, 68–70, 72, 76). Some analyses divided patients into those with and without nerve "grooving" or with "severe" *versus* nonsevere compression. This information was not collected prospectively in our patients, and we felt that a retrospective review of operative records would not be an adequate substitute for prospectively acquired data. No universally accepted criterion for severity of nerve compression exists. We did find that venous compression of the trigeminal nerve at MVD predicted a higher tic recurrence rate, as previously noted for both tic and hemifacial spasm (3, 69, 70, 77). We suggest that this may result from a tendency for tiny veins not seen at operation to enlarge after interruption of other venous drainage at MVD.

A prognostic factor for long-term success after MVD that seems to be previously unreported is the degree of immediate postoperative tic relief. Many patients with successful results from MVD awaken pain-free after surgery, and remain so. In others, tic resolves gradually over a week or two after operation. We found that incomplete pain relief during the first postoperative week predicted long-term tic recurrence.

COMPLICATIONS OF MVD FOR TRIGEMINAL NEURALGIA

Facial numbness can be considered as a complication after MVD, although it is a desired effect of percutaneous tic treatments. Our results show that numbness after MVD is more likely if a vein is found to compress the nerve and if compression by the superior cerebellar artery is not found. These operative findings are probably correlated with increased manipulation of the nerve, and possibly with inadvertent damage to the nerve root during electrocoagulation of veins in contact with the root. There was a clinically and statistically significant correlation between facial numbness and dysesthesia after MVD: Both burning and aching facial pain were between five and six times more likely in the presence of persistent facial numbness ($P = 0.001$ for both aching and burning pain). This suggests that damage to the trigeminal nerve at the root entry zone causes dysesthesias, just as damage at the level of the trigeminal ganglion does. We found no evidence that clinically evident damage to the trigeminal root was correlated with success of MVD for tic (as discussed more fully below). This argues for avoidance of intentional damage to the nerve root during MVD.

Some surgeons perform a partial trigeminal rhizotomy if there is only questionable vascular compression at MVD (61, 78). Although the number of patients in our series who had a partial rhizotomy in conjunction with MVD was small (2%), we found no evidence of a higher success rate in these patients. There is no published comparison between patients with comparable operative findings at MVD who did or did not undergo partial rhizotomy.

Other complications of MVD for TN are infrequent. Hearing loss has been minimized in our series by the use of intraoperative hearing monitoring, avoidance of retraction, and working primarily through the surgical corridor between the superior surface of the cerebellum and the tentorium, rather than between the lateral cerebellum and the petrous bone. Mortality from MVD is extremely unusual when the operation is performed as it is currently practiced at our institution, and the difference in mortality rates between MVD and percutaneous procedures, both performed by experienced hands, can no longer be measured.

CHOICE OF TREATMENT FOR MEDICALLY REFRACTORY TRIGEMINAL NEURALGIA

The choice between MVD and percutaneous procedures should be governed by the patient's own preference. Advantages of MVD include a long-term success rate that is consistently higher than all but a few reported series of percutaneous treatments and a substantially lower chance of facial numbness and dysesthesia than any percutaneous procedure except glycerol rhizolysis. Disadvantages include a longer recuperation period and a 1% chance of ipsilateral hearing loss. There is no compelling evidence that failure of MVD produces a higher failure rate if a later percutaneous treatment is used, or *vice versa.*

Trigeminal neuralgia is no longer a disease of the closing years of life, as it was in Harvey Cushing's day. Our patients had an average life expectancy of 32 years at the time of onset of symptoms. This is the time horizon that needs to be considered when a treatment is recommended. We feel that given this perspective, MVD represents the logical first choice of surgical treatment for TN in the majority of patients.

MICROVASCULAR DECOMPRESSION FOR HEMIFACIAL SPASM (HFS)

Methods

PATIENTS

All patients who had MVD for HFS performed at PUH between January 1, 1972 and March 1, 1992 were included in this study, which was reported in 1995 (3). Patients with "symptomatic" HFS, due to tumors (five patients: two lipomas, one epidermoid, one meningioma, and one trigeminal neurinoma), an arteriovenous malformation (AVM, 1 patient), or an aneurysm (1 posterior inferior cerebellar artery [PICA]) were excluded, as were patients with blepharospasm, facial myokymia, or Meige syndrome. Patients with HFS and ipsilateral TN (29 patients: 19 with atypical TN, and 10 with typical TN), or nervus intermedius neuralgia (three patients) were included, as were those with symptoms of HFS occurring on both sides of the face (11 sides in eight patients). Patients referred to PUH after one or more MVDs performed elsewhere (57 patients) were analyzed as a separate group. Overall, 782 operations were performed in 703 patients (705 sides).

Operations were performed according to a previously described technique (79).

CLINICAL EVALUATION

Operative findings, complications, and presence or absence of HFS at time of hospital discharge were prospectively recorded. Assessment of operative results was performed prospectively by annual question-naires, as described above for TN, using the following criteria for operative grading. A grade of "excellent" was assigned if HFS was completely absent, or if the patient reported 98% absence of spasm or greater. Some patients reported a sensation of facial twitching that was not visible to observers; these patients were graded as "excellent." A grade of "partial" relief was assigned if the spasm diminished by 75% or greater after operation. All other results were assigned a grade of "failure." If the patient was graded as an operative failure or partial success at the time of first postdischarge evaluation, the failure was considered to have occurred 1 month after operation. Statistical meth-ods were described previously (3).

Results

CLINICAL CHARACTERISTICS AND DEMOGRAPHIC VARIABLES

Six hundred and forty-eight first MVDs for HFS in patients without associated tumors, AVMs, or aneurysms were performed at PUH dur-ing the study period. Patients with less than 1 year follow-up (36 of 648 patients; 5.7%) were excluded from analysis of operative results, al-though they were included in the calculation of demographic variables, operative findings, and complications. (These patients had immediate postoperative results that were not statistically different from patients with more extended follow-up available [Mann-Whitney U test; P = 0.3]). Patients with prior MVDs performed elsewhere (57 patients) were excluded from demographic statistics, and were included in tab-ulations of operative findings and results as a separate group, as noted.

Demographics. Mean patient age was 52 years (range, 15 to 81 years). At time of operation, mean life expectancy, based on age- and sex-specific tables for the 1987 U.S. population as a whole (10), was 28 years (median 27 years). Sixty-five percent of patients were female, and 60% of patients had left-sided symptoms. Previous treatment with medication was common: 31% of patients had been treated with car-bamazepine and 21% with phenytoin. Only rarely did a patient report significant improvement of symptoms with either of these medications, in contrast to trigeminal neuralgia patients, who almost always achieved significant relief from carbamazepine and often from pheny-toin. Since 1985, an increasing proportion of patients (33 total) under-went botulinum toxin injections before referral, without satisfaction. Patients reported progressively decreasing control of symptoms with repeated injections, ptosis, disagreeable facial weakness, and require-ment for eye patching as objections to this therapy. Nineteen patients underwent extracranial procedures on the facial nerve that were intended to relieve HFS (alcohol injections, needle injuries to the tympanic portion of the nerve, extracranial partial section of the nerve) without relief or with later recurrence of spasm.

Symptoms: typical and atypical HFS. Patients were divided into two groups, "typical" and "atypical" HFS, based on their initial symptoms. Patients with typical HFS (92%) presented with initial twitching in the upper face (usually the lower eyelid) that progressed downward to involve the cheek and the corner of the mouth; finally, the platysma or frontalis muscle, or both, became involved. Patients with atypical HFS (8%) had initial twitching in the buccal muscles, with progressive spread upward into the cheek and orbicularis oculi. In both groups, after an initial period of clonic movements, a "tonus phenomenon" frequently became apparent, with hemifacial risus sardonicus and forced ipsilateral eye closure lasting several seconds. Patients with atypical HFS were more likely to be female (78%, compared with 63% of typical HFS patients; OR 2.1 [95% CI 1.05 to 4.2], $P = 0.03$), and tonus phenomenon was less likely to occur (59%, compared with 75% of typical HFS patients; OR 0.49 [95% CI, 0.27 to 0.88], $P = 0.02$). There were no significant differences in mean patient age, preoperative duration of symptoms, or right-to-left ratio between patients with typical and atypical HFS. Patients with atypical HFS were nine times more likely to have associated ipsilateral trigeminal or nervus intermedius neuralgia (12 of 51 atypical HFS patients [24%] compared with 20 of 597 typical HFS patients [3%]; OR 8.9 [95% CI 4.0 to 19], $P < 0.001$).

Mean age at onset of symptoms was 44 years (range, 7 to 75 years). Mean preoperative duration of symptoms was 7.4 years (range, 1 to 45 years). There was no significant difference in preoperative duration of symptoms between men and women, or between patients with and without tonus. Preoperative duration of symptoms showed a slight decline during the study period, equivalent to a decrease in preoperative symptom duration of 1.8 years between 1972 and 1991 (95% CI 0.12 to 3.6 years).

Bilateral HFS. Bilateral symptoms consistent with HFS on each side were noted in eight patients (1.2%). The twitches were asynchronous, and onset of symptoms in the two sides were typically separated by many years. Only three of these eight patients had sufficiently severe symptoms to require bilateral MVDs.

Neurological signs. Aside from the characteristic facial movements of HFS, there were few abnormal findings on physical examination. About half of patients (56%) had mild facial weakness on the side of the spasm, usually only detectable as a slightly deficient ability to bury the eyelashes on forced eye closure. Patients whose symptoms lasted 2 years or longer had a significantly greater chance of facial weakness on physical examination (OR 3.0 [95% CI 1.5 to 6.3, P < 0.003]). Synkinesis was noted in 10 patients, two of whom had a history of Bell's palsy. (The incidence of previous ipsilateral Bell's palsy in the entire group was 2%). There was no significant difference in preoperative duration of symptoms or likelihood of facial weakness between patients with and without synkinesis.

OPERATIVE FINDINGS

Operative findings are summarized in Table 7. The vessel most frequently found to compress the facial nerve was the PICA (68% of patients). Either the anterior inferior cerebellar artery (AICA) or the vertebral artery was found to compress the nerve in the majority of the remainder of patients. An unnamed small artery or arteriole was thought to be compressing the facial nerve in 11% of patients; veins were found in 20%, and thought to be the only source of compression in 3%. Either a vein, a small, unnamed artery, or both were found to compress the nerve, without additional compression by any named artery, in 6% of patients.

There were few significant associations between operative findings and demographic variables. Compression by a vertebral artery (11) was found more frequently in older patients (OR 1.03/year [95%; CI 1.01–1.04], P = 0.003), patients with typical onset of symptoms (OR 3.8 [95%; CI 1.4–9.8], P = 0.007), and on the left side (OR 4.3 [95%; CI 2.8–6.9], P < 0.001). Conversely, an unnamed small artery or vein as the sole compressing vessel was more likely in younger patients (OR 0.94/year [95%; CI 0.91–0.97], P < 0.001), with atypical onset of symptoms (OR 3.8 [95%; CI 1.6–9.2], P = 0.003) and longer preoperative duration of symptoms (OR 1.11/year [95%; CI 1.06–1.17], P < 0.001).

TABLE 7.
Operative findings in 648 consecutive first operations for hemifacial spasm

Compressing vessel	Patients	Percent (%) of total
PICA	442	68.2
AICA	229	35.3
Vertebral artery	155	23.9
Labyrinthine artery	19	2.9
SCA	4	0.6
Basilar artery	2	0.3
Unnamed small artery	71	11.0
Vein	132	20.4
Vein only	19	2.9
Unnamed small artery or vein only	38	5.9

OPERATIVE COMPLICATIONS

Operative complications for all patients are shown in Table 8. There was one operative death. This patient, who had undergone previous MVD elsewhere, presented to PUH with recurrent typical HFS, as well as a mild Chiari malformation. After undergoing reoperation at PUH, she developed progressive brainstem signs and required urgent suboccipital craniectomy and C1 laminectomy. Postoperatively she was conscious and easily extubated. Several hours later, she suffered a sudden respiratory arrest subsequent to narcotic administration. Despite resuscitation, she failed to regain consciousness, and supportive care was withdrawn.

Two brainstem infarctions occurred. One was noted after a first MVD, resulting in transient dysphagia. The second followed a reoperation and resulted in permanent facial weakness and arm and gait ataxia. Other serious complications included four cerebellar hematomas that required operative evacuation. One hematoma resulted in a temporary requirement for tracheostomy and gastrostomy in a man who has residual ataxia and has not returned to work. The other three patients returned to preoperative levels of function.

TABLE 8.
Operative complications after MVD for hemifacial spasm

Complication[a]	No. (%), 1st operation only (N = 648)	No. (%), all operations (N = 782)
Operative death	0 (0%)	1 (0.1%)
Brainstem infarct	1 (0.2%)	2[b] (0.3%)
Cerebellar hematoma	2[b] (0.3%)	4 (0.5%)
Facial weakness		
transient	25 (3.9%)	25 (3.2%)
mild, permanent	12 (1.9%)	14 (1.8%)
moderate, permanent	4 (0.6%)	7 (0.9%)
severe, permanent	6 (0.9%)	12 (1.5%)
Hearing loss		
mild, permanent	1 (0.2%)	1 (0.1%)
moderate, permanent	3 (0.5%)	3 (0.4%)
deaf ear	17 (2.6%)	21 (2.7%)
CSF leak	16 (2.5%)	19 (2.4%)
Wound infection	7 (1.1%)	9 (1.2%)
Wound hematoma	1 (0.2%)	1 (0.1%)
Pseudomeningocele	2 (0.3%)	4 (0.5%)
Bacterial meningitis	4 (0.6%)	4 (0.5%)

[a] Other complications included: transient hoarseness or dysphagia (11), transient sixth nerve palsy (2), permanent fourth nerve palsy (1), exacerbation of multiple sclerosis with transient quadriparesis (1), postoperative Guillain-Barré syndrome with persistent neurologic deficit (1), pneumonia (1), sepsis (1), and gastrointestinal hemorrhage (1).
[b] One cerebellar hematoma after first MVD and one brainstem infarction after reoperation resulted in permanent neurologic deficit.

Facial weakness. Facial weakness that was persistent and severe, or which resulted in persistent synkinesis, occurred in six patients (0.9%) after first MVDs for HFS. Since the introduction of intraoperative monitoring of facial nerve function and BSERs at PUH in 1980, this complication has occurred only twice in 480 operations (0.4%); the last 267 consecutive first MVDs for HFS were unmarred by permanent severe facial weakness. A logistic regression model showed that presence of any postoperative facial weakness (transient or permanent) was more frequent when the year of operation was before 1980 (OR 2.4 [95%; CI 1.3–4.4], P < 0.01) and if the vessel causing compression was the labyrinthine artery (OR 6.5 [95%; CI 2.3–18], P = 0.002). Patient age, sex, side of operation, presence of preoperative weakness, and typical *versus* atypical symptoms were not related to the chance of postoperative facial weakness.

Reoperations carried a fivefold greater risk of postoperative severe facial weakness (4.5% after reoperations compared with 0.9% after first operations, OR 5.0 [95%; CI 1.6–16], P < 0.01). This rate has decreased since the introduction of intraoperative monitoring, as for first operations, but the trend did not reach statistical significance.

Hearing loss. Postoperative hearing loss was more common than facial weakness. Seventeen of 648 patients without prior MVDs (2.6%) suffered total or severe permanent loss of hearing in the ipsilateral ear. This complication has become less common since the introduction of routine intraoperative monitoring of BSERs, but has not been eliminated. Before routine monitoring (1972 to 1979), 4.8% of first operations (8/167) were complicated by ipsilateral hearing loss; since the introduction of routine monitoring in 1980, the rate has been reduced to 1.9% (9 of 481). This downward trend did not reach statistical significance (P = 0.05). In a logistic regression analysis, hearing loss was significantly more probable in patients with atypical HFS (OR 3.8 [95%; CI 1.2–12]; P = 0.04). Patient age, sex, and side of operation were not related to probability of hearing loss. The rate of hearing loss was slightly higher following reoperations (4 of 134, 3.0%), but this trend did not reach statistical significance.

Other complications. Other complications are shown in Table 8. Transient hoarseness and dysphagia occurred in 1.4% of patients. All cerebrospinal fluid (CSF) leaks (21 patients, 2.7%) resolved after placement of a lumbar drain, except one CSF leak from a wound that required open repair and two CSF leaks from wounds that became superinfected; these required open repair. All wound complications and bacterial meningitides were satisfactorily managed without lasting sequelae.

OPERATIVE RESULTS

Follow-up. Follow-up rates for the entire population were high. For 648 patients who underwent first MVD for HFS at PUH, the 5-year actuarial follow-up rate was 92%, and the 10-year rate was 88%. Mean follow-up for the 612 patients followed for 1 year or more was 8 years. A total of 4,811 patient-years of follow-up information was accrued. Actuarial survival for the group as a whole (Kaplan-Meier estimator) was 93% at 10 years postoperatively and 80% at 20 years postoperatively.

Seventy patients (11%) were lost to follow-up (including loss before 1 year after operation) for reasons other than death. Lost patients had the same distribution of excellent and partially successful results immediately prior to loss as the population as a whole (Mann-Whitney U test, P > 0.8). A Cox proportional hazards model, defining loss to follow-up (excluding death) as failure, showed a significantly higher likelihood of loss for younger patients (P < 0.001) and for patients who lost hearing as a complication of operation (five of 16 patients, lost after 1.8, 4, 6, 8, and 11 years follow-up; P < 0.01). Patient sex, presence of trigeminal or nervus intermedius neuralgia, typical *versus* atypical symptoms, operating surgeon, immediate postoperative relief of spasm, and postoperative chemical meningitis or facial weakness were not related to chance of loss to follow-up.

Initial results. Initial success of MVD for HFS was high in previously unoperated patients, and there were few recurrences. Of the 612 patients followed for 1 year or more, 86% were graded "excellent" at 1 month, 5% were partial successes, and 9% were failures. At 10 years after operation, disregarding results of any but the initial procedure, 79% of all patients had excellent results, 5% partial success, and 16% were failures (Fig. 7).

Reoperations. If the initial operation failed to provide any relief from spasm in the first postoperative week, immediate reoperation was recommended. Of 12 such patients, 11 underwent reoperation in the first 30 days after the initial operation; 10 had long-term excellent results, and one patient remained an operative failure. An additional patient was not offered immediate reoperation and remained a partial success, despite a second exploration 17 months after the first MVD.

If the initial operation provided partial or complete relief from spasm, but the spasm later recurred, reoperation was usually recommended. Forty-nine patients underwent second operations more than 30 days after an initial operation at PUH. Second operations were less successful than initial procedures: immediate results were 61% excellent, 6% partial relief, and 33% failure. Five years after the second

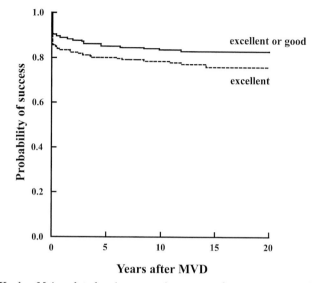

Fig. 7. Kaplan-Meier plot showing operative success for 648 patients after MVD for hemifacial spasm. *Dashed line*, chances of excellent relief of HFS after first MVD; *solid line*, chances of a good or excellent result. See text for grading of success.

operation, allowing for 10 patients who underwent third operations, results were 50% excellent, 22% partial success, and 28% failure (Fig. 8).

Long-term results. Including final results after one or two operations per patient (excluding patients with first operations elsewhere than PUH), results 10 years after operation were 84% excellent, 7% partial success, and 9% failure (Fig. 9). In the second postoperative decade, there were three recurrences in a total of 693 patient-years of follow-up (0.4% annual recurrence rate). The latest recurrence was 14 years after the original procedure. Fifty-eight patients were followed for 15 to 20 years without recurrence.

SUBGROUP ANALYSES: NO PRIOR TREATMENT, PREOPERATIVE VARIABLES

Variables tested in univariate analysis for possible influence on the chance of HFS recurrence after MVD included patient sex, side of symptoms, presence of ipsilateral paroxysmal facial pain (either trigeminal or geniculate in distribution), typical or atypical origin and progression of symptoms, history of Bell's palsy, presence of synkinesis or facial weakness on physical examination, and implant material used for MVD. Patient age and preoperative duration of symptoms were

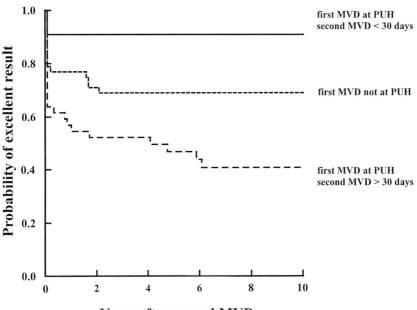

Years after second MVD

Fig. 8. Kaplan-Meier plot showing operative success after reoperation for HFS that recurred after a previous MVD. *Solid line*, probability of excellent result after an immediate second operation (less than 30 days after first MVD at PUH); *dashed line*, probability of excellent results after a delayed second operation (recurrence of spasm greater than 30 days after first MVD at PUH). The *dotted line* represents the probability of excellent results for a second MVD when the first MVD was performed elsewhere than PUH. Reoperations more than 30 days after first operation at PUH had worse results than immediate reoperations (logrank P < 0.01). Among patients whose second operations were more than 30 days after their first MVD, results were better after reoperations on patients whose first operations were not performed at PUH (logrank P = 0.014).

each stratified (more or less than 5 years of symptoms, older or younger than 65) and also tested as sole continuous covariates in a Cox proportional hazards model. For all Kaplan-Meier stratifications and Cox proportional hazards models, failure was defined as results less than "excellent." (When failure was defined as less than "partial success," the models lacked statistical power due to the smaller number of "failures.") Patients with prior MVDs elsewhere were excluded from these analyses.

Patient age, side and duration of symptoms, history of Bell's palsy, and presence of preoperative facial weakness or synkinesis were not statistically significant predictors of operative success.

The material used for the operative implant changed during the course of the study. Initially, Ivalon sponge implants (Unipoint Indus-

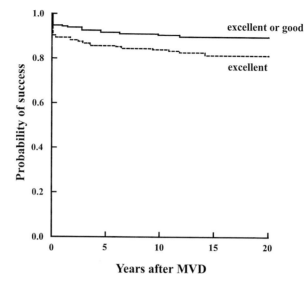

FIG. 9. Kaplan-Meier plot showing operative success for 648 patients after MVD for hemifacial spasm. Final results after one or two operations per patient are shown. *Dashed line*, chance of excellent results; *solid line*, chance of good or excellent results.

tries, High Point, NC) were used, followed by autologous muscle pledgets and shredded Teflon felt pledgets (C. R. Bard, Inc., Bard Implants Division, Billerica, MA) in turn. In a few patients early in the series, Gelfoam (Upjohn Co., Kalamazoo, MI), silicone sponge, or an unrecorded type of implant was used (Table 9). Comparison of Ivalon, muscle, and Teflon implants showed no statistically significant difference in results (logrank test, P = 0.15).

Presence of ipsilateral trigeminal or nervus intermedius neuralgia was a significant predictor of operative failure as a univariate strati-

TABLE 9.
Implant materials and other intraoperative techniques used in 648 consecutive first MVDs for hemifacial spasm

Material or technique	Patients	Percent (%) of total
Teflon	477	74
Muscle	76	12
Ivalon	63	10
Silicone	19	3
Gelfoam	6	1
Unrecorded	2	0.3
Vein coagulation and division	117	18

fying variable in a Kaplan-Meier model, but this resulted from confounding with atypical onset of HFS. In a Cox model incorporating both presence of pain and atypical onset of HFS symptoms, ipsilateral facial pain was not found to be a significant predictor of HFS recurrence.

Patient sex and type of onset of HFS (typical vs. atypical) were the only two variables that could be determined preoperatively that had statistically significant effects on the probability of operative success. Patients with atypical onset of symptoms had worse results than those with typical onset of symptoms, regardless of sex (59% compared with 88% probability of excellent results at 5 years, all operations per patient included; logrank P < 0.001; Fig. 10). Within the typical HFS group, male patients had a significantly higher chance of excellent results than female patients (93% compared with 83% 10 years after MVD, all operations per patient included; logrank P = 0.002; Fig. 11). The small size of the atypical subgroup prevented a meaningful comparison between male and female atypical HFS patients.

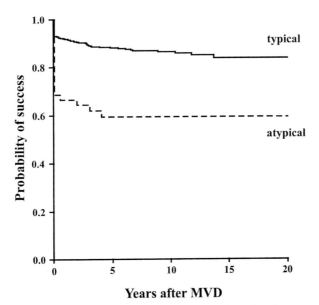

Years after MVD

FIG. 10. Kaplan-Meier plot showing success of MVD for hemifacial spasm stratified by onset of symptoms (typical vs. atypical). *Solid line,* chance of excellent results for patients with typical onset of symptoms; *dashed line,* chance of excellent results for patients with atypical onset of symptoms. Final results after one or two operations per patient are shown. The difference in results between typical and atypical subgroups is statistically significant (logrank P < 1×10^{-6}).

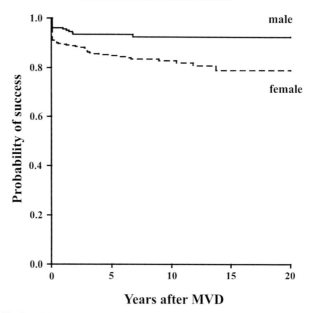

Years after MVD

FIG. 11. Kaplan-Meier plot showing success of MVD for typical hemifacial spasm stratified by patient gender. *Solid line*, chance of excellent results for male patients with typical HFS; *dashed line*, chance of excellent results for female patients with typical HFS. Final results after one or two operations per patient are shown. The difference in results between men and women is statistically significant (logrank P = 0.002).

SUBGROUP ANALYSES: OPERATIVE FINDINGS, IMMEDIATE POSTOPERATIVE RESULTS

The only operative finding significantly related to outcome was the finding of either a small, unnamed artery or a vein as the only compressing vessels. These patients had significantly higher rates of postoperative recurrence (logrank P < 0.001, for either first or all operations).

Relief of symptoms in the early postoperative period was another significant predictor of postoperative success. Patients with complete relief had significantly better results than those with some degree of postoperative spasm, even if it was only present briefly after operation (logrank P < 0.001, first operations only).

Presence or absence of postoperative chemical meningitis was not a significant predictor of success, either in the immediate postoperative period (Mann-Whitney U test, P > 0.5) or long term (logrank P > 0.5).

Cox proportional hazards models incorporating four variables (sex, typical *vs.* atypical onset of symptoms, postoperative relief of symptoms [complete, partial, or none], and unnamed small artery or vein as sole pathology) fit the observed data well. Two separate models were derived, one incorporating only results of first operations, and a second including all operations per patient. No additional variables (preoperative demographics, operative findings, or operative complications) entered into either model using a criterion of $P < 0.05$ for entry. Characteristics of the models are summarized in Table 10. The model including results of all operations per patient differs from the basic model in one significant way: lack of immediate postoperative relief after the first operation becomes less risky, perhaps because many of these patients are salvaged by reoperation and have excellent long-term results.

OPERATIVE RESULTS IN PATIENTS WITH PRIOR UNSUCCESSFUL TREATMENT FOR HFS

Thirty-three patients underwent prior treatment with botulinum toxin injection (one or more injection courses) at other centers. Operative results in these patients showed a very slightly higher failure rate than in patients who were not so treated. The difference did not reach statistical significance (logrank $P = 0.23$).

Patients who had undergone prior MVD procedures at other institutions (57 patients) had a success rate that was intermediate between patients with no prior intracranial procedures, and patients with prior MVD performed at PUH more than 30 days before. Five years after the

TABLE 10.

Cox proportional hazard model coefficients for four prognostic factors for success of MVD in relieving hemifacial spasm. Model I gives coefficients for probability of excellent results with first operation only; Model II incorporates final results of one or two operations per patient. Female sex, atypical onset of symptoms, unnamed artery or vein as sole compressing vessel at operation, and lack of immediate postoperative relief had higher risks of HFS recurrence. The table gives the relative risks of failure for each variable with 95% confidence intervals and P values.

Model	Variable	Relative risk (RR)	95% CI (RR)	P value
I	Female sex	2.2	1.4–3.4	<0.001
	Atypical onset	2.2	1.4–3.6	0.001
	Vein/arteriole as sole compressing vessel	2.6	1.6–4.2	<0.001
	Postoperative spasm relief (none/partial/complete)	3.1	2.3–4.3	<0.001
II	Female sex	2.3	1.4–4.0	0.002
	Atypical onset	2.7	1.6–4.6	<0.001
	Vein/arteriole as sole compressing vessel	3.7	2.2–6.3	<0.001
	Postoperative spasm relief (none/partial/complete)	1.7	1.2–2.4	0.003

PUH MVD, counting only results of the initial reoperation, 67% of patients had excellent results, 9% had partial success, and 24% were failures. Five patients were submitted to further operations; counting results of all operations, results for the group at time 5 years were 73% excellent, 13% partial success, and 14% failure. The difference between reoperative results in patients with first operations at PUH and elsewhere was statistically significant (results of first reoperations only, logrank P = 0.01; Fig. 8). Significantly more reoperated patients whose initial MVD was at another center were found to have compression of the facial nerve at the root exit zone by a PICA at reoperation than in the group previously operated at PUH (OR 7.2 [95%; CI 3.2–17], P < 0.001). This suggests that the true root exit zone of the facial nerve may not have been inspected at the first operation in some of these patients.

Discussion

MEDICAL TREATMENT OF HEMIFACIAL SPASM

Patients who present for evaluation for surgical treatment of HFS have often been treated with a long litany of medications. Among the most popular are carbamazepine, phenytoin, baclofen, clonazepam, and antianxiety agents (80, 81). In contrast to TN, in which patients consistently report dramatic relief from carbamazepine and sometimes from other medications, it is unusual to see a HFS patient who believes that any drug has provided significant relief of spasm, even for a short time. Although the natural history of HFS does not usually include long periods of complete freedom from symptoms, as are characteristic of TN, the severity of spasms does fluctuate from hour to hour and from day to day. There is no universally accepted grading scale for severity of HFS. Given these methodologic difficulties and the rarity of the disease, it is not surprising that no randomized, double-blind controlled trial of any medication has been reported in HFS. We do not recommend trial of any medication before proceeding to operative treatment of HFS.

BOTULINUM TOXIN INJECTIONS FOR HEMIFACIAL SPASM

A treatment for HFS that is growing in popularity among neurologists is the injection of botulinum toxin into the facial musculature. These injections reduce the intensity of facial spasm by blocking neuromuscular transmission and do not affect the abnormal neural impulses themselves. Therefore, when the botulinum toxin wears off, the spasm returns and the injections must be repeated.

Most reports of botulinum toxin injection for HFS have had short follow-up periods. In addition, each series tends to use outcome criteria that are idiosyncratic to the specific investigators, and outcome is generally evaluated by the treating physicians based on clinical follow-up. This may not be appropriate in a disorder that can fluctuate markedly in severity over a short period of time.

Botulinum toxin injections provide some degree of relief of HFS for most patients. Botulinum toxin investigators routinely use generous criteria for operative success: "objective or subjective reduction in spasm intensity lasting at least two weeks" (82), a two-point improvement on a five-point rating scale, lasting 6 weeks (83), or improvement by a single point on a 10-point subjective scale (two points being graded as "substantial" improvement) (84).

Using these criteria, the initial success rate of botulinum toxin injections for HFS ranges from about 80% to 100% (83–89). Some patients develop serum antibodies to botulinum toxin after treatment (90), although these are not said to result in loss of efficacy. Repeated injections are said to remain effective (82, 83), although some of our patients reported loss of efficacy over time. The average time to recurrence of symptoms after botulinum toxin injection is about 12 to 16 weeks (82, 83, 85, 91).

Complications of botulinum toxin injection are frequent but not disabling. The most common are excess facial weakness, facial bruising, dry eye, ptosis, diplopia, and difficulty swallowing. These occur with a low frequency per injection, but because each patient receives many injections over time, the cumulative frequency is high—60% to 75% over about 3 years of therapy (82, 91). As the toxin wears off, the complications resolve.

MICROVASCULAR DECOMPRESSION AND OTHER OPERATIVE TREATMENTS FOR HEMIFACIAL SPASM

In addition to MVD, many other operative procedures have been advocated for the treatment of HFS (92). These procedures involve damaging the facial nerve during its intratemporal or extracranial course (93–97). No long-term results have been published for these procedures.

MVD for HFS has been shown to be a safe and effective treatment in reports from centers throughout the world (3, 71, 92, 98–104). Success rates of between 80% and 97% have been reported, with few recurrences (5% to 10% in most large series). Most recurrences take place within 2 years of surgery (3, 98). Reoperations are less successful than first operations, and complications are more frequent.

Because operative failure is relatively uncommon in MVD for HFS, most series have lacked statistical power to demonstrate prognostic factors for operative success. Our analysis demonstrated that men have a higher chance of operative success than women and that patients with atypical HFS (in which the twitching starts in the lower face and progresses upwards) have worse results. In addition, patients with a vein or arteriole as sole compressing vessel and those with incomplete postoperative relief of spasm were at higher risk for long-term recurrence. Both we and others (99, 101) noted that relief of spasm is not immediate after operation in all patients, and spasm can subside as late as weeks to months postoperatively.

The most frequent complications after MVD for HFS are injury to the 7th and 8th cranial nerves. Permanent severe facial weakness or facial weakness with synkinesis occurred in less than 1% of the patients in our series, comparable to the rates reported by other groups (92, 98, 99, 101). In our series the likelihood of facial weakness was higher after repositioning of the labyrinthine artery and after reoperations. Permanent ipsilateral hearing loss occurred in 4.8% of our patients before the introduction of intraoperative BSERs, and in 1.9% of those operated since that time. Other surgeons have reported similar decreases in the rate of this complication after the introduction of intraoperative BSERs (105). In our series the rate of hearing loss was higher in patients with atypical HFS and after reoperations.

In the absence of effective medical treatment for HFS, the choice of treatment lies between botulinum toxin injections and MVD. Although permanent morbidity from botulinum injections is rare, the requirement for repeated treatments is a severe disadvantage. The life expectancy for our patients at onset of symptoms was 35 years (10). Over 100 thrice-yearly botulinum injections would thus be necessary for lifelong treatment of HFS in an average patient. This may be neither a simpler nor a more cost-effective treatment than MVD. We feel that all patients with HFS should be counseled by physicians familiar with the results of both treatments before deciding which is best for them.

MICROVASCULAR DECOMPRESSION FOR DISABLING POSITIONAL VERTIGO (DPV)

Methods

PATIENTS AND CLINICAL EVALUATION

Criteria for the diagnosis of DPV were reported elsewhere (5), and are summarized elsewhere in this volume. Between January 1983 and December 1990, 207 patients underwent MVD for DPV at the University of Pittsburgh. Of these, 177 had unilateral symptoms and 30 had bilateral symptoms. Eight unilateral patients and one bilateral patient were excluded from further analysis because they had undergone prior vestibular nerve sections elsewhere. Postoperative results were classified as successful (free of symptoms or markedly improved—returning to work, able to drive, and resuming normal activities), or unsuccessful (not meeting these criteria). This study, which was reported in 1993, was retrospective and relied on clinic records from follow-up visits.

Results

CLINICAL CHARACTERISTICS

Of 177 unilateral patients, 68% were women; mean age was 47 years (range, 19 to 74 years). Of 30 bilateral patients, 77% were women, and mean age was 41 years (range, 16 to 69 years). Mean preoperative duration of symptoms was 7 years. Eight patients with unilateral DPV had undergone vestibular nerve sections at other institutions prior to evaluation for MVD.

OPERATIVE RESULTS

In 163 patients who had unilateral MVD for DPV who had not had prior vestibular nerve sections at other institutions, 129 patients (79%) were markedly improved or symptom-free after surgery. These patients resumed work or normal activity. Thirty-four patients (21%) had no improvement after MVD. Six patients were lost to follow-up. There was no relationship between patient gender and the likelihood of operative success.

Of the 129 unilateral patients who were markedly improved after surgery, 14 patients (11%) had recurrences of symptoms between 1 and 3 years after MVD. All 14 underwent repeat MVD, after which 11 improved and three did not.

Eight patients had vestibular nerve sections prior to unilateral MVD for DPV. These patients had no improvement after MVD.

Of 26 patients with bilateral symptoms, 20 (77%) were improved postoperatively and six (23%) were not. One patient whose symptoms were refractory to MVD underwent a subsequent vestibular nerve section with poor results.

COMPLICATIONS

Ipsilateral hearing was lost in seven of the 169 patients who underwent unilateral MVD for DPV and in one of 14 patients who had reoperations. In 29 patients who underwent bilateral MVDs, one patient lost hearing unilaterally. In the complete series there was one transient unilateral vocal cord weakness, one transient trochlear palsy, and one patient with transient facial weakness.

MICROVASCULAR DECOMPRESSION FOR TINNITUS

Methods

PATIENTS AND CLINICAL EVALUATION

Seventy-four patients who underwent surgery for tinnitus at PUH between 1981 and 1990 were the subject of this study, which was reported in 1993 (4). Selection criteria were described previously (4) and are summarized elsewhere in this volume. Of the 74 patients, 72 underwent MVD and two had section of the 8th nerve close to the brainstem.

Results were classified as total relief, marked improvement (ability to assume daily activities and sleep), slight improvement, or no improvement. This study was retrospective and relied on clinic records from follow-up visits.

Results

Two patients were lost to follow-up, and the following results are based on the remaining 72 patients. Thirty-one patients (43%) were women and 41 (57%) were men. Mean age was about 50 years.

Thirteen patients (18%) were free of tinnitus postoperatively and 16 (22%) were markedly improved. The success rate (tinnitus-free or markedly improved) was higher for women (55%) than for men (29%). The mean preoperative duration of symptoms was shorter for patients with successful results: mean duration ranged from less than 3 years for patients with a successful result, to 5.2 years for those with slight improvement and 7.1 years for those with no change in symptoms after MVD.

Complications included four patients (5%) with hearing loss, two patients (3%) with worsened tinnitus after operation, and one patient with facial weakness, which occurred after a reoperation.

MICROVASCULAR DECOMPRESSION FOR GLOSSOPHARYNGEAL
NEURALGIA (GPN)

Methods

PATIENTS

All patients who had MVD for typical GPN performed at PUH between 1971 and 1994 were included in this study, which was reported in 1995 (6). Four patients had ipsilateral TN and one had ipsilateral disabling positional vertigo. Overall, 43 operations were performed in 40 patients (41 sides). Operative technique was described previously (6).

CLINICAL EVALUATION

Assessment of operative results was performed retrospectively, by review of clinic records and by questionnaires or telephone contact, using the following criteria for operative grading. A grade of "excellent" was assigned if the patient reported at least 95% relief of GPN without requirement for medication. Partial success was defined as at least 50% relief from GPN. All other results were assigned a grade of "failure."

Results

CLINICAL CHARACTERISTICS AND DEMOGRAPHIC VARIABLES

Forty-three MVDs on 41 sides, in 40 patients, were performed at PUH during the study period. Mean patient age was 55 years (range, 27 to 75 years). Forty-three percent of patients were female and 63% of patients had left-sided symptoms. One patient had bilateral symptoms. Mean duration of preoperative symptoms was 5 years; previous treatment with medications, including carbamazepine and phenytoin, was common.

OPERATIVE FINDINGS AND COMPLICATIONS

At operation, the root exit zones of the 9th and 10th cranial nerves were examined for vascular compression. In 39% of patients, the PICA was noted to cause neural compression at the root entry zone, and in 7% the vertebral artery was causing compression. Twelve percent of patients had compression due to two arteries, 27% had compression due to the combination of an artery and a vein, and 12% had compression due to a single vein.

There were two postoperative deaths (5%), both from sequelae of intraoperative hypertension. An additional two patients had transient postoperative hypertension. Three patients (8%) had permanent paresis of the 9th and 10th cranial nerves; of these, two are asymptomatic and a third has moderate dysphagia for liquids. Four additional patients (10%) had transient 9th and 10th cranial nerve palsies. Other complications were minor.

OPERATIVE SUCCESS

The single patient with bilateral GPN required a second MVD on each side in the first postoperative week because of poor postoperative symptom relief. Including the results of these second operations, 79% of patients had excellent immediate postoperative results and 10% had partial success; 10% were failures. At long-term follow-up (6 to 170 months after MVD), 76% of patients had excellent results, 15% partial success, and 8% were failures.

Discussion

MEDICAL TREATMENT OF GLOSSOPHARYNGEAL NEURALGIA

The close similarities between trigeminal and glossopharyngeal neuralgia have led physicians to try the same drugs in each. In addition, about 10% of patients in most series appear to have both GPN and ipsilateral TN (6, 106). Carbamazepine appears to be the most effective drug for GPN, as it is for tic. When the drug becomes ineffective or must be stopped because of side effects, the same group of agents described above as treatments for TN should be tried, especially phenytoin and baclofen. The likelihood of success for these drugs in GPN has not been well defined, and formal studies are difficult because of the rarity of the disease. Because operative treatments for glossopharyngeal neuralgia carry higher morbidity than do operations for tic, a more extensive trial of medications is warranted.

SURGICAL TREATMENTS FOR GLOSSOPHARYNGEAL NEURALGIA

Percutaneous radiofrequency lesioning of the glossopharyngeal nerve for GPN was described in small series of patients (24, 107, 108). The procedure seems to carry a high risk of persistent hoarseness and dysphagia (107). Extracranial section of branches of the nerve has been described (107, 109). This procedure has a high recurrence rate, similar to that seen after peripheral neurectomy for tic.

Intracranial section of the glossopharyngeal nerve and the upper rootlets of the vagus has a high success rate in relieving GPN (106, 107, 109, 110). Section of the glossopharyngeal nerve results in loss of taste sensation in the posterior third of the tongue, loss of ipsilateral posterior pharyngeal sensation and the ipsilateral gag reflex, and paralysis of the stylopharyngeus muscle. Section of the upper vagal fibers in addition increases the pharyngeal sensory deficit and may add paralysis of the ipsilateral vocal cord. In the series reported by Taha and Tew (107), subjective complaints after intracranial section of the glossopharyngeal and upper vagal nerves were not unusual (transient dysphagia, squeaky voice, and cough), but only two of 12 patients had persistent problems (dysphagia and cough, each in one patient). The authors did not consider posterior pharyngeal numbness to be a side effect unless it was bothersome to the patient. Pain relief was long-lasting (4 to 17 years).

Microvascular decompression of the glossopharyngeal and vagal nerves as a treatment for GPN was reported by our group (6) and by others (111–116). Long-term results were excellent in 76% of patients, and another 15% were partially relieved of pain (total 91%). Complications were more frequent and severe than after MVD for other cranial nerve disorders discussed in this chapter. Mortality was 5%, and permanent pareses of the 9th and 10th nerves occurred in three of 41 patients (only one patient had persistent symptomatic dysphagia for liquids; the other two patients were asymptomatic). The complication rate therefore seems to be comparable to, or lower than, that reported for intracranial section of the 9th and 10th nerves, with an equivalent or higher success rate. The advantage of MVD over intracranial section is the avoidance in most patients of permanent loss of ipsilateral posterior pharyngeal sensation and vocal cord function. In the 2% of GPN patients who develop bilateral symptoms, this is of obvious importance, although it would seem to be an advantage for other patients as well.

MECHANISM OF ACTION OF MICROVASCULAR DECOMPRESSION

Microvascular decompression has been shown to be a safe and effective treatment for many cranial nerve disorders, as reviewed in this chapter. However, the mechanism of action of MVD in some of these disorders has been questioned on theoretical grounds (117, 118).

The major criticism of the vascular compression hypothesis is the suggestion that MVD actually works by causing trauma to the nerve root, rather than by relieving vascular compression. It is well known that even minor trauma to the trigeminal nerve root will relieve tic, at least for a short time, and relief of HFS after lumbar puncture and after exploration of the facial nerve root (without MVD) has also been reported. We have observed in reoperations on some tic patients that the initial MVD, performed at other institutions, was directed at the 8th nerve, while the 5th nerve root entry zone had obviously not been exposed. Yet these patients had tic relief for some months after their inadvertent "sham" operations, presumably because of the minimal injury to the trigeminal nerve from retraction during the procedure.

MVD produces less numbness than percutaneous procedures, as shown in direct comparison studies (34) and in our own series (comparison of post-MVD patients to patients who had undergone percutaneous ablative procedures, Table 2). Yet MVD produces more durable tic relief than do the percutaneous procedures. It might be argued that damage to the trigeminal root is different from damage elsewhere in the trigeminal pathway, producing tic relief that is disproportionately durable because of some intrinsic quality of this portion of the nerve. To address this criticism directly, comparison of tic relief between patients with and without trigeminal numbness after MVD is necessary. Steiger (42) suggested a positive correlation between postoperative trigeminal numbness and tic relief after MVD in a group of 21 patients, although Burchiel et al. (62) found no difference in outcome between patients with or without numbness after MVD in a series of 40 patients.

The large size of our cohort of tic patients treated by MVD, with prolonged follow-up, allowed us to address this question with considerably greater statistical power than prior investigators. We studied tic relief in relation to trigeminal numbness in 480 patients who had undergone MVD for unilateral typical TN and who did not undergo any ablative procedures before or after MVD. Numbness was self-reported on a 5-point scale. We found no evidence that trigeminal numbness correlated positively with tic relief after MVD, even after adjustment for anatomic findings at operation. In fact, in patients with compressing SCAs and no compressing veins at MVD, tic relief was more durable in patients without postoperative numbness. As expected, postoperative trigeminal dysesthesia (burning and aching pain) correlated strongly with the presence of trigeminal numbness, suggesting that in this respect, damage to the trigeminal root entry zone causes the same consequences as does damage elsewhere in the trigeminal pathway.

Perhaps the damage to the trigeminal root takes place through postoperative fibrosis rather than being a direct consequence of intraoperative trauma. Patients who have particularly marked postoperative inflammatory responses, clinically manifest as "aseptic" or "chemical" meningitis, would therefore be expected to have better long-term tic or HFS relief. However, this variable was not significantly related to operative success after MVD for either tic or HFS in our series.

Our impression is that intraoperative nerve trauma is usually the result of dissection of small arteries and veins from their arachnoidal attachments to the 5th and 7th cranial nerves, rather than from lifting larger arteries off of them. Trigeminal numbness is positively correlated with the decompression of a vein at MVD and inversely correlated with the decompression of an SCA. However, relief of both tic and HFS is less durable after decompression of a vein in both tic and HFS, not more so. Finally, we note that reoperations are associated with more intraoperative nerve trauma both in tic and in HFS, as well as significantly higher rates of postoperative numbness and facial weakness respectively, yet the relief of these syndromes is markedly inferior after reoperations as compared with initial operations.

We believe that these are the first facts, as distinct from theories, to be introduced into the debate over the mechanism of action of MVD. There can be little doubt that MVD is an effective treatment for these disorders. The challenge for future surgeons is to further refine the methods used today in order to decrease the morbidity of MVD while maintaining, or improving, its efficacy. Because the best evidence suggests that MVD does not operate through nerve trauma, this is likely to be an achievable goal.

ACKNOWLEDGMENTS

The author wishes to thank Fred G. Barker II, MD, for his assistance with preparation of the manuscript and David J. Bissonette, PA-C, M.B.A., for assistance in data compilation and analysis.

REFERENCES

1. Barker FG 2nd, Jannetta PJ, Bissonette DJ, et al.: The long term outcome of microvascular decompression for trigeminal neuralgia. **N Engl J Med** 334:1077–1083, 1996.
2. Barker FG 2nd, Jannetta PJ, Bissonette DJ, et al.: Trigeminal numbness and tic relief after microvascular decompression for typical trigeminal neuralgia. **Neurosurgery** [in press].
3. Barker FG 2nd, Jannetta PJ, Bissonette DJ, et al.: Microvascular decompression for hemifacial spasm. **J Neurosurg** 82:201–210, 1995.
4. Møller MB, Møller AR, Jannetta PJ, et al.: Vascular decompression surgery for severe tinnitus: Selection criteria and results. **Laryngoscope** 103:421–427, 1993.
5. Møller MB, Møller AR, Jannetta PJ, et al.: Microvascular decompression of the eighth nerve in patients with disabling positional vertigo: selection criteria and operative results in 207 patients. **Acta Neurochir (Wien)** 125:75–82, 1993.
6. Resnick DK, Jannetta PJ, Bissonette D, et al.: Microvascular decompression for glossopharyngeal neuralgia. **Neurosurgery** 36:64–69, 1995.
7. Barker FG 2nd, Jannetta PJ, Babu R, et al.: Long term outcome after operation for trigeminal neuralgia in patients with posterior fossa tumors. **J Neurosurg** 84:818–825, 1996.
8. Jannetta PJ: Microvascular decompression of the trigeminal nerve root entry zone, in Rovit RL, Murali R, Jannetta PJ (eds): Trigeminal neuralgia. Baltimore, Williams & Wilkins, 1990, pp 201–22.
9. Pollack IF, Jannetta PJ, Bissonette DJ: Bilateral trigeminal neuralgia: A 14-year experience with microvascular decompression. **J Neurosurg** 68:559–565, 1988.
10. Vital statistics of the United States, 1987. Volume II—mortality. Part A. Hyattsville, MD, U.S. Dept. of Health and Human Services, 1990.
11. Linskey ME, Jho HD, Jannetta PJ: Microvascular decompression for trigeminal neuralgia caused by vertebrobasilar compression. **J Neurosurg** 81:1–9, 1994.
12. Barker FG 2nd: Analysis of the relationship between long-term operative success and a transient or delayed operative side effect. **Neurosurgery** 39:412–416, 1996.
13. Rovit RL, Murali R, Jannetta PJ, eds: Trigeminal neuralgia. Baltimore, Williams & Wilkins, 1990.
14. Zakrzewska JM: Trigeminal neuralgia. London, WB Saunders, 1995.
15. Masdeu JC: Medical treatment and clinical pharmacology, in Rovit RL, Murali R,

Jannetta PJ (eds): Trigeminal neuralgia. Baltimore, Williams & Wilkins, 1990, pp 79–93.

16. Patsalos PN: Medical management, in Zakrzewska JM (ed): Trigeminal neuralgia. London, WB Saunders, 1995, pp 80–107.

17. Taylor JC, Brauer S, Espir ML: Long-term treatment of trigeminal neuralgia with carbamazepine. **Postgrad Med J** 57:16–18, 1981.

18. McQuay H, Carroll D, Jadad AR, *et al.*: Anticonvulsant drugs for management of pain: A systematic review. **BMJ** 311:1047–1052, 1995.

19. Sweet WH, Wepsic JG: Controlled thermocoagulation of trigeminal ganglion and results for differential destruction of pain fibers. Part I: trigeminal neuralgia. **J Neurosurg** 40:143–156, 1974.

20. Håkanson S: Trigeminal neuralgia treated by the injection of glycerol into the trigeminal cistern. **Neurosurgery** 9:638–646, 1981.

21. Mullan S, Lichtor T: Percutaneous microcompression of the trigeminal ganglion for trigeminal neuralgia. **J Neurosurg** 59:1007–1012, 1983.

22. Murali R, Rovit RL: Are peripheral neurectomies of value in the treatment of trigeminal neuralgia? An analysis of new cases and cases involving previous radiofrequency gasserian thermocoagulation. **J Neurosurg** 85:435–437, 1996.

23. Murali R: Peripheral nerve injections and avulsions in the treatment of trigeminal neuralgia, in Rovit RL, Murali R, Jannetta PJ (eds): Trigeminal neuralgia. Baltimore, Williams & Wilkins, 1990, pp 95–108.

24. Tew JM Jr., Taha JM: Percutaneous rhizotomy in the treatment of intractable facial pain (trigeminal, glossopharyngeal, and vagal nerves), in Schmidek HH, Sweet WH (eds): Operative neurosurgical techniques. Philadelphia, WB Saunders, 1995, Vol. 2, pp 1469–1484.

25. Zakrzewska JM: Surgery at the level of the gasserian ganglion, in Zakrzewska JM (ed): Trigeminal neuralgia. London, WB Saunders, 1995, pp 125–156.

26. Rovit RL: Percutaneous radiofrequency thermal coagulation of the gasserian ganglion, in Rovit RL, Murali R, Jannetta PJ (eds): Trigeminal neuralgia. Baltimore, Williams & Wilkins, 1990, pp 109–136.

27. Taha JM, Tew JM Jr., Buncher CR: A prospective 15-year follow-up of 154 consecutive patients with trigeminal neuralgia treated by percutaneous stereotactic radiofrequency thermal rhizotomy. **J Neurosurg** 83:989–993, 1995.

28. Latchaw JP Jr., Hardy RW Jr., Forsythe SB, *et al.*: Trigeminal neuralgia treated by radiofrequency coagulation. **J Neurosurg** 59;479–484, 1983.

29. Broggi G, Franzini A, Lasio G, *et al.*: Long-term results of percutaneous retrogasserian thermorhizotomy for "essential" trigeminal neuralgia: considerations in 1000 consecutive patients. **Neurosurgery** 26:783–787, 1990.

30. Piquer J, Joanes V, Roldan P, *et al.*: Long-term results of percutaneous gasserian ganglion lesions. **Acta Neurochir Suppl** 39:139–141, 1987.

31. Onofrio BM: Radiofrequency percutaneous Gasserian ganglion lesions. Results in 140 patients with trigeminal pain. **J Neurosurg** 42:132–139, 1975.

32. Guidetti B, Fraioli B, Refice GM: Modern trends in surgical treatment of trigeminal neuralgia. **J Maxillofac Surg** 7:315–319, 1979.

33. Brisman R: Bilateral trigeminal neuralgia. **J Neurosurg** 67:44–48, 1987.

34. Zakrzewska JM, Thomas DGT: Patient's assessment of outcome after three surgi-

cal procedures for the management of trigeminal neuralgia. **Acta Neurochir** 122:225–230, 1993.

35. Sweet WH: Faciocephalic pain, in Apuzzo MLJ (ed): Brain surgery: Complication avoidance and management. New York, Churchill Livingstone, 1993, Vol. 2, pp 2053–2083.

36. Lunsford LD, Bennett MH: Percutaneous retrogasserian glycerol rhizolysis for tic douloureux: Part 1. Technique and results in 112 patients. **Neurosurgery** 14:424–430, 1984.

37. Lunsford LD: Percutaneous retrogasserian glycerol rhizotomy, in Rovit RL, Murali R, Jannetta PJ (eds): Trigeminal neuralgia. Baltimore, Williams & Wilkins, 1990, pp 145–164.

38. Burchiel KJ: Percutaneous retrogasserian glycerol rhizolysis in the management of trigeminal neuralgia. **J Neurosurg** 69:361–366, 1988.

39. North RB, Kidd DH, Piantadosi S, *et al.:* Percutaneous retrogasserian glycerol rhizotomy. **J Neurosurg** 72:851–856, 1990.

40. Slettebo H, Hirschberg H, Lindegaard KF: Long-term results after percutaneous retrogasserian glycerol rhizotomy in patients with trigeminal neuralgia. **Acta Neurochir** 122:231–235, 1993.

41. Sahni KS, Pieper DR, Anderson R, *et al.:* Relation of hypesthesia to the outcome of glycerol rhizolysis for trigeminal neuralgia. **J Neurosurg** 72:55–58, 1990.

42. Steiger HJ: Prognostic factors in the treatment of trigeminal neuralgia: Analysis of a differential therapeutic approach. **Acta Neurochir** 113:11–17, 1991.

43. Bergenheim AT, Hariz MI: Influence of previous treatment on outcome after glycerol rhizotomy for trigeminal neuralgia. **Neurosurgery** 36:303–310, 1995.

44. Tan LKS, Robinson SN, Chatterjee S: Glycerol versus radiofrequency rhizotomy—a comparison of their efficacy in the treatment of trigeminal neuralgia. **Br J Neurosurg** 9:165–169, 1995.

45. Young RI: Glycerol rhizolysis for the treatment of trigeminal neuralgia. **J Neurosurg** 69;39–45, 1988.

46. Bergenheim AT, Hariz MI, Laitinen LV, *et al.:* Relation between sensory disturbance and outcome after retrogasserian glycerol rhizotomy. **Acta Neurochir** 111:114–118, 1991.

47. Arias MJ: Percutaneous retrogasserian glycerol rhizotomy for trigeminal neuralgia. A prospective study of 100 cases. **J Neurosurg** 65:32–36, 1986.

48. Ischia S, Luzzani A, Polati E: Retrogasserian glycerol injection: A retrospective study of 112 patients. **Clin J Pain** 6:291–296, 1990.

49. Kondziolka D, Lunsford LD, Bissonette DJ: Long-term results after glycerol rhizotomy for multiple sclerosis-related trigeminal neuralgia. **Can J Neurol Sci** 21:137–140, 1994.

50. Mullan S: Percutaneous microcompression of the trigeminal ganglion, in Rovit RL, Murali R, Jannetta PJ (eds): Trigeminal neuralgia. Baltimore, Williams & Wilkins, 1990, pp 137–144.

51. Lobato RD, Rivas JJ, Sarabia R, *et al.:* Percutaneous microcompression of the gasserian ganglion for trigeminal neuralgia. **J Neurosurg** 72:546–553, 1990.

52. Lichtor T, Mullan JF: A 10-year follow-up review of percutaneous microcompression of the trigeminal ganglion. **J Neurosurg** 72:49–54, 1990.

53. Brown JA, McDaniel MD, Weaver MT: Percutaneous trigeminal nerve compression for treatment of trigeminal neuralgia: Results in 50 patients. **Neurosurgery** 32:570–573, 1993.

54. Kondziolka D, Lunsford LD, Flickinger JC, *et al.*: Stereotactic radiosurgery for trigeminal neuralgia: A multiinstitutional study using the gamma unit. **J Neurosurg** 84:940–945, 1996.

55. Jannetta PJ: Arterial compression of the trigeminal nerve at the pons in patients with trigeminal neuralgia. **J Neurosurg** 26:159–162, 1967.

56. Jannetta PJ: Treatment of trigeminal neuralgia by suboccipital and transtentorial cranial operations. **Clin Neurosurg** 24:538–549, 1977.

57. Jannetta PJ: Observations on the etiology of trigeminal neuralgia, hemifacial spasm, acoustic nerve dysfunction and glossopharyngeal neuralgia. **Neurochirurgia (Stuttg)** 20:145–154, 1977.

58. Jannetta PJ: Microsurgery of cranial nerve cross-compression. **Clin Neurosurg** 26;607–615, 1979.

59. Lovely TJ, Lowry DW, Jannetta PJ: Functional outcome and patient satisfaction following microvascular decompression. **Neurosurgery** 39:650, 1996 [Abstract].

60. Zakrzewska JM: Posterior fossa surgery, in Zakrzewska JM (ed): Trigeminal neuralgia. London, WB Saunders, 1995, pp 157–170.

61. Bederson JB, Wilson CB: Evaluation of microvascular decompression and partial sensory rhizotomy in 252 cases of trigeminal neuralgia. **J Neurosurg** 71:359–367, 1989.

62. Burchiel KJ, Clarke H, Haglund M, *et al.*: Long-term efficacy of microvascular decompression in trigeminal neuralgia. **J Neurosurg** 69:35–38, 1988.

63. Cutbush K, Atkinson RL: Treatment of trigeminal neuralgia by posterior fossa microvascular decompression. **Aust N Z J Surg** 64:173–176, 1994.

64. Hori T, Adachi S, Anno Y, *et al.*: Management of tic douloureux by percutaneous radiofrequency gasserian ganglion coagulation (PRGC) or microvascular decompression (MVD): Comparison of the follow-up results. **Stereotact Funct Neurosurg** 54+55:104–105, 1990 [Abstract].

65. Piatt JH Jr., Wilkins RH: Treatment of tic douloureux and hemifacial spasm by posterior fossa exploration: Therapeutic implications of various neurovascular relationships. **Neurosurgery** 14:462–471, 1984.

66. Mendoza N, Illingworth RD: Trigeminal neuralgia treated by microvascular decompression: A long-term follow-up study. **Brit J Neurosurg** 9:13–19, 1995.

67. Kolluri S, Heros RC: Microvascular decompression for trigeminal neuralgia. A five-year follow-up study. **Surg Neurol** 22:235–240, 1984.

68. Szapiro J Jr., Sindou M, Szapiro J: Prognostic factors in microvascular decompression for trigeminal neuralgia. **Neurosurgery** 17:920–929, 1985.

69. Hamlyn PJ, King TT: Neurovascular compression in trigeminal neuralgia: a clinical and anatomical study. **J Neurosurg** 76:948–954, 1992.

70. Klun B: Microvascular decompression and partial sensory rhizotomy in the treatment of trigeminal neuralgia: Personal experience with 220 patients. **Neurosurgery** 30:49–52, 1992.

71. Yamaki T, Hashi K, Niwa J, *et al.*: Results of reoperation for failed microvascular decompression. **Acta Neurochir** 115:1–7, 1992.

72. Apfelbaum RI: Surgery for tic douloureux. **Clin Neurosurg** 31:351–368, 1984.

73. Barba D, Alksne JF: Success of microvascular decompression with and without prior surgical therapy for trigeminal neuralgia. **J Neurosurg** 60:104–107, 1984.

74. Puca A, Meglio M, Cioni B, *et al.*: Microvascular decompression for trigeminal neuralgia: Prognostic factors. **Acta Neurochir Suppl** 58:165–167, 1993.

75. Meglio M, Cioni B, Moles A, *et al.*: Microvascular decompression versus percutaneous procedures for typical trigeminal neuralgia: personal experience. **Stereotact Funct Neurosurg** 54+55:76–79, 1990.

76. Breeze R, Ignelzi RJ: Microvascular decompression for trigeminal neuralgia: Results with special reference to the late recurrence rate. **J Neurosurg** 57:487–490, 1982.

77. Sun T, Saito S, Nakai O, *et al.*: Long-term results of microvascular decompression for trigeminal neuralgia with reference to probability of recurrence. **Acta Neurochir** 126:144–148, 1994.

78. Young JN, Wilkins RH: Partial sensory trigeminal rhizotomy at the pons for trigeminal neuralgia. **J Neurosurg** 79:680–687, 1993.

79. Jannetta PJ: Microvascular decompression of the facial nerve for hemifacial spasm, in Wilson CB (ed): Neurosurgical procedures: Personal approaches to classic operations. Baltimore, Williams & Wilkins, 1992, pp 154–162.

80. Alexander GE, Moses H III: Carbamazepine for hemifacial spasm. **Neurology** 32:286–287, 1982.

81. Sandyk R, Gillman MA: Clonazepine in hemifacial spasm. **Int J Neurosci** 33:261–264, 1987.

82. Dutton JJ, Buckley EG: Long-term results and complications of botulinum A toxin in the treatment of blepharospasm. **Ophthalmology** 95:1529–1534, 1988.

83. Taylor JDN, Kraft SP, Kazdan MS, *et al.*: Treatment of blepharospasm and hemifacial spasm with botulinum A toxin: A Canadian multicentre study. **Can J Ophthalmol** 26:133–138, 1991.

84. Yoshimura DM, Aminoff MJ, Tami TA, *et al.*: Treatment of hemifacial spasm with botulinum toxin. **Muscle Nerve** 15:1045–1049, 1992.

85. Elston JS: The management of blepharospasm and hemifacial spasm. **J Neurol** 239:5–8, 1992.

86. Cuevas C, Madrazo I, Magallon E, *et al.*: Botulinum toxin A for the treatment of hemifacial spasm. **Arch Med Research** 26:405–408, 1995.

87. Poungvarin N, Devahastin V, Viriyavejakul A: Treatment of various movement disorders with botulinum A toxin injection: An experience of 900 patients. **J Med Assoc Thailand** 78:281–288, 1995.

88. Price J, O'Day J: Efficacy and side effects of botulinum toxin treatment for blepharospasm and hemifacial spasm. **Austr N Z J Ophthalmol** 22:255–260, 1994.

89. Berardelli A, Formica A, Mercuri B, *et al.*: Botulinum toxin treatment in patients with focal dystonia and hemifacial spasm. A multicenter study of the Italian Movement Disorder Group. **Ital J Neurol Sci** 14:361–367, 1993.

90. Siatkowski RM, Tyutyunikov A, Biglan AW, *et al.*: Serum antibody production to botulinum A toxin. **Ophthalmology** 100:1861–1866, 1993.

91. Park YC, Lim JK, Lee DK, *et al.*: Botulinum A toxin treatment of hemifacial spasm and blepharospasm. **J Korean Med Sci** 8:334–340, 1993.

92. Wilkins RH: Facial nerve decompression for hemifacial spasm, in Apuzzo MLJ (ed): Brain surgery: Complication avoidance and management. New York, Churchill Livingstone, 1993, vol 2, pp 2115–2143.

93. Ludman H, Choa DI: Hemifacial spasm: Operative treatment. **J Laryngol Otol** 99:239–245, 1985.

94. Dobie RA, Fisch U: Primary and revision surgery (selective neurectomy) for facial hyperkinesia. **Arch Otolaryngol Head Neck Surg** 112:154–163, 1986.

95. Elmqvist D, Toremalm NG, Elner A, et al.: Hemifacial spasm: electrophysiological findings and the therapeutic effect of facial nerve block. **Muscle Nerve** 5:S89–S94, 1982.

96. Hori T, Fukushima T, Terao H, et al.: Percutaneous radiofrequency facial nerve coagulation in the treatment of facial spasm. **J Neurosurg** 54:655–658, 1981.

97. Fan Z: Intracranial longitudinal splitting of facial nerve: A new approach for hemifacial spasm. **Ann Otol Rhinol Laryngol** 102:108–109, 1993.

98. Payner TD, Tew JM Jr.: Recurrence of hemifacial spasm after microvascular decompression. **Neurosurgery** 38:686–690, 1996.

99. Illingworth RD, Porter DG, Jakubowski J: Hemifacial spasm: a prospective long-term follow up of 83 cases treated by microvascular decompression at two neurosurgical centres in the United Kingdom. **J Neurol Neurosurg Psychiatry** 60: 72–77, 1996.

100. Zhang KW, Shun ZT: Microvascular decompression by the retrosigmoid approach for idiopathic hemifacial spasm: Experience with 300 cases. **Ann Otol Rhinol Laryngol** 104:610–612, 1995.

101. Huang CI, Chen IH, Lee LS: Microvascular decompression for hemifacial spasm: Analyses of operative findings and results in 310 patients. **Neurosurgery** 30:53–57, 1992.

102. Fukushima T: Microvascular decompression for hemifacial spasm: Results in 2890 cases, in Carter LP, Spetzler RF (eds): Neurovascular surgery. New York, McGraw-Hill, 1995, pp 1133–1145.

103. Auger RG, Piepgras DG, Laws ER Jr.: Hemifacial spasm: Results of microvascular decompression of the facial nerve in 54 patients. **Mayo Clin Proc** 61:640–644, 1986.

104. Loeser JD, Chen J: Hemifacial spasm: Treatment by microsurgical facial nerve decompression. **Neurosurgery** 13:141–146, 1983.

105. Wilkins RH, Radtke RA, Erwin CW: The value of intraoperative brainstem auditory evoked potential monitoring in reducing the auditory morbidity associated with microvascular decompression of cranial nerves. **Skull Base Surg** 1:106–109, 1991.

106. Rushton J, Stevens C, Miller R: Glossopharyngeal neuralgia (vagoglossopharyngeal neuralgia): A study of 217 cases. **Arch Neurol** 38:201–205, 1981.

107. Taha JM, Tew JM Jr.: Long-term results of surgical treatment of idiopathic neuralgias of the glossopharyngeal and vagal nerves. **Neurosurgery** 36:926–931, 1995.

108. Isamat F, Ferran E, Acebes J: Selective percutaneous thermocoagulation rhizotomy in essential glossopharyngeal neuralgia. **J Neurosurg** 55:575–580, 1981.

109. White JC, Sweet WH: Pain and the neurosurgeon. A forty-year experience. Springfield, IL, Charles C Thomas, 1969.

110. Rovit RL, Murali R: Glossopharyngeal neuralgia: Section and decompression procedures, in Apuzzo MLJ (ed): Brain surgery: Complication avoidance and management. New York, Churchill Livingstone, 1993, Vol 2, pp 2153–2164.

111. Olds MJ, Woods CI, Winfield JA: Microvascular decompression in glossopharyngeal neuralgia. **Am J Otol** 16:326–330, 1995.

112. Sindou M, Henry J, Blanchard P: [Idiopathic neuralgia of the glossopharyngeal nerve. Study of a series of 14 cases and review of the literature]. **Neurochirurgie** 37:18–25, 1991 [Paris].

113. Sindou M, Mertens P: Microsurgical vascular decompression in trigeminal and glossopharyngeal neuralgias: A twenty-year experience. **Acta Neurochir Suppl** 58:168–170, 1993.

114. Morales F, Albert P, Alberca R, et al.: Glossopharyngeal and vagal neuralgia secondary to vascular compression of the nerves. **Surg Neurol** 8:431–433, 1977.

115. Wakiya K, Fukushima T, Miyazaki S: [Results of microsurgical decompression in 16 cases of glossopharyngeal neuralgia]. **Neurol Med Chir (Tokyo)** 29:1113–1118, 1989 [Jpn].

116. Yoshioka J, Ueta K, Ohmoto T, et al.: Combined trigeminal and glossopharyngeal neuralgia. **Surg Neurol** 24:416–420, 1985.

117. Adams CBT: The physiology and pathophysiology of posterior fossa cranial nerve dysfunction syndromes: Nonmicrovascular perspective, in Barrow DL (ed): Surgery of the cranial nerves of the posterior fossa. [Chicago], AANS, 1993, pp 131–154.

118. Adams CBT: Microvascular compression: An alternative view and hypothesis. **J Neurosurg** 70:1–12, 1989.

119. Cleveland WS: LOWESS: A program for smoothing scatterplots by robust locally weighted regression. **Am Statistician** 35:54, 1981.

22

Outcomes Assessment for Pallidotomy

G. REES COSGROVE, M.D., F.R.C.S.(C.), JOHN PENNEY, M.D.,
AND LESLIE SHINOBU, M.D.

Surgery for Parkinson's disease (PD) was introduced by Meyers in the late 1930s with open resection of the head of the caudate nucleus and other selected lesions within the basal ganglia (15). With the advent of human stereotactic frames, more accurate and reproducible lesioning of the basal ganglia was accomplished. Narabayashi began using chemopallidotomy for the treatment of Parkinson's disease in the early 1950s, and Guiot and Brion reported their success with thermocoagulation lesions of the pallidum in 1953 (6, 16). Irving Cooper popularized the procedure in the United States using a guidance device of his own design that utilized craniocerebral landmarks (3).

The initial surgical target in the pallidum was in the anterodorsal portion of the globus pallidus; however Leksell et al. reported less favorable outcomes with this target and moved to a more posterior and ventral location. This "posteroventral pallidotomy" resulted in more lasting improvement in rigidity, bradykinesia, and tremor (17). At the same time that Leksell and coworkers had demonstrated improvement in parkinsonian symptoms with pallidotomy, Hassler and Reichert reported that ventrolateral thalamotomy provided much more consistent and complete relief of the parkinsonian tremor, and therefore subsequent stereotactic procedures were directed at this thalamic target (8). Stereotactic surgery for PD became one of the most common neurosurgical interventions of the day, but with the introduction of dopamine [L-dopa] replacement therapy in the late 1960s, the surgical treatment for Parkinson's disease decreased precipitously.

Laitinen and coworkers rekindled interest in the posteroventral pallidotomy in 1992 by reporting their successful experience in 38 patients with medically refractory Parkinson's disease (11). These early results were eagerly received by patients and physicians throughout the world, and pallidotomy rapidly regained popularity as a surgical option in patients with medically refractory PD. Anecdotal reports in the media and personal endorsements have fueled enthusiastic acceptance of the procedure despite limited evidence in peer-reviewed literature.

Currently there exist numerous centers in the United States that perform pallidotomy even though the detailed and long-term assessment of outcome remains less than adequate. In the current health-care environment, it has become increasingly important to address the value of any surgical intervention and accurately assess its impact on the disease itself, as well as the functional capacity of the patient. This chapter will present the problems of assessing outcome for pallidotomy in a PD population and discuss the strengths and weaknesses of the existing Parkinson's disease rating scales, the importance of an accurate preoperative evaluation, the various methods of evaluation, and the timing of follow-up.

FACTORS AFFECTING PALLIDOTOMY OUTCOMES ASSESSMENT

There are a variety of both general and disease-specific factors that affect outcomes assessment for pallidotomy in PD patients. Parkinson's disease is a progressive neurodegenerative illness with considerable variations among affected individuals. These variations include the age of onset, initial presentation, clinical features, response to medication, along with severity and progression of the illness.

The onset of Parkinson's disease is usually insidious and occurs in most patients in their 50s and 60s, although it can present at a much earlier age. Older patients tend to have significant comorbidity, and this can affect outcomes and complication rates. Patients with tremor have a more benign course than those with primarily bradykinesia and gait disorder. A smaller subgroup of patients present with PD at a young age (30–40 years). These healthier, younger patients are generally considered to be the best candidates for pallidotomy and often respond dramatically. Surgical series with a predominance of younger patients will therefore typically have a better response rate to pallidotomy, whereas series comprising an elderly population will be less favorable.

The cardinal manifestations of PD include resting tremor, rigidity, and bradykinesia. Gait disturbance and postural imbalance are also prominent symptoms. After long-term (usually 5–10 years) dopamine replacement therapy, many patients begin to experience involuntary movements or drug-induced dyskinesias and may fluctuate suddenly between the on/dyskinetic state and the off/akinetic-rigid state (14). Although most patients have a combination of tremor, rigidity, and bradykinesia by the time a diagnosis is made, there is marked variability among patients. Some patients will have predominant tremor, whereas others will have rigidity and bradykinesia as the primary determinants of their functional disability. This clinical heterogeneity makes it difficult to compare outcomes across groups, and it may be more useful to focus on the impact of pallidotomy on specific symptoms or manifestations. Similarly, because certain parkinsonian symptoms (dyskinesias, dystonias) seem to respond better to pallidotomy, the selection of patients with a predominance of these symptoms will generally experience greater functional improvement.

Not only are there marked interindividual variations, but the symptoms of Parkinson's disease fluctuate on both a daily and even hourly basis in the same individual. Some of these fluctuations are medication-related, but others are related to diet, environment, mood, anxiety, and expectations. All of these variations make it difficult to obtain a stable baseline even in the same patient and can be a significant confounding variable for outcome assessment. For this reason, most centers attempt to obtain ratings in both the "best on" and the "worst off" states, with the most significant improvement seen in the "off" states.

Because PD is a progressive illness and pallidotomy simply alleviates symptoms without altering the underlying neurodegenerative process, the effects of pallidotomy cannot be expected to be permanent. Therefore, any benefit imparted by pallidotomy will eventually be overwhelmed by progressive illness. Patients who have milder forms of PD or who are in the earlier stages should sustain longer functional improvement, although they may also have less need of an operation. Conversely, patients with more severe disease or in the later stages of illness will likely experience a shorter duration of significant functional improvement. It is important, therefore, that the characteristics of the study population be considered along with the duration of follow-up when comparing pallidotomy outcomes. A final confounding variable is that the rate of progression varies widely among patients.

In most cases, the cause of PD is unknown, although parkinsonian-like conditions can be seen after neuroleptic or dopamine-depleting drugs; stroke; encephalitis; carbon monoxide, cyanide, MPTP = (1-methyl-4-phenyl-1,2,3,6-tetrahydropyridine) or manganese poisoning; hypoparathyroidism; hydrocephalus, or severe head trauma (18). Early on in the disease, the idiopathic forms of PD may be clinically indistinguishable from progressive supranuclear palsy or other striatonigral degenerative diseases. These disease states, the so-called Parkinson's plus syndromes, tend to be relatively insensitive to dopaminergic replacement, have an overall poorer prognosis, and tend not to improve after pallidotomy. Consequently, diagnostic accuracy is critical, and any series with a significant number of nonidiopathic PD patients will have an overall poor response rate.

As with any neurosurgical intervention for a disabling and frustrating disease, patients clearly want to improve and please their treating physicians. This introduces a significant positive bias in the analysis of results. Similarly, treating physicians want to have good results, and there may be a underreporting of negative outcomes. Finally, many patients treated at academic centers come from greatly distant geographic locations, and therefore complete and regular follow-up information is often difficult to obtain. In addition, patients who have had a poor outcome or less than satisfactory result may not return to the treating institution for follow-up and therefore not be included in the analysis of outcome.

Another major concern is that there is considerable variation between centers regarding the preoperative evaluation, selection criteria, operative technique, and postoperative evaluation. It is, therefore, extremely important to document the extent and severity of the disease in patients using validated clinical rating scales both preoperatively and postoperatively in order to make comparisons from one center to another. Consequently, a detailed, extensive presurgical evaluation is a prerequisite for valid assessment of outcome.

CLINICAL PD RATING SCALES

There is a wide variety of clinical rating scales that have been validated over many years in the study of PD. The majority of these scales have been utilized by the neurologic community initially to assess the extent and progression of PD among various populations and subsequently to evaluate the effectiveness of pharmacologic treatment.

A standard clinical rating scale that has been used for many years to stage PD in an individual patient is the Hoehn and Yahr Scale (Table 1). This five-point scale estimates the severity and extent of the clinical signs of parkinsonism in terms of unilateral or bilateral involvement,

TABLE 1
Hoehn and Yahr Scale

Stage 0.0 = No signs of PD
Stage 1.0 = Unilateral involvement only
Stage 1.5 = Unilateral and axial involvement
Stage 2.0 = Bilateral involvement without impairment of balance
Stage 2.5 = Mild bilateral involvement with recovery on retropulsion test
Stage 3.0 = Mild to moderate bilateral involvement; some postural instability but independent
Stage 4.0 = Severe disability; still able to walk or stand unassisted
Stage 5.0 = Wheelchair-bound or bedridden unless aided

the presence or absence of postural instability, and the ability to walk or stand independently (10). The higher the score, the more severely affected the patient is.

Another commonly used rating scale is the Schwab and England Activities of Daily Living Scale (Table 2). This scale estimates the percentage of functional disability and degree of independence experienced by patients as the result of their PD. Patients who are completely independent in all activities of daily life despite their illness receive a 100% score, while those who are bedridden obtain a 0% score. There can, however, be considerable interobserver variability in assigning scores because of the subjective nature of the scale.

A more comprehensive clinical rating scale is the Uniform Parkinson's Disease Rating Scale (UPDRS) which has been in use since the mid 1980s (5). This scale has been validated in numerous multicenter drug trials and produces consistent evaluations across centers and over time with high interobserver reliability. The UPDRS has been utilized as the primary clinical assessment scale in the majority of modern PD clinical studies.

The UPDRS is composed of four separate sections which evaluate (a) mentation, behavior, and mood, (b) activities of daily living, (c) motor examination and (d) complications of treatment. In the mentation,

TABLE 2
Schwab and England Activities of Daily Living Scale

%	Definition
100	Completely independent
90	Independent; able to do all chores with some degree of slowness, difficulty
80	Independent in most chores; takes twice as long
70	Not completely independent, more difficulty with chores; three to four times as long; must spend large part of day with chores
60	Some dependency; can do most chores but very slowly with much effort and some errors; some chores impossible
50	More dependent; help with half of chores; difficulty with everything
40	Very dependent; can assist with all chores but can do very few alone
30	With effort occasionally does or begins a few chores alone; needs much help
20	Nothing alone; can assist slightly with some chores; severe invalid
10	Totally dependent; helpless; complete invalid
0	Vegetative functions (swallowing, bladder and bowel incontinence); bedridden

behavior, and mood section, memory impairment, the presence of thought disorders, depression, and motivation/initiative are subjectively rated by the patient. In the activities of daily living section, the patient subjectively reports regarding speech, swallowing, nausea, anorexia, constipation, writing, tremor, walking, salivation, using utensils, dressing, personal hygiene, and turning over in bed. These responses are obtained for both the on and off states. In the motor examination section, an objective evaluation is performed by the examiner of speech, facial expression, rest tremor, action tremor, rigidity, finger taps, hand movements, pronation/supination, heel tapping, rising from a chair, posture, gait, and postural instability. The complications of therapy generally relate to side effects of medication and address wearing off, on/off phenomena, dyskinesias, freezing, and sleep.

Each section of the UPDRS has a maximum score, depending on the points accrued for each question. The response to each question is generally scored from 0 to 4, with 0 being normal and 4 reflecting marked/severe dysfunction. The *mentation, behavior, and mood* section has four questions for a total of 16 points; the *activities of daily living* (ADL) section has 13 questions for a total of 52 points; the *motor examination* section has 15 questions for a total of 108 points; the *complications of therapy* section has 11 questions for a total of 23 points with a total possible score of 199. Scores are obtained for both the on and off states, and the higher the score, the more severe the Parkinson's disease. The scores on each section of the UPDRS can be reported individually to identify specific functional changes in addition to the total overall score.

In 1992, a committee was formed to develop a core assessment program for intracerebral transplantation (CAPIT) to provide a common method for the preoperative diagnosis and postoperative evaluation of patients in centers performing intracerebral transplantation for Parkinson's disease (12). This comprehensive assessment program outlines accepted clinical diagnostic criteria for Parkinson's disease, practically defines the conditions of "best on" and "worst off," and provides the core methodology to evaluate patients pre- and postoperatively. These methods incorporate the clinical rating scales of UPDRS, the Hoehn-Yahr staging, a Dyskinesia Rating Scale, and four timed motor tests (pronation-supination, hand movement between two points, finger dexterity, and stand-walk-sit test). Recommendations regarding the use of pre- and postoperative imaging using magnetic resonance imaging (MRI) and positron emission tomography (PET) scans were also made. Additional suggestions concerning the timing and number of evaluations, medication adjustments, and pharmacologic testing were implied. The final recommendation was to have some method of self-reporting of the illness by the patient. This consisted of a diary recorded on an hourly basis on each day for at least 1 week prior to each evaluation.

ADDITIONAL ASSESSMENT TOOLS

A variety of general clinical outcome rating scales have been considered useful in assessing the overall success of a surgical intervention. The Clinical Global Improvement (CGI) scale is a five-point measure of outcome that grades the patient's overall response to surgery as excellent, good, moderate, poor, or worse (Table 3). Although this assessment is relatively nonspecific and certainly open to rater bias, it can provide a simplified measure of the overall success or failure of pallidotomy.

One of the most frequently used and broadly validated tools for evaluating functional outcome has been the Rand 36-item Health Survey 1.0 (SF 36). This questionnaire is completed by the patient and is an appropriate self-assessment tool for any kind of surgical intervention (9). Although not as detailed as the hourly diary suggested in the CAPIT program, it is easily obtained and provides more comprehensive information regarding the overall functional level of the patient.

Centers with experience in performing pallidotomies have also observed a variety of unusual symptoms that may also be improved with surgery. These include the amelioration of panic attacks, the abolition of severe diaphoretic episodes, and significant weight gain due to abolition of prolonged, violent dyskinesias. Inasmuch as dyskinesias and dystonias appear to be the features of PD that are most clearly improved after pallidotomy, it can be useful to examine these symptoms more closely. Specific dyskinesia scales or an estimation of hours in the day spent in the off, on, or dyskinetic state can be quite useful in demonstrating the impact of pallidotomy on these PD states.

Formal visual field testing can be performed both preoperatively and postoperatively to demonstrate the presence or absence of a visual field defect which has been reported in up to 14% of patients (11).

TABLE 3
Clinical Global Improvement Scale

Grade 5 = Excellent
Grade 4 = Good
Grade 3 = Moderate
Grade 2 = Poor/no response
Grade 1 = Worse

Because many patients with advanced PD may have associated cognitive decline it is important to evaluate their intellectual function in a standardized fashion. The Blessed Dementia Scale and a Mini-Mental Status Examination are standard questionnaires that evaluate patients for significant dementia but are relatively insensitive to minor cognitive changes (2). Detailed neuropsychologic testing can detect more subtle changes in cognitive function as a result of the PD or as a side effect of pallidotomy. Appropriate testing would encompass skill learning (mirror tracing, serial reaction time), frontal lobe functions (Stroop Color Naming, Wisconsin Card Sorting), memory testing (Wechsler Memory Scale, Warrington Visual Recognition of Faces and Stories, NYU stories), general intelligence/problem solving (Wechsler Adult Intelligence Scale, Ravens Colored Progressive Matrices), language (Boston Naming, Verbal Fluency), and spatial function (body scheme, Luria Mental Rotation, money road map, and matchsticks).

Because affective disorders frequently accompany Parkinson's disease, it is also appropriate to consider using some measure of the emotional state using either the Beck Depression Inventory or Hamilton Depression Scale (1, 7).

Newer methods of quantifying motor performance may be of particular importance in demonstrating the efficacy of pallidotomy. These methods include gait analysis, tremor analysis, and computerized evaluations of hand movement velocity, accuracy, and stability.

NEUROIMAGING

An MRI scan to exclude severe cortical atrophy, hydrocephalus, multiple lacunes, or other structural pathology is important in the presurgical evaluation of all patients undergoing pallidotomy. The study should be repeated in the acute postoperative setting to exclude complications and to verify accurate lesion placement. Some determination regarding the precise location and volume of the lesion should be made. This information is important in terms of correlation with eventual long-term outcomes.

In centers that use PET in their pallidotomy patients, it has been suggested that a preoperative PET scan can predict which patients will respond to surgical intervention (13). This observation may have increasing importance in the future as attempts are made to be more selective in choosing patients for surgery. It is too early to say whether advanced neuroimaging modalities, such as functional MRI or magnetic resonance spectroscopy, will be useful in the preoperative selection or the postoperative evaluation of pallidotomy patients.

METHODS OF ASSESSMENT

In order to obtain an accurate and unbiased assessment of outcome following pallidotomy, it is extremely important that the evaluation be performed by an independent, experienced, and unbiased observer. The same evaluator should perform the assessment at each visit to control for interobserver variability. The most appropriate evaluator is the movement disorder neurologist and not the operative neurosurgeon. However, even the neurologist is not completely unbiased, inasmuch as one involved in a successful program may bring a positive bias to the evaluation in the same way that a neurologist who is against this form of therapy might bring a negative viewpoint. Some centers have performed a blinded assessment of outcome using a videotaped demonstration of the patient (4). The patient is dressed in a hospital gown and hat to hide the patient's operative status from the observer and then performs a battery of simple tests. The videotaped segments are randomized and scored blindly. This type of rigorous assessment is laudable but is only applicable to a very small number of well-studied patients and only incorporates motor data.

The timing of postoperative evaluations is also important, and it is generally agreed that 3- to 6-month intervals are adequate. Another major issue is whether these evaluations are performed when the patient is in the best "on" or worst "off" state. The worst "off" state requires that the patient be off all medications for at least 12 hours before the evaluation, which can be difficult for a variety of reasons. A clinical determination of the patients on/off status during the evaluation is a less accurate situation. Currently it appears that the major benefit imparted to PD patients after pallidotomy is during the "off" state, although it is difficult to improve upon their level of functioning in their best "on" state. Therefore, it would be more difficult to demonstrate statistically significant improvement in a pallidotomy series with patients included who were evaluated presurgically in the "on" or partially "off" states.

SIDE EFFECTS AND COMPLICATIONS

A critical assessment of outcome for any surgical procedure must include the honest reporting of complications, both immediate and delayed. The acute complications can be detected by careful clinical examination and neuroimaging. These include intracranial hemorrhage, seizures, visual disturbance, postoperative dysarthria or dysphasia, confusional states, motor or sensory deficit, and cognitive impairment. Delayed complications can be much more difficult to detect and require regular follow-up and careful questioning.

STATISTICAL ANALYSIS

In order to provide a meaningful assessment of outcome, appropriate statistical analysis of the data must be performed wherever possible. In order to accomplish this the optimal situation would enroll all patients prospectively into a database in which complete preoperative and postoperative data would be entered and appropriate comparisons made. These comparisons must be made over the long term at 3- to 6-month intervals in order to demonstrate both the short- and long-term benefits or side effects of pallidotomy. Repeated measures using ANOVA and the paired t-test with correction of the significance level to control for multiple comparisons are generally considered the most appropriate statistical techniques to be used in analyzing the data.

MGH PALLIDOTOMY OUTCOMES ASSESSMENT

Although a wide variety of clinical and radiologic assessment tools are available, not all of them can be applied in a cost- and time-effective analysis. Any evaluation of outcome, however, must imply a detailed preoperative evaluation and examination of the patient in the baseline state. This requires a multidisciplinary effort to ensure diagnostic accuracy and select the best patients for surgery. The clinical rating scales and other evaluations must be obtained preoperatively in order to make accurate comparisons to the postoperative state. In the optimal situation, these clinical rating scales should be obtained both in the best "on" and worst "off" state. Although standardized testing cannot be mandated across centers, it is important that the responsible programs apply recognized, validated, and reproducible rating scales to their patient populations so that appropriate intercenter comparisons can be made.

As an example of what might be considered a reasonable approach, the MGH Pallidotomy Outcomes Assessment includes the following:

1. A detailed clinical examination in the "on" and "off" states
2. Videotaping of specific motor tasks
3. Hoehn and Yahr staging
4. Schwab and England Activities of Daily Living (ADL) Scale
5. UPDRS (mentation, ADL, motor, complication)
6. Clinical Global Improvement Scale
7. SF-36
8. Postoperative MRI (<24 hours and >3 months)
9. Fatigue Severity Scale
10. Other scales—Beck Depression Inventory, Dyskinesia Scale, hours on/off/dyskinetic, weight loss/gain, neuropsychological testing.

These tests are performed at 1.5, 3, 6, and 12 months postoperatively and then at 6-month intervals thereafter. The scores for each patient are then entered into a database for analysis. By obtaining accurate preoperative baselines, the effects of pallidotomy can be compared on an individual basis or averaged across the entire group.

RESULTS

While a detailed analysis of our results is not the subject of this chapter, it is appropriate to present certain data to illustrate some of the issues regarding pallidotomy outcomes assessment.

Between June 1993 and January 1996, we performed unilateral pallidotomies in 51 patients. The overall response to surgery for this initial group of patients using the CGI scale as rated by the neurologist at the time of last follow-up was excellent in 17, good in 13, moderate in 10, poor/no response in 4, and one patient became worse (Fig. 1). Although there is certainly some bias that enters into the rating, it does suggest that overall two-thirds of patients will experience a gratifying result from surgery. It is not clear using this scale, however, which of the symptoms of PD have been ameliorated or which dysfunction has been improved.

As stated previously, one can analyze the outcome after surgery on both an individual basis and a group basis. An example of a successful

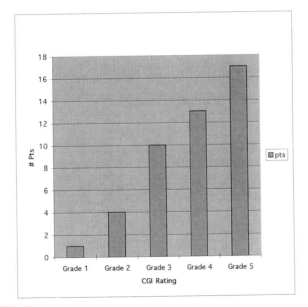

FIG. 1 CGI rating.

result in one patient is demonstrated with respect to hours in the day spent "off," "on," and dyskinetic (Fig. 2). This kind of analysis can clearly separate excellent results from poor results across a wide number of variables and distinguish surgical successes from failures. But in order to truly demonstrate the effectiveness of an intervention, one must document a statistical benefit across a population. Using the same variables of waking hours in the day spent in the "off," "on," and dyskinetic states, we can also see the benefit when the entire group is averaged (Fig. 3). This analysis was performed on a group of 75 patients who underwent pallidotomy with varying duration of follow-up. At the 3- and 6-month intervals, there was statistically significant ($P < .05$) improvement across the three conditions. There was a trend toward sustained improvement at the 12-month follow-up, but this did not reach statistical significance. This might be interpreted to mean that the effect of pallidotomy is temporary but more likely indicates that the number of patients analyzed (only 11 of 75) at this time period was too few to provide statistical power.

The final consideration is the difference in results when one compares scores obtained for patients in the "off" and "on" states. A comparison of UPDRS ADL scores in both the "off" and "on" states demonstrates a statistically significant ($P < .05$) improvement in ADL scores in the "off" scores but not in the "on" scores (Fig. 4). This improvement is significant when only the ADL section of the UPDRS

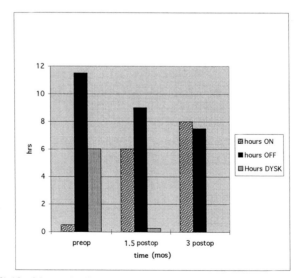

FIG. 2 Individual hours in the on/off/or dyskinetic state (DYSK).

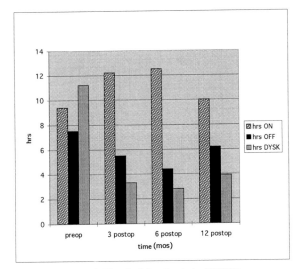

FIG. 3 Group hours in the on/off/or dyskinetic state (DYSK).

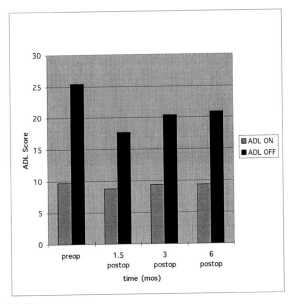

FIG. 4 UPDRS ADL scores.

is analyzed, but it is lost in the total UPDRS score when all of the sections are combined. This dilution of possible benefit can also be observed when motor scores are analyzed because while one can nearly abolish dyskinesias with pallidotomy, this represents only a negligible improvement in a total motor section score of 108 points. Nevertheless, the abolition of dyskinesias can have a substantial and worthwhile benefit to the patient's overall level of function.

CONCLUSIONS

The evaluation of the success or failure of pallidotomy in patients with medically refractory PD can only be made by the responsible reporting of patient outcomes using validated clinical rating scales. Currently available rating scales were not specifically developed for the evaluation of pallidotomy and therefore have some shortcomings. However, if results are reported in a clear and objective fashion, it is possible to make comparisons between centers and operative techniques. In this way, important observations can be made and new knowledge and insights can be gained regarding the optimal lesion location and size, the avoidance of complications, and the long-term success of pallidotomy.

REFERENCES

1. Beck AT, Ward CHH, Mendleson M, et al.: An inventory for measuring depression. **Arch Gen Psychiatry** 4:561–571, 1961.
2. Blessed G, Tomlinson BE, Roth M: Blessed-Roth dementia scale. **Psycholpharmacol Bull** 24:705–708, 1988.
3. Cooper IS, Bravo G: Chemopallidectomy and chemothalamectomy. **J Neurosurg** 15:244–250, 1958.
4. Eidelberg D, Moeller JR, Ishikawa T, et al.: Regional metabolic correlates of surgical outcome following unilateral pallidotomy for Parkinson's disease. **Ann Neurol** 39:450–459, 1996.
5. Fahn S, Elton RL, Members of the UPDRS Development Committee: Unified Parkinson's Disease Rating Scale, in Fahn S, Marsden CD, Calne DB, et al. (eds): *Recent Developments in Parkinsons Disease.* Florham Park, NJ, MacMillan Healthcare Information, 1987, vol 2, pp 153–163.
6. Guiot G, Brion S: Traitement des mouvements anormaux par la coagulation pallidale. Technique et resultats. **Rev Neurol** 89:578–580, 1953.
7. Hamilton M: Development of a rating scale for primary depressive illness. **Br J Soc Clin Psychol** 6:278–296, 1967.
8. Hassler R, Reichert T: Indikationen und Lokalisations-methode der gezielten Hirnoperationen. **Nervenarzt** 25:441–447, 1954.
9. Hays RD, Sherbourne CD, Mazel E: The RAND 36-item Health Survey 1.0. **Health Econ** 2:212–227, 1993.
10. Hoehn MM, Yahr MD: Parkinsonism: Onset, progression and mortality. **Neurology** 17:427–442, 1961.
11. Laitinen LV, Bergenheim T, Hariz MI: Leksell's posteroventral pallidotomy in the treatment of Parkinson's disease. **J Neurosurg** 76:53–61, 1992.

12. Langston JW, Widner H, Goetz CG, et al.: Core assessment Program for Intracerebral Transplantation (CAPIT). **Mov Disord** 7:2–13, 1992.

13. Lozano AM, Lang AE, Galvez-Jimenez N, et al.: Effect of Gpi pallidotomy on motor function in Parkinson's disease. **Lancet** 346:1383–1387, 1995.

14. Marsden CD, Parkes JD: Success and problems of long-term levodopa therapy in Parkinson's disease. **Lancet** 1:345–349, 1977.

15. Meyers R: Surgical procedure for postencephalitic tremor with notes on the physiology of the premotor fibers. **Arch Neurol Psychiatry** 4:455–459, 1940.

16. Narabayashi H, Okuma T: Procaine-oil blocking of the globus pallidus for the treatment of the rigidity and tremor of parkinsonism. **Proc Jpn Acad Sci** 29:134–137, 1953.

17. Svennilson E, Torvik A, Lowe R, Leksell L: Treatment of parkinsonism by stereotactic thermolesions in the pallidal region. A clinical evaluation of 81 cases. **Acta Psychiatr Neurol Scand** 35:358–377, 1960.

18. Weiner WJ, Lang AE: *Movement Disorders: A Comprehensive Survey.* Mount Kisco, NY, Futura, 1989.

23

Analysis of Outcome: Temporal Lobe Resection

WEBSTER H. PILCHER, M.D., PH.D., AND JOHN LANGFITT, PH.D.

There has been a dramatic expansion in the capacity to perform epilepsy monitoring and surgery in the United States over the past 20 years (11, 12). The number of comprehensive epilepsy centers has grown from a handful in the 1970s to nearly 150 in 1995, with a corresponding increase in the number of operative procedures performed. The introduction of sophisticated video-electroencephalogram (EEG) monitoring and neuroimaging techniques, and the accumulation of data regarding the neurobiology (28) and natural history of intractable temporal lobe epilepsy (TLE), has improved the accuracy of patient selection, as well as the outcome of surgery from the standpoint of seizure control (12).

Despite these significant technological, conceptual, and surgical advances, there remain major gaps in our understanding of the outcome of temporal lobe surgery from a number of perspectives. No randomized controlled trials have been performed addressing the efficacy of medical *versus* surgical therapy or the relative morbidity of alternative surgical approaches to nonlesional and lesional TLE. No multicenter outcome study has yet addressed the impact of epilepsy monitoring and surgery upon the quality of life (QOL) of afflicted patients, although such a study is currently underway. Finally, as we enter an era characterized by finite health-care resources and increasing scrutiny of costly medical interventions, no definitive cost-effectiveness studies are available that incorporate an assessment of QOL improvements and cost of surgical interventions for medically intractable TLE.

For many years the gold standard of outcome analysis in epilepsy surgery was provided by a simple assessment of postoperative seizure control (12, 37). It is increasingly recognized, however, that the disease of TLE is far more complex than a series of inconvenient epileptic attacks in afflicted patients. At the time of presentation for surgical consideration, seizures have often been present for as long as 2 decades, in many cases during critical stages of growth and development (Fig. 1). Some patients find engendered within themselves a disabling

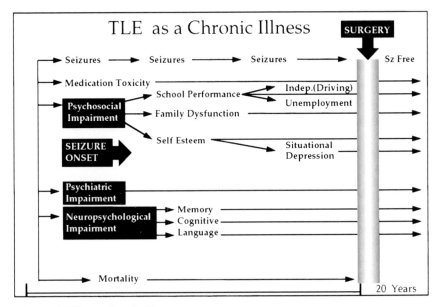

FIG. 1. TLE as a chronic illness.

array of psychosocial, neuropsychological and psychiatric impairments, all of which adversely impact their QOL. In a recent NIH-sponsored consensus conference on epilepsy surgery, neurosurgeons were challenged to develop more sophisticated and inclusive measures of outcome to describe the impact of surgical intervention upon patients with TLE (32). It was recommended that measures of outcome should address (a) the postoperative control of seizures, as well as the short-term and long-term neurological, neuropsychological, and psychobehavioral complications of surgery and (b) the impact of surgery upon both general health and recognized epilepsy-associated disabilities that adversely impact QOL. Finally, it was recommended that the outcome of intervention should be expressed in cost-effectiveness terms to facilitate comparisons of epilepsy monitoring and surgery with other expensive, high-technology health-care interventions available today (18, 32).

EPIDEMIOLOGY OF EPILEPSY

Epilepsy is a relatively common disease, with approximately 2 million patients currently afflicted in the USA. Of these patients, 330,000 are under 17 years of age (2, 11). The prevalence of active epilepsy is estimated at 0.6%, with a lifetime prevalence of 1.3%. It is estimated that as many as 100,000 individuals may be candidates for various forms of surgical intervention, with 5,000 new candidates generated each year (2, 11). In the population of surgical candidates, approximately two-thirds may be candidates for TLE.

SURGICALLY REMEDIABLE TLE SYNDROMES

Advances in our understanding of intractable TLE have contributed to the elucidation of specific surgically remediable syndromes (11, 36). These are conceived as medically intractable conditions with a known pathophysiology and natural history that may respond favorably to surgical intervention. The prototypical syndrome of *mesial TLE* incorporates the history of an early injury in childhood, such as a febrile seizure, meningitis, encephalitis, or closed-head injury. These patients may subsequently develop intractable seizures in adolescence and are at risk for developing irreversible psychosocial and neuropsychological disabilities. MRI reveals hippocampal atrophy and/or sclerosis and positron emission tomography (PET) scans suggest temporal lobe hypometabolism. The category of *lesional TLE* has been expanded by advances in neuroimaging and by neuropathologic correlations. These patients harbor temporal lobe neoplasms, vascular malformations, cortical dysplasias, migrational anomalies, or traumatic/ischemic injury, or they exhibit "dual pathology," in which a temporal lobe lesion is found in coexistence with hippocampal atrophy and sclerosis. *Cryptogenic TLE* incorporates patients with TLE by electrographic criteria but with normal imaging findings.

OUTCOME ASSESSMENT: SEIZURES

Classification Schemes

In the past, assessments of outcome of medical and surgical treatments of epilepsy focused primarily upon the impact of treatment upon seizure frequency. The classification scheme used by Rasmussen and colleagues at the Montreal Neurologic Institute emphasized seizure freedom in the highest outcome category and seizure frequency in subordinate categories (12, 37). Contemporary schemes, such as the Engel Outcome Classification (Fig. 2) define patterns of seizure outcome which correlate somewhat with improvements in the QOL of operated patients (11, 12, 16). For example, although Engel class I patients are free of "disabling seizures" for the 2 years before outcome classification, these patients may have had some seizures postoperatively. Engel class I patients may also have occasional auras, which are considered "nondisabling" ictal events, or even atypical generalized tonic clonic seizures with drug withdrawal. Thus, Engel class I pa-

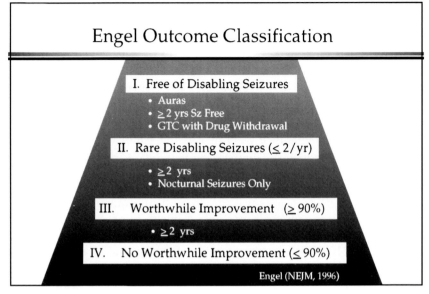

FIG. 2. Engel Outcome Classification.

tients are not necessarily seizure-free but are free of the "disabling seizures" that are likely to adversely impact QOL. Engel class II and III patients are felt to have variable degrees of "worthwhile" seizure improvement, although worthwhile is not explicitly defined. Engel class IV patients, with less than 90% improvement in seizure frequency, are believed to have experienced "no worthwhile improvement." Many class IV patients, however, feel that the reduction in seizure frequency and severity achieved is beneficial, despite their classification as "unimproved." Although such classification schemes provide useful descriptions of postoperative seizure control, they do not effectively address alterations in the quality, intensity, and severity of seizures that may significantly influence the postoperative result for many patients (18). Furthermore, these classification schemes do not incorporate general and epilepsy-specific QOL measures that are essential to any substantive assessment of the impact of surgery upon the psychosocial and neuropsychological disabilities which encumber these patients (18).

Postoperative Seizure Outcome

From the standpoint of seizure outcome, considerable progress has been made over the past several decades as the result of advances in patient selection and a convergence of surgical techniques in which the resection of mesial structures is emphasized (11, 13). In the 1986 Palm Desert International Conference on the Surgical Treatment of Epilepsies, data collected from 39 centers from 1949–1984 revealed a 55.5% seizure-free rate postoperatively (11, 12). These data were accumulated in a changing and less sophisticated clinical environment and included a mixture of lesional and nonlesional cases with considerable variability in patient selection methods and surgical techniques between centers. In the 1992 Palm Desert Conference, data accumulated from 107 centers from 1986–1990 revealed approximately 68% of patients to be seizure-free postoperatively with 90% of all patients experiencing greater than 90% improvement in seizure frequency (12, 37). Similar seizure outcomes were identified in patients with both lesional and nonlesional epilepsy, and seizure outcome appeared to be independent of the surgical approach used, including standard (anatomic), extended mesial, and tailored temporal lobe resections, as well as selective amygdalohippocampectomy (11, 12, 13).

Although the Engel Outcome Scale provides valuable information about postoperative seizure control in populations of patients, it does not reflect the dynamic fluctuations of seizure expression that may occur in individual patients (12, 16). Likewise, because only seizure control over the 2 years before assessment is analyzed, this scale does not identify which patients have been completely seizure-free since surgery. For example, a patient experiencing numerous seizures during the first 2 postoperative years, followed by seizure freedom, and a patient completely seizure-free for 5 years postoperatively would both be classified Engel class I at the 5-year assessment.

Despite the fluctuations in seizure expression that may occur in individual patients, contemporary data suggest a fairly stable pattern of seizure outcome in populations of patients over time after temporal lobe resection (10, 12, 40, 47). In a recent study, Sperling et al. followed 89 temporal lobe resection patients for 5–8 years postoperatively (40). These patients were selected with contemporary modalities, including scalp and invasive video-EEG, MRI, and neuropsychological criteria and were thus considered to be representative of outcomes achieved using a "modern era" approach. All patients underwent a standard temporal lobe resection for intractable nonlesional or lesional TLE. In this population, the percentage of patients in each seizure outcome category remained stable during the follow-up period, with 70% of patients Engel class I or "seizure-free" at 5 years. Many class I patients at the 5-year assessment had not been completely seizure-free since surgery but had experienced at least one unprovoked seizure during the follow-up period. Only 55% of all patients had been completely seizure-free during the entire first 5 years of follow-up; 42% experienced an initial unprovoked seizure during the first 2 years of follow-up, with 45% experiencing at least one seizure during the first 5 years. Thus, seizure freedom for 2 years postoperatively was highly predictive of subsequent seizure freedom during an extended follow-up period, confirming findings of earlier studies (10, 12, 39, 47).

Preoperative Predictors of Seizure Outcome

The comprehensive preoperative evaluation emphasizes the value of obtaining convergent data (i.e., interictal and ictal EEG, MRI, PET, neuropsychologic data) in individual patients who are selected as optimal surgical candidates. A particular effort has been directed at identifying those features of the preoperative evaluation which are predictive of seizure outcome postoperatively. In Spencer's analysis, for example, of the many features evaluated, only (a) mesial temporal sclerosis (MTS), (b) a known cause of epilepsy (i.e., a febrile seizure) and (c) the absence of secondarily generalized tonic clonic seizures significantly correlated with postoperative seizure outcome (39). A satisfactory postoperative seizure outcome occurred in 93% of patients when all three features were present; in 78–83% when two were present; in 53–61% when one was present and in 29% when none were present (39).

Lesional TLE

A wide variety of benign neoplasms, as well as vascular and cortical dysgenetic abnormalities, are associated with long-standing, medically intractable TLE (4, 14, 28, 39, 48). A distinct entity, referred to as "dual pathology," has been recognized in which a temporal lobe lesion is found in association with hippocampal sclerosis and/or atrophy. In contrast to the convergence of surgical approaches in nonlesional TLE that has been documented over the past decade, there is still uncertainty regarding the optimal surgical approach to patients with temporal lobe lesions and intractable TLE ("lesional TLE"). The principal debate with regard to the management of these patients is whether or not incorporating extralesional, presumably epileptogenic tissue, into the resection will improve the seizure outcome (4, 14, 23, 36, 38).

Lesional resection alone ("lesionectomy") in patients with intractable extratemporal lesional epilepsy has been demonstrated to relieve seizures effectively in more than 60% of patients (4, 5). In the series of Spencer et al., favorable outcomes were achieved in the temporal lobe with lesionectomy, as defined by frozen section margins (14, 38). In other series, however, the results of lesionectomy in patients with lesional TLE have been less favorable. In a Mayo Clinic series (30) stereotactic lesionectomy of temporal lobe lesions rendered 6/14 (43%)

of operated patients seizure-free, whereas standard temporal lobe resection inclusive of both the offending lesion and the mesial structures resulted in seizure freedom in 17/20 (85%) of operated patients. In a series of temporal lobe resections in lesional TLE, Jooma *et al.* reported 3/16 (19%) seizure-free after lesionectomy, whereas 13/14 (93%) patients undergoing combined lesional and standard temporal lobe resections achieved seizure freedom (23). In these comparative studies, reoperation to remove mesial structures after failed lesionectomy resulted in seizure freedom in selected patients, confirming the likelihood of extralesional epileptogenicity in patients with lesional TLE. Other series of patients undergoing combined lesional and temporal lobe resection (3, 36) reported more than 90% seizure-free with over one-half of operated patients seizure-free off medication. One theory advanced to explain the less favorable seizure outcome in temporal lobe lesionectomy is the possibility that extralesional mesial structures (*i.e.*, hippocampus, amygdala, and parahippocampal gyrus) are incorporated into the epileptogenic substrate (28), requiring their resection in selected cases if seizures are to be eliminated. The identification of hippocampal neuronal loss in patients with lesional TLE suggests that "dual pathology" may contribute to the persistence of seizures in selected patients who fail lesional resection (28).

Operative strategies have been proposed in which the decision to resect mesial structures, including the amygdala and hippocampus along with the lesion, is based upon (*a*) the lesion location (*i.e.*, mesial or lateral to the parahippocampal gyrus), (*b*) the presence or absence of hippocampal atrophy or sclerosis on MRI ("dual pathology"), and (*c*) the results of neuropsychologic assessment and the Wada test (14, 36). The important issue of the relative neuropsychologic morbidity of alternative approaches has not been definitively addressed.

Neuropathologic Substrate and Seizure Outcome

Neuroimaging and neuropathologic correlations have delineated a wide variety of pathological substrates associated with TLE which include mesial temporal sclerosis, lesional TLE and cryptogenic TLE (4, 13, 14, 39). Recent data suggest that long-term seizure outcome may be affected by the etiologic substrate as defined by histopathologic criteria (4, 39). In the series of Spencer *et al.*, continuous seizure freedom (2–10 years) is highest in patients with glial neoplasms (75%) and mesial temporal sclerosis (65%). In this series the highest relapse rate after 1 year of seizure freedom was noted in patients with cortical dysgenetic lesions (25%). Interestingly, patients with mesial temporal sclerosis experienced a 14% relapse rate after 1 year of seizure freedom, perhaps as an expression of the tendency of TLE to be a bilateral process.

COMPLICATIONS OF SURGERY

Although no multicenter prospective study of the complications of epilepsy surgery has been performed, on the basis of available data the rate of surgical complications of invasive monitoring and resective temporal lobe surgery is quite low, with mortality nearly nonexistent and significant morbidity in the 1–2% range (Fig. 3). The contributions of neuroimaging studies (MRI, PET, SPECT) in the realm of patient selection has reduced the requirement for preoperative invasive monitoring with a corresponding reduction in associated complications of these procedures (34, 35). The low morbidity and mortality rate of epilepsy surgery, when contrasted with the morbidity of intractable TLE and the excess mortality experienced by intractable epileptics argues for early surgical intervention (11, 17, 40).

POSTOPERATIVE NEUROPSYCHOLOGIC AND PSYCHOSOCIAL OUTCOME

Intellectual Abilities

Brenda Milner's seminal investigations at the Montreal Neurological Institute over many decades revealed that cognitive measures,

Invasive Monitoring			
	Depth Electrodes	Infection, Hemorrhage, Deficit	1-11%
	Subdural Strip Electrodes:	Infection	1-3%
	Subdural Grid Electrodes:	Infection	5-10%
		SDH	1-5%
		Neuro Deficit	1-2%
Resective Surgery		Death	<1%
	Infection		<1%
	Hematoma		<1%
	VFD	Mild	>50%
		Severe	2-4%
	III Palsy		<0.5%
	Death		<0.5%
Dominant TL (Language /Memory)			
	Anomia	Transitory	>20%
	Anomia	Persistent	1-3%
	Mild Memory Loss	STVM	40%
	Memory Loss	Global	1%
Neuro Behavioral			
	Transitory Psychosis/Depression		2-20%

Pilcher, et al (1993)

Fig. 3. Complications of epilepsy surgery. [Adapted from (34).]

including verbal, performance, and full-scale IQ scores, are relatively stable 5–20 years after temporal lobe resection (29). In fact, there was a suggestion that cognitive functions associated with the contralateral temporal lobe might actually improve when an ipsilateral seizure focus was removed. Her data revealed a trend toward improvement in VIQ after nondominant resection and in PIQ after dominant resection. These findings have been confirmed and extended by other investigators (31).

Language

Transient language deficits lasting several days to weeks may occur in as many as 20% of operated patients after dominant temporal lobe resections, with a persistent anomia appearing in as many as 1–3% of patients (34, 35). Persisting deficits in word-finding abilities have been reported after dominant temporal lobectomy in some studies (26, 41) but not others (7, 21). The different word-finding outcomes of different studies may reflect crosscenter differences in surgical technique, length of follow-up, and measures of word-finding used. Although extensive data harvested from language-mapping studies have demonstrated that cortical resections that encroach upon language sites are associated with measurable deficits postoperatively (15), no randomized trial has demonstrated the increased efficacy of awake temporal lobe resection with language mapping *versus* a measured resection from the standpoint of language function postoperatively.

Memory

Global memory deficits after temporal lobe resection, although dramatic and disabling, are fortunately quite rare, perhaps as a reflection of careful preoperative neuropsychologic evaluations, including the Wada test, that identify patients at risk for these deficits (29, 31, 34, 35).

In contrast, measurable short-term verbal memory deficits after dominant temporal lobe resection may occur more frequently (31, 34, 35). Although these deficits are often subtle, they are increasingly recognized as a potential source of morbidity (31). In the recent follow-up study of Sperling et al., a trend toward deterioration in measures of short-term verbal memory after dominant resections was documented (40). In another study, statistically meaningful declines in verbal memory in 20% of dominant temporal lobe resections were reported (6). The actual morbidity represented by this deterioration in verbal memory performance, in terms of day-to-day function and QOL, has not yet been addressed. In our clinical experience, when seizure improvement was achieved postoperatively, all patients interviewed felt that the loss of verbal memory was worth the trade-off. Recent data suggest that patients with high verbal memory scores preoperatively are particularly vulnerable to postoperative verbal memory impairment (19, 31). Although ipsilateral material-specific memory functions may decline postoperatively, there may also be a contralateral improvement, particularly when seizure freedom is obtained (31).

Postoperative Employment Status

The 5-year follow-up study by Sperling et al. of 89 patients undergoing temporal lobe resections revealed significant postoperative improvement in employment status (40). In this study unemployment declined postoperatively from 24 to 11%. Full-time employment increased from 34% preoperatively to 63% postoperatively. Of the variables analyzed, seizure outcome was most intimately linked to employment status. At post-op year 5, 71% of seizure-free patients had full-time employment, whereas only 3% were unemployed. Of the 23 patients not seizure-free, 44% worked full time, whereas 30% were unemployed. Importantly, some improvements in vocational status took up to 6 years to occur, perhaps accounting for the more favorable outcomes in this longer-term study. Numerous earlier reports from other centers had suggested minimal improvement in employment outcome, even when seizures were improved or eliminated (1, 8, 39).

QOL in Epilepsy

In 1947 the WHO defined health as ". . . not only the absence of infirmity and disease, but also a state of physical, mental and social well-being" (20). As QOL research has burgeoned over the past several decades, numerous domains have been recommended for objective analysis in QOL assessments. These include symptoms of disease, functional status, role activities, social functioning, emotional status, cognition, sleep and rest, energy and vitality, health perceptions, and general life satisfaction (20). A number of generic health profiles have been developed for use in QOL assessments in patients suffering from various diseases or undergoing treatment. Prominent among these is the Rand Corporation 36 Item Health Survey, which consists of multiple scales designed to assess these QOL domains in a comprehensive fashion. Such generic instruments may be combined with disease-specific instruments that provide additional measures that are sensitive to specific disabilities associated with a particular illness (18, 20, 44). These disease-specific instruments facilitate the assessment of outcome of treatment of a particular disease but not across diseases.

For many years, physicians caring for patients with intractable epilepsy have recognized the adverse impact of seizures upon their patients, and concern regarding the psychosocial status of patients with TLE has been long-standing (8, 42). However, it is only recently that systematic objective analyses of the effect of seizures and their reduction by medical or surgical treatment upon QOL have been undertaken (18, 20).

The first multidimensional instrument specifically aimed at assessing elements of QOL in patients with epilepsy undergoing temporal lobe resection was the Washington Psychosocial Seizure Inventory, developed by Dodrill *et al.* in 1980 (8). This inventory emphasizes adjustment to epilepsy in the domains of family background, emotional adjustment, financial status, adjustment to seizures, medical management, and overall adjustment. Although this inventory represents an important contribution to outcome analysis, it assesses a relatively narrow range of QOL measures and is not sufficiently generic to permit QOL comparisons with other disease states (20, 24). In medically managed epileptics the impact of seizure frequency upon psychosocial profiles was recently addressed in a community study of epileptic patients in the United Kingdom (22). In this report, seizure-free patients scored higher than patients with varying degrees of seizure frequency on a battery of psychosocial measures of depression, anxiety, adverse impact of epilepsy, and unemployment.

Over the past decade, considerable efforts have been directed at developing measures that can objectively assess the impact of relief of seizures upon the QOL of surgical patients (18, 20). Inventories have been designed that incorporate both epilepsy-specific measures along with established generic health profiles that have been extensively used and validated in outcome research in other disease states. These composite profiles are exemplified by the ESI-55 (44).

The ESI-55 ("Epilepsy Surgery Inventory-55"), developed by Vickrey (44), is a self-report measure of 11 domains of health-related QOL that incorporates the Rand Corporation 36 Item Health Survey, along with 19 epilepsy-specific items. The generic Rand Corporation 36 Item Health Survey has been validated in numerous QOL studies of patients with other medical diseases; its integration into the ESI-55 facilitates comparisons of postoperative QOL improvements in TLE patients with QOL states of patients with other, unrelated medical illnesses. In a study of 170 epilepsy surgery patients, Vickrey used the ESI-55 to assess QOL in postoperative patients in relation to seizure outcome. In this study, seizure-free patients scored significantly higher than patients with auras only or with persistent seizures, suggesting that postoperative TLE seizures and auras significantly impact QOL in these patients (46).

Using the Rand 36 Item generic core of the ESI-55 survey, Vickrey contrasted the QOL of patients with hypertension, cardiac disease, and diabetes with that of postoperative TLE patients with varying degrees of seizure freedom postoperatively (45). The results showed TLE patients with persistent seizures postoperatively scored lower than those of hypertensive, cardiac, and diabetic patients in many domains. On the other hand, when seizure freedom was achieved postoperatively, TLE patients scored higher than comparison groups on the majority of ESI-55 subscales. This study documents the QOL impairment attributable to intractable TLE, as well as the favorable impact of postoperative seizure freedom to the extent that QOL in seizure-free patients exceeds that of patients with other common chronic illnesses.

ECONOMIC EVALUATIONS PERTINENT TO EPILEPSY SURGERY

Estimates of the Cost of Epilepsy

In Begley's analysis of 1990 incidence data, 300,000 persons experienced a newly recognized seizure in 1990. Of these individuals 147,000 were ultimately diagnosed with epilepsy, with 5,000 projected to be potential surgical candidates (2, 11).

Epidemiologic data, expert opinion on resource use, and representative unit cost estimates were used to estimate the lifetime cost of epilepsy from a societal perspective of all individuals diagnosed with epilepsy in 1990. In creating this model, they envisioned the natural history of all 147,000 newly diagnosed epileptic patients as falling into six prognostic groups, with groups 1–3 experiencing early remission of seizures and groups 4–6 experiencing intractable seizures. Patients with intractable epilepsy (groups 4 and 5) comprised only 6 and 8% of the total population, respectively. These two groups, however, accounted for the preponderant burden of unemployment and excess mortality experienced by all epileptics. Direct medical costs (treatment, rehabilitation, etc.) and indirect costs (productivity losses resulting from underemployment, unemployment, and excess mortality) were assigned to each of the six cohorts. Group 5, comprising patients with frequent intractable seizures (only 8% of the total population), accounted for 40% of the total direct cost and 72% of the total indirect cost of epilepsy, or a total of 1.7 billion dollars of lifetime cost. The lifetime cost of epilepsy for all epileptics diagnosed in 1990 (from a societal perspective) was estimated at 3 billion dollars. The discounted lifetime cost per patient in group 5, the group from which most surgical patients are drawn, was $138,000. This small cohort of patients, which includes most candidates for temporal lobe resection, accounts for a significant proportion of the overall lifetime cost of all individuals with newly diagnosed epilepsy (2).

Cost-Effectiveness of Epilepsy Surgery

Decision analysis modeling was used by Wiebe and colleagues at the University of Western Ontario to assess the relative cost and effectiveness of epilepsy monitoring and surgery, as compared to continued best medical management of patients with intractable TLE (49). In this analysis the costs of presurgical evaluation, temporal lobe surgery, and 35 years of postoperative care for 30 consecutive patients undergoing temporal lobe resections from 1992 to 1993 were estimated. Similarly, the discounted direct costs of medical management of patients with varying levels of seizure control for 35 years was estimated by an expert panel. Probability estimates of clinical outcomes, patient management decisions, and sequelae of treatment were provided by an exhaustive literature review and analyses by an expert panel. Using a "decision-to-treat" approach, the relative cost-effectiveness of temporal lobe surgery *versus* continued medical management was determined.

In this study, although costs were initially higher in the surgical group, the overall costs of surgery and medical management equalized at 8.5 years and at the 35-year termination of the analysis, preoperative evaluation and surgery were both less costly and more effective than best medical management.

Extensive sensitivity analyses were conducted to account for the numerous assumptions required by decision analysis methodology regarding natural history, effectiveness of alternative treatments, and costs. Only when assumptions strongly favoring medical management outcomes were used (*i.e.*, 47% seizure-free with surgery and 30% seizure-free with medical management) was surgical therapy determined to be more costly in the long run. Otherwise, surgery was always less costly and more effective (*i.e.*, the "dominant choice").

Economic evaluations of health care are distinctly affected by the "perspective" of the study (*i.e.*, societal, payer, provider) and the costs considered in the analysis (*i.e.*, "direct," "indirect," or "intangible") (9). In this analysis, only discounted direct costs of epilepsy were considered, which embrace only the actual costs of hospital and outpatient care. Indirect costs attributed to productivity losses (*i.e.*, unemployment, underemployment, excess mortality) that are considered to be particularly relevant to the disease of intractable TLE were excluded. Incorporation of these indirect costs into the analysis likely would have made the evaluation and surgery strategy even less costly in the long run.

CLINICAL NEUROSURGERY

Cost Utility Studies

Although cost-effectiveness studies such as that of Wiebe provide useful comparisons between medical and surgical treatment of intractable TLE, such studies are limited by their relatively proximal outcomes (*i.e.*, seizure control) (20). The limitations of cost-effectiveness analyses become most apparent when an outcome assessment is required that incorporates a measure of the impact of surgical treatment upon the more distal outcomes (*i.e.*, QOL) or when comparisons between unrelated health-care technologies are desired.

Comparisons of unrelated health-care technologies are facilitated when outcomes of various treatments are expressed in terms of "quality adjusted life years" (QALYs) gained as a result of health-care intervention (33). In QALY analysis, the lifetime of an individual can be considered to consist of two major components: (*a*) quantity of life in years and (*b*) quality of life, expressed for each year of life on a valuation scale of 0–1, with 0 representing death and 1.0 representing a perfect QOL for that individual. A variety of valuation scales may be used to rate the quality of each year of life (33, 43).

In Figure 4, the impact of surgical intervention and subsequent seizure freedom in a patient with intractable TLE is depicted. In this patient, as a result of seizure onset at age 10, the QOL valuation

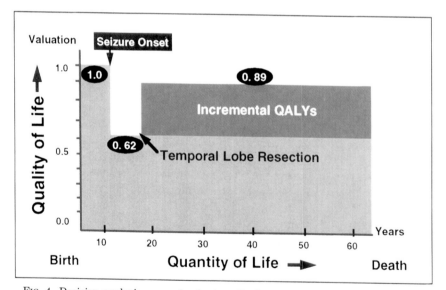

FIG. 4. Decision analysis comparing best medical management versus evaluation for temporal lobe resection in patients with intractable TLE. Probabilities of clinical events and outcomes were derived from an extensive literature review. [Adapted from (25).]

declines from 1.0 to 0.62. With successful temporal lobe resection resulting in seizure freedom, the QOL valuation increases to 0.89. If the patient lives an additional 45 years, the "incremental QALYs" resulting from treatment may be calculated. If the cost, in dollars, of the medical treatment is known, the "cost per QALY gained" may also be calculated.

Cost Utility Analysis of Temporal Lobe Resection versus Best Medical Management for Intractable TLE

To date, no cost-effectiveness studies are available comparing the competing management strategies of preoperative evaluation and surgery (EVAL/SURG) with best medical management (MEDMAN) in the United States. Furthermore, no cost-utility assessments have been attempted, although the burgeoning QOL data related to TLE and epilepsy surgery provides useful tools to derive valuation measures of QOL in various seizure states.

Langfitt, at the University of Rochester, undertook a cost-utility assessment of preoperative epilepsy monitoring and temporal lobe resection (EVAL/SURG) *versus* best medical management (MEDMAN) in Rochester, New York (25). Using a decision analysis paradigm, all conceivable clinical outcomes and associated probabilities were modeled on the basis of an extensive literature review (Fig. 5). An intention-to-treat paradigm was used in which discounted costs and seizure outcomes associated with all patients undergoing preoperative monitoring were encompassed into the surgical group (EVAL/SURG), regardless of whether or not a definitive operation was ultimately performed. Local (Rochester, NY) discounted costs were calculated for the process of preoperative evaluation and in-hospital surgery. Follow-up costs were based on estimates of lifetime use of epilepsy-related healthcare services for patients with different levels of seizure control (2), using local unit-cost estimates. Utilities for seizure outcome states in operated and nonoperated patients were estimated from mean patient scores on the ESI-55 (25, 44):

Seizure State	Quality Adjustment
Preoperative	0.62
Persisting seizure	0.72
Auras	0.81
Seizure-free	0.89

Multiplication of the expected survival in years by the quality adjustment factor for each patient in the MEDMAN and EVAL/SURG groups yielded the QALYs achieved by each group. With appropriate discounting of QALYs to adjust for the differential timing of costs and outcomes

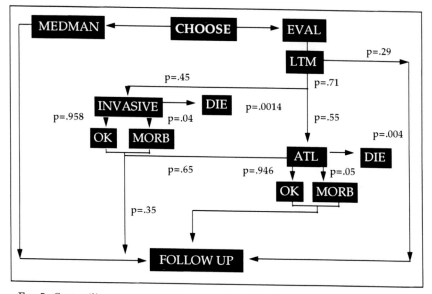

Fig. 5. Cost-utility assessment of preoperative epilepsy monitoring and temporal lobe resection (EVAL/SURG) *versus* best medical management (MEDMAN).

(25, 27, 33, 43), the cost-effectiveness ratio (CER) was calculated for each treatment arm:

$$\frac{\text{Cost (EVAL/SURG} - \text{MEDMAN)}}{\text{QALYs (EVAL/SURG} - \text{MEDMAN)}} = \$15,581 \text{ per QALY}$$

A CER of \$15,581 per QALY gained was calculated for "base case" assumptions. These assumptions may be conservative regarding effectiveness of epilepsy surgery, because they were based on older case series. This suggests that the surgical approach was more effective but also somewhat more costly than best medical management. One-way and multiway sensitivity analyses were performed to establish the range of possible outcomes and to sample "best-case" and "worst-case" scenarios. When clinical parameters of patient selection and surgical outcome were optimized, EVAL/SURG was a "dominant choice," *i.e.*, both more effective and less expensive than continued medical management.

Cost utility studies such as this one (25) produce a cost-effectiveness endpoint, which provides an attractive point of departure for critical comparisons of competing high-cost, high-technology medical interventions. Using the CER of temporal lobe resection represented by the base case assessment, anterior temporal lobe resection compares favorably with other health-care interventions available today (Fig. 6). In this era of finite health-care resources, it has been recommended that such comparisons should be used by government agencies and health-care payors in their analyses of new health-care technologies (27). Fig. 7 depicts a decision tree by which the relative value of health-care technologies may be addressed. Any new health-care technology that is more effective and less costly than existing treatments is a "dominant choice" and should be adopted immediately. A technology that is less effective and more costly should be discarded. However, the majority of new health-care technologies are somewhat more effective than existing technologies and also somewhat more costly. In this situation, it has been recommended that if the Cost/QALY is greater than $50,000, the new technology may be considered "not worth the cost" (27). It must be recognized, however, that these analyses are limited by the validity of the numerous assumptions required, including (a) discounting of cost and QALYs (b) QOL valuation scales; (c) exclusion of indirect and intangible costs of illness; (d) the "perspective" of the study (provider or societal) as well as (e) specific assumptions about medical issues such as the stability of seizure outcome (25).

Cost Effectiveness of Medical Treatment

Treatment	CER's (1995 US $/QALY)
Lifetime TB screening (every 10 years)	324,537
Post menopausal estrogen (all women)	196,363
MRI vs. CT in dx. of dementia	146,400
HDC/ABMT vs. standard chemo	113,530
TB screening (once at age 50)	79,526
Stenting vs. balloon angioplasty (CAD)	29,893
Asymp. intracranial aneurysm repair	28,441
Antibiotic Tx. in dental procedures in artificial joint patients	22,903
Early AAA repair vs. watchful waiting	20,454
ATLX vs. medical management for MIE	15,581
Post-menopausal Estrogen (severely osteoporotic women)	5,727
Pap screening in low-income elderly women	Saves $2,502 per case

FIG. 6. Cost-effectiveness ratios of various medical treatments. [Adapted from (25).]

Economic Assessment of New Technologies

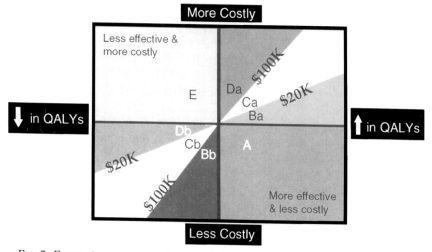

FIG. 7. Economic assessment of new technologies. [Adapted from (27).]

Economic modelling studies of preoperative evaluation and temporal lobe resection in the treatment of intractable TLE suggest that it is a relatively cost-effective use of health care resources. Prospective data are clearly needed to confirm these initial results. It is essential that all epilepsy centers begin to express the outcome of surgery in a fashion that reflects the impact of surgery not only upon seizure control but also upon the myriad neuropsychological, psychosocial, and psychiatric disabilities that encumber our patients. Ultimately, an assessment of QOL improvement and cost of treatment will be required if we are to establish the value to society of the surgical treatment of patients with TLE.

REFERENCES

1. Batzel LW, Fraser RT: Resection surgery for epilepsy: Outcome and quality of life. **Neurosurg Clin N Am:** 1993.
2. Begley CE, Annegers JF, Lairson D, *et al.*: Cost of epilepsy in the United States: A model based on incidence and prognosis. **Epilepsia** 35(6):1230–1243, 1994.
3. Berger M, Ghatau A, Haglund M, *et al.*: Low-grade gliomas associated with intractable epilepsy: Seizure outcome utilizing electrocorticography during tumor resection. **J Neurosurg** 79:62–69, 1993.
4. Cascino GD, Boon P, Fish DR: Surgically remediable lesional syndromes, in Engel J (ed): *Surgical Treatment of the Epilepsies.* New York, Raven Press, 1993, ed 2, pp 77–86.

5. Cascino GD, Kelly P, Sharbrough FW, *et al.:* Long-term follow-up of stereotactic lesionectomy in partial epilepsy: Predictive factors and EEG results. **Epilepsia** 33:639–644, 1992.

6. Chelune GJ, Naugle R, Luders H, *et al.:* Individual change following epilepsy surgery: Practice effects and base rate information. **Neuropsychology** 7:41–52, 1993.

7. Davies KG, Maxwell RE, Beniak TE: Language function after temporal lobectomy without stimulation mapping of cortical function. **Epilepsia** 36:130–136, 1995.

8. Dodrill CB, Batzel LW, Fraser R: *Psychosocial Changes after Surgery for Epilepsy,* in Kyders G (ed): *Epilepsy Surgery.* New York, Raven Press, 1991; pp 661–668.

9. Drummond MF, Stoddart GL, Torrance GW: *Methods for the Economic Evaluation of Health Care Programs.* New York, Oxford Press, 1997.

10. Elwes RDC, Dunn G, Binnie CD, *et al.:* Outcome following resective surgery for temporal lobe epilepsy: A prospective follow-up study of 102 consecutive cases. **J Neurol Neurosurg Psychiatry** 54:949, 1991.

11. Engel J: Current concepts: Surgery for seizures. **N Engl J Med** 334(10):647–648, 1996.

12. Engel J, VanNess P, Rasmussen T, *et al.:* Outcome with respect to epileptic seizures, in Engel J (ed): *Surgical Treatment of the Epilepsies.* New York, Raven Press, 1993, ed 2.

13. Fried I: Anatomic temporal lobe resections for temporal lobe epilepsy. **Neurosurg Clin N Am** 4(2):233–242, 1993.

14. Fried I, Cascino GD: Lesional surgery, in *Surgical Treatment of the Epilepsies.* New York, Raven Press, 1993, ed 2, pp 501–509.

15. Haglund MM, Ojemann G: Extratemporal resective surgery for epilepsy. **Neurosurg Clin N Am** 4(2):283–292, 1993.

16. Haglund MM, Ojemann LM: Seizure outcome in patients undergoing temporal lobe resections for epilepsy. **Neurosurg Clin N Am** 4(2):337–344, 1993.

17. Hauser WA, Annegers JF, Elveback LR: Mortality in patients with epilepsy. **Epilepsia** 21:399–412, 1980.

18. Hays RD, Vickrey BG, Engel J: Postscript: Epilepsy surgery outcome assessment, in Engel J (ed): *Surgical Treatment of the Epilepsies.* New York, Raven Press, 1993, ed 2, pp 685–688.

19. Helmstaedter C, Elgen C: Cognitive consequences of two-thirds anterior temporal lobectomy on verbal memory in 144 patients: A three month follow-up study. **Epilepsia** 37:171–180, 1996.

20. Hermann BP: Quality of life in epilepsy. **J Epilepsy** 5(3):153–165, 1992.

21. Hermann BP, Wyler AR, Somes G: Language function following anterior temporal lobectomy. **J Neurosurg** 74:560–566, 1991.

22. Jacoby A, *et al.:* The clinical course of epilepsy and its psychosocial correlates: Findings from a U.K. community study. **Epilepsia** 37(2):148–161, 1996.

23. Jooma Y, Privitera G: Lesionectomy versus electrophysiologically guided resection for temporal lobe tumors manifesting with complex partial seizures. **J Neurosurg** 83:231–236, 1995.

24. Langfitt JT: Comparison of psychometric characteristics of three quality of life measures in intractable epilepsy. **Qual Life Res** 4:101–114, 1995.

25. Langfitt JT: Cost-effectiveness of anterotemporal lobectomy for medically-intractable complex partial epilepsy. *Epilepsia,* in press, 1997.
26. Langfitt JT, Rausch R: Word-finding deficits persist after left anterotemporal lobectomy. **Arch Neurol** 53:72–76, 1996.
27. Laupacis L, Feeny D, Detsky, *et al.*: How attractive does a new technology have to be to warrant adoption and utilization? Tentative guidelines for using clinical and economic evaluation. **Can Med Assoc J** 146:473–481, 1992.
28. Mathern G, Babb T, Pretorius J, *et al.*: The pathophysiologic relationships between lesion pathology, intracranial Ictal EEG onsets, and hippocampal neuron losses in temporal lobe epilepsy. **Epilepsy Res** 21:133–147, 1995.
29. Milner B: Psychological aspects of focal epilepsy and its neurosurgical management. **Adv Neurol** 8:299, 1975.
30. Moore J, Cascino G, Trenerrary M, *et al.*: A comparative study of lesionectomy versus corticectomy in patients with TLE. **J Epilepsy** 6:239–242, 1993.
31. Naugle RI: Neuropsychological effects of surgery of epilepsy, in Luders H (ed): *Epilepsy Surgery.* New York, Raven Press, 1992, pp 637–646.
32. NIH Consensus Development Conference Statement: Surgery for epilepsy, March 19–21, 1990. **Epilepsia** 31:806–812, 1990.
33. Nord E: Methods for quality adjustment of life years. **Soc Sci Med** 34(5):559–569, 1992.
34. Pilcher WH, Ojemann GA: Surgical evaluation and treatment of epilepsy in brain surgery: Complication avoidance and management, in *Surgical Evaluation and Treatment of Epilepsy.* New York, Churchill Livingston, 1993.
35. Pilcher WH, Roberts D, Flanigin H, *et al.*: Complications of epilepsy surgery. **Surg Treatment Epilepsies** 48:565–581, 1993.
36. Pilcher WH, Silbergeld D, Berger M, *et al.*: Intraoperative electrocorticography during tumor resection: Impact on seizure outcome in patients with gangliogliomas. **J Neurosurg** 78:891–902, 1993.
37. Primrose CD, Ojemann GA: Outcome of resection surgery for temporal lobe epilepsy, in *Epilepsy Surgery.* New York, Raven Press, 1991.
38. Spencer DD, Spencer SS, Mattson RH, *et al.*: Intracerebral masses in patients with intractable partial epilepsy. **Neurology** 34:432–436, 1984.
39. Spencer SS: Long-term outcome after epilepsy surgery. **Epilepsia** 37(9):807–813, 1996.
40. Sperling MR, O'Connor MJ, Syakin A, *et al.*: Temporal lobectomy for refractory epilepsy. **JAMA** 276(6):470–475, 1996.
41. Stafniak P, Saykin AJ, Sperling MR, *et al.*: Acute naming deficits following dominant temporal lobectomy: Prediction by age at 1st risk for seizures. **Neurology** 40:1509–1512, 1990.
42. Taylor DC: Psychiatric and social issues in measuring the input and output of epilepsy surgery, in Engel J (ed). **Surgical Treatment of the Epilepsies.** New York, Raven Press, pp 485–503.
43. Torrance GW: Utility approach to measuring health-related quality of life. **J Chron Dis** 40(6):593–600, 1987.
44. Vickrey BG, *et al.*: A health-related quality of life instrument for patients evaluated for epilepsy surgery. **Med Care** 30(4):299–317, 1992.

45. Vickrey BG, *et al.*: Quality of life of epilepsy surgery patients as compared with outpatients with hypertension, diabetes, heart disease, and/or depressive symptoms. **Epilepsia** 35(3):597–607, 1994.

46. Vickrey BG, *et al.*: Outcomes in 248 patients who had diagnostic evaluations for epilepsy surgery. **Lancet** 346:1445–1449, 1995.

47. Walczak TS, *et al.*: Anterior temporal lobectomy for complex partial seizures: Evaluation, results and long-term follow-up in 100 cases. **Neurology** 40:413–418, 1990.

48. Weber J, Silbergeld D, Winn R: Surgical resection of epileptogenic cortex associated with structural lesions. **Neurosurg Clin N Am** 4(2):327–336, 1993.

49. Wiebe S, Gafni A, Blume WT, *et al.*: An economic evaluation of surgery for temporal lobe epilepsy. **J Epilepsy** 8:227–235, 1995.

50. Wieser HG, *et al.*: Surgically remediable temporal lobe syndromes, in Engel J (ed): *Surgical Treatment of the Epilepsies*. New York, Raven Press, 1993, ed 2.

24

Analysis of Outcome in Carotid Endarterectomy Trials

MARC R. MAYBERG, M.D.

Clinical trials have achieved a growing role in the contemporary practice of medicine, due in part to the advent of improved methodology for multicenter studies, increasing public awareness of clinical trials, the role of clinical trials in determining reimbursement policies, and a general consensus in the medical community that any treatment administered should be proven effective according to rigorous scientific criteria. More recently, emphasis has been placed on the need to document the efficacy of surgical procedures through clinical trials.

The effect of clinical trials on clinical practice has been especially notable in the field of cerebrovascular surgery. The ECIC Bypass trial (9) introduced the concept of multicenter prospective randomized trials to the neurosurgical community. The widespread recognition of this trial and its consequences led in part to the development of several studies designed to test the efficacy of carotid endarterectomy. With the growing emphasis on clinical trials in cerebrovascular disease, it has become important for the practicing physician to be familiar with the methodology of clinical research. In this manner, clinical decisions based on these trials will be based on a better understanding of their strengths and weaknesses. This chapter will focus on specific outcome measures used in the contemporary clinical trials for carotid endarterectomy. A significant volume of data from retrospective and prospective nonrandomized studies in cerebrovascular disease has been published; the focus of this chapter on prospective randomized trials does not discount the validity of these earlier studies. Nevertheless, prospective randomized trials have several distinct methodologic advantages in demonstrating causality, or the cause-and-effect relationship, between treatment (*e.g.,* surgery) and outcome (*e.g.,* stroke, death, *etc.*). In this regard, the validity and reproducibility of outcome measures are essential components of a rigorous clinical trial, especially because such trials have become the standard by which surgical procedures are judged and ultimately applied in clinical practice.

METHODOLOGY OF CLINICAL TRIALS

The design of clinical trials is important in determining their validity, applicability to broader populations, and ultimate clinical usefulness. A clinical trial should be designed to provide internal validity, or conclusions that are not the result of erroneous observations, as well as external validity, *i.e.*, inferences that relate observations in the study sample to broader populations. To accomplish this, the methodology should be constructed to minimize random error (because of chance occurrences) and systematic error (because of bias of some type). In addition, the study must pose a research question that is novel, relevant to clinical practice, feasible, ethical, and important. Failure to encompass one or more of these criteria can seriously limit the extent to which findings from a clinical trial may be applied to clinical practice.

Defining the Study Population

External validity for any clinical trial is determined in large part by the parameters used to define the population being studied. Inclusion criteria set forth parameters that determine the key predictive variables to be studied, *e.g.*, carotid stenosis and transient ischemic attacks as risk factors for subsequent cerebral infarction. Exclusion criteria, on the other hand, define a set of variables that might otherwise confound the analysis, *e.g.*, atrial fibrillation. These criteria define a cohort or subset of patients who are followed over time to analyze risk factors and/or describe the natural history of the condition being studied. A careful balance between inclusionary and exclusionary criteria must be determined to provide a cohort that is selective and relatively uniform, yet large enough to provide adequate sample size (see below) and general enough to be applicable to larger populations. Extreme care must be taken to ensure that the study population is not biased by undefined selection criteria. For example, the ECIC Bypass Trial (9) was widely criticized (20, 29) for including only a portion of all qualified patients at participating centers. In this study, referral bias may have produced a subset of patients with a stroke risk that was different from that of the general population. To assess this issue, most subsequent clinical trials in carotid endarterectomy have incorporated follow-up of nonrandomized qualified patients to ensure against this potential deficit.

Data Acquisition and Precision

The means by which data is collected in any clinical trial contributes to its accuracy and ultimate validity. This concept is at the core of outcomes analysis. The precision of observations is defined as the consistency of repeated measurements. Consistency is diminished by random errors from the observer, the subject, and the instrument used to gather data. Precision can be enhanced by several methods, including training the observer, blinding the observer to the treatment group, and standardizing the data collection instrument. The sensitivity of an outcome instrument is defined as the [number of positive observations/total number of true positive occurrences]; conversely, specificity is defined as the [number of negative observations/total number of true negative occurrences]. Variables can be continuous (e.g., serum glucose), discrete (e.g., number of earlier TIAs), or categorical (e.g., stroke). The precision of categorical variables can be further enhanced by using preestablished outcome scales, as discussed below.

Types of Cohort Trials

Retrospective cohort trials identify a given population and analyze the existence of potential predictive variables at an earlier time. For example, Sundt et al. (30) used retrospective analysis to define perioperative risk factors in patients undergoing carotid endarterectomy. The advantage of retrospective trials is their relative simplicity, short duration, and low cost. The major disadvantages are uncontrolled patient selection, potential bias in determining predictors, and the lack of evidence for sequential cause and effect. Although retrospective trials may compare outcome data to that derived from other trials or cross-sectional studies, conclusions are weakened by potential differences in the populations studied. Prospective cohort trials, on the other hand, define one or more predictive variables (or treatments) in a given population and measure outcomes over time. By reducing bias and controlling subject selection, true causality can be inferred with a much greater level of confidence, compared to that of retrospective trials. The disadvantages of prospective trials include complexity, duration, cost, and potential ethical concerns. The validity of prospective trials can be further enhanced by randomization, stratification, and blinding. Randomization eliminates bias from confounding variables by ensuring that treatment groups are comparable in every regard. Although certain variables may be analyzed retrospectively in prospective trials (post hoc analysis), additional validity can be obtained by stratification of subgroups (e.g., TIA versus amaurosis fugax versus completed stroke) in which separate randomization occurs for each group. Blinding of treatment to observer (single-blind) or to both patient and observer (double-blind) can reduce bias from unintended treatment or imprecision of outcome determination. In certain settings (*e.g.,* surgical procedures) blinding is difficult or impossible. The validity of outcome analysis is enhanced by maximizing the follow-up of patients entered in a prospective trial. Considerable effort must be made to follow as many patients as possible for the entire duration of the trial and to minimize crossover from one treatment group to another. Intent-to-treat analysis follows outcome in all randomized patients, regardless of whether they receive the intended treatment. This technique minimizes variability from unexpected occurrences such as crossover between groups but can produce seemingly inaccurate outcome determinations (*e.g.,* a patient randomized to carotid endarterectomy who has a stroke before surgery).

OUTCOME MEASURES IN STROKE TRIALS—OVERVIEW

As described above, the scientific rigor of any clinical trial depends in large part upon the precision, validity and general applicability of the outcome measures chosen. In most trials, outcomes are generally designated as primary or secondary. Primary outcomes are the important measures which form the basis of the trial hypothesis, *e.g.,* stroke, death, stroke-related death, *etc.* Sample size is calculated from estimates based upon predicted incidence of primary outcome events. Secondary outcomes, on the other hand, can include various measures which are potentially related to the treatment studied, (*e.g.,* surgical complications, myocardial infarction, length of stay, *etc.*) but not essential to the basic research question.

Primary Outcome Measures

Most trials for surgical treatment of cerebrovascular disease have measured ipsilateral stroke, death within a defined interval after randomization, and death resulting from stroke as primary outcomes (19). Although seemingly straightforward, these outcomes are difficult to measure with precision (21). For example, death seems to be an incontrovertible observation. However, death can result from a variety of causes that may or may not be related to the treatment, especially in a cohort with a limited life expectancy because of associated vascular and pulmonary disease. For example, in the V.A. Asymptomatic Stenosis Trial (18), nearly 30% of both medical and surgical cohorts died during the 5-year follow-up. Similarly, differentiating stroke-related death may be difficult to identify, as in the case of fatal pulmonary complications because of prolonged disability after stroke.

Stroke creates even more problems as an outcome measure, because stroke is a heterogeneous and dynamic disease process. Any analysis of stroke must encompass the severity, the presumed pathologic mechanism, the vascular distribution, the radiographic correlates, the duration of symptoms and signs, and some measure of the ultimate disability produced. The neurologic examination is inherently subjective and prone to considerable interobserver and intraobserver variability. This dilemma has led to the establishment of several stroke scales (21), each of which includes one or more of the features listed above. Stroke scales can be broadly classified as those measuring primarily (a) physical deficit, (b) functional performance, or (c) global outcome. Physical deficit stroke scales (NIH, Scandinavian, Toronto) use a standardized format to quantitate various aspects of the neurologic exam, e.g., motor, sensory, speech, or vision deficits. Disability scales (Barthel, Rankin, Glasgow Outcome), on the other hand, measure the functional ability to perform activities of daily living. Global scales (Glasgow) define outcome according to broad categories rating overall patient status. In all three types of scales, numerical assignments for each index of the scale are totaled to provide continuous (ordinal) variables, which can then be compared by statistical means.

Secondary Outcome Measures

A variety of secondary outcomes have been tabulated in carotid endarterectomy trials (19). Measurements of the carotid artery have been anatomic (angiographic stenosis) or physiologic (flow velocity). Similarly, secondary outcomes related to the brain have been both anatomic (CT/MRI) or physiologic (CBF). Several nonneurologic clinical outcome measures have been included in carotid endarterectomy trials, including a variety of medical events (myocardial infarction (MI), pulmonary insufficiency, etc.), surgical complications (hematoma, cranial nerve palsy), or nonneurologic death. Secondary outcome measures related to neurologic status have included disability, quality-of-life assessment, cognitive function, and measures of disability. Finally, several analyses have used data from carotid endarterectomy trials to measure indices of cost and cost-effectiveness, including total hospital charges, length of stay, and total direct and indirect cost of treatment.

OUTCOME MEASURES IN TRIALS FOR CAROTID ENDARTERECTOMY

Trials for Asymptomatic Carotid Stenosis

The CASANOVA Study (8) randomized patients with asymptomatic carotid stenosis (greater than 50% but less than 90%) to either immediate carotid endarterectomy ($N = 206$) or no immediate surgery, including some patients who underwent delayed surgery after developing ischemic symptoms, progressive severe stenosis, bilateral stenosis, or contralateral stenosis ($N = 204$). At 3-year follow-up, using death or new stroke as primary endpoints, there was no difference in primary outcome (ipsilateral stroke or death) between the immediate surgery group and the other group of patients (10.7 *versus* 11.3%). However, nearly one-half of the patients in the "no-immediate-surgery" group eventually did have an endarterectomy for one of the reasons stated above. The unusual study design for this trial considerably lessens its statistical validity.

The VA Asymptomatic Stenosis Trial (18, 31, 32) randomized patients with asymptomatic carotid stenosis (greater than 50%) to operative ($N = 211$) or nonoperative therapy ($N = 233$). At a mean follow-up of 4 years, the combined outcomes encompassing ipsilateral neurologic ischemic events (transient ischemic attack (TIA) and stroke) reduced the incidence for the surgical group (8%), compared to that of the medical group (20.6%) ($P < .001$). However, the sample size was not sufficiently large enough to show a statistically significant difference in stroke alone. For the outcome measure ipsilateral stroke, the incidence for the surgical group was 4.7% (including perioperative strokes) in contrast to 9.4% in the medical group ($P = .056$). However, when perioperative mortality (1.9%) was included with surgical stroke rate, the difference between the two groups was not statistically significant (Fig. 1).

The Asymptomatic Carotid Atherosclerosis Study (ACAS) trial (1) substantiated the hypothesis that carotid endarterectomy may prevent stroke in certain patients with asymptomatic carotid stenosis. Among 1662 individuals randomized with high-grade carotid stenosis (>60%

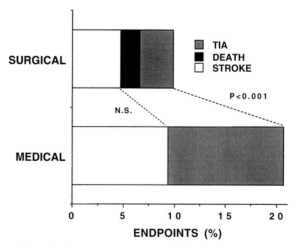

FIG. 1. Comparison of primary outcome events (TIA, death, or stroke) between surgery and nonsurgery groups in the VAAST.

diameter reduction by ultrasound and/or angiography), there was a projected overall 53% relative risk reduction in the primary outcome measure ipsilateral stroke over 5 years (mean follow-up was 2.7 years) in patients receiving carotid endarterectomy (5.1%), compared to that of unoperated patients (11.0%) (Fig. 2). Although 9% of patients were not treated according to their randomization status, the stroke risk reduction was comparable for analysis by intent to treat or actual treatment. The stroke risk reduction was more prominent in men and was apparently independent of degree of stenosis or contralateral carotid artery disease. A substantial portion of the surgical risk was attributable to angiography (a 1.2% stroke rate), and the initial risk for surgery plus angiography was offset by a constant risk of ipsilateral stroke at approximately 2.2% per year in the nonsurgical group. The surgical benefit was apparent after 10 months and was statistically significant at 3 years.

Trials for Symptomatic Stenosis

The European Carotid Surgery Trial (ECST) (11) entered patients with mild (defined as less than 30%), moderate (30–69%), or severe (70–99%) carotid stenosis, who were randomized to surgical or non-surgical treatment. Interim analysis of 2200 patients (mean follow-up = 2.7 years) led to premature termination of the trial for mild and severe stenosis groups. For mild stenosis, among 374 randomized patients there was no significant difference in ipsilateral stroke between the surgical and nonsurgical groups. There were more treat-

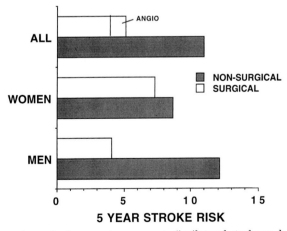

FIG. 2. Comparison of primary outcome events (ipsilateral stroke or death within 30 days) between nonsurgical and surgical patients in the ACAS trial.

ment failures in the surgery group, which was attributed to the 2.3% risk of death or disabling stroke during the first 30 days after surgery. For severe stenosis, however, surgery was shown to be beneficial in preventing stroke (Fig. 3). There was a 7.5% risk of ipsilateral stroke or death within 30 days of surgery. At 3 years of follow-up, there was an additional 2.8% risk of stroke in the surgery group (total = 10.3%), compared to 16.8% in the nonsurgery group ($P < .0001$). Importantly for the outcome measures, death or ipsilateral disabling stroke, the incidence was reduced from 11% in the nonsurgery group, compared to 6% in the surgery group. ECST used a different criterion for determining carotid stenosis than North American Symptomatic Carotid Endarterectomy Trial (NASCET), V.A. Symptomatic Stenosis (VASST), or ACAS. When re-analyzed using NASCET criteria, patients in ECST with >70% stenosis had a stroke risk and achieved benefit from surgery at rates comparable to those with NASCET or the V.A. Symptomatic Stenosis Trial (VASST). Patient entry for patients with moderate stenosis (30–69%) continues in this trial.

The North American Symptomatic Carotid Endarterectomy Trial (NASCET) (25) prematurely stopped randomizing patients with carotid stenosis greater than 70% because of the overwhelming stroke risk reduction observed in the surgical group. A total of 659 patients in this category of stenosis were randomized to surgical ($N = 331$) or nonsurgical ($N = 328$) therapy. At a mean follow-up of 24 months, the primary outcome measure ipsilateral stroke was noted in 26% of nonsurgical patients, compared to 9% of patients with endarterectomy, for

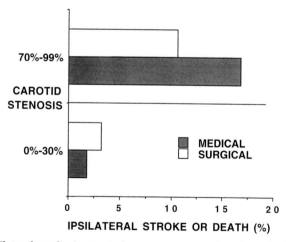

FIG. 3. Ipsilateral stroke in surgical *versus* nonsurgical patients in the ECST for low-grade (<30%) and high-grade (>70–99%) carotid stenosis.

an overall risk reduction of 17% (relative risk reduction = 71%). The benefit for surgical patients was highly significant ($P < .001$) for a variety of outcome measures, including stroke in any territory, major strokes and major stroke or death from any cause (Fig. 4). A perioperative morbidity/mortality of 5.8% was rapidly surpassed in the nonsurgical group, such that surgical benefit was apparent at 3 months. In addition, the protective effect of surgery was durable over time, with few strokes noted in the endarterectomy group beyond the perioperative period. The secondary outcome functional disability (assessed by a standardized disability scale) was significantly less in the surgery group over time ($P < .001$) (17). Multivariate analysis demonstrated that surgical benefit was independent of a variety of concurrent demographic variables such as age, sex, or risk factors for stroke. There was a direct correlation between surgical benefit and the degree of angiographic stenosis. NASCET continues to randomize symptomatic patients with carotid stenosis 30 to 69%; the benefit of carotid endarterectomy in this group of patients remains indeterminate.

Enrollment in the VASST was discontinued in early 1991 based on preliminary data consistent with the NASCET findings. Subsequent analysis demonstrated a statistically significant reduction in the primary outcome measures ipsilateral stroke or crescendo TIA for patients with carotid stenosis >50% (22). A total of 193 men (ages 35 to 82 years, mean = 64.2 years) were randomized to surgical ($N = 91$) or nonsurgical ($N = 98$) treatment. The complication rate of cerebral angiography was low, with no permanent residual deficits and transient complications in 5% (2% local vascular, 2% transient neurologic, and 1% minor allergic). Two-thirds of randomized patients demon-

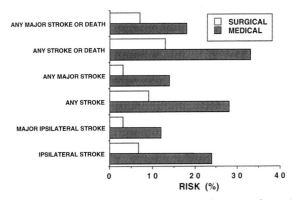

FIG. 4. Treatment failure in surgical *versus* nonsurgical patients for various outcomes in patients with >70% carotid stenosis in the NASCET.

strated angiographic internal carotid artery stenosis greater than 70%. Secondary outcome measures describing complications of surgery were relatively infrequent, including respiratory insufficiency requiring extended intensive care monitoring (5%), minor-to-moderate wound hematoma (5%), cranial nerve deficit (5%), myocardial infarction (2%), and pulmonary embolism (1%).

At a mean follow-up of 11.9 months there was a significant reduction in stroke or crescendo TIA (Fig. 5) in patients receiving carotid endarterectomy (7.7%), compared to that of nonsurgical patients (19.4%), or a risk reduction of 11.7% (relative risk reduction = 60%, P = .028). Among stratified subgroups, the benefit of surgery was most prominent in TIA patients, compared to patients with TMB or stroke, although these differences were not statistically significant. The benefit for surgery was apparent as early as 2 months after randomization and persisted over the entire period of follow-up. The efficacy of carotid endarterectomy was durable with only one ipsilateral stroke beyond the 30-day perioperative period. Discounting one preoperative stroke, a perioperative morbidity of 2.2% and mortality of 3.3% (total = 5.5%) was achieved over multiple centers among relatively high-risk patients.

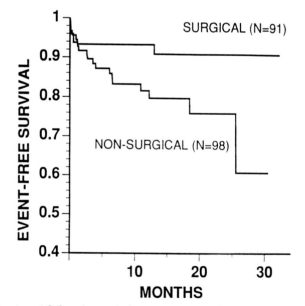

FIG. 5. Treatment failure in surgical *versus* nonsurgical patients with >50% stenosis in the VAAST. [Reproduced with permission from (22).]

COST-EFFECTIVENESS OF CAROTID ENDARTERECTOMY

Data from the ACAS (1) and VAAST (18) trials provides strong evidence that the risk of ipsilateral stroke can be lessened by endarterectomy in selected asymptomatic patients with >50–60% carotid stenosis. However, controversy remains about the external validity of these trials (23). In both studies, patients, surgeons, and institutions were selected for low surgical risk. Women were not studied in the VASST, and the surgical benefit for women was less prominent in ACAS. Nonwhites represented only 5% of patients studied in the ACAS trial. In both studies, medically treated asymptomatic carotid stenosis was associated with a relatively low annual incidence of ipsilateral stroke (approximately 2% per year), compared to that observed for symptomatic high-grade stenosis (greater than 10% per year). Using these data, 19 endarterectomies in patients with asymptomatic stenosis would be necessary to prevent one stroke, compared to 5 or 6 procedures that would be required to prevent one stroke in symptomatic patients.

On the other hand, NASCET, ECST, and VASST unequivocally showed that carotid endarterectomy reduced stroke risk, compared to medical therapy in patients with high-grade (>70%) symptomatic carotid stenosis. However, these data should also be viewed critically when selecting patients for surgery. First, a major determinant for surgical benefit in all three studies was the low surgical complication rate observed. This underscores the fact that this procedure should be done only by surgeons with experience in the operation on and low morbidity for endarterectomy. Second, the patients in these studies were carefully selected to include a highly specific cohort within well-defined clinical parameters. In a nonselected population, the benefit of surgery in reducing stroke risk is less predictable. Finally, although there is clear benefit of carotid endarterectomy in patients with severe carotid stenosis, the fate of symptomatic patients with moderate carotid stenosis has not been resolved. NASCET and ECST continue to randomize patients with 30 to 70% stenosis.

Several features common to the symptomatic stenosis trials can be generalized to broader medical populations. First, carotid endarterectomy provided a profound protection against subsequent ipsilateral stroke or crescendo TIA in patients with high-grade symptomatic stenosis. The stroke risk reduction was realized early after surgery, persisted over extended periods of time, and was independent of other risk factors. Second, stroke in the nonsurgical group considerably exceeded those reported from earlier prospective and retrospective studies. Symptomatic patients receiving aspirin in earlier prospective multicenter trials had annual stroke rates ranging from 3 to 7% (3, 6, 7), compared to rates between 15 and 20% in unoperated patients from NASCET and VASST. Third, the inaccuracy of carotid duplex ultrasonography noted in both NASCET and VASST (see below) suggested that symptomatic patients with intermediate degrees of stenosis, as indicated by duplex ultrasonography, should have definitive assessment by angiography before determination of therapy.

SECONDARY OUTCOME MEASURES IN ENDARTERECTOMY TRIALS

Following publication of the three major trials for symptomatic carotid stenosis, a number of post hoc analyses have been performed. These reports provide additional data regarding accuracy of diagnostic measures for carotid stenosis and specific clinical factors that increase stroke risk in patients with symptomatic carotid stenosis.

Accuracy of Diagnostic Measures

Angiograms from the NASCET trial were examined by three groups of observers to test the accuracy of subjective assessments of stenosis (mild, moderate, severe, or occluded) against measured stenosis. Using a 70% stenosis cutpoint, the sensitivity among groups was 84–95% and specificity was 78–88% (26). Bruits were a relatively poor predictor of high-grade stenosis in NASCET patients, with a sensitivity of 63% and a specificity of 61% (26). Similarly, ulcers documented at surgery were poorly detected by angiography (sensitivity = 46%, specificity = 74%) (28). Two studies examined the accuracy of Doppler noninvasive testing, compared to that of angiography. In NASCET, for a 70% stenosis cutpoint, the specificity was 60% and the sensitivity was 88% (16). In VASST, duplex sensitivity compared to angiography varied from 24% in the 30–49% range to 71% for 50–79% stenosis and 91% for occlusion. Using a cutpoint of 50% stenosis, duplex sensitivity was 90%, and specificity was 76%; the degree of stenosis was underestimated in nearly one-half of patients with moderate (30–49%) stenosis (27). A meta-analysis (5) showed that duplex, Doppler, and magnetic resonance angiography have equivalent sensitivity (82–86%) and specificity (89–94%) for detecting high-grade carotid stenosis. These data are in contradistinction to single-center retrospective analyses showing much greater duplex accuracy (15) and point out the important differences observed in retrospective, compared to prospective, studies.

Other Risk Factors for Stroke

Subgroup analysis for ECST and VASST was limited by relatively small patient samples. For NASCET, however, a number of factors were identified in nonsurgical patients that contributed to stroke risk.

Angiographic ulceration nearly doubled the stroke risk for patients with high-grade (>70%) stenosis (10). These data must be interpreted in light of the poor accuracy of angiography for detecting ulcers (above) (28). Hemispheric ischemia (stroke or TIA) produced a stroke risk three times higher than that observed for amaurosis fugax (4). Although increased age was associated with higher stroke risk, surgery provided benefit independent of age. Contralateral carotid occlusion was a strong risk factor for stroke; contralateral stenosis was not (4). Evidence of earlier asymptomatic stroke demonstrated by means of CT scan also increased stroke risk (4). Carotid endarterectomy was uniformly beneficial in reducing stroke risk independent of these associated risk factors. Sundt et al. (30) previously established a scale for estimating surgical risk for endarterectomy based on preoperative medical and radiographic risk factors. A retrospective meta-analysis of surgical risk at 12 academic medical centers identified the following factors as significant: ipsilateral carotid occlusion or siphon stenosis, intraluminal thrombus, or age (increased myocardial infarction but not stroke) (14). On the other hand, degree of carotid stenosis or ulcers, symptom type, sex, race, cardiac history, and contralateral stenosis were not associated with increased surgical risk. Timing of surgery in patients with completed stroke in NASCET did not affect surgical risk (13). In combination, these data may allow the determination of stroke risk and surgical risk profiles based on demographic, symptomatic, and diagnostic criteria, which will identify cohorts most likely to benefit from carotid endarterectomy.

SUMMARY

The trials for carotid endarterectomy have had a major impact on the practice of medicine. Beyond demonstrating the efficacy of this procedure for stroke prevention in certain patient cohorts, these studies have set a standard for the evaluation of surgical procedures by carefully planned, scientifically rigorous, prospective randomized controlled trials. In addition, data from these trials have been used to develop clinical guidelines (2, 12, 24), determine reimbursement policies, and establish criteria for perioperative morbidity. Concordance of methodology (especially primary outcome measures) among the various trials has enabled important valid comparisons between different patient cohorts. The benefit provided by carotid endarterectomy in most trials was so profound that the relative imprecision of stroke-related outcome measures did not significantly affect the findings. New outcome measures for stroke that evolved during these studies are being applied to ongoing trials for a variety of stroke therapies (21).

REFERENCES

1. Asymptomatic Carotid Atherosclerosis Study, Executive Committee: Endarterectomy for asymptomatic carotid artery stenosis. **JAMA** 273:1421–1428, 1995.
2. Adams HP Jr, Brott GH, Crowell RM, et al.: Guidelines for the management of patients with acute ischemic stroke. **Circulation** 90:1588–1601, 1994.
3. Barnett HJM: A randomized trial of aspirin and sulfinpyrazone in threatened stroke. **N Engl J Med** 299:53–59, 1978.
4. Barnett HJM: Status report on the North American Symptomatic Carotid Surgery trial. **J Mal Vasc** 18:202–208, 1993.
5. Blakeley DD, Oddone Z, Hasselblad V, et al.: Noninvasive carotid artery testing: A meta-analytic review. **Ann Intern Med** 122:360–367, 1995.
6. Bousser MG, Eschwege E, Hagvenau M, et al.: "AICLA" controlled aspirin and dipyridimole in the secondary prevention of atherothrombotic cerebral ischemia. **Stroke** 14:5–14, 1983.
7. Candelise L, Landi G, et al.: A randomized trial of aspirin and sulfinpyrazone in patients with TIA. **Stroke** 13:175–179, 1982.
8. CASANOVA Study Group: Carotid surgery versus medical therapy in asymptomatic carotid stenosis. **Stroke** 22:1229–1235, 1991.
9. The ECIC Bypass Study Group: Failure of extracranial-intracranial arterial bypass to reduce the risk of ischemic stroke: Results of an international randomized trial. **N Engl J Med** 313:1191–1200, 1985.
10. Eliasziw M, Streifler JY, Fox AJ, et al.: Significance of plaque ulceration in symptomatic patients with high-grade carotid stenosis: North American Symptomatic Carotid Endarterectomy Trial. **Stroke** 25:304–308, 1994.
11. European Carotid Surgery Trialists' Collaborative Group: European Carotid Surgery Trial: Interim results for symptomatic patients with severe (70–99%) or with mild (0–29%) carotid stenosis. **Lancet** 337:1235–1243, 1991.
12. Feinberg WM, Albers GW, Barnett HJM, et al.: Guidelines for the management of transient ischemic attacks. **Stroke** 25:1320–1335, 1994.
13. Gasecki AP, Ferguson GG, Eliasziw M, et al.: Early endarterectomy for severe carotid artery stenosis after a nondisabling stroke: Results from the North American Symptomatic Carotid Endarterectomy Trial. **J Vasc Surg** 20:288–295, 1994.
14. Goldstein LB, McCrory DC, Landsman PB, et al.: Multicenter review of preoperative risk factors for carotid endarterectomy in patients with ipsilateral symptoms. **Stroke** 25:1116–1121, 1994.
15. Hames TK, Ratliff DA, Humphries KN, et al.: The accuracy of duplex scanning in the evaluation of early carotid disease. **Ultrasound Med Biol** 11:819–825, 1985.
16. Haynes RB, Taylor DW, Sackett DL, et al.: Poor performance of Doppler in detecting high-grade carotid stenosis. **Clin Res** 40:184A, 1992.
17. Haynes RB, Taylor DW, Sackett DL, et al.: Prevention of functional impairment by endarterectomy for symptomatic high-grade carotid stenosis: North American Symptomatic Carotid Endarterectomy Trial Collaborators. **JAMA** 271:1256–1259, 1994.
18. Hobson R, Weiss D, Fields W, et al.: Efficacy of carotid endarterectomy for asymptomatic carotid stenosis. **N Engl J Med** 328:221–227, 1993.

19. Howard VJ, Toole JF, Grizzle J, et al.: Comparison of multicenter study designs for investigation of the efficacy of carotid endarterectomy. **Stroke** 23:583–593, 1992.

20. Langfitt T, Goldring S, Zervas N: The extracranial-intracranial bypass study: A report of the committee appointed by the American Association of Neurologic Surgeons to examine the study. **N Engl J Med** 316:817–820, 1987.

21. Lyden PD, Gabriel TL: A critical appraisal of stroke evaluation and rating scales. **Stroke** 22:1345–1352, 1991.

22. Mayberg MR, Wilson SE, Yatsu F, et al.: Carotid endarterectomy and prevention of cerebral ischemia from symptomatic carotid stenosis. **JAMA** 266:3289–3294, 1991.

23. Mayberg MR, Winn HR: Carotid endarterectomy for asymptomatic stenosis: Controversy resolved. **JAMA** 273:1459–1461, 1995.

24. Moore WS, Barnett HJ, Beebe HG, et al.: Guidelines for carotid endarterectomy: A multidisciplinary consensus statement from the Ad Hoc Committee, American Heart Association. **Stroke** 26:188–201, 1995.

25. North American Symptomatic Carotid Endarterectomy Trial Collaborators: Beneficial effect of carotid endarterectomy in symptomatic patients with high-grade stenosis. **N Engl J Med** 325:445–453, 1991.

26. Sauv'e JS, Thorpe KE, Sackett DL, et al.: Can bruits distinguish high-grade from moderate symptomatic carotid stenosis? The North American Symptomatic Carotid Endarterectomy Trial. **Ann Intern Med** 120:633–637, 1994.

27. Srinivasan J, Weiss D, Mayberg MR: Duplex accuracy compared to angiography in the Veterans Affairs Cooperative Studies Trial for symptomatic carotid stenosis. **Neurosurgery** 36:648–655, 1995.

28. Streifler JY, Eliasziw M, Fow AJ, et al.: Angiographic detection of carotid plaque ulceration: Comparison with surgical observations in a multicenter study. North American Symptomatic Carotid Endarterectomy Trial. **Stroke** 25:1130–1132.

29. Sundt TM Jr: Was the international randomized trial of extracranial-intracranial arterial bypass representative of the population at risk? **N Engl J Med** 316:814–816, 1987.

30. Sundt TM Jr, Sandok BA, Whisnant JP: Carotid endarterectomy: Complications and preoperative assessment of risk. **Mayo Clin Proc** 50:301–306, 1975.

31. Towne JB, Weiss DG, Hobson RW: First phase report of cooperative Veterans Administration Asymptomatic Carotid Stenosis Study—Operative morbidity and mortality. **J Vasc Surg** 11:252–259, 1990.

32. Veterans Administration Cooperative Study: Role of carotid endarterectomy in asymptomatic carotid stenosis. **Stroke** 17:534–539, 1986.

25

Outcomes Analysis: Intracranial Pressure Monitoring

JACK E. WILBERGER, JR., M.D.

Surgery and its microcosm of neurosurgery have been uniquely ineffective in translating its ever-expanding knowledge of anatomy and pathophysiology into surgical treatments that can be proven definitively to positively affect the outcome of the disease process in question.

Whether we agree or not, however, neurosurgery is increasingly called on to prove the value of our interventions. As cogently argued by Spencer Vibbert in his book, *What Works?* (26):

> The terms of the debate about outcomes and guidelines are becoming clear. Those opposed, say the United States is rushing to impose an unproven system and perhaps also an unnecessary burden on physicians and hospitals just because there is political pressure to do something— anything—about the health care crisis. Those in favor maintain that the reason we are in that crisis in the first place is that we have paid untold millions of dollars in exchange for unnecessary—perhaps even harmful—medical tests, treatments, and procedures. Meanwhile, the question that started the whole controversy is in danger of being forgotten.
>
> The question is a simple one: What works?

Typically, we will witness the introduction of a new neurosurgical procedure or treatment concept—oftentimes accompanied by great fanfare and advocacy—which in many cases may be based on sound, anatomic, and pathophysiologic principles. The procedure or treatment may be widely adopted and performed with little or no previous controlled clinical studies. A large number of anecdotal case series are then accumulated—some of which are reported in the literature and many of which are accepted by practitioners at face value. Occasionally, an investigator will attempt to critically evaluate the procedure/ treatment through a controlled clinical trial. However, the obstacles to doing so are oftentimes insurmountable—funding, adequate patient number for the sample size, ethical concerns—and the procedure/ treatment becomes ingrained in our neurosurgical textbooks and patient care armamentarium, with its validity and appropriateness rarely, if ever, questioned again (1, 24).

The field of neurotrauma is no better and no worse than any other area of neurosurgery in determining what works. The development of the *Guidelines for the Management of Severe Head Injury* by the Joint Section on Neurotrauma and Critical Care has uniquely brought to our attention that there is little (if any) scientific evidence to support some of the most strongly held principles we advocate (8). The entire document contains only three standards: procedures or interventions that have been demonstrated to have benefit (or lack thereof) in prospective randomized controlled trials in improving outcome and procedures that should be followed in the treatment of all patients. The remaining 34 guidelines and options are only slightly better than the expert opinions ingrained in our textbooks for decades.

One particular issue in neurotrauma management uniquely highlights the problem of how to determine if what we do works—intracranial pressure (ICP) monitoring.

ICP MONITORING OVERVIEW

Even though ICP monitoring was introduced by Lundberg in the 1960s, the debate over its value did not begin in earnest until several decades later with the publications of the Traumatic Coma Databank (TCDB) (13–15, 23). In the first coordinated effort to describe the demographics, treatment, and outcome from severe head injury (HI), the TCDB reported a 36% overall mortality, compared to that of the best of earlier studies with 50% mortalities. Because the percentage of time ICP was more than 20 mm Hg was one of the strongest predictors of outcome, the concept of ICP monitoring became entrenched—albeit primarily in academic centers.

Recent studies on the effect of cerebral perfusion pressure (CPP) management have served to heighten the debate. Because CPP = mean blood pressure − ICP and the occurrence of significant hypotension has been associated with as much as a 50% increase in mortality, the need for ICP monitoring becomes essential to ensure adequate cerebral perfusion and thereby optimize outcome (3, 11). It has thus become the consensus of expert opinion and the textbook "standard" that ICP monitoring is necessary in the management of severe HI (5). However, a recent study of trauma centers would suggest that this is not a "standard" in the daily practice of neurotrauma. Ghajar et al. surveyed 219 trauma centers, finding ICP monitoring routinely used in only 35%, whereas 7% never used monitoring in the overall management of severe HI.

To date, there has been no prospective randomized trial of the impact of ICP monitoring on outcome. Many are convinced that such an undertaking may not be ethical. Others would argue that the heterogeneity and pathophysiology of HI preclude our ability to focus on any single therapeutic intervention with clarity sufficient to definitively determine its impact on outcome. Recent experience in randomized controlled pharmacologic trials tend to support this argument. However, purely from a scientific standpoint, to prove that mortality is decreased by 10% by ICP monitoring with a statistical significance at the $P < .05$ level would require at least 349 patients in each treatment arm.

OUTCOME ANALYSIS: PROCESS

In outcomes analysis, it is essential that the available scientific literature support the validity of the proposed intervention on improving outcome. Thus, in the context of the current discussion, is there sufficient evidence to support the use of ICP monitoring per se for its impact on outcome? This question is complicated by the associated, but separate, issue of the correlation between elevated ICP and outcome.

For this review, a MedLine search for the last 20 years was carried out, using the following key terms and their various combinations: cerebral perfusion pressure, head injury, intracranial pressure, intracranial hypertension, intracranial pressure monitoring, outcome. A total of 1051 articles were cited on MedLine. Ultimately, 41 articles with clinical relevance to the issue at hand were thoroughly evaluated. The protocol for the development of the *Guidelines for the Management of Severe Head Injury* was used to classify the strength of these publications. Class I evidence involved prospective randomized controlled trials; class II evidence included clinical studies in which the data were collected prospectively and retrospective analyses that were based on reliable data; observational studies, cohort studies, and prevalence studies, as well as case control studies, were also included in this category. With class III evidence, most studies were based on retrospectively collected data; this includes clinical series, databases, registries, case reviews, case reports, and expert opinion (8).

The effect of an intervention on positively improving outcome is most clearly supported by class I evidence. However, strong class II evidence may likewise support the benefit of an intervention, especially if the issue does not lend itself to a prospective, randomized, controlled clinical trial.

SCIENTIFIC LITERATURE ON ICP AND OUTCOME

A clear correlation between the level of intracranial hypertension and poor outcome has been claimed by a number of investigators (Table 1).

One has to keep in mind, however, that the information from most of these studies is not purely observational. Treatment of intracranial hypertension has gone hand in hand with its measurement.

ICP has been touted as a strong predictor of outcome. Patients with normal ICP have the best outcomes, whereas those with elevated ICP responding to therapy do less well and those with high ICPs, unresponsive to treatment, do the worst.

Early studies by Miller in 1977 and 1981 prospectively managed a group of 225 severe HI patients with a uniform protocol including ICP monitoring. Overall, 56% had a favorable recovery. Normal ICP (<20 mm Hg) was observed in 54% of these patients whereas in 40%, ICP was above that level. When ICP was normal throughout the hospital course, 74% had a favorable recovery, whereas if the ICP was raised and not reducible by aggressive medical management, mortality was 92% (16, 17).

Narayan, 10 years later, found very similar results in a group of 207 patients. When ICP was consistently normal (<20 mm Hg), favorable outcomes were seen in 72%; when elevated, but reducible, favorable outcome was reduced to 43%; and when elevated, but not reducible, mortality was 95% (18, 19).

Marmarou in his analysis of TCDB data, estimated outcome probability in any given patient related to the proportion of ICP measurements greater than 20 mm Hg (ICP > 20 mm Hg) (14). As ICP > 20 mm Hg increases, favorable outcomes become less probable while unfavorable outcomes increase in likelihood ($P < .001$) (Fig. 1).

TABLE 1
Relationship between Intracranial Hypertension and Outcome

Outcome Analysis: ICP and Outcome		
Series (yr)	n	Outcome/Mortality
Miller (II) (1977)	160	ICP < 20, 33% mortality
		ICP > 20, 75% mortality
Miller (II) (1981)	225	ICP < 20, 77% favorable
		ICP > 20, 47% favorable
Marshall (II) (1979)	100	ICP < 15, 77% favorable
Narayan (II) (1982)	207	ICP < 20, 77% favorable
		ICP > 20, controlled 43% favorable
		ICP > 20, uncontrolled 5% favorable
Marmarou (II) (1991)	428	ICP > 20, increased mortality

OUTCOME = VEG/DEAD

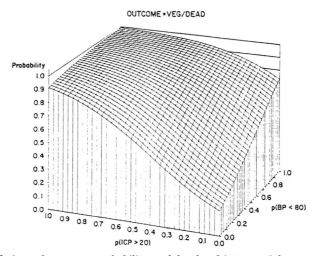

FIG. 1 Estimated outcome probability and levels of intracranial pressure. Three-dimensional surface of estimated outcome probability versus the proportion of intracranial pressure (ICP) measurements greater than 20 mm Hg (p(ICP > 20)) and the proportion of blood pressure measurements less than 80 mm Hg (p(BP < 80)) for the vegetative/dead outcome group. To simplify the presentation, the other modeled factors were fixed at the following values: age = 30 years, admission motor score = 3 (flexion), and abnormal pupils = 1. The substantial effect of hypotension is readily evident from the front-to-back upward sloping of the surface. The impact of ICP elevation is apparent from the right-to-left upward sloping of the surface.

There are several studies proposing that the empiric treatment for suspected intracranial hypertension in the absence of ICP monitoring provides for just as good outcomes while avoiding the potential complications of monitoring (Table 2).

The complications of ICP monitoring have been well-described and include infection, hemorrhage, and direct neurologic injury. Additionally, monitors may potentially provide inaccurate readings because of obstruction, malposition, or electronic malfunction. A recent review of 584 patients who had a total of 712 catheters implanted were documented as having a 10.4% incidence of ventriculitis (9).

Stuart et al. prospectively studied 100 severe HI patients in whom ICP monitoring was not undertaken, with outcomes very similar to those in a contemporary series advocating ICP monitoring (34% mortality, 49% favorable recovery). This series has primarily been criticized over potential significant patient selection bias, as the authors themselves noted that "mortality rates decreased with increasing distance of transfer and this probably represents both natural and medical selection. Many of the most severely injured do not survive long

TABLE 2
Treatment of ICP and Outcome

Outcome Analysis: ICP Monitoring/Outcome		
Series (yr)	n	Outcome
Stuart (II) (1983)	100	Empiric rx 34% mortality 46% favorable
Smith (I) (1986)	80	rx ICP > 25: 35% mortality Empiric rx: 42% mortality

enough to reach a major center and medical officers are reluctant to send a patient a long distance if the prognosis is helpless (22)."

In 1986, Smith et al. reported a prospective randomized trial of ICP-directed *versus* empiric treatment after severe HI. In one group, varying treatment was tailored to specific levels of intracranial hypertension based on data from ICP monitoring with a mortality of 35%. In the second group, empiric treatment with mannitol was undertaken without ICP monitoring, and there was a resultant 42% mortality. Thus, although there was a trend toward improved outcome in the ICP monitored group, the difference was not statistically significant. However, this study included only 40 patients per group, well below the numbers needed to judge efficacy or the lack thereof (21).

However, there are many more studies in which ICP monitoring played a central role in patient management and, thereby, improved outcome (Table 3).

A study by Saul and Ducker, while being prospective, evaluated two consecutive groups of patients using an ICP treatment threshold of 20 mm Hg in one and 15 mm Hg in the second. Mortality in the 127 patients in the former group was 46%, compared to 28% in the latter ($P < .05$). It is, however, important to keep in mind that the groups were studied in two different time periods (20).

Eisenberg's randomized trial of pentobarbital, albeit small in size, provides some of the clearest evidence that knowledge of ICP levels gained from monitoring directs appropriate treatment that does affect outcome. Patients were randomized in two treatment groups when ICP became refractory (>40 mm Hg) to all other measures: the control group ($n = 36$) and the high-dose pentobarbital group ($n = 32$). Ultimately, however, 32 of the 36 controls were crossed over into the active treatment group at certain "ICP treatment failure" levels. Of patients who responded to the barbiturates, the likelihood of survival at 1 month was 92%, compared to 17% for nonresponders. By 6-month

TABLE 3
Evidence for ICP Monitoring

Outcome Analysis: ICP Monitoring/Outcome			
Series (yr)	Treatment	n	Outcome/Mortality (%)
Saul, Ducker (II) (1982)	ICP rx > 20	127	46
	ICP rx > 15	106	28
Eisenberg (I) (1988)	Barb responders	19	10.5
	Barb nonresponders	44	86.3
TCDB (II) (1991)	TIL	428	36
Ghajar (II) (1993)	CSF drainage ICP > 15	34	12
	No monitoring	15	53

follow-up, 36% of responders and 90% of nonresponders were vegetative or dead (4).

In 1991, TCDB, using ICP monitoring as a central tenet of patient management, reported a drop in mortality rate to 36% from previously reported rates of over 45% (14, 15).

Presently, mortality rates are being seen in the 20% range. In recently reported results from the Pegorgotein study, mortality in the control group was 22% with ICP monitoring guiding medical management (25). Similarly, current advocates of CPP management—which mandates ICP monitoring—are reporting extremely favorable results. In Rosner's 1995 series of 158 patients, mortalities ranged from 52% in patients with Glasgow Coma Scores of 3–12% when the Glasgow Coma Score was 7, with an overall mortality rate of 29%. More importantly, favorable outcome ranged from 35% (GCS 3) to 75% (GCS 7). Only 2% of all the patients in the series remained vegetative, and for those patients who survived, the likelihood of having a favorable recovery was almost 80%. These results are significantly improved over those of virtually all other reported series across GSC categories in a comparison of death rates, survival-*versus*-death, or vegetative or favorable *versus* nonfavorable outcome classifications ($P < .001$) (11).

CONCLUSIONS

Thus, as can be seen, there is limited class I data and an abundance of class II data that the absolute level of ICP affects outcome and the ability to therapeutically reduce ICP improves outcome. However, does monitoring ICP per se have a direct impact on outcome? This issue remains unproven and most likely will. As noted earlier, this would require a multicenter randomized prospective trial of treatment targeted to specific ICP values in monitored patients versus empiric treatment in nonmonitored patients. The empiric treatment alone would be problematic, *i.e.*, when, if ever, would barbiturates be instituted? More than 700 patients would be required at an estimated cost of more than 5 million dollars. Indeed, such a trial was proposed to the National Institutes of Health several years ago, but funding was withheld.

There is, however, presently an ongoing randomized trial of CPP-directed management *versus* ICP-directed management in treatment of severe HI. If the CPP-directed arm were to result in superior outcomes, the necessity of ICP monitoring would be supported definitively by class I data.

Until such a time, the carefully considered ICP monitoring recommendations of the *Guidelines for the Management of Severe Head Injury* are appropriate:

> Standards—There are insufficient data to support a treatment standard for indications for intracranial pressure monitoring.
>
> Guidelines—ICP monitoring is appropriate in patients with severe head injury with an abnormal admission CT scan. Severe head injury is defined as a Glasgow Coma Score of 3–8 after cardiopulmonary resuscitation. An abnormal CT scan of the head is one that reveals hematomas, contusions, edema, or compressed basal cisterns.
>
> ICP monitoring is appropriate in patients with severe head injury with a normal CT scan when two or more of the following features are noted at admission: age over 40 years, unilateral or bilateral motor posturing, or systolic blood pressure of less than 90 mm Hg.
>
> ICP monitoring is not routinely indicated in patients with mild or moderate head injury. However, a physician may choose to monitor ICP in certain conscious patients with traumatic mass lesions.

REFERENCES

1. American Medical Association: *Office of Quality Assurance and Health Care Organizations Attributes to Guideline Development of Practice Parameters.* Chicago, American Medical Association, 1990.
2. Becker DP, Miller JD, Ward JD, *et al.:* The outcome from severe head injury with early diagnosis and intensive management. (Class II). **J Neurosurg** 47:491–502, 1977.
3. Chesnut R, Marshall LF, Klauber MR: The role of secondary brain injury in determining outcome from severe head injury. (Class III). **J Trauma** 34(2):216–222, 1993.
4. Eisenberg HM, Frankowski RF, Contant CF, *et al.:* High dose barbiturates control

elevated intracranial pressure in patients with severe head injury. (Class I). **J Neurosurg** 69:15–23, 1988.

5. Ghajar JB, Hariri R, Narayan RK, *et al.*: Survey of critical care management of comatose head injured patients in the United States. **Crit Care Med** 23:560–567, 1995.

6. Ghajar JB, Hariri RJ, Patterson RH: Improved outcome from traumatic coma using only ventricular CSF drainage for ICP control. (Class III). **Adv Neurosurg** 21:173–177, 1993.

7. Gopinath SP, Contant CF, Robertson CS, *et al.*: Critical thresholds for physiological parameters in patients with severe head injury. (Class II). Vancouver, British Columbia, Canada, Congress of Neurological Surgeons Annual Meeting, 1993.

8. *Guidelines for the Management of Severe Head Injury.* American Association of Neurological Surgeons, 1995.

9. Holloway KL, Barnes T, Choi S, *et al.*: Ventriculostomy infections: the effect of monitoring duration and catheter exchange in 584 patients. (Class II). **J Neurosurg** 85:419–424, 1996.

10. Jennette B, Teasdale G, Galbraith S, *et al.*: Severe head injury in three countries. (Class III). **J Neurol Neurosurg Psychiatry** 40:291–295, 1977.

11. Johnson AH, Rosner MJ, Rosner SD: Cerebral perfusion pressure: Management protocol and clinical results. (Class II). **J Neurosurg** 83:949–962, 1995.

12. Johnston IH, Johnston JA, Jennette WB: Intracranial pressure following head injury. (Class II). **Lancet** 2:433–436, 1970.

13. Lundberg N, Troupp H, Lorin H: Continuous recording of ventricular fluid pressure in patients with severe acute traumatic brain injury. (Class II). **J Neurosurg** 22:581–590, 1965.

14. Marmarou A, Anderson RL, Ward JD, *et al.*: Impact of ICP instability and hypotension on outcome in patients with severe head trauma. (Class II). **J Neurosurg** 75:S95–S66, 1991.

15. Marshall LF, Gautille T, Klauber MR, *et al.*: The outcome of severe closed head injury. (Class II). **J Neurosurg** 75:S28–S36, 1991.

16. Miller JD, Becker DP, Ward JD, *et al.*: Significance of intracranial hypertension in severe head injury. (Class II). **J Neurosurg** 47:503–576, 1977.

17. Miller JD, Butterworth JF, Gudeman SK, *et al.*: Further experience in the management of severe head injury. (Class II). **J Neurosurg** 54:289–299, 1981.

18. Narayan RK, Greenberg RP, Miller JD, *et al.*: Improved confidence of outcome prediction in severe head injury: A comparative analysis of the clinical examination, multimodality evoked potentials, CT scanning, and intracranial pressure. (Class II). **J Neurosurg** 54:751–762, 1981.

19. Narayan RK, Kishore PR, Becker DP, *et al.*: Intracranial pressure: To monitor or not to monitor? A review of our experience with severe head injury. (Class II). **J Neurosurg** 56:650–659, 1982.

20. Saul TG, Ducker TB: Effect of intracranial pressure monitoring and aggressive treatment on mortality in severe head injury. (Class II). **J Neurosurg** 56:498–503, 1982.

21. Smith HP, Kelly DL, McWhorter JM, *et al.*: Comparison of mannitol regimens in

patients with severe head injury undergoing intracranial pressure monitoring. (Class I). **J Neurosurg** 65:820–824, 1986.

22. Stuart GG, Merry GS, Smith JA, *et al.:* Severe head injury managed without intracranial pressure monitoring. (Class II). **J Neurosurg** 59:601–605, 1983.

23. Troupp H: Intraventricular pressure in patients with severe brain injuries. (Class II). **J Trauma** 5:373–378, 1965.

24. Woolfe SH: Practice guidelines: A new reality in medicine. **Arch Intern Med** 153:2646–2655, 1993.

25. Young B, Runge JW, Waxman KS, *et al.:* Effects of Pegorgotein on neurologic outcome of patients with severe head injury. (Class I). **JAMA** 276:538–543, 1996.

26. Vibbert S: *What Works?* Chicago, Academic Press, 1994.

IV

General Scientific Session IV Treatment Of Posterior Fossa Tumors

26

Tentorial Meningiomas

MICHAEL J. HARRISON, M.D., AND OSSAMA AL-MEFTY, M.D.

Few lesions in neurosurgery have attracted so much attention as meningiomas. Even in debilitated patients with tumors strategically situated in adverse locations, their benign histology tantalizes us with the prospect of a cure with restoration of normal neurologic function. Among meningiomas, an inordinate amount of literature has been directed toward the rarest of lesions. This is particularly true of tentorial meningiomas. Despite the fact that tumors in this location represent less than 3% of all meningiomas, their frequent involvement with dural venous sinuses, deep venous structures such as the vein of Galen and internal cerebral veins, plus the brainstem and cranial nerves, has led to interest far exceeding their rate of occurrence (8, 13, 15, 22, 31, 34, 38).

Attempts at categorizing tentorial meningiomas based solely on radiologic studies is artificial. Radiologic studies contribute invaluable information but often can not determine the site of origin for these lesions. On neuroradiologic evaluation, tumors of the free edge of the tentorium blend with lesions classified as petrous pyramid tumors, petroclival lesions, and those considered cavernous sinus meningiomas (22, 28). Even among lesions which could be classified as little else but tentorial meningiomas, neurosurgeons have segregated certain tumors such as torcular and pineal region tumors into separate categories based on unique problems attendant their surgical management (17, 19).

CLASSIFICATION

To discuss the surgical management of tentorial meningiomas appropriately, one must categorize based on their site of origin. As recognized by Aoygi and Kyuno, these lesions arise from arachnoid cell clusters within the dura (9). This site of origin is of paramount importance in determining the ease of resectability. In the modern era with advanced neuroimaging techniques, we have the capacity to visualize minute detail regarding the location and extent of these lesions. However, in the case of tentorial meningiomas, once they have reached a moderate size, they can not be distinguished from petroclival meningiomas on the basis of neuroimaging. The technical difficulties germane to each lesion are contingent on the structures the tumor abuts, engulfs, or invades. The location of the dura from which they arise will determine this. Numerous authors have attempted to lend order to these lesions by assigning a classification (5, 8, 13, 22, 32, 34, 38). The scheme we find most beneficial was proposed by Yasargil (Fig. 1) (38). In his schemata, tentorial meningiomas arise from (a) the inner ring (free edge), (b) the outer ring along the transverse sinus (occipital), or (c) the intermediate ring, which is the intervening dural surface between the inner and outer rings. Within these groups exist subcategories that influence surgical approach and potential risks. For example, an anteriorly situated tumor along the inner ring will involve the nerves controlling extraocular motions and may invade the cavernous sinus, whereas lesions situated posteriorly along the inner ring will be situated in the pineal region and will have an avid association with the basal veins of Rosenthal, the vein of Galen, and straight sinus. Likewise, tumors posteriorly situated along the outer ring will involve the torcular, whereas lesions more laterally placed will involve only the transverse sinus. Torcular meningiomas are often addressed separately from other tentorial meningiomas. Additionally, it must be noted that within this classification there will be lesions whose extension is primarily supratentorially, infratentorially, or both. Each of

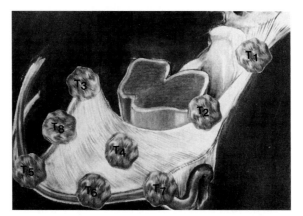

FIG. 1 Schematic classification representing the various locations for tentorial tumors. Under Yasargil's classification, T1–T3 lesions are inner ring lesions or lesions of the incisura—anterior, lateral, and posterior. T4 and T8 are intermediate ring lesions with T8 tumors involving the falcotentorial junction. T5–T7 lesions are posterior ring tumors involving the torcular, transverse sinus, and transverse-sigmoid junction respectively.

these variations on the theme will alter the flavor of the tumor and contribute variables that must be understood if successful surgery is to be undertaken.

Again, we would like to emphasize that it is difficult to distinguish tentorial meningiomas from petroclival meningiomas on the basis of neuroimaging studies once the tumors have attained a large size (Fig. 2). Yet, this distinction will play a critical role during surgical resection. Both sets of lesions appear to fill identical compartments and compress the brainstem upon expansion. It is only the rare instance of a small tumor detected early in its development in which an origin can be ascertained by radiologic examination (Fig. 3). These categories are helpful in anticipating potential pitfalls and complications and are essential in the selection of surgical approaches. Additionally, there are anatomic considerations with tumors that arise from the tentorium, segregating them from cavernous sinus and petroclival tumors and aiding in their resection. These differences will be delineated later.

SPECIAL ANATOMIC CONSIDERATIONS FOR INNER RING TUMORS

Despite their similar radiographic appearance, tentorial meningiomas differ dramatically from petroclival and sphenopetroclival meningiomas in terms of operative difficulty and surgical outcome. Upon expansion, these lesions look identical with compression of the same structures and, as previously noted, often can not be separated on the basis of preoperative imaging. Yet, at surgery, these tumors are distinctly different. The surgical difference resides in the layers of arachnoid investing the various tumors and is analogous to differences previously reported for anterior clinoidal meningiomas (1). Petroclival meningiomas originate medial to cranial nerve V. Because of this origin there will be only one arachnoid layer separating them from the brainstem. They invaginate into the prepontine cistern before contacting the brainstem (21, 37). By virtue of this anatomic relationship, there may be significant adherence to the midbrain, pons, and medulla, precluding total resection. Additionally, there may be invasion of the clival bone and erosion into the sphenoid sinus, presenting further difficulties during resection. Tentorial meningiomas on the other hand arise from the tentorial edge, where there is a convergence of the interpeduncular, crural, and ambient cisterns (Fig. 4) (21, 37). With expansion from the tentorium into the brainstem, they push multiple layers of arachnoid ahead of them. This provides a clear demarcation between tumor, brainstem, and cranial nerves. By developing a plane within these layers of arachnoid, tentorial meningiomas can often be totally resected without coming in direct contact with the brainstem.

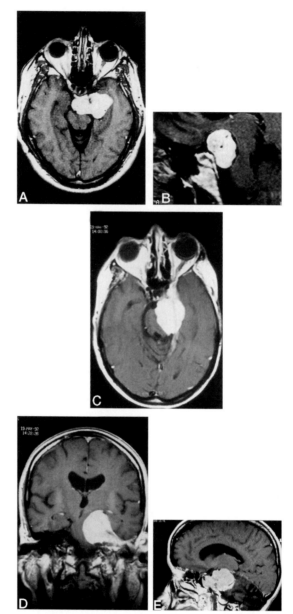

FIG. 2 Once anterior and lateral inner ring meningiomas have reached even moderate size, they cannot be distinguished from one another or from petroclival meningiomas based on preoperative neuroimaging studies. Contrast-enhanced, T1-weighted MRI in axial (**A**) and sagittal (**B**) planes of an anterior inner ring meningioma (Yasargil T1). T1-weighted, contrast-enhanced MRI in axial (**C**), coronal (**D**), and sagittal (**E**) planes, depicting a typical lateral inner ring meningioma (Yasargil T2).

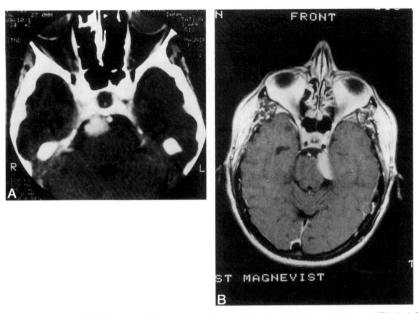

FIG. 3 (**A**) Axial CT scan with contrast of a small petroclival meningioma. (**B**) Axial MRI with contrast of a small lateral inner ring meningioma (Yasargil T2). These are rare examples of lesions detected while still small enough to determine their site of origin accurately.

At the end of resection, an intact layer of arachnoid may cover the brainstem, such that it is not visualized. This is true of both T1 and T2 lesions (anterior and lateral incisural lesions). The vital arterial structures that must be dissected from the tumor with T1 and T2 lesions include the posterior communicating, anterior choroidal, posterior cerebral, and superior cerebellar arteries. Depending on the extent of the tumor, the basal vein of Rosenthal may be involved. Cranial nerves III through VI will all be involved with tumor and must be dissected free. Depending on the extension into posterior fossa, cranial nerves VII and VIII and potentially the lower cranial nerves will abut the tumor. Still, multiple layers of arachnoid will separate the nerves from tumor and facilitate establishment of a plane for dissection and removal. Additionally, this same barrier created by arachnoid precludes invasion of bone along the clivus.

For posteriorly situated tumors along the inner ring the considerations are similar. These are referred to as T3, or pineal region, meningiomas. The arachnoid layer draping the basal veins of Rosenthal, precentral cerebellar veins, and vein of Galen is exception-

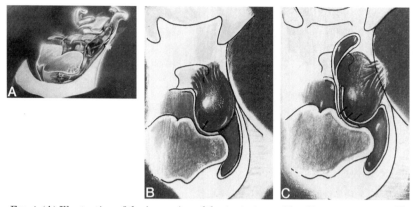

FIG. 4 (**A**) Illustration of the inner ring of the tentorium with adjacent structures. This illustration depicts the convergence of interpeduncular, ambient, and crural cisterns with their multiple overlapping layers of arachnoid (*arrow*). (**B**) When tumors arise from the petroclival region, only one layer of arachnoid separates the tumor from the brainstem, which can lead to a tumor more adherent to the brainstem and more difficult to resect (*arrow*). (**C**) When meningiomas arise from the tentorium, multiple layers of arachnoid separate the tumor from the brainstem, arteries, and nerves, providing a cleavage plane that facilitates dissection (*arrows*).

ally dense. This affords a barrier between these critical structures and the tumor, thus facilitating removal. The venous structures will be the greatest deterrent to complete removal, but the fourth cranial nerves and posterior cerebral and superior cerebellar arteries must be identified as well and preserved during dissection.

The differentiation of petroclival lesions and tentorial lesions based on these extra layers of arachnoid is a novel concept that has not been previously described. This variation in arachnoid layers has been noted during the removal of many petroclival and tentorial meningiomas. It is a distinction of paramount importance with tremendous implications for the ease of resection and can only be determined intraoperatively. This finding should stimulate surgeons to attempt and develop the arachnoid planes along the tumor interface to their maximum. In this fashion planes of cleavage between tumor, vascular, and neural structures are dissected with minimal trauma to structures essential for preservation.

CLINICAL PRESENTATION

As with all meningiomas, tentorial tumors are more common in females in middle- to older-age groups. Because of the diffuse area covered by the tentorium, coupled with the ability of these lesions to extend supratentorially, infratentorially, or both, meningiomas arising from it affect numerous structures and have protean manifestations (13, 15, 27). The most frequent signs and symptoms are nonspecific and include headaches, visual changes, and papilledema. Tumors arising along the anterior medial tentorium can compress the brainstem or engulf cranial nerves involved in facial sensation or ocular motility. Meningiomas of this region can also present with trigeminal neuralgia or tic convulsif, which is the combination of trigeminal neuralgia with hemifacial spasm (25, 35). If there is compression of the dominant temporal lobe, seizures or speech difficulties can result. Tumors in the pineal region can present with Parinaud's syndrome or hydrocephalus. We have reported the case of a pineal region meningioma that presented along with hearing loss (12). Lesions extending into the posterior fossa can present with cerebellar signs, and peritorcular lesions can compress the calcarine cortex and produce visual field deficits. Additionally, peritorcular lesions obstructing venous outflow can produce dramatic rises in intracranial pressure disproportionate to what is expected from their mass.

RADIOLOGIC EVALUATION

Radiologic studies have evolved dramatically over the last 2 decades. With the advent of computerized tomography in the early 1970s, a revolution has occurred with neuroimaging techniques. CT images still provide superior bony detail and are invaluable where tumors invade bone, but MRI with multiplanar images provides the greatest detail of soft tissues and can visualize subtleties unseen on CT scan, including edema within the brain and brainstem. This can have significant prognostic value when one is contemplating total surgical resection. If one is restricted to a single imaging modality, MRI would be the diagnostic test of choice. By altering acquisition sequences, MR angiography and venography can provide details about the involvement of arteries with tumor, the blood supply to the lesion, the position of the vein of Labbé, and the patency of the sinuses. However, where sinus patency is in question, formal angiography at present provides superior resolution (Fig. 5). Even with catheter angiography, involvement of sinus by tumor can be missed in a large percentage of studies (15, 31). Additionally, catheter angiography can provide the opportunity for embolization of meningiomas, although this is rarely done by the senior author (O. A-M.) (26).

SURGERY

Great strides have been made in the treatment of all tumors involving the nervous system as a result of advances in neuroimaging modalities, neuroanesthesia, the operative microscope, microsurgical an-

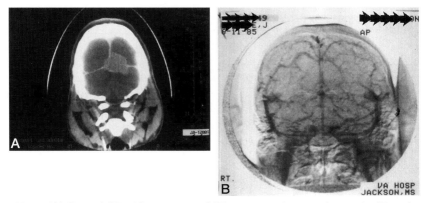

FIG. 5 (**A**) Coronal CT with contrast and (**B**) a venous-phase angiogram in AP projection of a torcular meningioma (Yasargil T5) with occlusion of the torcular.

atomic knowledge, and the routine use of microsurgical technique. These advances are also mirrored in the results seen with the management of tentorial meningiomas. Yet, much of the data in the literature must be viewed as historical (5, 8, 13, 15, 29, 30, 31). Articles appearing, for example, in 1995 and spanning a period of 30 years present patients managed in the 1960s. This was an era that predated even rudimentary computerized tomography by a decade and was in the premicrosurgical era. For example, an article on Guidetti's series of 61 tentorial meningiomas, published in 1988, covers patients who underwent surgery as early as 1951 (15). Even series reporting superb results must be analyzed with this bias. Much of what is published today in no way reflects the capabilities of the modern neurosurgeon. This is acknowledged by Sekhar in his commentary on the recently published series of tentorial meningiomas by Gokalp *et al.* (13). Samii published an article about a series in 1996 of 25 tumors involving the tentorial notch operated on in the microsurgical era (28). In that this series dealt solely with medially situated tumors against the brainstem and involved essential vascular structures and cranial nerves, a higher complication rate might well be expected than in a series including all tentorial meningiomas. However, there were no mortalities in this series; 88% underwent a Simpson grade 1 or 2 resection, and 80% of the patients on long-term follow-up have resumed normal life activities. This is more reflective of the capacity of modern neurosurgery to address these lesions.

SURGICAL INDICATIONS

The best management of patients with tentorial meningiomas is aggressive surgical resection. An asymptomatic lesion or minimally symptomatic lesion in an elderly patient must give us pause to consider the options (36). It is well-documented that meningiomas in elderly patients frequently lie dormant and do not produce additional problems. However, a patient's best and often only true chance of cure occurs at first operation. It is our belief that aggressive surgical resection with total removal of the tumor and simultaneous preservation or restoration of function must always be the objective. Modern microsurgical anatomic knowledge and surgical technique provide this ability. The only situation in which total resection may be precluded is that in which a vital patent venous sinus is involved with tumor. Only in malignant or recurrent tumors in which poor medical status precludes secondary resection would we use radiation therapy (4, 20) or consider the use of hormonal therapy (6, 14, 23) (which is still experimental) to stem expansion of the lesion.

CHOICE OF SURGICAL APPROACH

T1 and T2 Lesions (Anterior and Lateral Inner Ring Tumors)

Meningiomas of the anterior and medial incisura should be approached through a cranioorbital-zygomatic osteotomy (COZ). This approach has been previously described in detail (11). By removing the orbital rim and roof in continuity with a frontotemporal craniotomy and performing a zygomatic osteotomy, excellent exposure of these lesions is obtained while minimizing the need for retraction. The COZ provides several advantages over the pterional approach: (a) It brings deep-seated lesions closer to the surgeon, providing the shortest possible distance for dissection. (b) It creates numerous potential corridors for attacking the lesion (subfrontal, transsylvian, and subtemporal). (c) Avenues along the base of the skull intercept the vascular supply to the lesion at the onset of tumor resection, thus minimizing blood loss. (d) A single bone flap is created, thus minimizing the need for reconstruction and maximizing cosmetic results. (e) Brain retraction is minimized by the removal of this additional bone. If the tumor is larger, with significant extension into the posterior incisura or inferiorly into the posterior fossa, a petrosal approach or an extended petrosal approach including zygomatic osteotomy is included (2, 3). The superior petrosal sinus is ligated, and the tentorium is cut along the petrous bone while one guards against injury to the trochlear nerve that runs along the tentorial free margin up to its entry into the cavernous sinus. The tentorium is coagulated and cut circumferentially around the tumor to devascularize the lesion, and the tumor is internally decompressed with a suction or ultrasonic aspirator until significant room has been created for dissection of the tumor capsule from the nerves, brainstem, and vascular structures (Fig. 6).

T3 and T8 Lesions (Falcotentorial Lesions of the Pineal Region and Straight Sinus)

A low occipital craniotomy fashioned to expose the superior sagittal sinus, torcular, and transverse sinus is created. The patient is approached via a posterior interhemispheric transtentorial approach from the nondominant side and is positioned in three-quarter prone position, with the nondominant hemisphere-dependent. This position allows gravity to "retract" the occipital lobe. The vascular supply to the tumor emanates from the tentorium, which should be divided around the edge of the tumor. The tumor must then be enucleated and dissected from the venous anatomy feeding into the straight sinus. The rate-limiting factor in complete removal of these tumors is invasion of a still-patent straight sinus or avid adherence to the great veins draining into the sinus. It is mandatory that these structures be preserved. In general there will be dense arachnoid around the basal veins and vein of Galen that affords a plane of dissection along the anterior aspect of the tumor. Where these veins can not be separated

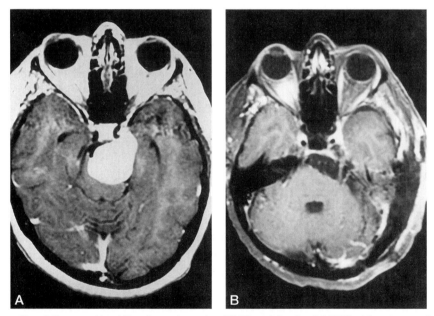

FIG. 6 Preoperative (**A**) and postoperative (**B**) T1-weighted axial MRI with contrast of an anterior inner ring meningioma (Yasargil T1), displaying total resection of the tumor.

from the tumor or the straight sinus is invaded, yet still patent, it is safest to leave residual tumor and return if the lesion becomes symptomatic or occludes the sinus (Fig. 7).

T4 Lesions (Tumors of the Intermediate Ring)

Tumors that arise from the intermediate ring of the tentorium, that do not involve the medial structures, and that do not invade the dural venous sinuses are theoretically the easiest of the tentorial meningiomas to manage. Depending on its extension supratentorially, infratentorially, or both, an occipital, suboccipital, or combination approach may be used. Where a tumor has only minimal extension into either the supratentorial or infratentorial compartment, it can be resected via an approach solely on the side of the sinus with maximum tumor. A 2-cm margin of tentorium peripheral to the tumor attachment should be resected where possible to diminish the risk of recurrence (Fig. 8) (18, 24, 33).

T5–T7 Lesions (Tumors of the Posterior Ring Affecting the Venous Sinuses)

Lesions afflicting the torcular and lateral sinuses add a very powerful variable to the equation. Tumors involving the venous sinuses must be assessed preoperatively for patency of the involved sinus and the adequacy of collateral drainage for potential sacrifice of the sinus. Adequate exposure supra- and infratentorially plus medial and lateral to the involved sinus must be obtained. As with any surgery involving vascular structures, adequate proximal and distal control is essential.

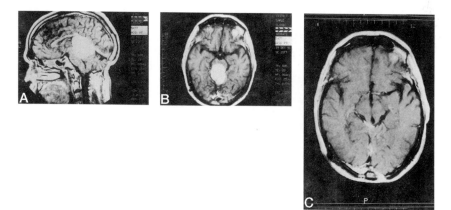

FIG. 7 Preoperative T1-weighted MRI with contrast in sagittal (**A**) and axial (**B**) projections of a pineal region meningioma (Yasargil T3) and postoperative MRI with contrast in axial plane depicting the resection (**C**).

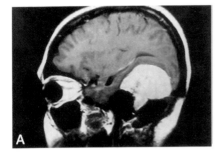

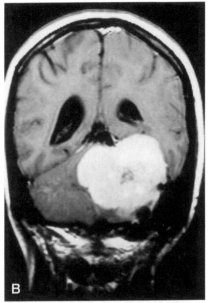

FIG. 8 Sagittal (**A**) and coronal T1-weighted MRIs (**B**) with contrast of a patient with a typical intermediate ring tentorial meningioma (Yasargil T4) with both supra- and infratentorial extension. (**C**) A postoperative axial MRI study displaying total resection.

Tumors of the torcular region require exposure of what has been referred to as all "four quadrants" (10). This includes visualization of the superior sagittal sinus, torcular Herophili, both transverse sinuses, and the occipital sinus proximal and distal to what is involved with tumor. Where tumor invades only part of one wall of a sinus, it is possible to resect the wall with simultaneous repair, using direct suture technique. Where more than one wall is involved, a decision must be made, based on preoperative radiologic studies, as to whether to sacrifice the sinus. Attempts at repair of more than one wall, as well as venous bypass grafts, have a high incidence of failure, and the risk is probably unwarranted if the sinus is essential for adequate drainage of the brain (16). An attempt at resection and bypass of a patent torcular is fraught with risk. It is our practice to leave some residual tumor in the sinus when a vital segment of sinus is involved and await future occlusion by tumor.

When total occlusion of either the torcular or lateral sinus occurs, hemodynamic changes can occur that influence surgical resection. With occlusion of the torcular, venous outflow must seek a different route, and dense venous collaterals frequently develop along the occipital cortex and in the occipital and suboccipital dura (Fig. 9). These collaterals are as essential as a patent torcular for the drainage of the brain and must be preserved. Thus, formal angiography should be undertaken for all lesions involving the torcular. Dural resection around the tumor must spare these collaterals, and adequate assessment is only available at present by catheter angiography. Where the lateral sinus has been occluded at the junction with the sigmoid sinus, another variable is introduced. Development of venous collateral drainage is usually not an issue. Instead, occlusion at this point has been reported to produce dural anteriovenous malformations (39). Without angiography this may well be missed, leading to unexpected difficulties at surgery and potentially persistent symptoms postoperatively.

COMPLICATIONS AND OUTCOME

As noted by numerous authors, the morbidity and mortality affiliated with resection of tentorial meningiomas has steadily declined over the years. Reports in the 1950s and 1960s documented mortality ranging from 20 to 29% (5, 7). Series in the 1980s and early 1990s revealed mortality of about 7–10% (8, 15, 31). Many of the complications encountered in earlier series, such as brain swelling and vascular injuries, can be directly attributed to older surgical methodologies that did not include modern skull base approaches and the lack of micro-

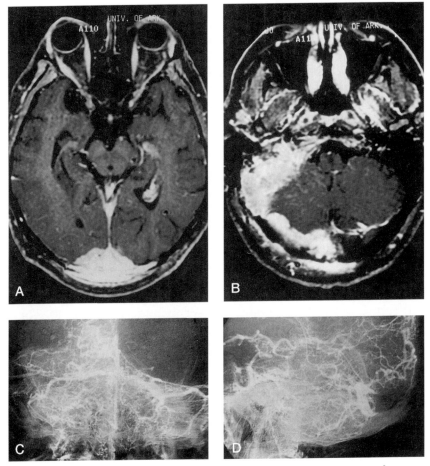

Fig. 9 (**A** and **B**) T1-weighted axial MRI examinations with contrast of a more extensive torcular meningioma with occlusion of the sinuses and venous-phase angiography in AP (**C**) and lateral projections (**D**), displaying the extensive venous collaterals that have developed after occlusion of the torcular.

surgical technique. With the use of skull base approaches that limit brain retraction, complications have steadily declined.

The two most recent series, those of Gokalp *et al.* (13) in 1995 and Samii *et al.* (28) in 1996, report a mortality of 2.7% and 0%, respectively. As noted in the introduction, the latter series is the only one in the literature in which all patients were operated on with access to computed tomography and using modern microsurgical technique. Thus, although tentorial meningiomas represent a formidable operative challenge, contemporary focus is directed toward minimizing morbidity. With universal use of microsurgical technique and increasing frequency of the application of skull base approaches to these lesions, morbidity will continue to fall. To improve results further, we must advance our microsurgical anatomic knowledge, most specifically with regard to the arachnoidal cisterns enveloping each tumor. The knowledge of arachnoid planes and the development of these planes at surgery represent the next step in eliminating morbidity during surgery for tentorial meningiomas.

REFERENCES

1. Al-Mefty O: Clinoidal meningiomas. **J Neurosurg** 73:840–849, 1990.
2. Al-Mefty O, Fox JL, Smith RR: Petrosal approach for petro-clival meningiomas. **Neurosurgery** 22:510–517, 1988.
3. Al-Mefty O, Smith RR: Clival and petroclival meningiomas, in Al-Mefty O (ed): *Meningiomas*. New York, Raven Press, 1991, pp 517–537.
4. Barbaro Nm, Gutin PH, Wilson CB, *et al.*: Radiation therapy in the treatment of partially resected meningiomas. **Neurosurgery** 20:525–528, 1987.
5. Barrows HS, Harter DH: Tentorial meningiomas. **J Neurol Neurosurg Psychiatry** 25:40–44, 1962.
6. Black PMcL: Meningiomas. **Neurosurgery** 32:643–657, 1993.
7. Castellano F, Ruggiero G: Meningiomas of the posterior fossa. **Acta Radiol [Suppl] (Stockh)** 104:26–69, 1953.
8. Ciric I, Landau B: Tentorial and posterior cranial fossa meningiomas—Operative results and long-term follow-up: experience with twenty-six cases. **Surg Neurol** 39:530–537, 1993.
9. Cushing H: The meningiomas (dural endotheliomas): Their source and favoured seats of origin. **Brain** 45:282–316, 1922.
10. Cushing H, Eisenhardt L: *Meningiomas*. Springfield, IL: Charles C Thomas, 1938, pp 506–537.
11. DeMonte F, Al-Mefty O: Anterior clinoidal meningiomas. **Neurosurg Oper Atlas** 3:49–61, 1993.
12. DeMonte F, Zelby AS, Al-Mefty O: Hearing impairment resulting from a pineal region meningioma. **Neurosurgery** 32:665–668, 1993.
13. Gokalp HZ, Arasil E, Erdogan A, *et al.*: Tentorial meningiomas. **Neurosurgery** 36:46–51, 1995.
14. Grunberg SM, Weiss MH, Spitz IM, *et al.*: Treatment of unresectable meningiomas with the antiprogesterone agent mifepristone. **J Neurosurg** 74:861–866, 1991.
15. Guidetti B, Ciapetta P, Domenicucci M: Tentorial meningiomas: Surgical experience with 61 cases and long-term results. **J Neurosurg** 69:183–187, 1988.
16. Hakuba A: Reconstruction of dural sinus involved in meningiomas, in Al-Mefty O (ed): *Meningiomas*. New York, Raven Press, 1991, pp 371–382.
17. Harsh GR IV, Wilson CB: Meningiomas of the peritorcular region, in Al-Mefty O (ed): *Meningiomas*. New York, Raven Press, 1991, pp 363–369.
18. Kinjo T, Al-Mefty O, Kanaan I: Grade zero removal of supratentorial convexity meningiomas. **Neurosurgery** 33:394–399, 1993.

19. Konovalov AN, Spallone A, Pitzkhelauri DI: Meningioma of the pineal region: A surgical series of 10 cases. **J Neurosurg** 85:586–590, 1996.
20. Kupersmith MJ, Warren FA, Newall J, et al.: Irradiation of meningiomas of the intracranial anterior visual pathway. **Ann Neurol** 21:131–137, 1987.
21. Liliequist B: The subarachnoid cisterns: An anatomic and roentgenologic study. **Acta Radiol [Suppl] (Stockh)** 185:5–108, 1959.
22. Malis L: Surgical approaches to tentorial meningiomas, in Wilkins RH, Rengachary SS (eds): *Neurosurgery Update I: Diagnosis, Operative Technique, and Neuro-Oncology*. New York, McGraw-Hill, 1990, pp 399–408.
23. Markwalder T-M, Gerber HA, Waelti E, et al.: Hormonotherapy of meningiomas with medroxyprogesterone acetate: Immunohistochemical demonstration of the effect of medroxyprogesterone acetate on growth fractions of meningioma cells using the monoclonal antibody Ki-67. **Surg Neurol** 30:97–101, 1988.
24. Mirimanoff RO, Dosoretz DE, Linggood RM, et al.: Meningioma: Analysis of recurrence and progression following neurosurgical resection. **J Neurosurg** 62:18–24, 1985.
25. Ogasawara H, Oki S, Kohno H, et al.: Tentorial meningioma and painful tic convulsif: Case report. **J Neurosurg** 82:895–897, 1995.
26. Rodesch G, Lasjaunias P: Embolization and meningiomas, in Al-Mefty O (ed): *Meningiomas*. New York, Raven Press, 1991, pp 285–297.
27. Rostomily RC, Eskridge JM, Winn HR: Tentorial meningiomas. **Neurosurg Clin N Am** 5:331–348, 1994.
28. Samii M, Carvalho GA, Tatagiba M, et al.: Meningiomas of the tentorial notch: Surgical anatomy and management. **J Neurosurg** 84:375–381, 1996.
29. Schechter MM, Zingesser LH, Rosenbaum A: Tentorial meningiomas. **AJR** 104:123–131, 1968.
30. Sekhar LN: Commentary on Gokalp HZ, Arasil E, Erdogan A, et al.: Tentorial meningiomas. **Neurosurgery** 36:51, 1995.
31. Sekhar LN, Jannetta PJ, Maroon JC: Tentorial meningiomas: Surgical management and results. **Neurosurgery** 14:268–275, 1984.
32. Sen C: Surgical approaches to tentorial meningiomas, in Wilkins RH, Rengachary SS (eds): *Neurosurgery*. New York, McGraw-Hill, 1996, ed 2, pp 917–924.
33. Simpson D: Recurrence of intracranial meningiomas after surgical treatment. **J Neurol Neurosurg Psychiatry** 20:22–39, 1957.
34. Sugita K, Suzuki Y: Tentorial meningiomas, In Al-Mefty O (ed): *Meningiomas*. New York, Raven Press, 1991, pp 357–361.
35. Taub E, Argoff CE, Winterkorn JMS, et al.: Resolution of chronic cluster headache after resection of a tentorial meningioma: Case report. **Neurosurgery** 37:319–321, 1995.
36. Umansky F, Ashkenazi E, Gertel M, et al.: Surgical outcome in an elderly population with intracranial meningioma. **J Neurol Neurosurg Psychiatry** 55:481–485, 1992.
37. Yasargil MG: *Microneurosurgery*. Stuttgart, Thieme, 1984, vol I, pp 12–26.
38. Yasargil MG: *Microneurosurgery*. Stuttgart, Thieme, 1996, vol IVB, pp 134–161.
39. Yokota M, Tani E, Maeda Y, et al.: Meningioma in sigmoid sinus groove associated with dural arteriovenous malformation: Case report. **Neurosurgery** 33:316–319, 1993.

27

Foramen Magnum Meningiomas

CARLOS A. DAVID, M.D., AND ROBERT F. SPETZLER, M.D.

Meningiomas constitute the majority of tumors arising at the foramen magnum. This location leads to often unrecognized, insidious progressive symptomatology, which may even have a remitting pattern. The deep treacherous location of these tumors, which are surrounded by some of the most critical structures of the nervous system, together with their potential for cure, makes these tumors a formidable surgical challenge.

Meningiomas of the foramen magnum were first reported in 1874 by Hallopeau (8), and the first successful removal was performed by Elsberg and Strauss (4) in 1929. Despite the eventual success of this case, the early surgical attempts at removal frequently resulted in catastrophe. With the advent of a classification scheme by Cushing and Eisenhardt (3), these tumors could be divided into two groups with distinctly different presentations and surgical difficulty: *craniospinal* and *spinocranial*. The former refer to lesions originating in the basilar groove anterior or anterolateral to the medulla and the latter to those posterior or posterolateral to the medulla. More recently, the term foramen magnum meningioma has been used to include both of these locations.

Traditionally, these lesions have been approached posteriorly, and occasionally via an anterior route such as the transoral or transcervical approach. The initial results were dismal, with significant damage to the lower cranial nerves and brainstem during dissection and tumor removal. Many patients died intraoperatively and those who survived were left with marked disabilities. Improved knowledge of the surgical anatomy with the concurrent development of lateral approaches to the skull base has significantly improved the results of surgical extirpation of these lesions.

EPIDEMIOLOGY

In a review of several series of meningiomas throughout the neuraxis, Scott and Rhoton (18) estimated that the incidence of foramen magnum meningiomas was about 1.8%. Comprising 6–7% of all posterior fossa meningiomas, these lesions are the most common tumor of the foramen magnum (18). Meningiomas constitute 70% of benign tumors arising at the foramen magnum (15, 26). Similar to meningiomas at other locations, meningiomas of the foramen magnum show a predilection for females, with an estimated range of 2:1 to 3.6:1 female to male ratio (2, 6, 13, 23, 26).

Age at presentation varies between the fourth and sixth decade. These tumors are extremely rare in the pediatric population, with only 2% of meningiomas occurring in children (10). Due to the rarity of these tumors in children, the clinical features and growth characteristics are unknown but assumed to be similar to that in the adult population.

CLINICAL FEATURES

The clinical symptomatology associated with foramen magnum meningiomas is often insidious and disparate. The symptoms can be so varied and diverse that the entity was frequently overlooked in the past. Patients' presentations were mistakenly attributed to spondylosis, multiple sclerosis, or even hysteria. Although there is no classical syndrome of foramen magnum meningiomas, a group of typical findings with variable clinical courses can be discerned. In the early stages, patients complain of pain involving the suboccipital and cervical regions. This pain is usually described as a deep, aching sensation that is aggravated by neck movement, coughing, and straining. The pathophysiologic basis for this pain has been an area of significant speculation. It is believed to stem from the fact that the innervation of the dura covering the anterior aspect of the posterior fossa is derived from the first three cervical nerves (18).

As the tumor progresses, sensory and motor deficits develop. The deficits may develop slowly in a relapsing-remitting pattern reminiscent of multiple sclerosis. The most commonly described sensory changes have been dysesthesias, which may be a cold sensation or more typically burning (6). Dysesthesia may progress to hypesthesia, diminished temperature sensation, and loss of tactile and position sense. Astereognosis, stereoanesthesia, and even Lhermitte's sign have also been described by some (7). Rarely, trigeminal sensory loss in an onionskin pattern, hyperesthesia, and frank trigeminal neuralgia have been noted (2).

Perhaps the most typical finding is a progressive spastic quadriparesis, classically termed an "asymmetrical pyramidal quadriparesis" (23). Weakness and spasticity first develop in the ipsilateral arm and subsequently progress to involve the ipsilateral leg, then the contralateral leg, and finally the contralateral arm. The most severe involvement is the ipsilateral side. This pattern of quadriparesis is seen with anterolaterally growing tumors. With anterior tumors, the quadriparesis may be more symmetrical, or the patient may develop Bell's cruciate paralysis. Approximately 25–44% of patients have atrophy and weakness of the sternocleidomastoid and trapezius muscles from involvement of the accessory nerve (2, 7, 13, 23). Another peculiar finding, wasting of the distal upper extremity and intrinsic hand muscles, has been attributed to venous outflow obstruction with subsequent infarction at lower levels (19). Late findings include the development of a spastic or ataxic gait, sphincter disturbances, and respiratory dysfunction from compression of the medullary respiratory centers.

RADIOGRAPHIC FEATURES

The imaging characteristics of foramen magnum meningiomas are no different from their counterparts in other areas of the neuraxis. Plain and contrast-enhanced computed tomography (CT) detects up to 95% of meningiomas (16). Plain CT typically shows a well-circumscribed ovoid to lobulated, iso- to slightly hyperdense mass that has intense and uniform enhancement. Axial images in conjunction with sagittal and coronal reconstructions can yield important information regarding the tumor extent, its relationship to the brainstem, and surgical planning. Magnetic resonance imaging (MRI) has become the gold standard for imaging lesions of the foramen magnum. Accurate evaluation of a tumor location, attachment, and extension, as well as its involvement with neurologic structures and blood vessels can be clearly delineated. On T1-weighted images, meningiomas appear isointense to slightly hypointense and enhance markedly with gadolinium. T2-weighted images can be quite helpful by showing a variable heterogeneous iso- to hyperintense signal (16).

Angiography can be a helpful adjunct in the workup of foramen magnum meningiomas. The vascular supply to the tumor can be delineated, and the position of major vessels with respect to the tumor can be determined. Particularly, the positions of the anterior spinal artery, posterior spinal artery, posterior inferior cerebellar artery (PICA), and vertebral artery, which may be encased by tumor, should be noted. Occasionally, arteries feeding the tumor may be amenable to embolization which can decrease the hemorrhagic potential of some very vascular meningiomas. In addition to study of the posterior fossa arteries, the venous drainage patterns, dominance, and extent of involvement by tumor should be defined. This information can be critical if sacrifice of the sigmoid sinus or jugular vein is considered during a transpetrosal approach.

SURGICAL MANAGEMENT

Anatomic Considerations

Detailed descriptions of the anatomy of the foramen magnum and posterior fossa region are available elsewhere (17, 18). Only the pertinent surgical anatomy is reviewed here. The region of the foramen magnum is occupied by the caudal medulla, rostral spinal cord, cerebellar tonsils, and the accompanying neural and vascular structures. The spinal cord is anchored to the lateral dura by the bilaterally located dentate ligaments. The most rostral dentate ligament forms an important surgical landmark in approaches to the foramen magnum. The lateral attachment of this dentate ligament is associated with the vertebral artery as it enters the dura with the posterior spinal artery and dorsal root of C1 (Fig. 1).

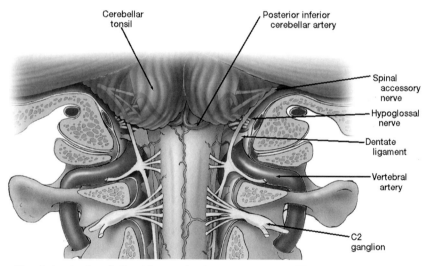

Cerebellar tonsil

Posterior inferior cerebellar artery

Spinal accessory nerve

Hypoglossal nerve

Dentate ligament

Vertebral artery

C2 ganglion

FIG. 1 Anatomic relationships at the foramen magnum. The cerebellar tonsils are located superior to the level of the foramen magnum. The accessory nerve can be seen arising from the spinal cord and traveling in a rostral direction between the dentate ligaments and dorsal roots. The vertebral artery can be seen passing through the dura ventral to the most rostral dentate ligament. This most rostral dentate ligament attaches laterally at the level of the foramen magnum and marks the entrance of the vertebral artery as it enters, giving rise to the posterior spinal artery and dorsal root of C1. The hypoglossal nerve rootlets can be seen draping over the dorsal surface of the vertebral artery in their characteristic manner. (Reproduced with permission from the Barrow Neurological Institute.)

After piercing the dura, the vertebral artery travels rostrally joining the opposite vertebral artery to form the basilar artery at the level of the pontomedullary sulcus. Once intradural, the vertebral artery gives rise to the PICA at variable sites at or above the level of the foramen magnum.

Characteristically, cranial nerves IX–XI arise as a series of rootlets along the anterolateral medulla and spinal cord and travel rostrally to the jugular foramen. The accessory nerve has a spinal component that arises from the spinal cord as a series of rootlets between the dentate ligaments and dorsal spinal roots. This component courses rostrally through the foramen magnum to join the rootlets of the lower cranial nerves before exiting via the jugular foramen. The rootlets of the hypoglossal nerve arise from the anterior medulla and characteristically pass behind the vertebral artery, draping over its dorsal surface on the way to the hypoglossal canal, which is located anteriorly at the rostral limit of the occipital condyles.

Selection of a Surgical Approach

Meningiomas of the foramen magnum can occur anywhere along its circumference. Most commonly, they are found anterolaterally within the foramen magnum (2, 6, 13, 23). Approximately 20% will occur posteriorly or posterolaterally. Rarely, they grow in a purely anterior location or extend rostrally to involve the lower clivus (Fig. 2).

The choice of surgical approach primarily then must reflect the location of the meningioma (Fig. 3). In addition, the anterior-posterior displacement of the medulla and spinal cord, the size of the tumor, and the rostral-caudal extent of the lesion are also determinants. For example, large anterior or anterolaterally placed tumors that have displaced the brainstem posteriorly provide a window in which to remove the tumor obviating a more aggressive and complex anterolateral approach. Rostral extension requires the addition of a petrosal approach.

Traditionally, meningiomas of the foramen magnum have been approached via a posterior or lateral suboccipital craniectomy. Although this approach works well for posterior or posterolateral tumors, it does not provide the visualization and exposure needed for anterolateral and anterior tumors. Anterior approaches via the transcervical or transoral routes have been employed but have not gained wide acceptance. In an effort to obtain better exposure of more anterior lesions, lateral modifications of the posterior approaches were developed (1, 5, 9, 21), (i.e., far lateral and extreme lateral approaches). These modified approaches provide good visualization of the foramen magnum and can be combined with various transpetrosal approaches (Table 1) to pro-

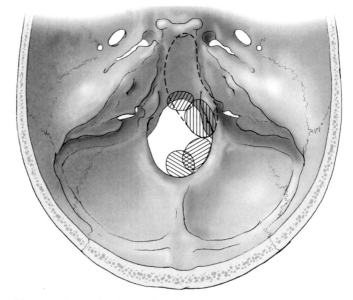

Fig. 2 Diagram illustrating the various locations of foramen magnum meningiomas. Seventy to eighty percent occur anterolaterally and 20% posteriorly. They are rarely in purely anterior locations. In addition, rostral extension along the clivus is common. (Reproduced with permission from the Barrow Neurological Institute.)

vide a panoramic view of the entire petroclival region to the foramen magnum and upper cervical region (Fig. 4**A** and **B**).

SURGICAL TECHNIQUES

Posterior Suboccipital Approach

The posterior suboccipital craniotomy and cervical laminotomy are most commonly used for meningiomas that are directly posterior or slightly posterolateral. Some surgeons advocate this approach even for lesions that are ventral to the brainstem (18). In our opinion, however, a more lateral approach should be used if a considerable amount of the tumor is present ventrally.

POSITION

The position used for the suboccipital approach depends on the tumor's location and the surgeon's preference. Typically, either the prone or the three-quarter prone position is most useful. Rarely has the sitting or semisitting position been used. The prone position is the preferred position at our institution. The patient is placed in a rigid three-point skull fixator such as the Mayfield head holder. The head is

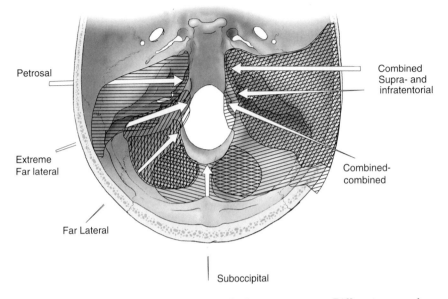

Petrosal

Combined
Supra- and
infratentorial

Extreme
Far lateral

Combined-
combined

Far Lateral

Suboccipital

FIG. 3. The various surgical approaches to the foramen magnum. Different approaches
can be combined in order to reach more extensive tumors. (Reproduced with permission
from the Barrow Neurological Institute®.)

TABLE 1.
Approaches to the Foramen Magnum and Adjacent Regions

Location of Lesion	Surgical Approach
Posterior foramen magnum	Suboccipital craniotomy
Anterior foramen magnum	Far lateral or extreme lateral approach
With middle/lower clivus extension	Far lateral with petrosectomy
With entire clivus involvement	Far lateral combined supra- and infratentorial approach

maintained straight prone and neutral. A small degree of flexion is
sometimes helpful but should be used with caution to avoid a compressive injury to the already tenuous brainstem. For eccentric tumors, the
head can be turned slightly toward the side of the tumor; this maneuver facilitates visualization of the more ventral aspects of the tumor.

SKIN INCISION AND CRANIOTOMY

A vertical skin incision along the midline is usually adequate for
posterior or posterolateral tumors. Alternatively, a hockey stick incision may be useful for tumors extending laterally. The incision is made

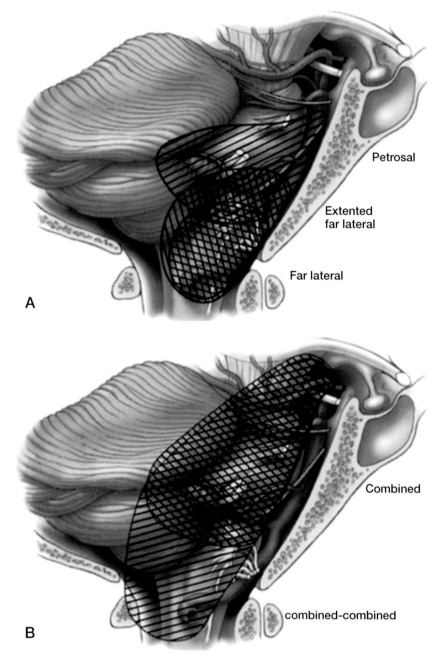

FIG. 4 The area of visualization for the different approaches to the foramen magnum and lower clivus. (**A**) Far lateral, extended far lateral, and petrosal routes. (**B**) Combined supra- and infratentorial transpetrosal routes and combined-combined. (Reproduced with permission from the Barrow Neurological Institute®.)

through the subcutaneous tissues, exposing the underlying fascia and suboccipital musculature. These tissues are separated from the subcutaneous tissues to expose the insertion on the superior nuchal line and inion. The muscles and fascia are divided in a T-shaped manner, and a muscular cuff is left attached along the superior nuchal line to facilitate closure (Fig. 5A). Dissection proceeds along the midline raphé exposing the suboccipital region, foramen magnum, and arches of the atlas and axis. Exposure continues laterally depending on the laterality of the tumor. Careful subperiosteal dissection is used along the sulcus arteriosus of C1 until the extracranial vertebral artery is delineated at its point of entry into the atlantooccipital membrane. A C1 laminectomy is completed using a high-speed drill with a B1 footplate (Midas Rex, Inc., Fort Worth, TX). A suboccipital craniotomy including the rim of the foramen magnum is performed with the drill footplate attachment. Bone edges are waxed meticulously to avoid a postoperative cerebrospinal fluid (CSF) leak.

INITIAL INTRADURAL EXPOSURE

A tiny dural-arachnoid opening into the cisterna magna is made, and CSF is allowed to escape. Once enough CSF has drained to relax the

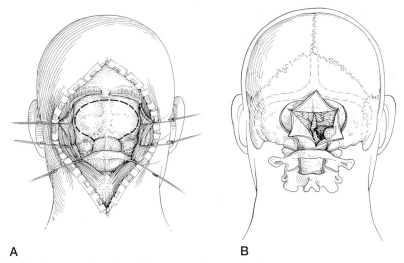

A   **B**

FIG. 5 The posterior suboccipital approach to posterior foramen magnum meningiomas. (**A**) A midline incision is used, the subcutaneous tissues are separated from the underlying fascia, and the muscle is divided in a T-shaped manner with a muscular cuff being left for later closure. (**B**) After a suboccipital craniotomy is completed, the dura is opened exposing the tumor. Posterior lesions tend to displace the neural structures ventrally and are usually easily peeled off and removed. (Reproduced with permission from the Barrow Neurological Institute®)

brain adequately, the dura is widely opened in a Y-shaped manner. The occipital marginal sinus is gently coagulated, and dural tack-up sutures are placed in the usual manner. The remaining intradural work is performed under the operating microscope with microsurgical technique.

Posterior or posterolateral lesions are quite evident upon intradural exposure. They tend to displace the neural structures ventrally and hence are easily removed, frequently peeling easily from the medulla (Fig. 5**B**). Occasionally, large tumors are more adherent and encase vital neurovascular structures. Such tumors are best debulked internally before attempting to separate them from the brainstem. Care must be exercised to avoid transmitting undue pressure on the attached neural structures. The small arteries on the ventral aspect of the tumor should be preserved if possible because they may provide critical blood supply to the already attenuated spinal cord.

More laterally situated tumors present a different problem. These tumors frequently displace the medulla and spinal cord posteriorly. Consequently, the ventral spinal roots and the spinal root of the accessory nerve are frequently draped along the dorsal surface of the tumor. These rootlets must be carefully dissected free from the tumor and rarely need to be sacrificed. With this dissection completed, the dentate ligaments should be identified and sectioned, thereby releasing the spinal cord and providing a wider region in which to work. Intratumoral debulking alternates with piecemeal dissection as the surgeon works between the spinal and accessory rootlets.

The surgeon must always be vigilant of the location of the vertebral artery and PICA, both of which are often encased by tumor, particularly in the more laterally situated tumors. When the tumor has been removed, the dural base should be excised if possible. Alternatively, aggressive coagulation will suffice.

CLOSURE

The dura is closed in a water-tight manner either primarily or with a dural graft or harvested fascia. The suboccipital craniotomy and arch of C1 are replaced and secured with miniplates. The wound is then closed in multiple layers, with the muscular and fascial layers reapproximated in a water-tight manner.

Far Lateral Suboccipital Approach

The difficulty encountered when attempting to remove more anterior lesions via the standard approaches outlined above led to a search for better surgical routes. Transoral and transcervical routes created deep difficult exposures associated with high risks of infectious complications. A true lateral approach was limited by the vertebral artery and occipital condyle. Refinements in surgical technique, however, modified the lateral suboccipital approach into the far lateral approach. This approach controls the extracranial vertebral artery and partially removes the occipital condyle to provide a much better lateral view of anterior lesions. This improved exposure is obtained by bone removal and obviates the need for significant brain retraction.

POSITION

The patient is placed in a modified park bench position (Fig. 6A and B). The patient is positioned laterally with the operative side facing upward and the axilla protected with a foam roll. The dependent arm is allowed to hang over the end of the table, cradled with foam padding. The head is fixated in a Mayfield three-pin head holder after it is flexed in the anteroposterior plane, rotated 45° contralaterally, and then bent laterally approximately 30° toward the contralateral shoulder (Fig. 6B). This series of maneuvers allows the ipsilateral mastoid process to be the highest point and significantly opens the occipitocervical space. At this point the ipsilateral shoulder is taped down; the knees and body are well padded and also secured to the operating table with tape, thus providing the greatest possible working room for the surgeon and full rotation of the operating table.

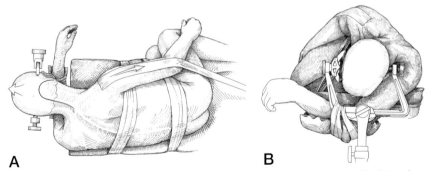

A   **B**

FIG. 6 (**A**) Illustration depicting the patient positioning for a right far lateral or extended far lateral approach as viewed from above. The right shoulder is pulled down and secured. The patient is also secured to the operating table to allow rotation as needed throughout the surgical procedure. (**B**) Position as viewed from the cranial vertex. Note the final head position obtained after performing the maneuver described in the text. (Reproduced with permission from the Barrow Neurological Institute®.)

INCISION AND EXPOSURE

An inverted hockey-stick incision begins at the mastoid process and courses toward the midline just below the superior nuchal line (Fig. 7**A**). At the midline, the incision continues downward staying in the midline to the level of C3 or C4. The muscles are then divided just below the superior nuchal line, and a cuff of the muscle and nuchal ligament is left for later reapproximation during closure. Dissection proceeds along the midline avascular plane exposing the spinous processes of the upper cervical vertebrae. Subperiosteal dissection continues laterally exposing the suboccipital region and ipsilateral lamina of C1 and C2. The myocutaneous flap is then secured with fishhooks on a Leyla bar (22).

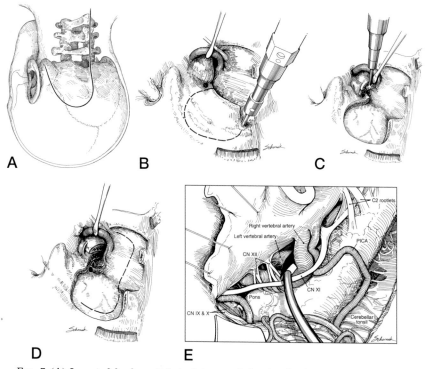

FIG. 7 (**A**) Inverted hockey-stick incision used for the far lateral and extended far lateral approaches. Note the incision extends from the mastoid tip along the nuchal line and down the midline to the level of C3 or C4. (**B**) Illustration of C1 laminectomy and suboccipital craniotomy being performed. (**C**) Illustration of the drilling of the occipital condyle. (**D**) Drawing depicting the posterior fossa dural opening. (**E**) Intradural exposure obtained with the far lateral approach. [**A,** reproduced with permission from the Barrow Neurological Institute; **B, C, D,** and **E,** reproduced with permission from (1).]

Subperiosteal dissection proceeds along the sulcus arteriosus of C1 revealing the vertebral artery and its surrounding venous plexus. Dissection continues from lateral to medial exposing the vertebral artery along its entire course from the transverse foramen to its entry point at the atlantooccipital membrane. Soft tissues are further removed from the edge of the foramen magnum and the atlantooccipital joint in preparation for bone removal.

BONE REMOVAL

A hemilaminectomy of C1 is performed first with a high-speed drill and footplate (Midas Rex, Inc., Fort Worth, TX) and later replaced at the completion of the procedure. A suboccipital craniotomy begins just lateral to the midline at the foramen magnum and extends upward toward the transverse and sigmoid sinuses and then downward as far laterally as possible to the foramen magnum just medial to the dural entry point of the vertebral artery (Fig. 7**B**). The dimensions of the craniotomy should be tailored to the lesion in question. In addition, it may be combined with a transpetrosal approach to provide access to extensive lesions along the clivus as discussed later in the chapter.

With the craniotomy completed, the remaining ipsilateral rim of the foramen magnum is removed with a rongeur. With a small dissector, the vertebral artery is retracted and protected away from the region of the occipital condyle while it is drilled and removed (Fig. 7**C**). The inner portion of the condyle is drilled out as well as the medial portion of the superior lateral mass and facet of C1, leaving a thin cortical shell of bone which can be removed with curettes and bone rongeurs. To maintain stability, only the posterior one-third to one-half of the occipital condyle should be removed. This point is usually 1 cm deep to the dural entry point of the vertebral artery and is marked by brisk bleeding from the condylar emissary vein. The bleeding is easily controlled with bone wax or other hemostatic material (Gelfoam, Surgicel). The occipital condyle can be removed more extensively as part of the extended far lateral (transcondylar/transjugular) approach, which is discussed in the next section.

INTRADURAL EXPOSURE

The dura is opened in a curvilinear manner with the base hinged laterally (Fig. 7**D**). The initial opening is performed at the midline just above C1 to allow egress of CSF from the cisterna magna in order to relax the brain before the dura is opened completely. The opening is completed upward toward the cerebellar hemisphere and sigmoid sinus and downward below and lateral to the vertebral artery. The dural flap is retracted laterally over the edge of the craniotomy, providing a direct view of the anterior foramen magnum and lower clivus (Fig. 7E).

Using the operative microscope, arachnoidal adhesions are dissected, and the upper dentate ligaments can be sectioned as already described to provide a greater view of the premedullary space and to reduce traction on the spinal cord during tumor removal. Tumor removal proceeds as described: the capsule is coagulated and opened, and internal debulking and tumor removal proceeds in a piecemeal fashion. Again, the surgeon must be vigilant of the vertebral artery and PICA, which are frequently encased by tumors growing in this location. If not easily separable, a small tuft of tumor should be left attached to these vessels rather than risk injury to these critical arteries.

CLOSURE

The closure is similar to other intracranial operations. The cervical and posterior fossa dura are closed in a water-tight fashion either primarily or with grafts if needed. The suboccipital bone and C1 hemilamina are replaced and secured using small bone plates and screws. The wound is closed in multiple layers in a water-tight manner.

Extended Far Lateral Approach

This modification of the far lateral approach, sometimes referred to as the extreme lateral or the extreme transcondylar or transjugular (20, 21) approach, improves medial exposure along the lower clivus. The increased exposure is accomplished by completely isolating and mobilizing the vertebral artery from C2 to its dural entry point and by completely resecting the occipital condyle and skeletonizing the hypoglossal canal (Fig. 8). In addition, the jugular bulb may be obliterated, providing access to tumors that involve this structure.

Patient positioning, the skin incision, and initial exposure are performed as already described. The vertebral artery is isolated completely, and the transverse foramen of C1 is opened and the artery displaced medially. This bone is then resected. The suboccipital craniotomy is also performed as described but includes a partial mastoidectomy up to but not unroofing the facial nerve. The sigmoid sinus and jugular bulb are skeletonized. The occipital condyle is removed completely. If needed, the sigmoid sinus and jugular vein are ligated, for example, if extensive extradural tumor is present or the jugular foramen is involved.

The dura is opened in a similar manner but is circumferentially cut around the entry point of the vertebral artery, thus allowing complete medial retraction of the vertebral artery and a direct unimpeded view of the foramen magnum and lower clivus from a completely lateral perspective.

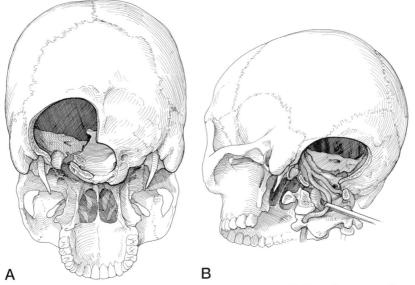

A   B

FIG. 8 Extended far lateral approach—condyle resection (**A**). Note the extent of bony removal providing a more lateral vantage point to the anterior foramen magnum (**B**). (Reproduced with permission from the Barrow Neurological Institute®.)

After the tumor has been removed, the closure requires filling the dead space with autologous fat. An occipitocervical fusion is also needed due to the instability associated with complete condyle removal.

The extended far lateral approach provides greater access and working room for resecting tumors along the anterior foramen magnum and lower clivus, but it should be reserved for extensive tumors with large extradural components and bone invasion. The morbidity associated with this approach is significantly greater than that associated with the far lateral approach due to the displacement of the vertebral artery, risk of CSF leak, and instability associated with condyle removal. We have found that the majority of tumors in this location can be removed via the far lateral approach or in combination with a transpetrosal approach and have found the extended far lateral approach unnecessary for meningiomas of the foramen magnum.

Combined Approaches

Occasionally, meningiomas of the foramen magnum can extend upward along the clivus making their removal via a single approach impossible. Improved visualization can be achieved by combining the far lateral approach with an isolated transpetrosal approach or with the combined supra- and infratentorial approach referred to as the "combined-combined" approach. These exposures can provide extremely wide venues of the entire clival region down to the upper cervical region. Again, the choice of approach is based on the location and extent of the tumor (Figs. 3 and 4).

COMBINED FAR LATERAL-TRANSPETROSAL APPROACH

Combining the far lateral approach with an isolated transpetrosal approach can be useful for tumors that extend into the cerebellopontine angle and involve the lower to midclivus. The options associated with petrosectomy include a retrolabyrinthine resection that preserves hearing but provides a very small avenue in which to work. The translabyrinthine technique sacrifices hearing and provides a somewhat larger working area, and the transcochlear technique provides the largest working area via maximal petrous resection but sacrifices hearing and transposes cranial nerve VII (Fig. 9).

The combined far lateral-petrosal approach is performed as already described for the far lateral approach. The skin incision, which is modified to include the exposure needed for the petrosal approach, is extended superiorly over the pinna and down toward the root of the

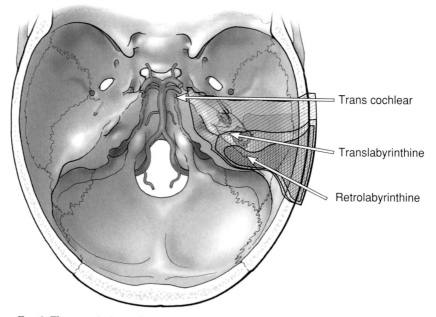

FIG. 9 Three variations of petrosal approaches. See text for details. (Reproduced with permission from the Barrow Neurological Institute®.)

zygoma (Fig. 10). A cuff of muscle and fascia is left along the superior nuchal line as described, and the soft tissues are dissected to expose the lateral temporal bone, zygoma, mastoid region, and external auditory meatus.

The petrosectomy is performed and is followed with the far lateral exposure. The dura is opened parallel to the petrosal and sigmoid sinuses with these two incisions meeting at the sinodural angle. A second incision is made as described earlier for the far lateral aspect of the craniotomy, thus providing two avenues around the sigmoid sinus in which to remove tumor. On occasion the sigmoid sinus can be divided, connecting these two regions and providing increased exposure of the region.

The closure is as previously outlined with the addition of packing the eustachian tube and filling the petrous defect with a fat graft. In addition, temporary lumbar drainage of CSF can be used if there is a high risk of CSF leakage.

FAR LATERAL COMBINED SUPRA- AND INFRATENTORIAL APPROACH (COMBINED-COMBINED APPROACH)

The combined-combined approach is useful when lesions extend from the entire clivus to the foramen magnum. It is performed in a similar manner to the combined far lateral petrosal approach with the addition of a temporal craniotomy. The temporal craniotomy can be performed as part of the suboccipital craniotomy or as a separate section.

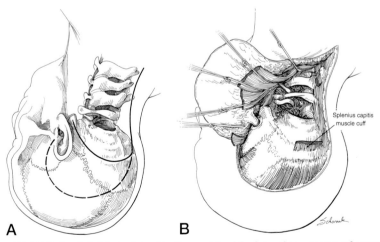

A   **B**

FIG. 10 (**A**) Extended skin incision for the combined far lateral transpetrosal approach or combined-combined approach. (**B**) Initial exposure after soft tissue dissection. [Reproduced with permission from (1).]

The dural incision is begun with an opening over the temporal lobe parallel to the middle fossa floor that extends across the superior petrosal sinus to join a second incision made anterior to the sigmoid sinus. The petrosal sinus is clipped and cauterized before division. The dural incision continues through the tentorium behind cranial nerve IV to the tentorial incisura, connecting the supra- and infratentorial spaces. The dural opening for the far lateral approach is also performed (Fig. 11**A**). If the sigmoid sinus is to be sacrificed, the two dural incisions are joined (Fig. 11**B** and **C**), providing a panoramic view of the entire clivus and anterior brainstem (Fig. 12). Closure follows the same principles described for the other approaches.

SIGMOID SINUS SACRIFICE

Ligation and division of the sigmoid sinus can increase the exposures described. This maneuver can be performed safely only after confirming that it communicates freely with the contralateral transverse sigmoid sinus and superior sagittal sinus via the torcula. Intraoperative pressure monitoring can help determine if it is safe to sacrifice the sigmoid sinus.

After the petrosal sinus has been ligated, a 25-gauge needle is used to measure sigmoid sinus pressure after temporary ligation. The sigmoid sinus can be divided only if the pressure does not increase more than 10 mm Hg.

Transoral and Transcervical Approaches

The transoral approach is useful for extradural anterior foramen magnum lesions; however, its use for intradural lesions is severely limited by the high incidence of CSF fistulae and meningitis. It provides a midline exposure and is the most direct route to anterior foramen magnum meningiomas. Although this approach had various proponents (7, 14), it did not gain widespread acceptance and has since been abandoned for intradural lesions.

The transcervical route is based on Henry's extensile approach and is performed via the anterior fascial planes of the neck (7, 24). It provides a similar exposure to the transoral route without the risks of CSF fistulae and meningitis; however, the extensive dissection with mandibular dislocation and the depth of the exposure have not made it practical. It should no longer be considered for approaching intradural lesions of the foramen magnum.

SURGICAL OUTCOME

Early surgical series typically reported poor results with foramen magnum meningiomas. Mortality rates ranged from 13.2 to 46% (12, 25).

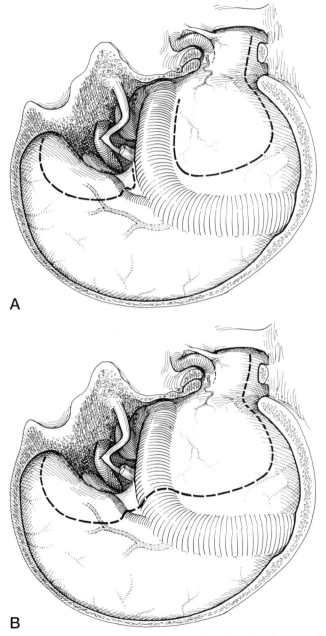

A

B

FIG. 11 Dural incisions and exposure in the combined-combined approach. (**A**) Preservation of the sigmoid sinus. (**B** and **C**) Dural incision and exposure with sacrifice of the sigmoid sinus. [**A,** reproduced with permission from the Barrow Neurological Institute; **B** and **C,** reproduced with permission from (1).]

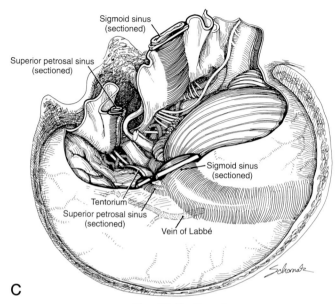

C

FIG. 11 Continued

Refined surgical techniques have improved outcomes. In 1988, Guidetti (7) reported an operative mortality rate of 11%. The large series from the Mayo Clinic (13) had a 5% operative mortality rate; 75% of these patients had excellent outcomes that were largely determined by their preoperative neurologic status and the duration of their symptoms.

RADIATION THERAPY

Complete resection without serious morbidity or death is difficult if the tumor adheres to the cranial nerves, brainstem, and critical vessels such as the PICA or vertebral arteries. In this case, radiotherapy for residual meningiomas can serve as an important adjunct and can be used for patients who are medically unsuitable for surgical intervention. Radiotherapy can be delivered via external beam or stereotactically with the Gamma Knife or LINAC systems. Control of regrowth has been reported at 95% 2 years after treatment by Kondziolka and Lundsford (11).

CONCLUSIONS

Foramen magnum meningiomas are relatively rare tumors that present with a relatively indolent course. At the time of diagnosis the

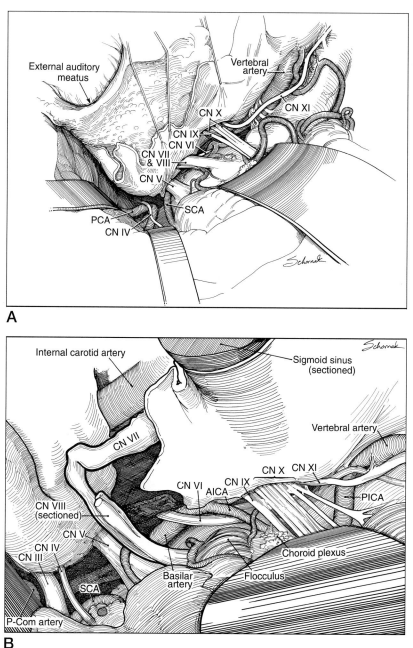

FIG. 12 (**A**) Intradural exposure of a combined-combined approach with retrolabyrinthine petrosectomy and (**B**) transcochlear petrosectomy. [Reproduced with permission from (1).]

tumors are usually quite large. Their location makes removal a complex surgical problem and frequently necessitates a combination of surgical approaches. Refinements in imaging, anesthesia, and surgical technique have significantly improved the dismal results obtained in the past. Continued vigilance on the part of the clinician will permit earlier diagnosis and will optimize functional recovery, which is primarily determined by the patient's preoperative neurologic status.

REFERENCES

1. Baldwin HZ, Miller CG, van Loveren HR, *et al.*: The far lateral/combined supra- and infratentorial approach: A human cadaveric prosection model for routes of access to the petroclival regions and ventral brain stem. **J Neurosurg** 81:60–68, 1994.
2. Castellano F, Ruggiero G: Meningiomas of the posterior fossa. **Acta Radiol (Suppl)** 104:1–177, 1953.
3. Cushing H, Eisenhardt L: *Meningiomas. Their Classification, Regional Behaviour, Life History, and Surgical End Results.* New York, Hafner, 1962.
4. Elsberg CA, Strauss I: Tumors of the spinal cord which project into the posterior cranial fossa. Report of a case in which a growth was removed from the ventral and lateral aspects of the medulla oblongata and upper cervical cord. **Arch Neurol Psychiatry** 21:261–273, 1929.
5. George B, Dematons C, Cophignon J: Lateral approach to the anterior portion of the foramen magnum. Application to surgical removal of 14 benign tumors: Technical note. **Surg Neurol** 29:484–490, 1988.
6. Guidetti B, Spallone A: Benign extramedullary tumors of the foramen magnum. **Surg Neurol** 13:9–17, 1980.
7. Guidetti B, Spallone A: Benign extramedullary tumors of the foramen magnum, in Kepes H (ed): *Advances and Technical Standards in Neurosurgery.* New York, Springer-Verlag, 1988, p 83.
8. Hallopeau MH: Note sur deux faits de tumeurs du mésocéphale; communiquée á la société de biologie. **Gazette Medicale Paris** 3:111–112, 1874.
9. Heros RC: Lateral suboccipital approach for vertebral and vertebrobasilar artery lesions. **J Neurosurg** 64:559–562, 1986.
10. Kepes H: *Meningiomas. Biology, Pathology, and Differential Diagnosis.* New York, Masson, 1982.
11. Kondziolka D, Lundsford LD: Radiosurgery of meningiomas. **Neurosurg Clin N Am** 3:219–230, 1992.
12. Love JG, Thelen EP, Dodge HW Jr: Tumors of the foramen magnum. **J Internat Coll Surg** 22:1–17, 1954.
13. Meyer FB, Ebersold MJ, Reese DF: Benign tumors of the foramen magnum. **J Neurosurg** 61:136–142, 1984.
14. Miller E, Crockard HA: Transoral transclival removal of anteriorly placed meningiomas at the foramen magnum. **Neurosurgery** 20:966–968, 1987.
15. Mullan S, Naunton R, Hekmat-Panah J, *et al.*: The use of an anterior approach to ventrally placed tumors in the foramen magnum and vertebral column. **J Neurosurg** 24:536–543, 1966.

16. Osborn AG: *Diagnostic Neuroradiology.* St. Louis, Mosby, 1994, p 579.

17. Rhoton AL Jr, de Oliveira E: Microsurgical anatomy of the region of the foramen magnum, in Wilkins RH, Rengachary SS (eds): *Neurosurgery Update I. Diagnosis, Operative Technique, and Neuro-Oncology.* New York, McGraw-Hill, 1990, p 434.

18. Scott EW, Rhoton AL Jr: Foramen magnum meningiomas, in Al-Mefty O (ed): *Meningiomas.* New York, Raven Press, 1991, p 543.

19. Scott M: The surgical management of meningiomas of the cerebellar fossa. **Surg Gynecol Obstet** 135:545–550, 1972.

20. Sen C, Sekhar LN: Extreme lateral transcondylar and transjugular approaches, in Sekhar LN (ed): *Surgery of Cranial Base Tumors.* New York, Raven Press, 1993, p 389.

21. Sen CN, Sekhar LN: An extreme lateral approach to intradural lesions of the cervical spine and foramen magnum. **Neurosurgery** 27:197–204, 1990.

22. Spetzler RF: Two technical notes for microneurosurgery. **BNI Q** 4:38–39, 1988.

23. Stein BM, Leeds NE, Taveras JM, *et al.:* Meningiomas of the foramen magnum. **J Neurosurg** 20:740–751, 1963.

24. Stevenson GC, Stoney RJ, Perkins PK, *et al.:* A transcervical transclival approach to the ventral surface of the brain stem for removal of a clivus chordoma. **J Neurosurg** 24:544–551, 1966.

25. Yasargil MG, Mortara RW, Curcie M: Meningiomas of the basal posterior cranial fossa, in Krayenbühl H (ed): *Advances and Technical Standards in Neurosurgery.* Wien, Austria, Springer-Verlag, 1980, p 3.

26. Yasuoka S, Okazaki H, Daube JR, *et al.:* Foramen magnum tumors. Analysis of 57 cases of benign extramedullary tumors. **J Neurosurg** 49:828–838, 1978.

28

Cranial Base Chordomas

ARNOLD H. MENEZES, M.D., BRUCE J. GANTZ, M.D., VINCENT C. TRAYNELIS, M.D., AND TIMOTHY M. McCULLOCH, M.D.

Chordomas are rare, slow-growing infiltrative neoplasms of presumed notochordal origin that arise along the vertebral axis and show a proclivity for the sphenooccipital and sacral regions (10, 14, 22–24, 28, 33). The location of these tumors in close proximity to the brainstem, cervicomedullary junction, cavernous sinus, hypothalamus, pituitary gland and the lower cranial nerves make complete tumor resection of cranial chordomas difficult. Subtotal tumor resection has inevitably resulted in local tumor recurrence (10, 29, 36, 39). The diagnosis of chordomas in the past was dependent on plain radiographs, pneumo-encephalography, myelography, angiography, radioisotope scanning and, subsequently, computerized tomography (CT). Thus, tumors at the skull base posed both a diagnostic and a surgical challenge.

The advent of high-resolution CT associated with CT myelotomog-raphy and, subsequently, magnetic resonance imaging (MRI) has com-pletely changed the neuroimaging of skull base chordomas. Likewise, the improved neurosurgical instrumentation and extensile exposures of the cranial base, together with the use of proton beam radiation, have opened new vistas for treatment of patients with cranial base chordomas. This chapter will deal with the management of skull base chordomas in the present setting, using the newer techniques avail-able since 1985 with a critical appraisal of treatment outcome.

PRESENTATION

Chordomas of the clivus and craniovertebral junction are the most common of the extradural neoplasms that involve this region. The overall incidence of chordomas is 0.2–0.5 per 100,000 persons per year and accounts for approximately 0.15% of all intracranial tumors (10, 24). About 25% of chordomas occur at the base of the skull, arising from the clivus. Although usually midline, the notochord may have distal projections that extend to the clinoid processes of the petrous bones. The location of the chordoma within the clivus, in its pathology and the nature of its growth, and the structures that are involved anatomically determine the clinical symptoms and signs. Intracranial chordomas may arise along the basisphenoid or the basiocciput or below the sphenooccipital synchondrosis. Most patients experience symptoms referable to the tumor for over a year before diagnosis (24). The frequent complaints are headaches and visual disturbances; however, as with most intracranial tumors, the specific symptoms with which each patient presents depends on the location of the neoplasm. The headaches are commonly occipital and occipitocervical in location, aggravated by changes in neck position as well as by assuming an upright stance. The latter condition results from involvement of the occipital condyles, and patients with such involvement benefit from a stabilization procedure in addition to the tumor resection. Not uncommonly, the second cranial nerve root is compromised.

Basisphenoid lesions tend to cause dysfunction of the upper cranial nerves and of the endocrine system. In contrast, chordomas that arise from the basiocciput are likely to affect the lower cranial nerves, the ascending and descending tracts, and the cerebellum. Lateral extensions of these tumors can give rise to unilateral symptoms, such as hypoglossal nerve palsy, and the larger tumors have the potential to cause both upper and lower cranial nerve palsies and a variety of problems secondary to brainstem compression. It is not uncommon for chordomas to cause symptoms from local growth into the nasal cavity, pharynx, and paranasal sinuses.

Chordomas usually occur in adults, with a peak incidence occurring in the 4th decade of life (5, 14, 15). Fewer than 5% of these tumors arise in children, and they have a tendency to arise predominantly in the sphenooccipital region. The presentation in children is one of intracranial hypertension secondary to hydrocephalus and long tract signs. Occasionally, local nasal mass symptoms bring the child to medical attention.

Physical examination often reveals optic nerve dysfunction or extraocular palsies in lesions that are parasellar and involve the upper clivus. Forty percent of individuals have detectable lower cranial nerve palsies, and over one-half of these patients have a palpable retropharyngeal mass (23, 24). Patients with chordomas of the middle and lower clivus are frequently found to have cortical spinal tract dysfunction and sensory deficits.

PATHOLOGY

Chordomas have been divided into (a) the classic chordoma, (b) chondroid chordomas, and (c) atypical chordomas (19, 24, 28). The gross appearance of a classic chordoma is a lobulated gelatinous tumor that typically infiltrates bone but may grossly appear as somewhat demarcated. Tumor is pinkish-gray in color and has a pseudocapsule. This accounts for approximately 80–85% of tumors. Histologically, chordomas exhibit a variable mix of sheets and cords or clusters of small polygonal cells with eosinophilic cytoplasm and hyperchromatic nuclei. There is a myxoid matrix present. Cytological atypia is absent or minimal.

A subpopulation of what has been considered chordomas arises largely in the sphenoocciput and exhibits cartilaginous differentiation. Such tumors have been ascribed a more indolent clinical course. The extent of its cartilaginous presence varies from minimum to extensive, and these tumors have been termed "chondroid" chordomas to distinguish them from the classic chordomas. Some authors dispute the existence of chondroid chordomas, preferring to regard these cartilage-containing neoplasms as chondrosarcomas. A better survival rate has been ascribed to these chondroid chordomas. This survival rate is 15.8 years *versus* 4.1 years for typical classic chordoma (15, 19). Chondroid chordomas occur in 5–15% of all chordomas.

The third variety of chordomas is termed "atypical." This is because of a sarcomatoid appearance. There are round cells and epithelial cells, or spindle cells present with large areas of necrosis. These are solid tumors that are aggressive with frequent recurrence and account for 1.3–8% of all chordomas.

Immunohistochemical studies and electron microscopy are useful diagnostic adjuncts in evaluating chordomas because of their ability to confirm a notochord pattern of differentiation by means of analogy through human fetal notochord (5, 6, 28, 33). The immunohistochemical profile of reactivity with antibodies to vimentin, cytokeratin, epithelium membrane antigen (EMA), and S-100 protein generally distinguishes a chordoma from other sarcomatoid round cell or myxoid neoplasms. Chondrosarcomas are negative for cytokeratin, epithelium membrane antigen (EMA), and carcinoembryonic antigen (CEA). Vimentin and S-100 protein are present in both. Immunostaining from keratins has no prognostic value (28). Chondrosarcomas have been lumped together with chordomas because of supposed parallel lines of occurrence, location and aggressive behavior. Only chordomas will be considered in this presentation.

IMAGING CHARACTERISTICS OF CRANIAL CHORDOMAS

Cranial base chordomas are clearly defined by the use of high-resolution CT, with which they appear as solitary or multiple areas of decreased attenuation within the clivus. This is important information in deciding the extent of tumor and bone involvement. The T2-weighted image on MRI is likewise important to see the extent of bright marrow signal in the skull base signifying replacement of bone by tumor (24, 27, 28). In most instances, these tumors are relatively avascular. However, at times carotid and vertebral angiography are essential to recognize the intimate relationship with the vessel. Frequently, tumor removal necessitates manipulation of the internal carotid artery with its potential risk of injury (15, 17). Thus, a balloon test occlusion of the artery should also be done as part of the angiographic evaluation. This test itself has inherent risks; however, the information it provides about the circulatory reserve is important in formulating the treatment strategy (12, 15).

SELECTING THE OPERATIVE APPROACH

It is difficult to cure a patient with chordoma with the use of surgical resection alone. No single operative approach serves for all cranial chordomas. The findings of the clinical history, the examination, and the radiography usually allow a diagnosis of chordoma to be highly suspect. Simple biopsy via the transoral or transsphenoidal route has been advocated by Derome and others, who claim that this is a safe and technically simple procedure that can identify the occasionally incurable carcinoma that is best treated with methods other than aggressive surgical resection (11). We believe that most cases are best approached with initial intent to perform resection of the tumor rather than just biopsy (24, 25). Location of the tumor is the single most important factor in determination of the approach. No single approach is indicated for all chordomas, and in some cases several different approaches are necessary for adequate excision (24, 25). The factors taken into consideration are (a) the location of the tumor, (b) surgical familiarity of the particular approach and team experience, and (c) craniocervical instability.

Most cranial base chordomas are extradural in location until there is infiltration and violation of the dura, when they spread along the subarachnoid space with compression of the brainstem and cerebellum and cervicomedullary junction. Midline tumors are best approached via the midline route, such as the transoral-transpalatopharyngeal route, the sphenoethmoidal route, and the transmaxillary and transfacial approaches (5, 18, 21, 26, 37, 39). Sphenooccipital lesions are approached via an anterolateral, lateral, or posterolateral route; and infratemporal fossa approach; a presigmoid transpetrosal approach; and in combination with transtentorial middle fossa approach (4, 16,

25, 34, 35). The location in the clivus is of great importance. The transoral route does not traverse above the middle of the clivus, (26) whereas the midline skull base approach of Derome et al. has difficulty in reaching the foramen magnum from above (11). It is best to approach the intradural aspects of tumors via a route that does not traverse the oral cavity or the nasal cavity (6, 25). In most instances, the internal carotid artery involvement is with the tumor surrounding it or because of displacement, rather than true infiltration (17, 35). In the series from the University of Pittsburgh (15), the clivus was invaded in 93%; there was cavernous sinus invasion in 75%; and 63% had invasion of the petrous bone with extension into the cerebellopontine angle. The various series actually reflect the bias of the individual surgical teams and their referral pattern for such tumor involvement (5, 11, 15, 21). We believe that hearing preservation is important, and this needs to be kept in mind when planning either a translabyrinthine or presigmoid approach to the clivus.

The tumor involvement of the occipital condyles is of major concern. Apart from craniovertebral instability, this may be a source of tumor recurrence, hence resection is kept in mind and stabilization accomplished (24).

Recent Surgical Series Involving Resection of Cranial Base Chordomas

Watkins et al. describe a significant series of 38 patients treated at the National Hospital of Neurology and Neurosurgery, Queen Square, London (39). The presentation and results of treatment were reviewed between 1958 and 1988. The surgical approaches used were craniotomy in 28 of 38 patients and transoral or transmaxillary route in 10 other patients. All received postoperative external beam radiotherapy comprised of 50–60 Gy. A recurrence was seen in 23 of 38 patients, and 13 of 38 patients died within 5 years. Twelve patients were lost to follow-up. The conclusions of this series were that two groups existed, one with indolent disease and the other with aggressive growth and poor outcome.

Gay et al. reviewed the management of chordomas and chondrosarcomas involving the cranial base between 1984 and 1993 at the University of Pittsburgh (15). This is an impressive series of patients, and the authors recommend an aggressive approach to achieve a high rate of long-term recurrence-free survival. The extent of resection and recurrences was determined radiologically. In this series there were 46 chordomas and 14 chondrosarcomas. Fifty percent of patients had undergone previous surgery before referral, and 22% had previous external beam radiation therapy. The surgical approach used was essentially a subtemporal infratemporal fossa approach with, at times, a transpetrous approach. In other instances, an extended subfrontal approach was used, and in a few the lateral transcondylar approach was made. There was a high tendency to stay between the infratemporal fossa subtemporal approach and the extended subfrontal approach. Using this technique, this group of experienced neurosurgeons describe a 67% total or "near total resection." Eighteen percent died in an average of 5-year follow-up. Twenty percent of patients received postoperative radiation, which was comprised of either external beam, proton beam, or gamma knife therapy (15, 20). There was an overall 5-year recurrence-free survival of 84% in the patients who had undergone total resection and 64% recurrence free survival in those with partial resections. However, the morbidity was fairly severe. Thirty percent cerebrospinal fluid leaks were present in the group, and 10% experienced meningitis as a major complication. There was an 80% immediate new cranial nerve deficit present, though the majority supposedly improved. Forty percent of patients had a permanent functional deterioration in the Karnofsky score.

Chordomas in children are a rare occurrence, and 27 have been reported (5, 8, 40). A classic chordoma is seen in 28%, whereas atypical chordoma in 72% was seen. Thus, the prognosis reflects the atypical lesions. All children with atypical lesions died in a mean of 6 months. Classic chordomas treated within the last 10 years have survived with a mean of 70 months. Metastasis occurs in approximately 60% of children below the age of 5 years. It is in the form of both metastasis that occurs along the site of surgical resection and distant metastasis to lung, bone, and liver. This is a constant feature in 90% of children with atypical chordomas. Metastasis occurs in 9% of children past the age of 5 years and in 20% of individuals above the age of 20 years (5, 7, 8, 39, 40).

Forsyth et al. reviewed 51 intracranial chordomas who were surgically treated between 1960 and 1984 at the Mayo Clinic and Mayo Foundation, Rochester, Minnesota (14). The median age at presentation was 46 years, and 19 tumors were classified as "chondroid" type. Eleven patients underwent a biopsy, and subtotal removal was made in 40. Thirty-nine patients received postoperative radiation therapy. A 5-year survival rate of 51% and a 10-year survival rate of 35% was noted. Univariate analysis showed that patients undergoing resection lived longer in the biopsy patients with a 5-year survival rate of 36%, whereas 55% survived among the 40 patients who received resection. Patients who underwent postoperative radiation therapy tended to have longer disease-free survival times. The disease-free survival data were the same for patients with chondroid chordomas as for those with typical chordomas. Tumor mitotic activity tended to be associated with shorter disease-free survival. The overall impression was that the prognosis in chordomas was not favorable; surgical resection was beneficial; and postoperative radiation prolonged disease-free survival.

We are reporting here on our experience with 36 patients at the University of Iowa Hospitals and Clinics between 1985 and 1995, using the team approach to the cranial base. There were 20 males and 16 females. Thirty-three percent of patients had undergone a previous craniotomy or an attempt at tumor resection via a skull base approach. Twenty-six percent of individuals had previous radiation therapy, and of the 36 individuals, 4 had previously undergone proton beam therapy. The patients reported here all had typical chordoma and underwent detailed histologic and immunohistochemical analysis of the tumor. The primary approaches to these tumors consisted of the transpalatopharyngeal route in 11, transmaxillary route in 7, transphenoethmoidal route in 5, infratemporal fossa approach in 4, lateral extrapharyngeal approach in 4, and a transfacial approach in 5 others. Of 36 individuals, 8 required occipitocervical stabilization. Of these eight, four patients underwent a posterolateral transcondylar approach for resection of remaining tumor, at which time a dorsal occipitocervical fixation was also made. Gross total tumor resection or near total tumor resection was accomplished in 62% of individuals. Fourteen percent (five patients) died in follow-up within a mean of 5 years. Of these five patients, three had previously undergone proton beam therapy and had extensive tumor recurrences. In one other individual, a vertebral artery "blowout" occurred 3 weeks after ventral and dorsal decompression and resection with fusion. In this individual, external beam radiation therapy had been completed before our evaluation, at which time the tumor seemed to have "explosive characteristics," bringing the patient to our attention with massive airway obstruction. Surgical resection was near total with recovery of neurologic deficits. However, a vertebral artery blowout caused her death. Another individual succumbed to a myocardial infarction in the postoperative period. Twenty-two percent of individuals received postoperative radiation for incomplete tumor resection or because of tumor location. Of these, four received proton beam therapy and four conventional radiation therapy. Tumor relapse was seen in seven individuals within 2 years. Three patients had previously undergone proton beam therapy with widespread recurrences and subsequently succumbed. These patients have been included in the mortality already described. Four of the seven patients who had relapses underwent rescue operations and have been tumor progression-free for 2 years. There were no cases of postsurgical cerebrospinal fluid leakage nor meningitis nor new cranial nerve deficits.

RADIATION THERAPY

External Beam Conventional Photon Radiation

In our review of conventional external beam radiotherapy for chordomas, there has been consistent movement toward achieving a higher dosage (1, 8, 9, 24, 30, 31, 32, 36, 38, 39). Radiation therapy accumulating less than 40 Gy has resulted in a progression-free survival rate of 0% over a 5-year period. However, radiation therapy providing more than 48 Gy had a progression-free survival of 75% over a 5-year span. Radiation therapy itself has severe risks that include tumor recurrences, the possibility of brain radiation necrosis, and radiation vasculitis. This author has seen the devastating effects of such therapy and, hence, an aggressive surgical approach has been advocated for such lesions.

Proton Beam Therapy

The combined series of patients treated at the Massachusetts General Hospital proton beam facility has been summarized.(2, 3, 13, 29) This is actually a combination of proton and photon beam irradiation achieving a median dosage of 70.1 cobalt gray equivalent (CGE). The median follow-up was 54 months (range, 8–158 months). Two hundred and four chordomas were reported, of which 153 were cranial base chordomas and 51 pertaining to the upper cervical spine. These were grouped together, showing a relapse rate of 31% (63 of 204 patients). Of these 63 relapses, 95% were local recurrences, and 20% had distant metastasis. The survival for these patients with relapses was 44% over a 3-year span and 5% over a 5-year span. Thus, it should be stated that a good prognosis was recognized in approximately 69% of patients. A poor prognosis was seen when the tumor volume was more than 75 ml, when there was more than 10% of tumor necrosis, and when the cervical spine was also involved. The authors must bring up the question of hormonal interference, because females did not fare as well as male patients. There was no histologic correlation with poor prognosis.

Eighteen children were treated under this protocol with proton beam therapy, ranging in age from 4–18 years. The median tumor dose was 69 CGE with a 72-month median follow-up. Over a 5-year period, the actuarial survival was 68%, whereas the 5-year disease-free survival rate was 63%. This parallels the adult population, in which the disease-free survival rate was 69% over a 5-year period in combination with the primary surgical resection.

CLINICAL MATERIAL

Case 1

This 36-year-old female presented with slurred speech, occipital headaches, and dizziness of 9 months' duration. She had progressive gait difficulties, and 1 month before our evaluation was unable to swallow, necessitating placement of a feeding gastrostomy. At our evaluation her main neurologic deficits were absent gag responses bilaterally. She had low-volume slow speech with bilateral tongue atrophy. Her grips were weak, and she was spastic in her lower extremities with a mincing gait with truncal and appendicular dystaxia. MRI revealed a large isointense mass on T1-weighted images, based on the lower clivus with invagination into the ventral posterior fossa at the pontomedullary junction (Fig. 1A). There was compression and distortion, with circumferential engulfing of the right vertebral artery and prominent masses extending laterally toward the jugular foramen (Fig. 1B). Iohexol CSF-enhanced CT scanning of the posterior fossa structures in such a manner as to include the upper cervical spine (Fig. 2A and B). It revealed destruction of the lower clivus and the occipital condyles, extending upward to the level of the jugular foramen. There appeared to be extradural tumor, mainly in the lower clivus, whereas the midclivus showed tumor that had eroded into the subarachnoid space with severe compression and distortion of the right lateral aspect of the medulla (Fig. 2A and B). CT-reformatted imaged in the sagittal and coronal plane showed destruction of the odontoid process and the inferior clivus, with indentation of the ventrolateral medulla (Fig. 3A). Frontal reformatted CT reconstructions through the plane of the odontoid process revealed complete destruction of both occipital condyles by the tumor mass (Fig. 3B). Because of the large amount of midline and bilateral tumor extension from jugular foramen to jugular foramen in its lateral dimension and from the junction of the upper and middle clivus to the middle aspect of the dens, a transoral-transpalatopharyngeal route for tumor resection and decompression was performed. The tumor was pinkish-gray, lobulated, and gelatinous in appearance and presented immediately when the longus colli muscles were separated. Tumor resection was carried into the subarachnoid space lateral to the tectorial membrane and to the level of the jugular foramen laterally. The right vertebral artery was encased in tumor that could easily be removed with preservation of the anterior spinal artery branch. Dural reconstruction was performed, using fascia

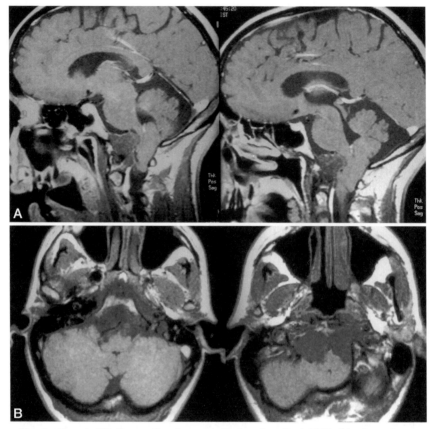

Fig. 1. *Case 1:* (**A**) Composite of parasagittal and sagittal MRI of brain and upper cervical spine with gadolinium enhancement. A large mass is seen replacing the anterior atlas arch, the inferior clivus, and the odontoid process occupying the anterior one-half of the sagittal diameter of foramen magnum with invagination into the pontomedullary junction. A Chiari I malformation is also seen, with the cerebellar tonsils at the C1-C2 interspace and the cervicomedullary buckle present at the level of the midaxis body. (**B**) Composite of axial T1-weighted MRI through the level of the vertebral arteries above foramen magnum on the left and through the midpontine level on the right. The chordoma is well-visualized in the prevertebral space, encasing both vertebral arteries. This chordoma extends from one jugular foramen to the other, and the irregularity in the ventral posterior fossa abuts the vasculature.

harvested from the external oblique aponeurosis that was held in place by reconstituted plasma glue. Postoperative cerebrospinal fluid lumbar drainage was maintained for 5 days and discontinued after that. Intravenous antibiotic therapy was maintained for this period of time,

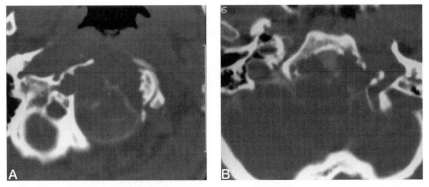

FIG. 2. (**A**) CSF iohexol-enhanced axial CT through the plane of the foramen magnum. Note the destruction of the inferior clivus and the occipital condyles by the extradural mass. (**B**) CSF iohexol-enhanced axial CT through the level of the upper medulla. The jugular foramen is visualized bilaterally. The destruction of the inner table of the clivus is seen by the chordoma, which has now moved to an intraarachnoid location, displacing and rotating the right and anterolateral aspect of the medulla.

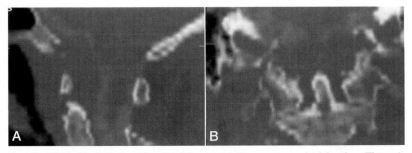

FIG. 3. (**A**) Reformatted midsagittal image of the craniocervical border. There is a large prevertebral mass that has replaced the inferior clivus as well as the odontoid process. (**B**) Coronal reformatted CT of the craniocervical junction through the plane of the odontoid process. Note the destruction of the occipital condyles bilaterally.

using metronidazole, cefotaxime, and nafcillin. There was no evidence of cerebrospinal fluid leakage, and postoperative MRI was made before posterior decompression and dorsal occipitocervical fixation (Fig. 4**A** and **B**). Note that the MRI, studies on midsagittal T1-weighted images show marked upward migration of the cerebellar tonsils and the medulla with gross decompression (Fig. 4**A**). Axial T2-weighted MRIs are demonstrated in composite fashion to better define the extent of ver-

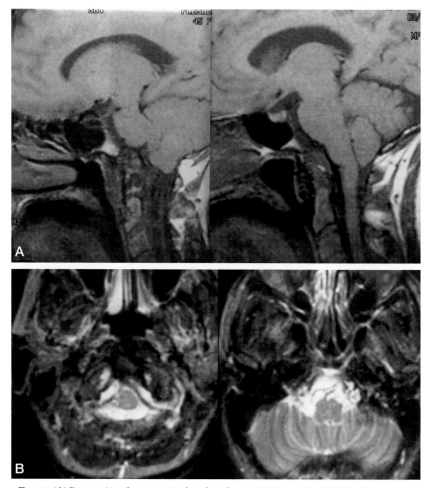

Fig. 4. (**A**)Composite of parasagittal and midsagittal T1-weighted MRI of the posterior fossa and upper cervical spine made 2 weeks after transpalatopharyngeal resection of the extradural and intradural classic chordoma. The cerebellar tonsils have ascended up above the level of the posterior arch of C1. The tumor is no longer visible, and the medulla has assumed its normal contour. The tumor resection led has postoperative changes. (**B**) Composite of T2-weighted axial MRI through the plane of the occipital condyles (*left*) and 1.5 cm above it. The chordoma has been resected. The vertebral arteries are free of encasement, and there is a normal contour to the cervicomedullary junction and the medulla.

tebral artery decompression and that of the medulla (Fig. 4**B**). She recovered her lower cranial nerve deficits, the strength in her hands, and her gait was normal.

Case 2

This 45-year-old male presented with difficulty breathing and swallowing. Physical examination revealed bilateral anosmia with loss of taste and a large mass seen in the nasal cavity that was pinkish in appearance and was friable. Frozen section biopsy diagnosis of this nasal mass was consistent with chordoma. MRI defined a lobulated mass with high signal intensity replacing the entire clivus and filling the nasopharynx. This mass extended laterally to the cavernous sinus and anteriorly to the pterygopalatine fossae bilaterally with encasement of both carotid arteries (Fig. 5A–C). He underwent a LeForte I dropdown maxillotomy with near total resection of tumor. He presented 2 years later with tumor medial to the internal carotid artery, as well as with recurrent tumor in the sphenoid and ethmoid sinuses and complete replacement of tumor in his clivus. This was approached via a right lateral rhinotomy and dropdown maxillotomy with removal of the medial orbit and walls of the maxillary sinuses with gross total resection of the tumor in the paranasal sinuses, as well as the entire clivus. He has done well postoperatively (Fig. 6A and B).

CASE 3

This 62-year-old individual presented with difficulty swallowing, increasing ataxia, and slurred speech of 3–4 years' duration. This condition had gotten worse in the immediate 4 weeks before our evaluation. He had a diagnosis of sphenooccipital chordoma and had previously undergone three operative procedures for this. His first presentation was at age 45 years, when a chordoma was resected from the clivus, sella, and down to the C6 vertebral body in the prevertebral space. He subsequently underwent an attempt at removal of the right middle fossa and posterior fossa components via separate craniotomies. At the time of this evaluation the patient was mildly cachectic with slurred speech. He had involvement of cranial nerves V through XII on the right, with spastic quadriparesis more pronounced in the legs than in the arms and marked difficulty with his balance. MRI (Fig. 7A–C) identified tumor replacing the right half of the clivus, displacing the right internal carotid artery ventrally with encasement and destruction of the petrous apex and intradural tumor into the ventral aspect of the posterior fossa on the right invaginating into the pons and the medulla. There was gross tumor present also in the deep temporal fossa. He underwent right retroauricular infratemporal fossa subtemporal transzygomatic exposure of the lesion after facial nerve rerout-

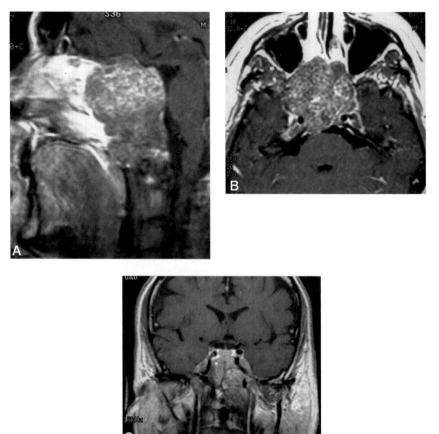

FIG. 5. *Case 2:* (**A**) Midsagittal gadolinium-enhanced MRI of the anterior skull base to include the posterior fossa. The sella and parasellar region, including the dorsum sellae and clivus, is replaced by a lobulated mass that also invaginates into the nasal cavity. (**B**) Axial gadolinium-enhanced MRI through the plane of the cavernous sinus and medulla. Note the position of tumor replacing the clivus as well as encasing the two carotid arteries. The lesion is just above the maxillary sinuses and the pterygopalatine fossa bilaterally. (**C**) Coronal gadolinium-enhanced MRI through the plane of foramen of Monro and cavernous sinus. Note the encasement of both carotid arteries in the cavernous sinus with replacement of the clivus. The lesion extends to the tip of the odontoid process.

ing. The tumor was encountered both medially and laterally to the carotid artery and through the petrous apex into the posterior fossa through the dura. Here the tumor was removed from the pons and the medulla. There was preservation of the trigeminal, as well as the facial

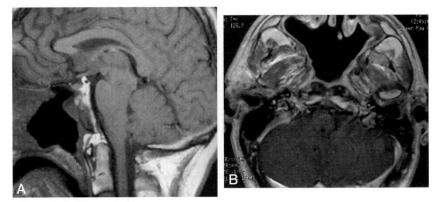

Fig. 6. (**A**) Postoperative midsagittal MRI of brain and posterior fossa made 2 weeks after transfacial transmaxillary resection of the clivus chordoma. Note the absence of tumor in the entire clivus and nasal cavity. (**B**) Postoperative axial MRI through the plane of the condyles and the mandible and midclivus. There is thickening of the mucosa of the maxillary sinus and the high nasopharynx. No tumor can be detected.

and auditory, nerves. Gross tumor resection was accomplished. The dural resection bed was lined with external oblique aponeurosis fascia and then covered with fat and vascularized sternomastoid muscle to fill the defect. Postoperatively he recovered strength and sensation in his upper and lower extremities with improvement in this gait. However, his swallowing dysfunction persisted, and a feeding gastrostomy was installed. He has been tumor-free for the past 3½ years (Fig. 8**A** and **B**).

CONCLUSIONS AND RECOMMENDATIONS FOR CRANIAL BASE CHORDOMAS

We strongly believe that gross surgical resection or near total resection should be the goal *if* possible. The overall management morbidity must be taken into consideration and weighed against recurrence rates and the extent of tumor resection. A close follow-up with postoperative imaging is essential and may need to be done every 3 months for the first year. This is especially true of aggressive lesions. We have preferred to perform reoperation in patients before subjecting them to radiation therapy. In this manner, the neurologic and functional status of the patient can be stabilized for many years. We believe that proton beam therapy should be considered in atypical lesions and in recurrences that are not amenable to a rescue surgical operation. In such individuals as well as in children, proton beam therapy should be entertained after reduction in tumor volume.

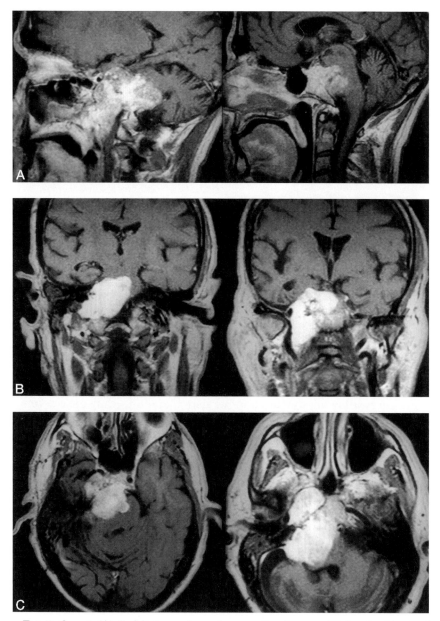

Fig. 7. *Case 3:* (**A**) Gadolinium-enhanced composite of parasagittal and midsagittal MRI of the brain in a 62-year-old male with a previous history of basisphenoid chordoma. Tumor is present in the pterygopalatine fossa and the paraclival regions replacing the petrous bone and clivus, invaginating into the pons and medulla. (**B**) Frontal projection of gadolinium-enhanced MRI through the plane of foramen of Monro (*right*) and 2 cm anterior to it. The clivus chordoma on the right has replaced the dorsum sellae and

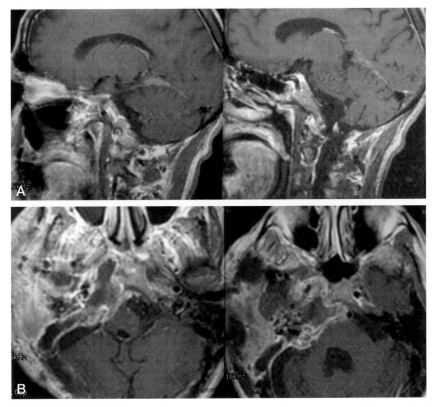

FIG. 8. (**A**) Composite of gadolinium-enhanced parasagittal and near midline sagittal MRI in Case 3 made 1 month postoperatively after retroauricular infratemporal fossa and subtemporal resection of the tumor. (**B**) Postoperative gadolinium-enhanced axial MRI made 2 months after resection of the clivus-petrous-basiocciput chordoma. Note the tumor resection bed, where the dura is enhanced and the indentation into the pons and medulla is now absent. There is a fat pad with muscle in the infratemporal fossa. The fourth ventricle is dilated and migrated toward the right.

invaginated into the midbrain and pons with lateral displacement of the petrous and cavernous and carotid artery. (**C**) Axial MRI with gadolinium enhancement obtained through the plane of the pons and medulla (*right*). The chordoma has replaced the dorsum sella, clivus, and petrous apex with intradural location into the ventrolateral posterior fossa, invaginating into the pons and medulla. There is tumor present medial to the carotid artery.

REFERENCES

1. Amendola BE, Amendola AM, Oliver E, *et al.*: Chordoma: Role of radiation therapy. **Radiology** 158:839–843, 1986.
2. Austin JP, Urie MM, Cardenosa G, *et al.*: Probable causes of recurrence in patients with chordoma and chondrosarcoma of the base of skull and cervical spine. **Int J Radiat Oncol Biol Phys** 25:439–444, 1993.
3. Benk V, Liebsch NJ, Munzenrider JE, *et al.*: Base of skull and cervical spine chordomas in children treated by high-dose irradiation. **Int J Radiat Oncol Biol Phys** 31:577–581, 1995.
4. Blevins NH, Jackler RK, Kaplan MJ, *et al.*: Combined transpetrosal-subtemporal craniotomy for clival tumors with extension into the posterior fossa. **Laryngoscope** 105:975–982, 1995.
5. Borba LAB, Al-Mefty O, Mrak RE, *et al.*: Cranial chordomas in children and adolescents. **J Neurosurg** 84:584–591, 1996.
6. Bouropoulou V, Bosse A, Roesner A, *et al.*: Immunohistochemical investigation of chordomas: Histogenetic and differential diagnostic aspects. **Curr Top Pathol** 80:183–203, 1989.
7. Chambers PW, Schwinn CP: Chordoma. A clinicopathologic study of metastasis. **Am J Clin Pathol** 72:765–776, 1979.
8. Coffin CM, Swanson PE, Wick MR, *et al.*: Chordoma in childhood and adolescence: A clinicopathologic analysis of 12 cases. **Arch Pathol Lab Med** 117:927–933, 1993.
9. Cummings BJ, Hodson DI, Bush RS: Chordoma: The results of megavoltage radiation therapy. **Int J Radiat Oncol Biol Phys** 9:633–642, 1983.
10. Dahlin DC, MacCarty CS: Chodroma: a study of fifty-nine cases. **Cancer** 5:1170–1178, 1952.
11. Derome P, Visot A, Monteil JP, *et al.*: Management of cranial chordomas, in Sekhar LN, Schramm VL (eds): *Tumors of the Cranial Base.* M. Kisco, NY, Futura, 1987, pp 607–662.
12. Erba SM, Horton JA, Latchaw RE, *et al.*: Balloon test occlusion of the internal carotid artery with stable xenon/CT cerebral blood flow imaging. **AJNR** 9:533–538, 1988.
13. Fagundes MA, Hug EB, Leibsch NJ, *et al.*: Radiation therapy for chordomas of the base of skull and cervical spine: Patterns of failure and outcome after relapse. **Int J Radiat Oncol Biol Phys** 33:579–584, 1995.
14. Forsyth PA, Cascino TL, Shaw EG, *et al.*: Intracranial chordomas: A clinicopathological and prognostic study of 51 cases. **J Neurosurg** 78:741–747, 1993.
15. Gay E, Sekhar LN, Rubinstein E, *et al.*: Chordomas and chondrosarcomas of the cranial base: Results and follow-up of 60 patients. **Neurosurgery** 36:887–897, 1995.
16. George B, Dematons C, Cophignon J: Lateral approach to the anterior portion of the foramen magnum: Application to surgical removal of 14 benign tumors—Technical note. **Surg Neurol** 29:484–490, 1988.
17. Goel A: Chordoma and chondrosarcoma: Relationship to the internal carotid artery. **Acta Neurochir (Wien)** 133:30–35, 1995.
18. Gormley WB, Beckman ME, Ho KL, *et al.*: Primary craniofacial chordoma: Case report. **Neurosurgery** 36:1196–1199, 1995.
19. Heffelfinger MJ, Dahlin DC, MacCarty CS, *et al.*: Chordomas and cartilaginous tumors at the skull base. **Cancer** 32:410–420, 1973.

20. Kondziolka D, Lunsford LD, Flickinger JC: The role of radiosurgery in the management of chordoma and chondrosarcoma of the cranial base. **Neurosurgery** 29:38–46, 1991.
21. Lalwani AK, Kaplan MJ, Gutin PH: The transsphenoethmoid approach to the sphenoid sinus and clivus. **Neurosurgery** 31:1008–1014, 1992.
22. Lanzino G, Sekhar LN, Hirsch WL, *et al.*: Chordomas and chondrosarcomas involving the cavernous sinus: Review of surgical treatment and outcome in 31 patients. **Surg Neurol** 40:359–371, 1993.
23. Mabrey RE: Chordoma: A study of 150 cases. **Am J Cancer** 25:501–517, 1935.
24. Menezes AH, Traynelis VC: Tumors of the craniovertebral junction, in Youmans J (ed): *Neurological Surgery*. Philadelphia, W.B. Saunders, 1995, ed 4, pp 3041–3072.
25. Menezes AH, Traynelis VC, Gantz BJ: Surgical approaches to the craniovertebral junction. **Clin Neurosurg** 41:187–203, 1994.
26. Menezes AH, VanGilder JC: Transoral-transpharyngeal approach to the anterior craniocervical junction—10 Year experience of 72 patients. **J Neurosurgery** 69:895–903, 1988.
27. Meyers SP, Hirsch WL, Curtin HD, *et al.*: Chordomas of the skull base: MR features. **AJNR** 13:1627–1636, 1992.
28. Mitchell A, Scheithauer BW, Unni KK, *et al.*: Chordoma and chondroid neoplasms of the spheno-occiput: An immunohistochemical study of 41 cases with prognostic and nosologic implications. **Cancer** 72:2943–2949, 1993.
29. O'Connell JX, Renard LG, Liebsch NJ, *et al.*: Base of skull chordoma: A correlative study of histologic and clinical features of 62 cases. **Cancer** 74:2261–2267, 1994.
30. Pearlman AW, Friedman M: Radical radiation therapy of chordoma. **AJR** 108:333–341, 1970.
31. Raffel C, Wright DC, Gutin PH, *et al.*: Cranial chordomas: Clinical presentation and results of operative and radiation therapy in twenty-six patients. **Neurosurgery** 17:703–710, 1985.
32. Romero J, Cardenes H, la Torre A, *et al.*: Chordoma: Results of radiation therapy in eighteen patients. **Radiother Oncol** 29:27–32, 1993.
33. Rosenberg AE, Brown GA, Bhan AK, *et al.*: Chondroid chordoma—a variant of chordoma: A morphologic and immunohistochemical study. **Am J Clin Pathol** 101:36–41, 1994.
34. Sekhar LN, Janecka IP, Jones NF: Subtemporal-infratemporal and basal subfrontal approach to extensive cranial base tumors. **Acta Neurochir (Wien)** 92:83–92, 1988.
35. Sen CN, Sekhar LN: The subtemporal and preauricular infratemporal approach to intradural structures ventral to the brain stem. **J Neurosurg** 73:345–354, 1990.
36. Sen CN, Sekhar LN, Schramm VL, *et al.*: Chordoma and chondrosarcoma of the cranial base: An 8-year experience. **Neurosurgery** 25:931–941, 1989.
37. Swearingen B, Joseph M, Cheney M: A modified transfacial approach to the clivus. **Neurosurgery** 36(1):101–105, 1995.
38. Tai PTH, Craighead P, Bagdon F: Optimization of radiotherapy for patients with cranial chordoma: A review of dose-response ratios for photon techniques. **Cancer** 75:749–756, 1995.
39. Watkins L, Khudodas ES, Kaleoglu M, *et al.*: Skull base chordomas: A review of 38 patients, 1958–1988. **Br J Neurosurg** 7:241–248, 1993.
40. Yadav YR, Kak VK, Khosla, *et al.*: Cranial chordoma in the first decade. **Clin Neurol Neurosurg** 94:241–246, 1992.

CHAPTER

29

Epidermoid and Dermoid Cysts of the Posterior Fossa

CHARLES S. COBBS, M.D., LAWRENCE H. PITTS, M.D., AND CHARLES B. WILSON, M.D.

Epidermoid cysts are congenital nonneoplastic, slowly growing lesions. They arise from displaced epithelial remnants during closure of the neural tube, starting in the 3rd and continuing into the 5th week of embryonic life (39). Epidermoids are composed entirely of epidermal elements; dermoids have not only epidermal but also dermal structures, such as hair and sebaceous glands. Enlargement of epidermoids may occur by desquamation of normal cells into a cystic cavity. In the case of dermoid cysts, enlargement may also be caused by secretion of dermal elements.

These lesions may occur anywhere along the neuraxis, because they are thought to be formed by inclusions of ectoderm during closure of the neural tube. The variations among the types of lesions seen with dermoids and epidermoids are many and may range from simple, small calvarial lumps to intracranial masses of considerable size to direct cutaneous/central nervous system connections. With respect to age and distribution, dermoids were originally thought to occur more frequently among children, but more recent series have shown that both types of cysts occur at a mean age of 36 years, with a roughly equal distribution in men and women (21, 44).

Epidermoid and dermoid cysts involving the central nervous system account for 0.7–1.8% of all intracranial tumors (although they are not neoplastic *per se*) (5, 7, 16, 32). Intracranial epidermoid cysts are most commonly located in the cerebellopontine angle (CPA) and in the parasellar region (7, 16, 17, 33, 37, 43, 44). Intracranial dermoids usually occur in the posterior fossa and generally originate near the midline (14). Incidence ratios comparing epidermoids to dermoids show that epidermoids are 4–10 times as common as dermoids (44).

HISTORICAL BACKGROUND

Epidermoid cysts were first fully described by the French pathologist, Cruveilhier, in 1829 as "tumeur perlee" because of their pearly appearance (10). For the next 100 years they were known as Cruveilhier's pearly tumors (12). Muller described them as cholesteatomas in reference to three cases he reported, from the cholesterol crystals he noted in the cysts (27). In 1897 Bostroem suggested that these cysts were formed by ectopic inclusions of dermis and epidermis during embryologic development and called them dermoids and epidermoids (8).

This theory was further supported by Bailey in 1920 and, in 1928, Critchley and Ferguson extended the hypothesis by proposing that epidermoids and dermoids were the result of fetal inclusion of epidermal cells, depending on the depth of the layer or according to the embryologic age (4, 9). Manno *et al.* then proposed that dermoids arose when displaced epithelial cells occurred early in fetal life, because they were more pluripotent cells, and that epidermoids were formed if the misplaced cells occurred later in fetal life, because they would be differentially unipotent (25). Since that time, many different names have been attributed to these cysts, including cholesteatoma and pial epidermoid. "Epidermoid" and "dermoid" cysts are now the accepted terms for these lesions.

EMBRYOLOGY

With the advent of modern embryology, it became apparent that inclusion of ectodermal elements at the time of the closure of the neural groove at the 3rd to 5th weeks of embryonic life would explain why these misplaced cells caused midline dermoids and epidermoids (Fig. 1) (36). Investigators furthermore hypothesized that epidermoids more frequently lay away from the midline because of epithelial misplacement during development of the secondary otic and optic vesicles in the forebrain and metencephalon in the 4th or 5th week of development (12, 31). This hypothesis supports the theory that epidermoids may form earlier in development than dermoids, because earlier misplacement of the tissue results in epithelium alone seen in epidermoids, while later in life, misplaced epithelium and mesenchyme contain organizing substances that result in squamous epithelium and skin appendages seen in dermoids (12, 41).

HISTOPATHOLOGY

Grossly, dermoids are well-defined, opaque, oval, or rounded multilobular masses that are generally well demarcated from surrounding

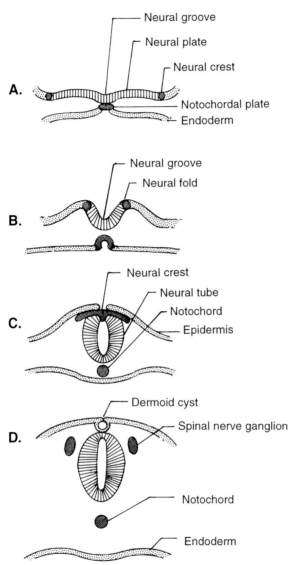

FIG. 1 Schematic diagram illustrating the development and differentiation of the neural plane and tube during the 3rd to 5th weeks of embryonic life. Note that dermal elements may become sequestered and form a dermoid cyst, as represented in **D**. If only epidermal tissue is sequestered, an epidermoid cyst forms.

structures by a wall of fibrous material that varies in its thickness and adherence (21). These cysts may be densely adherent to adjacent brain

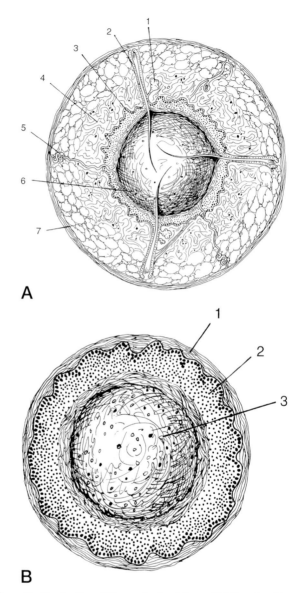

Fig. 2 Schematic illustration of the contents of dermoid (**A**) and epidermoid (**B**) cysts. Dermoid cysts are characterized by normal dermal elements, including sebaceous glands (*1*), hair follicles (*2*), stratified and keratinized squamous epithelium (*3*), connective tissue (*4*), sweat glands (*5*), grumous contents with numerous cholesterol crystals and glandular secretory products (*6*), and a connective tissue capsule (*7*). Epidermoid cysts contain a connective tissue capsule (*1*), keratinized stratified squamous epithelium (*2*), and grumous contents rich in cholesterol crystals (*3*).

tissue; often, there is a layer of reactive gliosis in the surrounding neural tissue. Dermoids may be associated with dermal sinuses to the skin, focal change in skin pigmentation, tufts of external hair and, in the spinal cord, spina bifida (Fig. 2**A**) (5). Calcification may be seen in the wall of the cyst. The material inside the cyst can vary from a dense cheesy substance to a brown, mucoid, oily fluid. Hairs are usually found in the cystic contents.

Epidermoid cysts are usually more cauliflower-shaped than dermoids. They have a thinner wall that does not usually cause as much reactive fibrosis as the wall of a dermoid (Fig. 2**B**). Hence, these cysts often have a mother-of-pearl sheen. The inner contents of the cyst usually have the appearance of a flaky, translucent substance. This grumous substance is formed by the desquamated keratinized squamous epithelial cells, the breakdown products of which form a laminated material rich in cholesterol crystals (21). This inner substance may be either a waxy material or a thick brown oily liquid.

Microscopically, the lining of dermoid and epidermoid cysts recapitulates the normal histology seen in skin. In the case of dermoids, the cyst wall may consist of areas of only stratified squamous epithelium, as well as areas containing normal dermal elements, such as sweat glands, sebaceous glands, and hair follicles (Fig. 3). Thus, the contents of dermoids may contain not only hair but also sebaceous material. Should a dermoid cyst rupture, the cyst contents, especially cholesterol, can incite a very reactive aseptic granulomatous meningitis with giant cell foreign body reaction (21).

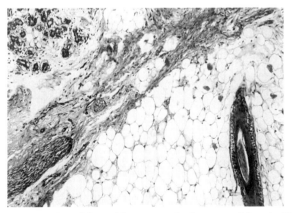

FIG. 3 Microscopic section of dermoid cyst reveals elements of dermis. Note sebaceous gland in upper left, stratified squamous epithelium and fat in center, and hair follicle in lower right.

In the case of epidermoids, only the epidermal layer of skin is seen in the cyst wall, which includes a basal cell layer and the overlying stratified squamous epithelium. The capsule may contain foci of calcification (12). Progressive exfoliation of desquamated keratinized squamous epithelium causes accumulation of grumous material in the center of the cyst and slowly produces the pearly, flaky material. As with dermoid cysts, rupture of epidermoids can result in a granulomatous meningitis. Repeated episodes of such an aseptic meningitis may lead to communicating hydrocephalus in patients with dermoids and epidermoids (44).

Malignant Changes

Malignant change is extremely rare in dermoids and epidermoids but does occur (15, 23). Most patients in whom this occurs die within 1 year from squamous cell carcinoma that arises from the normal squamous epithelial layer of the cysts (21). Of the 13 reported cases of carcinomatous degeneration in an intracranial epidermoid cyst, 10 cases examined either at autopsy or at first operation revealed evidence of a benign epidermoid cyst with histologic transition to malignant degeneration. In only three of the cases was a benign epidermoid cyst subtotally removed initially, with the later operation for recurrence revealing malignant transformation. It has been suggested that protracted chronic inflammation from dermoids and epidermoids may predispose to the development of squamous cell carcinoma, as this form of cancer is seen in long-standing ulcers and draining sinuses (1).

CLINICAL PRESENTATION

Duration of Symptoms

Intracranial epidermoid and dermoid cysts are usually slow in clinical presentation because of their indolent rate of growth. As opposed to neoplastic growth, these cysts are thought to have a linear growth pattern similar to that of skin (3). In general, symptoms may be present for several years, and the sudden onset of symptoms is unusual (28). Before modern imaging techniques were available, patients often suffered such symptoms for years before a diagnosis was possible. One early series reported patients with intracranial epidermoids whose symptoms persisted as long as 29 and 53 years (42). In a more modern series of patients with CPA epidermoids, the average length of onset of symptoms was 4 years (7). Rarely, these cysts will present in a period shorter than a few weeks. Mechanisms of rapid onset of symptoms include tension hydrocephalus, rupture of cystic components leading to chemical meningitis, acute brain swelling, and vascular compromise (28).

Tumor Location

Depending on the location of the cyst, a variety of symptoms may occur. One report describes a patient who presented with painful ophthalmoplegia and a 6th nerve palsy that was subsequently found to have an epidermoid invading the cavernous sinus (22). Other unusual presentations of epidermoids and dermoids include monocular oscillopsia related to chewing in a patient with an orbital epidermoid and a mistaken diagnosis of multiple sclerosis in a woman with diplopia and unsteady gait who had a fourth ventricular epidermoid (37).

When they occur in the posterior fossa, signs and symptoms of a slowly enlarging posterior fossa mass occur. Presenting signs typically include cranial nerve abnormalities, such as trigeminal neuralgia, hemifacial spasm, hearing loss, vertigo, ataxia, hemiparesis, and hemi-anesthesia (2, 13, 44). In four reports describing posterior fossa dermoid and epidermoid cysts, cranial nerve (CN) VII, VIII, and V abnormalities were among the most common presenting signs (Table 1). Other common CN abnormalities included CN VI, as well as CNs IX–XII. Three series reported that more than 80% of patients with posterior fossa dermoids and epidermoids presented with cerebellar signs, including nystagmus and ataxia.

One of the most frequently occurring presenting symptoms in these patients is hearing loss. Other common presenting symptoms include tinnitus, gait disturbance, and vertigo. Trigeminal neuralgia was also seen frequently in three of the series. Interestingly, headache was not one of the most frequent presenting complaints of patients with epidermoids and dermoids of the posterior fossa. This is likely a result of the extremely slow growth rate of these cysts and rarity of acute hydrocephalus in these patients. If not treated, posterior fossa dermoids and epidermoids can eventually lead to dementia related to hydrocephalus, seizures, and dysarthria (42).

A review of patients on the adult services at UCSF in the last 22 years who presented with posterior fossa dermoid and epidermoid cysts is consistent with the existing literature. In our patient series, there were 14 females and 14 males. Of patients with epidermoid cysts, there were 12 female and 13 male patients. There were two female patients and one male patient with dermoid cysts. The ages of patients with epidermoid cysts ranged from 27–65 years (average age = 40), whereas the ages of the patients with dermoid cysts were 20, 51, and 76 years.

Of these 28 patients, the most common presenting sign was 6th cranial nerve palsy, and the most common symptom was trigeminal neuralgia (Table 2). Most patients had more than one presenting sign

TABLE 1

Most Common Presenting Symptoms in Posterior Fossa Dermoid and Epidermoid Cysts

Series Author	Presenting Sign (%)		Presenting Symptom (%)	
Yamakawa *et al.* (43)	CN VIII	(93)	Hypacusis	(67)
(*n* = 15, CPA location)	CN VII	(80)	Gait disturbance	(67)
	Ataxia	(80)	Tinnitus	(60)
	CN V	(73)	Facial palsy	(40)
	CN IX and X	(47)	Diplopia	(27)
	Choked disc	(27)	Dysarthria	(27)
	CN XII	(27)	Facial spasm	(13)
	Pyramidal sign	(27)	Vertigo	(13)
	CN XI	(7)	Tic douloureux	(13)
Sabin *et al.* (33) (*n* = 10,	CN, IX, X, XI, XII	(70)	Diplopia	(60)
CPA location)	Nystagmus	(80)	Deafness	(50)
	Ataxia	(70)	Tinnitus	(50)
	CN VIII	(50)	Weakness	(50)
	CN V	(50)	Vertigo	(40)
	CN III, IV, VI	(40)	Gait ataxia	(40)
	Limb paresis	(40)	Headache	(40)
Yasargil *et al.* (46)	Cerebellar Signs	(95)	Dysequilibrium	(42)
(*n* = 26, "infratentorial"	CN V	(50)	Headache	(35)
location)	CN VIII	(46)	Hypoacusis	(27)
	CN VII	(35)	Vertigo	(27)
	CN VI	(23)	Diplopia	(26)
	CN IX-X	(22)	Tic douloureux	(15)
	Hemiparesis	(15)	Facial numbness	(12)
Samii *et al.* (35) (*n* = 40,	CN VIII	(55)	Hearing loss	(55)
CPA location)	CN V	(43)	Dizziness	(40)
	CN VII	(18)	Gait disturbance	(18)
	CN VI	(10)	Tic douloureux	(13)
	CN IX	(10)	Tinnitus	(11)
	Seizure	(3)	Diplopia	(10)

or symptom. The variety of symptoms was diverse, with problems ranging from pontine to cervicomedullary CN palsies to signs of compression of the cerebral peduncles to cerebellar ataxia.

The duration of symptoms before surgery also varied, with some patients having symptoms for more than 5 years before diagnosis and treatment were initiated (Table 3). The average duration for most of the common presenting signs and symptoms was in the range of 1–4 years. However, the range of duration of symptoms was broad.

The locations of dermoid and epidermoid cysts within the posterior fossa were typical in the UCSF series, with the majority occurring in the CPA. Interestingly, all three dermoid cysts also were found to lie in a lateral CPA location, despite the fact that they usually are found in the midline (Table 4).

TABLE 2
Symptoms and Signs in 25 Patients with Epidermoid Cysts and 3 Patients with Dermoid Cysts at UCSF

	Presenting Sign (%)		Presenting Symptom (%)	
UCSF Series	VI nerve palsy	(14)	Tic douloureux	(29)
(1974–1996)	Ataxia	(14)	Headache	(18)
	Visual loss	(11)	Dizziness	(14)
	Hearing loss	(14)	Diplopia	(11)
	Nystagmus	(11)	Nausea	(7)
	VII nerve palsy	(7)	Vomiting	(7)
	Hemifacial spasm	(7)	Fatigue	(7)
	Meningismus	(7)	Back pain	(4)
	Hemisensory loss	(7)	Dysphagia	(4)
	Hemiparesis	(4)	Drop attacks	(4)
	Dysarthria	(4)	Tinnitus	(4)
	Facial numbness	(4)	Aphasia	(4)
	Fever	(4)	Swallowing problems	(4)

TABLE 3
Preoperative Duration of Presenting Symptoms in UCSF Patients

Symptom or Sign	Duration (yr)	Average (yr)
Tic douloureux	3 mo, 1, 1, 2, 3, 4, 5, 10	3.2
VI nerve palsy	6 wk, 6 mo, 2, 10	3.1
Ataxia	2, 2, 2, 6	3.0
Hearing loss	1, 1, 2, 5	2.2
Dizziness	1, 1, 2, 5	2.2
Headache	6 wk, 4 mo, 6 mo, 1, 5	1.4

TABLE 4
Dermoid and Epidermoid Cyst Location in UCSF Patients

Location of Lesion	No. of Cases
R[a] CPA	7[b]
L CPA	8[b]
R prepontine paramedian	3
L CPA/middle fossa	2[b]
Midline pontomedullary region	2
Intramedullary	1
R CPA/midline/middle fossa	1

[a] R, right; L, left.
[b] Includes one patient with a dermoid cyst. The exact posterior fossa location of 4/28 epidermoid cysts was not described.

RADIOGRAPHIC FEATURES

Before the era of MRI imaging, the radiographic diagnosis of dermoid and epidermoid cysts was quite difficult. Because other lesions appeared similar on plane skull films and CT scans, a distinction between such lesions as meningioma, arachnoid cyst, acoustic neuroma, and others could not be made accurately. MRI imaging now provides almost certain diagnosis of these cysts preoperatively (12).

The first radiographic descriptions of an intracranial epidermoid were made by Cushing in 1922, who noted that these lesions had discrete, sharply demarcated areas of bony destruction with raised edges of increased density (11, 21). Plane films, however, were of little use in diagnosis of CPA epidermoid and dermoids. In the pre-CT scan era, Pantopaque myelograms were used, in which CPA epidermoids exhibited the characteristic lobulated or scalloped border, in contrast to the contour of a meningioma or acoustic neuroma (12). The CT scan era increased the reliability of radiographic diagnosis of posterior fossa dermoids and epidermoids. In one of the earliest reports comparing CT scans to plan skull films in the diagnosis of CPA epidermoids, CT scans were helpful in diagnosing eight of the nine cases, whereas skull radiographs were normal in four and nonspecific in five (26). Both epidermoids and dermoids present with low attenuation (-22 to $+32$ Hounsfield units) on CT scan, with the variation reflecting the content of low-density lipid and high-density keratin in the lesion (21). Occasionally, the CT appearance will show hyperdense areas, and only rarely will the cysts have areas of enhancement (34). The CT scan appearance can be misleading, because the density of these cysts is similar to that of cerebrospinal fluid, and the cysts can, therefore, be easily confused with arachnoid cysts. Occasionally, on bone window program CT, bone absorption of the petrous bone by the cyst may be a clue to the presence of posterior fossa epidermoids (12).

MRI has superseded CT for accurate preoperative evaluation and planning, especially in posterior fossa cysts (21). MRI is especially useful for determining the full extension of the cyst, particularly in the posterior fossa and in the sagittal plane (44). Epidermoid cysts have a fairly characteristic appearance on MRI. Generally, they have decreased relaxation times (low signal intensity) on T1-weighted images and increased relaxation times (high signal intensity) on T2-weighted images (20, 38). This causes them to typically appear isointense or slightly hyperintense relative to cerebrospinal fluid on both T1 or T2-weighted MR images (Fig. 4) (28, 35). However, these cysts may vary considerably in MRI appearance, and may display inhomogeneous areas of low T1 signal or increased T1 signal (Fig. 5) (38, 44).

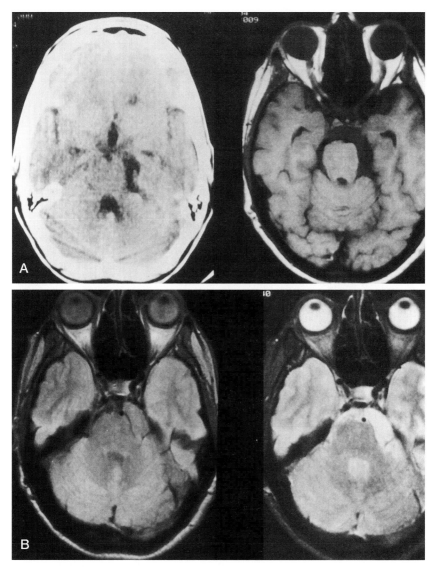

FIG. 4 Axial CT (**A,** *left*) and T1-weighted MR image (**A,** *right*) of an epidermoid cyst in the left prepontine cistern in a 38-year-old woman who presented with a 4-year history of left second division trigeminal neuralgia. **B** shows axial proton density T2 (*left*) and second echo T2-weighted images (*right*) of the same patient. Note that on CT, the cyst appears homogeneous and isodense to CSF, and on T1-weighted image appears slightly hyperintense to CSF. On proton density T2-weighted MR image, the cyst appears hyperintense to CSF, whereas second echo T2 appears isointense to CSF.

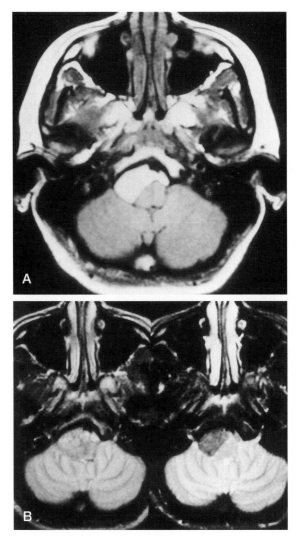

Fig. 5 Axial T1-weighted MR image (**A**) of a patient with a right cerebellopontine epidermoid cyst that compresses the pons and extends to the left of the midline. In **B**, the axial proton density image (*left*) and an axial second echo T2-weighted image (*right*) of the same patient. Note that the T1-weighted image is hyperintense, the proton density image is heterogeneous, and the second echo T2 image is hypointense relative to CSF.

Cystic epidermoids with dense capsules may have bright signal on T1 and T2-weighted images as a result of high lipid content, whereas classical pearly cysts may be hypointense on T1-weighted images (12). The dermoid cysts show variable relaxation times, depending on the

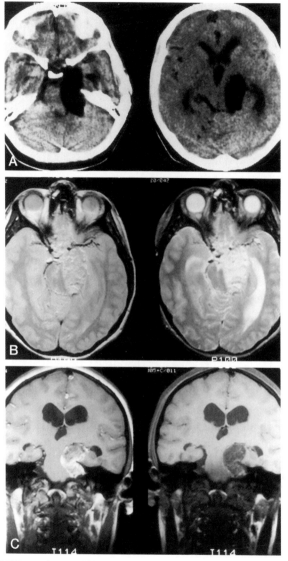

FIG. 6 Axial CT scan images (**A**) of a 20-year-old female who presented with a 4-month history of headache and had a ruptured dermoid cyst. Unenhanced CT reveals a large left cerebellopontine hypodense lesion that extends into the left middle fossa. Axial proton density MR image (**B**, *left*) reveals the large left cerebellopontine mass, heterogeneous and isointense to brain. In the axial T2-weighted image (**B**, *right*), the lesion is hyperintense. A coronal T1-weighted image reveals a heterogeneous hyperintense lesion compressing the left cerebral peduncle (**C**, *left*). Note in this image that the lesion has caused hydrocephalus, and there are multiple small hyperintense areas in the subarachnoid space. A fat saturation T1-weighted image (**C**, *right*) shows that the lesion becomes hypointense, consistent with fat.

amount of fat present, but usually a pattern of short T1 and prolonged T2 is seen (Fig. 6) (19, 44). Epidermoid cysts do not enhance with the administration of gadolinium contrast (12).

Diffusion-weighted MR imaging has recently become the best and most useful radiographic modality for discriminating between epidermoid cysts and arachnoid cysts in the posterior fossa. This imaging technique represents a physiologic MR cisternogram and is not only useful in distinguishing between CSF and epidermoid cysts but is the only method that can distinguish between epidermoid cyst and encephalomalacia (35, 40).

SURGICAL TREATMENT

Ideally, epidermoid and dermoid cysts should be entirely excised, because they will recur and are not chemo- or radiosensitive. However, in practice it is usually difficult to obtain a gross total resection without incurring injury to involved neurovascular structures, as the cyst capsule often is adherent to these structures. If total removal is possible, however, a cure is attainable. Recurrent tumors are difficult to treat and are virtually never surgically curable (24).

The technical aspects involved in operating on posterior fossa dermoids and epidermoids are fairly straightforward. As stated, the cerebellopontine angle is the most common place for infratentorial epidermoids to occur. In our UCSF series, most patients were positioned in the lateral decubitus position, and a vertical paramedian retromastoid incision was used to expose the occipital bone squama. Next, a suboccipital craniectomy was performed to achieve the optimal exposure of the cyst, depending on its rostrocaudal extent. Because of the way these cysts grow throughout the subarachnoid spaces, it is not uncommon for them to grow into the region of the 6th nerve and the trigeminal canal, as well as around into the interpeduncular space (24). They may also extend both above and below the tentorium, assuming a transtentorial configuration (35). Thus, the extent of the tumor should be considered when making the bony opening.

Samii *et al.* recently suggested that it is useful conceptually to divide the posterior fossa into four compartments or "floors" when surgically approaching CPA epidermoids. According to their scheme, the first floor lies between the tentorium and the fifth nerve, the second floor between the fifth nerve and the seventh and eighth nerve complexes, the third floor lies from there down to the lower cranial nerves, and the fourth floor from these nerves down to the foramen magnum. They propose that approaching resections in this way permits easier identification of the cranial nerves near their bony or dural entrance, where their anatomy is most normally preserved (35).

Once the capsule is observed upon opening the dura, the cyst should be immediately entered, and removal of the soft cyst contents should be first achieved to create "working space." This will help to avoid manipulation of neighboring neural structures during the rest of the resection (44). Once the cyst contents are debulked, a meticulous dissection of the external capsule should ensue. Because the cyst capsule of dermoids and epidermoids may be firmly attached to nerves and vessels, a complete removal of the capsule at any price is unwise and should be avoided (35). The capsules of dermoid cysts in particular often display dense reactive involvement of the arachnoid and, occasionally, of the pia mater (44). In such cases tedious and patient dissection is required; complete and total removal is usually possible.

The most favorable outcomes of a modern series on resection of posterior fossa dermoid and epidermoid cysts was by Yasargil et al. in 1989 (44). Their series reported results from resection of 22 CPA epidermoids and one infratentorial dermoid. A total resection was obtained in all but one patient. Patient mortality was zero, and there were no recurrences in the 5.7-year follow-up period. Samii et al. in 1996 reported a series of 40 patients with cerebellopontine angle epidermoids (35). Total resection was achieved in 30 (75%) of these patients, although parts of the cyst capsule were left behind in 10 patients because of adherence to the brainstem and adjacent structures. In both series, more than 85% of patients had good or excellent outcomes.

COMPLICATIONS AND RECURRENCES

Only one complication is unique to epidermoid and dermoid cysts. These cysts occasionally present with a meningitis-like syndrome after spontaneous rupture of the contents into the subarachnoid space or the ventricle (6, 24). Care must be taken during surgery to avoid spilling the contents of the cyst, because a severe syndrome of aseptic meningitis may result. This syndrome is signaled by high temperature and intense local pain (1, 24). Patients may become confused and have impaired levels of consciousness. Lumbar puncture demonstrates cloudy fluid with neutrophils and lymphocytes, but the culture will be negative (24). If meningitis occurs, CSF cultures should be taken, and both broad spectrum antibiotics and dexamethasone (4 mg every 6 hours) started. If CSF cultures are negative, the antibiotics can be stopped. Adhesive arachnoiditis in the areas surrounding the CNs in the area of surgery can be a late complication, particularly if there is spillage of cyst contents during surgery (24).

Other common complications after posterior fossa dermoid and epidermoid resections include transient CN deficits. Of the 28 patients reviewed at UCSF, 18 patients had at least some new deficits postoperatively, whereas only 5 patients had deficits that persisted for more than a few days. The most common postoperative CN deficits included VII, VIII, VI, and IV. Long-term deficits were diverse and included CN VIII palsy, aseptic meningitis leading to hydrocephalus, ataxia, aphasia, and trigeminal neuralgia. We had no postoperative deaths. In their review of the literature, Samii *et al.* report that the operative mortality from posterior fossa epidermoid surgeries performed since 1950 is in the range of 6% (35).

The diagnosis of recurrence is made by the appearance of new neurologic deficits or by MRI (24). A review of nine major reports on epidermoid cysts of the cerebellopontine angle by Samii *et al.* showed that cyst recurrences after surgery occurred in from 0–30% of patients (35). In this series of articles the follow-up time of the patients was from 4.5 to 9 years. The higher rates of recurrence seen in earlier studies in this series are likely related to incomplete removal of the cyst, unrecognized at the time, rather than to regrowth of small remnants of the cyst lining known to be left behind, according to the authors. Of the four patients in the UCSF series who required reoperation, two patients required operations 6 years after their original procedures, and two patients had reoperations 1 year after the original procedure. All four of these patients had their original surgeries in the pre-MRI era, and it is possible that the lack of adequate imaging contributed to their incomplete original resection.

CONCLUSION

Dermoid and epidermoid cysts of the posterior fossa are uncommon benign lesions that produce a variety of slowly progressive symptoms mainly referable to CN dysfunction. They often can be completely removed by carefully planned surgery if they are relatively small when they are diagnosed. Because their growth is very slow (on the order of decades), incomplete removal of these tumors is warranted, rather than aggressive surgical extirpation if the latter would be accompanied by significant postoperative morbidity.

REFERENCES

1. Abramson RC, Morawetz RB, Schlitt M: Multiple complications from an intracranial epidermoid cyst: Case report and literature review. **Neurosurgery** 24:574–578, 1989.
2. Altschuler EM, Jungreis CA, Sekhar LN, *et al.*: Operative treatment of intracranial epidermoid cysts and cholesterol granulomas. **Neurosurgery** 26:606–614, 1990.
3. Alvord EC: Growth rates of epidermoid tumors. **Ann Neurol** 2:367–370, 1977.

4. Bailey P: Cruveilhier's "tumeurs perlees." **Surg Gynecol Obstet** 31:390–401, 1920.

5. Baxter JW, Netsky MG: Epidermoid and dermoid tumors: Pathology, in Wilkins RH, Rengachary SS, (eds): *Neurosurgery*. New York, McGraw-Hill, 1985, vol 1, pp 655–661.

6. Becker WJ, Watters GV, de Chadarevien JP, *et al.*: Recurrent aseptic meningitis secondary to intracranial epidermoids. **Can J Neurol Sci** 11:387–389, 1984.

7. Berger MS, Wilson CB: Epidermoid cysts of the posterior fossa. **J Neurosurg** 62:214–219, 1985.

8. Bostroem E: Ueber dei pialen epidermoide, dermoide und lipome ud duralen dermoide, centralbl allg. **Path Path Anat** 8:1–98, 1897.

9. Critchley M, Ferguson FR: The cerebrospinal epidermoids (cholesteatoma). **Brain** 51:334–384, 1928.

10. Cruveilhier J: *Anatomie Pathologique du Corps Humain*. Paris, J.B. Baillere, 1829–1835, block 2,341.

11. Cushing H: A large epidermoid cholesteatoma of the parietotemporal region deforming the left hemisphere without cerebral symptoms. **Surg Gynecol Obstet** 34:557–566, 1922.

12. De La Cruz A, Doyle KJ: Epidermoids of the cerebellopontine angle, in Jackler RK, Brackmann DE (eds): *Neurotology*. St. Louis, Mosby-Year Book, 1994, pp 823–833.

13. DeSouza CE, Menezes CO, DeSouza RA, *et al.*: Profile of congenital cholesteatomas of the petrous apex. **J Postgrad Med** 35:93–97, 1989.

14. Fenstermaker RA, Ganz E, Roessmann U: Giant invasive dermoid tumor with subependymoma-like reaction: Case report. **Neurosurgery** 25:646–648, 1989.

15. Garcia CA, McGary PA, Rodriguez F: Primary intracranial squamous cell carcinoma of the right cerebellopontine angle. **J Neurosurg** 34:824–826, 1981.

16. Grant FC, Austin GM: Epidermoids: Clinical evaluation and surgical results. **J Neurosurg** 7:190–198, 1950.

17. Guidetti B, Gagliardi FM: Epidermoid and dermoid cysts: Clinical evaluation and late surgical results. **J Neurosurg** 47:12–18, 1977.

18. Horowitz BL, Chari MV, James R, *et al.*: MR of intracranial epidermoid tumors: Correlation of in vivo imaging with in vitro ^{13}C spectroscopy. **AJNR** 11:299–302, 1990.

19. Hudgins RJ, Rhyner PA, Edwards MS: Magnetic resonance imaging and management of a pineal region dermoid. **Surg Neurol** 27:558–562, 1987.

20. Ishikawa M, Kikuchi H, Asato R: Magnetic resonance imaging of the intracranial epidermoid. **Acta Neurochir** 1:108–111, 1989.

21. Johnston FG, Crockard HA: Dermoid, epidermoid and neurenteric cysts, in Kaye AH, Laws ER (eds): *Brain Tumors*. New York, Churchill Livingstone, 1995, ed 1, pp 895–905.

22. Kline LB, Galbraith JG: Parasellar epidermoid tumor presenting as painful ophthalmoplegia. **J Neurosurg** 54:113–117, 1981.

23. Lewis AJ, Cooper PW, Kassel EE, *et al.*: Squamous cell carcinoma arising from a suprasellar epidermoid cyst. **Neurosurgery** 59:538, 1983.

24. Long DM: Intracranial epidermoid tumors, in Apuzzo MLJ (ed): *Brain Surgery*. New York, Churchill Livingstone, 1993, pp 669–688.

25. Manno NJ, Uihlein A, Kernohan JW: Intraspinal epidermoids. **J Neurosurg** 19: 754, 1962.

26. Mikhael MA, Mattar AG: Intracranial pearly tumors: The roles of computed tomography, angiography and pneumoencephalography. **J Comput Assist Tomogr** 2:421–429, 1978.

27. Muller J: *Ueber den Feineren Bau und Die Formen der Krankhaften Geschwultse.* Berlin, G Reimer, 1838, vol 1, p 51.

28. Netsky MG: Epidermoid tumors: Review of literature. **Surg Neurol** 29:477–483, 1988.

29. Obana WG, Wilson CB: Epidermoid cysts of the brainstem. **J Neurosurg** 74:123–128, 1991.

30. Knight RT, St. John JN, Nakada T: Chewing oscillopsia—A case of voluntary visual illusions of movement. **Arch Neurol** 41:95–96, 1984.

31. Rand CW, Reeves DL: Dermoid and epidermoid tumors (cholesteatomas) of the central nervous system. **Arch Surg** 46:350–376, 1943.

32. Robbins SL, Angell M, Kumar V: *Basic Pathology.* Philadelphia, W.B. Saunders, 1981, vol 3, pp 126–127.

33. Sabin HI, Bordi LT, Symon L: Epidermoid cysts and cholesterol granulomas centered on the posterior fossa: Twenty years of diagnosis and management. **Neurosurgery** 21:798–805, 1987.

34. Salazar J, Vaquero J, Suacedo G, *et al.*: Posterior fossa epidermoid cysts. **Acta Neurochir (Wien)** 85:34–39, 1987.

35. Samii M, Tatagiba M, Piquer J, *et al.*: Surgical treatment of epidermoid cysts of the cerebellopontine angle. **J Neurosurg** 84:14–19, 1996.

36. Scholtz E: Einege bemerkungen ueber das meningeale cholesteatom in anschluss an einen fall von cholesteatom des III ventrikels. **Virchow's Arch Pathol Anat** 184:225–273, 1906.

37. Schraeder PL, Cohen MM, Goldman W: Bilateral inter-nuclear ophthalmoplegia associated with 4th ventricular epidermoid tumor: Case report. **J Neurosurg** 54: 403–405, 1981.

38. Tampieri K, Melanson K, Ethier R: MR imaging of epidermoid cysts. **AJNR** 10:351–356, 1989.

39. Tan T: Epidermoids and dermoids in the central nervous system. **Acta Neurochir (Wein)** 26:13–24, 1972.

40. Tsuruda JS, Chew WM, Moseley ME, *et al.*: Diffusion-weighted MR imaging of the brain: Value of differentiating between extraaxial cysts and epidermoid tumors. **AJR** 155:1059–1065, 1990.

41. Tytus JS, Pennybacker J: A report upon pearly tumors in relation to the central nervous system. **J Neurol Neurosurg Psychiatry** 19:241–259, 1956.

42. Ulrich J: Intracranial epidermoids: A study in their distribution and spread. **J Neurosurg** 21:1051–1058, 1964.

43. Yamakawa K, Shitara N, Genka S, *et al.*: Clinical course and surgical prognosis of 33 cases of intracranial epidermoid tumors. **Neurosurgery** 24:568–573, 1989.

44. Yasargil MG, Abernathy CD, Sarioglu AC: Microneurosurgical treatment of intracranial dermoid and epidermoid tumors. **Neurosurgery** 24:561–567, 1989.

30

Vestibular Neurilemmomas
(Honored Guest Lecture)

PETER J. JANNETTA, M.D., D.Sci.

The management of vestibular neurilemmomas remains a considerable challenge to neurosurgeons and neurootologists. Improved access to high-resolution imaging has greatly increased the number of asymptomatic or minimally symptomatic individuals harboring these challenging lesions. Furthermore, advances in stereotactic radiosurgery continue to challenge and redefine the role of microsurgery.

As outlined by Moskowitz and Long (19) and House (11), the surgery for vestibular neurilemmomas has proceeded through a number of distinct eras. Initially, patients presented in extremis, and excision with survival was the goal. Later, with the advent of microsurgery and better imaging, preservation of facial nerve function became paramount (24, 31). Next, as surgical techniques and imaging were refined, hearing preservation was sought in selected patients (5, 13). Finally, in the present era, radiosurgery is increasingly viewed as a legitimate alternative to microsurgery in selected patients (14, 21, 23). For microsurgeons, radiosurgery must serve as an impetus to strive for excellent results while minimizing patient morbidity and discomfort.

Over the past 25 years, 691 vestibular neurilemmomas have been resected at the University of Pittsburgh, with the majority performed by this author. Through the presentation and analysis of this broad experience, I hope to share some technical pearls and pitfalls. More importantly, I hope to challenge future generations to improve on these results. This chapter will consist of three sections: Selection Criteria, Technical Aspects of Microsurgical Resection, and Outcome Assessment, followed by Conclusions.

SELECTION CRITERIA

Many factors must be weighed in considering a patient for microsurgical resection of a vestibular neurilemmoma. These include the patient's age, symptomatology, general health (and life expectancy, where appropriate), tumor size, baseline cranial nerve function, and the presence or absence of neurofibromatosis type II (NF2). One additional factor that cannot be overlooked is patient expectation. If the patient is unwilling to accept any risk of morbidity or mortality, radiosurgery or observation alone should be selected. Each of the above variables for patient selection will be examined in some detail.

Age

The mean age in our series is 49 years (range, 15–86 years) with a slight female preponderance. Throughout this series, the mean patient age has remained unchanged (Table 1). This is somewhat surprising, as one might expect a decline in the mean age for two reasons: (*a*) earlier detection of younger patients and (*b*) increased use of radiosurgery for older patients. In terms of an age beyond which microsurgery will not be offered, if a patient is up to 75 years old and in excellent health, he or she will be considered a candidate for resection. It should be noted that patients older than 75 will be considered for at least subtotal resection if they are symptomatic from brainstem compression. This is similar to the strategy described by Lownie and Drake (15).

Tumor Size

During the period from 1971 to 1996, there has been a shift toward smaller tumors (Table 1). Although the mean age of patients has remained constant, the presence of a higher percentage of small- and medium-sized lesions suggests that earlier detection and treatment of small lesions is occurring secondary to increased availability of high-resolution imaging. For patients with small tumors (largest diameter, ≤1.5 cm) and good hearing, excision with hearing preservation is the goal. In this series, of the 38 patients with small tumors resected via the retromastoid route and Gardner-Robertson (5) class 1 hearing, 10

TABLE 1
Demographic Information

Yrs	No. of Patients	Average Symptom Duration (yr)	Mean Age (yr)	Male/Female	Small Tumors (%)	Medium Tumors (%)	Large Tumors (%)
1971–1975	49	5.4	50		6 (12)	11 (22)	32 (65)
1976–1980	105	3.7	49		16 (15)	37 (35)	52 (50)
1981–1985	162	5.6	50		35 (22)	70 (43)	57 (35)
1986–1990	188	4.0	50		58 (31)	84 (45)	46 (24)
1991–1996	187	2.8	47		75 (40)	73 (39)	39 (21)
Total	691	4.0	49	44%/56%	190 (27)	275 (40)	226 (33)

of 38 (26%) had class 2 or better hearing postoperatively. There are technical factors that may improve the ability to preserve hearing (13). They will be reviewed in a subsequent section.

Hearing preservation is possible but considerably less likely with medium (largest dimension between 1.5 and 3 cm) and large tumors (largest dimension, >3 cm); this is the experience in this series as well as other reports (5). Of great importance with medium or large tumors is the status of adjacent cranial nerves. Anatomic and functional loss of cranial nerve VII rises sharply with tumor size in both this and other series (4, 6–9, 16, 19, 20, 22, 28, 30). For these lesions, patients must be made aware of the risk of temporary or permanent facial and trigeminal dysfunction. Patients harboring large tumors with hydrocephalus and brainstem distortion may benefit from preoperative CSF diversion. In our experience, 44 of 691 patients (6.4%) required permanent CSF diversion. In the majority of patients, this was performed before their microsurgical resection. The effects of chronically raised intracranial pressure can be significant. One patient in our series had a large tumor with moderate ventriculomegaly, significant brainstem distortion, and chronic papilledema. The patient's symptoms were believed to be primarily the result of brainstem distortion; therefore, tumor resection was completed before cerebrospinal fluid diversion. In the postoperative period, the patient experienced rapid visual decline to legal blindness and has only made a partial recovery.

Presenting Symptoms

The vast majority of patients in this series presented with gradual hearing loss (79%), tinnitus (51%), and dysequilibrium (41%). The average duration of symptoms was 4 years. Ten percent of patients presented with rapid hearing loss; this group tended to be younger and to have large tumors. Trigeminal dysfunction was less common, with sensory symptoms occurring in 19% and typical trigeminal neuralgia occurring in 5%. Preoperative facial weakness was seen in 9% and correlated strongly with poor postoperative facial nerve function. A summary of presenting symptoms is supplied in Table 2.

Neurofibromatosis Type II (NF 2)

The presence of NF2 in our series is 5%. As expected, the mean age of members of this group was younger than in the overall series (27 versus 49 years). In addition, this group had shorter symptom duration, higher morbidity, more recurrences, and worse facial nerve and hearing outcomes. In this difficult group of patients, the goals of surgery and expectations are influenced by several important factors: (a) the presence of bilateral tumors with a high probability of bilateral

TABLE 2
Summary of Presenting Symptoms[a]

Symptomatology	No. of Patients (%)	Average Symptom Duration (yr)
Hearing loss		
Gradual	386 (79)	4.5
Sudden	49 (10)	2.0
Tinnitus	249 (51)	4.0
Dysequilibrium	202 (41)	3.6
Facial numbness	92 (19)	4.1
Headache	76 (15)	4.0
Facial weakness	44 (9)	6.0
Trigeminal neuralgia	25 (5)	8.8

[a] Complete data available for 491 patients.

hearing loss, (b) the presence of other tumors of the neuraxis, and (c) the growth rate and tenacity of vestibular neurilemmomas in patients with NF2. This last factor leads to a much higher incidence of cranial nerve loss and recurrence, compared to that of patients without NF2. In terms of hearing preservation, neither microsurgery nor radiosurgery (14) has been dramatically successful. Therefore, treatment for bilateral vestibular neurilemmomas may be delayed unless one is faced with obvious radiographic progression or brainstem compromise.

TECHNICAL ASPECTS OF MICROSURGICAL RESECTION

Microsurgical resection of vestibular neurilemmomas may be performed using a variety of positions and approaches. Choice of position and approach is dictated by several important factors: (a) Tumor size (purely intracanalicula, small, medium, or large), (b) tumor orientation (rostral to porus, caudal to porus, extending far laterally in porus), (c) the surgeon's familiarity and comfort with an approach and position, and lastly, (d) the goals of operation. A detailed discussion of the merits and shortcomings of each approach is unfortunately beyond the scope of this chapter. For virtually all of the variants listed above, the author favors a retromastoid approach. In the overall series, the vast majority of resections were performed via this route (Table 3). For each tumor size (small, medium, and large), I will discuss my surgical technique with an emphasis on optimal results and complication avoidance. First, I will review some features of intraoperative monitoring and anesthetic techniques.

Intraoperative Monitoring

Virtually all patients in this series were monitored with bilateral brainstem evoked responses (BSER). Even in patients with absent or

TABLE 3
Positioning and approaches for 691 patients (1971–1996)

Position	No. of Patients (%)	Approach	No. of Patients (%)
Sitting	124 (18)	Retromastoid	560 (81)
Supine	131 (19)	Translabyrinthine	125 (18)
Lateral	436 (63)	Middle fossa	6 (1)
Total	691		691

severely attenuated BSERs on the operative side, the author has found contralateral BSERs to be valuable for providing information on the status of the brainstem during tumor dissection and manipulation. Subdermal needle electrodes are used for recording both spontaneous and evoked electromyographic (EMG) activity. Recordings are made from the orbicularis oculi, orbicularis oris, and mentalis muscle groups. A bipolar recording montage is used to allow facial nerve activity to be localized to a specific muscle group. These data are also coupled to an auditory circuit, allowing both the surgeon and neurophysiologist to have real-time auditory feedback when the facial nerve is manipulated, which is similar to the method previously described by Delgado et al. (3). This allows one to alter surgical technique immediately to avoid maneuvers that irritate the facial nerve. In addition to facial nerve monitoring, trigeminal nerve activity is recorded from the muscles of mastication on a fourth channel. This allows for more precise identification of cranial nerves, as trigeminal irritation can often be mistaken for facial activity because of the proximity of the muscle groups supplied by the two nerves.

Direct stimulation and recording of evoked EMG is performed using a constant voltage monopolar stimulator. With this type of stimulator, current passage is independent of changes in shunting because of variable amounts of fluid in the operative field. The facial nerve stimulator uses a low impedance source (1000 ohms) of impulses (duration, 100 μsec), presented a rate of 5 Hz. An insulated monopolar electrode with a 2- to 4-mm exposed tip is coupled to a return needle electrode that is placed in adjacent soft tissue. This technique facilitates direct identification of the facial nerve and allows one to determine a stimulus threshold for any portion of the nerve (18).

In patients with serviceable preoperative hearing, direct cochlear monitoring is used as a supplement to BSERs. In its current form, this system uses a small-pledget electrode that is placed in the lateral recess of the fourth ventricle, overlying the cochlear nucleus. This receiving electrode is coupled to a monopolar stimulating electrode, allowing monitoring of compound action potentials and threshold determination for the cochlear portion of the eighth nerve (13, 17).

Anesthetic Technique

The delivery of anesthesia is more challenging for the surgery of vestibular neurilemmomas because paralytic agents cannot be used because they would abolish essential facial EMG monitoring. Balanced anesthetic techniques are used, consisting of intravenous narcotic infusion and inhalation agents. Additional anesthetic challenges for this type of surgery involve the specter of air embolism with the sitting position as well as, sometimes, dramatic pulse (asystole) and blood pressure changes with tumor capsule manipulation. In several patients early in the current series, resection had to be interrupted after massive air embolus or repeated asystole with tumor manipulation. Because of these considerations, patients should have a central venous catheter and arterial line, regardless of tumor size or approach used; it is obligatory for the sitting position.

Operative Techniques

SMALL TUMORS (<15 MM LARGEST DIAMETER)

Preferred approach. Retromastoid.

Patient Positioning. Lateral with head flexed, nose turned 10–15% toward the floor, slight vertex down. This position permits excellent visualization of cisternal tumor, as well as tumor in the lateral portion of the porus acousticus (Fig. 1).

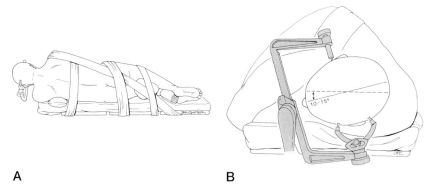

A **B**

Fig. 1 Schematic of patient in lateral position. (**A**) Posterior view. (**B**) View from patient's head. Table is reversed to allow surgeon's knees to fit beneath patient's head.

Incision. Linear, lazy S, positioned slightly more medially than for a microvascular decompression. This will permit the necessary medial bone resection to allow visualization of the petrous bone en face.

Bone Work. Craniectomy must expose the junction of the transverse and sigmoid sinuses. In addition, bone must be removed low and lateral along distal sigmoid sinus to allow visualization of caudal pole of tumor and brainstem with minimal cerebellar retraction. As mentioned above, additional medial bone removal will allow better visualization of the petrous bone for drilling and dissection of the porus acousticus. For medial bone removal and dural incision, it is important to remember that the medial transverse sinus is often more caudally located than the transverse-sigmoid junction. Failure to anticipate this can result in injury to the transverse sinus at the superior and medial aspect of the craniectomy.

Dural opening. Dura is usually opened in a flap based on the sigmoid sinus. Additional relaxing incisions are added to this primary incision at the medial superior and medial inferior poles.

Dissection Sequence. For small tumors, the double arachnoid layer is opened longitudinally after coagulation of the posterior porus dura. Next, the poles of the tumor are identified. At the rostral pole, the petrosal venous complex is identified and divided early in the dissection if necessary. This is done to prevent avulsion of the complex off of the superior petrosal sinus with subsequent retraction. Next, the posterior aspect of the capsule is stimulated to ensure that the facial nerve is not on its surface. If the facial nerve is not present, the lateral aspect of the tumor capsule may be coagulated to devascularize the lateral portion of the tumor. At this point, the rostral and caudal lips of the porus are identified with a 45° microhook (Fig. 2). Next, the dura over the porus is coagulated and removed. In addition to favoring the retromastoid approach, the author performs drilling of the porus relatively early in the dissection sequence, rather than drilling toward the end of the procedure. This is preferred because it permits early distal identification of the facial nerve. Then, with both proximal and distal facial nerve identified, one can work relatively quickly to free the facial nerve along its entire course.

The porus is then drilled using a small round cutting burr. Drilling is performed laterally for approximately 10 mm until a thin shell of bone remains. This is removed using a small curette. Although a diamond burr is favored by some, it is my belief that a cutting burr works more quickly and generates less heat. Copious irrigation is used to minimize heat transmission to adjacent structures. After bone removal is completed, dura is opened with an no. 11 blade. The distal

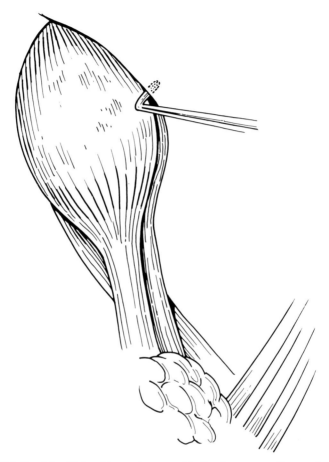

FIG. 2 Relationship of lateral tumor to porus. Limits of porus are discerned using a 45° microhook.

aspect of the tumor is identified and carefully dissected medially. After stimulating to identify the seventh cranial nerve (and the cochlear portion of the eighth cranial nerve if hearing preservation is being attempted), the tumor is dissected from laterally to medially. Once identified, one or both vestibular nerves are sharply divided distal to the point of obvious tumor involvement. This is done to prevent inadvertent traction on inner ear structures with potential hearing loss. Once tumor dissection has reached the lip of the porus, the tumor is opened. The tumor is then internally debulked to allow manipulation of the capsule. As reviewed below, if hearing preservation is the goal, internal debulking and excessive tumor manipulation are to be avoided because they may result in cochlear nerve damage (6). After this, the tumor is carefully dissected off of the brainstem, allowing identification of the entry zones of cranial nerves VII and VIII. At this point, dissection proceeds from medial to lateral and vice versa until all tumor has been removed from the seventh nerve. Similarly, if the cochlear portion of the eighth nerve is not invaded by tumor, tumor is carefully removed from it.

Closure. After tumor has been completely removed, a facial nerve threshold is obtained at the brainstem and at the porus. After irrigation, several Valsalva maneuvers are performed to ensure that hemostasis has been achieved. The drilled portion of the porus is then carefully waxed and covered by surgical cellulose. Great care must be taken to prevent bone wax from compressing the remaining nerves within the porus. The dura mater is then closed in watertight fashion. After rewaxing any exposed mastoid air cells, a methylmethacrylate cranioplasty is fashioned to fill the bone defect. This has been used in the past several years because it provides a better cosmetic closure and appears to minimize chronic incisional pain and headache by preventing direct scar formation between muscle and dura. Muscle, fascia, and skin are then closed in layers.

MEDIUM TUMORS (15–30 MM LARGEST DIAMETER)

Approach. Retromastoid.

Position. Same as for small tumors.

Incision. Linear of lazy S, extending slightly more inferior to allow for more bone removal inferiorly.

Bone Work. Same as for small tumors with perhaps a bit more caudal and medial bone removal.

Dural Opening. Same as for small tumors.

Dissection Sequence. Obtain caudal egress of CSF and identify tumor poles. If tumor bulk is excessive, perform limited lateral and internal debulking after confirming absence of facial nerve on the back of tumor capsule. After removing some tumor bulk, the porus can be more easily drilled. The remainder of the dissection sequence is identical to that followed for small tumors.

Closure. Same as for small tumors.

LARGE TUMORS (>30 MM LARGEST DIAMETER)

Approach. Retrosigmoid.

Positioning. Although large tumors can be resected in the lateral position, the author prefers the modified sitting or "sitting slouch" position (Fig. 3). In this position, the table is flexed at its midportion, allowing the legs to be elevated. The patient's head is placed in three-point head fixation and positioned as follows: The neck is gently distracted and maximally flexed. The head is then turned 15–20° *toward* the side of the tumor. This provides an excellent view of the petrous bone for management of the intracanalicular portion of the tumor.

The sitting position is chosen for large tumors because it allows one to perform two-handed tumor dissection with continuous irrigation, as described by Samii *et al.* (25, 26). This technique is described in detail in the following sections.

Incision. The author favors a laterally based, C-shaped incision extending from the top of the pinna back to the midpoint between mastoid and inion, and finally down to a point 2–3 cm behind the mastoid process. The resulting myocutaneous flap is then retracted laterally with fishhooks. One additional fishhook is laced on the medial border of the incision to ensure adequate medial visualization. With this incision, care must be taken to avoid excessive caudal muscle dissection as this may result in vertebral artery injury.

Bone Work. A large craniectomy is performed to expose the sigmoid sinus from the transverse-sigmoid junction down almost to the jugular bulb. The craniectomy then proceeds caudally to within several millimeters of the foramen magnum and for a distance of approximately 5 cm medially.

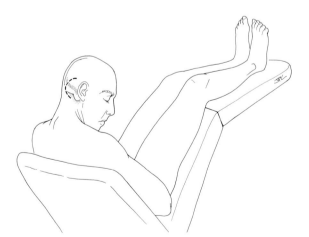

FIG. 3 Schematic of modified sitting position. Patient's head must be placed on stretch, maximally flexed, and turned 15–20° *toward* the operative side. C-shaped incision is indicated.

Dural Opening. Dura is opened along the transverse and sigmoid sinuses, leaving a 3- to 5-mm cuff to facilitate closure. The caudal aspect of the dura is then incised parallel to the foramen magnum. This creates a large dural flap, which is then placed over the cerebellum for protection.

Dissection Sequence. After obtaining egress of CSF from the caudal cistern, a broad retractor blade is used to elevate and retract the cerebellum. This provides the additional benefit of protecting a large area of cerebellum during drilling and dissection. As with medium tumors, the lateral tumor is coagulated and debulked to provide access to the porus. After completing the drilling and dissection of the porus, the technique for dissection for large tumors diverges from the technique used for small- and medium-sized lesions. With an assistant providing generous irrigation, dissection proceeds as follows. Using a fine forceps in the left hand and a grasping forceps in the right hand, the tumor is gently teased away from its intimate arachnoid capsule. As this technique can result in some slow, steady bleeding, copious irrigation is essential to visualize the proper plane of dissection. By continually working around the tumor in the proper plane, all essential neurovascular structures, including the facial nerve, will remain undisturbed in the adjacent outer arachnoid layer. In the sitting position, gravity allows for drainage of blood and irrigation, leaving one with a clear operative field. An additional benefit of gravity is that it can facilitate tumor dissection. This position and dissection strategy are used for all large tumors resected by the author.

Closure. Dura is closed in water tight fashion, using a retractor to gently reduce the cerebellum to prevent injury. The remainder of the closure proceeds in the same manner as for small- and medium-sized lesions.

Staging

In patients with large tumors, there is often extensive brainstem distortion with an indistinct plane between tumor capsule and pia of the brainstem. This makes for tedious dissection with a real risk of brainstem infarction, as well as cranial nerve loss. For this difficult subgroup, we have found staged resection to be beneficial. We have used this strategy in 84 patients with no deaths. In this group of staged resections, the average patient age was 41 years, with a slight female preponderance. Ten patients (12%) had neurofibromatosis type 2. Anatomic preservation of cranial nerve VII was achieved in 73%, with an average House-Brackmann (10) grade of 3 at longest follow-up (mean, 43 months). Gross total resection was achieved in 90% of lesions, with two documented recurrences (2.4%). Facial reanimation was performed in 19 of 23 patients with transected seventh cranial nerves. Complications for this staged group included cerebrospinal fluid fistula in 11 patients (13%), with 8 of 11 resolving after lumbar drainage. The remaining three patients (3.6%) required reexploration. Six patients had meningitis (bacterial in 3, aseptic in 3). Two patients developed wound infections, and 10 patients developed exposure keratitis (2, 27).

Hearing Preservation—Technical Features

Regardless of tumor size, hearing preservation may be attempted; however, the likelihood of success falls dramatically with increasing tumor size (5, 12, 13). One factor that appears to play a role is the presence of caudal *versus* rostral eccentricity seen on preoperative imaging in coronal sections. In tumors with predominantly rostral orientation, the author feels more optimistic about the ability to save hearing. Conversely, tumors with significant caudal extension below the porus appear to be more difficult from a hearing preservation standpoint (M. Samii, personal communication). One explanation for this observation involves the status of the cochlear nerve. In rostrally growing tumors, the nerve proceeds from brainstem to porus without significant distortion. In caudally growing tumors, the nerve is likely displaced and thinned, making it more vulnerable to operative injury.

In addition to this general radiographic assessment of the ability to preserve hearing, there are several important technical considerations that are essential for attempts at hearing preservation. First, as mentioned above, once identified, the superior and inferior vestibular nerves must be sharply sectioned to prevent transmission of traction forces to inner ear structures. Second, direct lateral-to-medial retraction of the cerebellum is to be avoided, as it may result in stretching and damage of the cochlear nerve. However, gentle rostral-caudal retraction of the cochlear nerve is generally well tolerated. Third, internal debulking and blunt dissection of the tumor from adjacent cranial nerves is to be avoided, because it may cause traction injury (13).

OUTCOME ASSESSMENT

Long-term follow-up data is available on 379 (55%) patients with a mean follow-up of 29 months. Although this number is somewhat low, there is no reason to believe that the patients followed are not representative of the whole surgical series. Furthermore, this represents more extensive follow-up than has been reported in other published series (8, 9, 15, 19). This part of the chapter will highlight some of the basic outcome measures of vestibular neurilemmoma resection, namely, anatomic and functional status of the cochlear and facial nerves, recurrence rates and, finally, complications.

Facial Nerve

Better operative techniques and monitoring equipment remain the mainstay of facial nerve preservation. This series, as well as other published reports, demonstrates a clear relationship between maximum tumor size and facial nerve salvage (4, 6–9, 16, 19, 20, 22, 28, 30). Table 4 demonstrates an anatomic preservation rate of 94% for small lesions, 88% for medium lesions, and 75% for large tumors. As expected, this results in a functional disparity between small and large tumors. Whereas the majority of patients with small tumors have House-Brackmann grades 1–2 at longest follow-up, 54% of patients with larger tumors retain grade 3 or better function at longest follow-up. These anatomic and functional results are similar to those seen in other published series (Table 5), and they should serve as a reminder that large vestibular neurilemmomas are extraordinarily difficult lesions to treat. The high morbidity associated with these lesions has prompted the use of alternative microsurgical options, such as staged resection.

Cochlear Nerve

One of the more controversial aspects of analysis of outcome data for vestibular neurilemmoma surgery concerns the concepts of hearing preservation or functional hearing. Although definitions of functional hearing differ widely, the concept remains the same. Functional hearing in an ear should provide the individual with useful binaural hearing. In patients with contralateral deafness, useful hearing may serve to warn the individual of impending danger without providing appre-

TABLE 4
Facial Nerve Anatomic and Functional Results

Tumor Size	Anatomic Preservation of Facial Nerve (%)	House-Brackmann Grade at Longest Follow-up (%)	Mean Duration of Follow-up (Mo)
Small (<15 mm)	94	Grades 1 + 2: 82 Grades 3 + 4: 14 Grades 5 + 6: 4	22.2
Medium (15–30 mm)	88	Grades 1 + 2: 56 Grades 3 + 4: 31 Grades 5 + 6: 13	26.4
Large (>30 mm)	75	Grades 1 + 2: 30 Grades 3 + 4: 36 Grades 5 + 6: 34	27.0

TABLE 5.
Comparison of Data with Published Series[a]

Author/yr (Ref)	Series Size	Mortality (%)	CSF Fistula (%)	Gross Total Resection	VII Preservation (%)	Patients Available for Follow-up (%)	Mean Follow-up (Mo)	Recurrences (%)
Jannetta, 1996	691	7 (1)	17% total, 15(%) retrosig., 21(%) translab.	83 (94% S,[a] 85% M, 70% L)	94% S, 88% M, 75% L	379 (55%)	29	13 (3.4)
Ojemann 1992 (21)	410	2 (0.5)	8	80	95–100% S,[b] 75% M, 56% L	N/A	≤12	12 (3)
Ebersold 1992 (4)	255	2 (0.8)	11	97	92.6	160 (63%)	12	N/A
Hardy 1989 (7)	100	3 (3)	31	97	82	97 (100%)	N/A	N/A
Shiobara 1988 (28)	125	2 (1.6)	8.8	87	80	N/A	N/A	N/A
Glasscock 1986 (6)	568	4 (0.7)	14	99	94% S, 92% M, 55% L	N/A	N/A	2 (0.4)
Welch 1985 (30)	77	4 (5)	3 (3.9)	84	100% S, 78% M, 34% L	N/A	N/A	N/A

[a] Tumor sizes: S, small; M, medium; L, large.
[b] Functional preservation.

ciable speech discrimination. The current series uses the 50/50 rule of Wade and House (29), which corresponds to Gardner-Robertson class 1 or 2 (5). In a small series, we used a scheme that we devised and that may give more useful information about the true status of hearing (13). Hearing preservation may be accomplished for small tumors, but as this and other series demonstrate, is quite difficult for medium- or large-sized lesions. Table 6 details the dramatic decline in hearing preservation rates for larger tumors in the present series.

Recurrence

Recurrence remains one of the most frustrating outcomes for both patient and surgeon. After careful dissection and initially negative postoperative imaging, a recurrence is detected. In this large series, many patients have had their resection performed at the University of Pittsburgh and, subsequently, are followed by their referring physician. Our recommendation for follow-up imaging is to obtain an MRI 1–2 months after resection, which should then be followed by imaging at 6 months and 1 year. Images are then obtained at yearly intervals until year 5 postop. At that point, the scanning interval should be increased to every 24 months. The follow-up is completed at 10 years postop.

In this series, there have been 13 documented recurrences (3.4%) with a mean interval from OR to recurrence of 49.8 months (range, 11–77 months). For the NF2 patient group there have been three recurrences, a rate of 8%. Two patients with recurrence have been successfully treated with stereotactic radiosurgery and currently have stable disease. As a result of incomplete follow-up (371/691), the actual

TABLE 6
Details of Hearing Preservation

	Preoperative	Postoperative	Totals
Small tumors (≤15 mm)			
Class 1 hearing	38	8	
Class 2 hearing		2	
Class 1 + class 2	38	10	10/38 = 26%
Medium tumors (15 mm–30 mm)			
Class 1	40	3	
Class 2		1	
Class 1 + 2		4	4/40 = 10%
Large tumors (>3 mm)			
Class 1	14	0	
Class 2		0	
Class 1 + 2			0/14 = 0%

[a] Class refers to Gardner-Robertson classification (5).

recurrence rate may be somewhat higher. However, even if one assumes that the actual recurrence rate is doubled (*i.e.*, 6.8%), the results of this series remain comparable to those of other published reports (1, 20).

Complications

The microsurgical resection of vestibular neurilemmomas can result in major or minor complications. Such complications are related to (*a*) complications of closure, (*b*) brainstem events secondary to arterial or venous injury, or (*c*) cranial nerve injury during dissection. A survey of complications, as well as their frequency, is contained in Table 7.

The occurrence of CSF fistula after microsurgical resection of a vestibular neurilemmoma is a source of great concern for surgeon and patient. Such leaks typically occur on postoperative days 2–4 and often present as ipsilateral clear rhinorrhea. Less commonly, a leak will occur directly through the wound. In the current series, the initial CSF fistula rare is 15% for retrosigmoid resection. This figure is higher for translabrynthine resections (21%), primarily because of the incomplete dural closure afforded by this technique. Fortunately, more than two-thirds of CSF fistulas resolved after several days of closed lumbar drainage. For the remaining patients, reexploration was required to obliterate the fistula. Typically such reexploration consisted of fat packing of the middle ear. This can result in substantial conductive hearing loss in patients with otherwise useful hearing. Therefore, all patients are given a trial of closed lumbar drainage. It is also important to note that the occurrence of CSF fistula predisposes the patient to bacterial meningitis. In the current series, virtually all cases of bacterial meningitis were preceded by a CSF leak.

The risk of mortality in this series is 1% (7/691) with most deaths occurring after brainstem damage from primary vascular event or hematoma. The occurrence of primary vascular injury can be minimized by using staged resection, as well as meticulous dissection techniques. The incidence of hematoma/contusion was 2.6% in this series. This represents an important avoidable complication. Frequent retractor relaxation, optimal patient positioning, adequate bony exposure, and maintenance of clear CSF flow during the procedure can all help to limit the occurrence of retraction injury and hematoma. In addition, one should be prepared to resect the lateral one-third of the cerebellar hemisphere if contusion and swelling are believed to be present. This will result in no detectable functional impairment and may prevent significant morbidity or mortality.

Air embolism (AE) is a much-feared complication associated with sitting or modified sitting positions. The incidence of significant AE

TABLE 7.
Complications

Complication	Total of 691 Cases [Number (%)]	Retrosigmoid: 548 Cases [Number (%)]	Translabyrinthine: 131 Cases [Number (%)]	Middle Fossa: 4 Cases [Number (%)]	Combined Approach: 8 Cases [Number (%)]
CSF fistula (total)	115 (17)	82 (15)	28 (21)	0	5 (63)
CSF fistula (reexploration required)	33 (4.8)	21 (3.8)	12 (9.2)	0	0
Exposure to keratitis	45 (6.5)	36 (6.6)	9 (6.9)	0	0
Aseptic meningitis	34 (5)	32 (5.8)	2 (1.5)	0	0
Bacterial meningitis	21 (3)	15 (2.7)	5 (3.8)	1 (25)	0
Hematoma/contusion	18 (2.6)	14 (2.6)	4 (3.1)	0	0
Wound infection	17 (2.5)	12 (2.2)	5 (3.8)	0	0
Air embolism	11 (1.6) 10 sitting 1 lateral	11 (2)	0	0	0
Pneumonia	11 (1.6)	11 (2)	0	0	0
Swallowing problems	11 (1.6)	11 (2)	0	0	0
Pulmonary embolus	7 (1)	7 (1.3)	0	0	0
Death	7 (1)	6 (1)	1 (0.7)	0	0

was 2% for the entire series. Although one procedure had to be aborted after an AE, no major morbidity occurred with this or any other patient. In the author's view, the risk of AE is far outweighed by the benefits afforded by the modified sitting position. This position permits the rapid and safe removal of large tumors.

One final complication that deserves mention is exposure keratitis (EK). The appearance of EK in 6.5% of patients underscores the need for aggressive eye care and follow-up in the postoperative period. Early gold weight placement is currently preferred over tarsorraphy, because it facilitates eye care while providing superior cosmesis. Regardless of the method of surgical eye protection used, prompt recognition and treatment of corneal exposure are crucial to prevent corneal ulceration and infection with resultant scarring and visual loss.

CONCLUSIONS

The microsurgical resection of vestibular neurilemmomas remains one of the greatest challenges to neurosurgeons and neurootologists. Patients often present with subtle symptoms and high expectations. Even in the most experienced hands, microsurgical resection has real risks, including death. By using a meticulous technique and attending to every detail, one can minimize and even eliminate most adverse effects.

In the current era of radiosurgery, microsurgeons are further challenged to maintain the same high tumor control rates and low morbidity seen with focused irradiation techniques. Although at times adversarial, the disciplines of microsurgery and radiosurgery should be complementary. Through proper patient evaluation and selection, both techniques may be used against these difficult lesions.

ACKNOWLEDGMENTS

The author wishes to thank Christopher H. Comey, M.D. for his assistance with preparation of the manuscript.

REFERENCES

1. Cerullo CJ, Grutsch JF, Heifermann K, et al.: The preservation of hearing and facial nerve function in a consecutive series of unilateral vestibular nerve schwannoma surgical patients (acoustic neuroma). **Surg Neurol** 39:485–493, 1993.
2. Comey CH, Jannetta PJ, Sheptak PE, et al.: Staged removal of acoustic tumors: Techniques and lessons learned from a series of 83 patients. **Neurosurgery** 37: 915–921, 1995.
3. Delgado TE, Buchheit WA, Rosenholtz HR, et al.: Intraoperative monitoring of facial muscle evoked responses obtained by intracranial stimulation of the facial nerve: A

more accurate technique for facial nerve dissection. **Neurosurgery** 4:418–421, 1979.

4. Ebersold MJ, Harner SG, Beatty CW, *et al.*: Current results of the retrosigmoid approach to acoustic neurinoma. **J Neurosurg** 76:901–909, 1992.

5. Gardner G, Robertson JH: Hearing preservation in unilateral acoustic neuroma surgery. **Ann Otol Rhinol Laryngol** 97(1):55–56, 1988.

6. Glasscock ME, Kveton JF, Jackson CG, *et al.*: A systematic approach to the surgical management of acoustic neuroma. **Laryngoscope** 96:1088–1094, 1986.

7. Hardy DG, MacFarlane R, Baguley D, *et al.*: Surgery for acoustic neurinoma: An analysis of 100 translabyrinthine operations. **J Neurosurg** 71:799–804, 1989.

8. Harner SG, Beatty CW, Ebersold MJ: Retrosigmoid removal of acoustic neuroma: Experience 1978–1988. **Otolaryngol Head Neck Surg** 103:40–45, 1990.

9. Harner SG, Ebersold MJ: Management of acoustic neuromas, 1978–1983.**J Neurosurg** 63:175–179, 1985.

10. House JW, Brackmann DE: Facial nerve grading system. **Otolaryngol Head Neck Surg** 93:146–147, 1985.

11. House WF: Acoustic tumor surgery: An historical perspective. **Semin Hearing** 10(4):293–305, 1989.

12. Jannetta PJ: Acoustic neurinomas: Neurosurgical approaches and results, in Sekhar LN, Schramm VL Jr (eds): *Tumors of the Cranial Base: Diagnosis and Treatment.* Mt. Kisco, NY, Futura, 1987, pp 563–586.

13. Jannetta PJ, Moller AR, Moller MB: Technique of hearing preservation in small acoustic neuromas. **Ann Surg** 200:513–523, 1984.

14. Linskey ME, Lunsford LD, Flickinger JC: Radiosurgery for acoustic neurinomas: Early experience. **Neurosurgery** 26:736–745, 1990.

15. Lownie SP, Drake CG: Radical intracapsular removal of acoustic neurinomas: Long-term follow-up review of 11 patients. **J Neurosurg** 74:422–425, 1991.

16. Mangham CA: Complications of translabrynthine vs. suboccipital approach for acoustic tumor surgery. **Otolaryngol Head Neck Surg** 99:396–400, 1988.

17. Moller AR, Jannetta PJ: Monitoring auditory function during cranial nerve microvascular decompression operations by direct recording form the eighth nerve. **J Neurosurg** 59:493–499, 1983.

18. Moller AR, Jannetta PJ: Preservation of facial function during removal of acoustic neuromas: Use of monopolar constant voltage stimulation and EMG. **J Neurosurg** 61:757–760, 1984.

19. Moskowitz N, Long DM: Acoustic neurinomas: Historical review of a century of operative series. **Neurosurgery** 1:2–18, 1991.

20. Noren G, Arndt J, Hindmarsh T: Stereotactic radiosurgery in cases of acoustic neurinoma: Further experiences. **Neurosurgery** 13:12–22, 1983.

21. Ojemann RG: Management of acoustic neuromas (vestibular schwannomas) (Honored Guest Presentation). **Clin Neurosurg** 40:498–535, 1992.

22. Penzholz H: Development and present state of cerebellopontine angle surgery from the neuro- and otosurgical point of view. **Arch Otorhinolaryngol** 240:167–174, 1984.

23. Pollock BE, Lunsford LD, Kondziolka D, *et al.*: Outcome analysis of acoustic neu-

roma management: A comparison of microsurgery and stereotactic radiosurgery. **Neurosurgery** 36:215–229, 1995.

24. Rand RW, Kurze T: Microsurgical resection of acoustic tumors by a transmeatal posterior fossa approach. **Bull LA Neurol Soc** 30:17–20, 1965.

25. Samii M: Microsurgery of acoustic neurinomas with special emphasis on preservation of seventh and eighth cranial nerves and the scope of facial nerve grafting, in Rand RW (ed): *Microneurosurgery.* St. Louis, Mosby, 1985, ed 3, pp 366–388.

26. Samii M, Turel KE, Penkert G: Management of seventh and eighth nerve involvement by cerebellopontine angle tumors. **Clin Neurosurg** 32:242–272, 1984.

27. Sheptak PE, Jannetta PJ: The two-stage excision of huge acoustic neuromas. **J Neurosurg** 51:37–41, 1979.

28. Shiobara R, Ohira T, Kanzaki J, *et al.*: A modified extended middle cranial fossa approach for acoustic nerve tumors: Results of 125 operations. **J Neurosurg** 68: 358–365, 1988.

29. Wade PJ, House W: Hearing preservation in patients with acoustic neuromas via the middle fossa approach. **Otolaryngol Head Neck Surg** 92:184–193, 1984.

30. Welch MAR, Dawes JDK: Suboccipital approach in the removal of acoustic neuromas. **J Laryngol Otol** 99:1217–1223, 1985.

31. Yasargil MG, Fox JL: The microsurgical approach to acoustic neurinomas. **Surg Neurol** 2:393–398, 1974. AU: 1986 correct? See ref. 6.

31

Brainstem Gliomas

HAROLD J. HOFFMAN, M.D., B.Sc. (MED.), F.R.C.S.C., F.A.C.S.

In the past brainstem gliomas were regarded as inoperable tumors. Matson, in 1969, in his pediatric neurosurgery book, stated that "should any patient still be alive 18 months after diagnosis, reinvestigation and surgical exploration is indicated, as some other lesion is probably present." He further stated that regardless of specific histology, all brainstem gliomas must be regarded as malignant tumors, because their location in itself renders them inoperable. Furthermore, he stated that exploration for confirmation of diagnosis should be avoided because such surgery is useless (9).

In 1939 Bailey *et al.* described the treatment of brainstem gliomas as "a pessimistic chapter" in the history of neurosurgery (2). Traditionally, all tumors involving the brainstem were considered infiltrative with diffuse gliomatous proliferation.

Before the advent of modern neuroimaging, brainstem tumors were diagnosed by means of air and contrast x-ray techniques. These studies gave a very poor view of the brainstem but certainly allowed neurosurgeons to recognize tumors in the brainstem and to operate on them.

Olivecrona, in 1967, described 26 patients with tumors in the medulla, of which 7 survived for 10–25 years after an operation that comprised either partial removal or biopsy and decompression (11). Apparently, these patients did not receive radiotherapy.

In 1968, Pool reported three cases of confirmed astrocytomas in the brainstem, in which the lesions were intrinsically solid and cystic and the patients survived for long periods of time (13). Pool ascribed this long-term survival to the effects of radiotherapy. In 1971, Lassiter *et al.* described five patients with brainstem masses that were largely cystic and contained mural nodules (8). These patients were treated by uncapping of the cyst, biopsy of the nodule, and postoperative radiotherapy. Again, there were long-term survivors among these patients. Villani, in writing about brainstem gliomas in 1975, stated that during the previous 30 years, no important progress has been achieved in this field (17).

Brainstem gliomas are a relatively common tumor in children. Russell and Rubinstein stated that 77% of brainstem gliomas occur in patients less than 20 years of age (14). Matson stated that 18.7% of posterior fossa tumors were in the brainstem (9). Koos and Miller found that 13.4% of their posterior fossa tumors were in the brainstem (7), and in my own institution 28.7% of posterior fossa tumors are located in the brainstem.

There are a number of classifications of brainstem gliomas. In our institution, 20% of brainstem gliomas are dorsally exophytic into the fourth ventricle; 50% of brainstem gliomas are diffuse intrinsic tumors that start in the pons and spread throughout the brainstem; 20% of brainstem tumors are focal in the brainstem, and 10% are located at the craniocervical junction.

DORSALLY EXOPHYTIC BRAINSTEM TUMORS

In 1980 at our own institution we encountered a small but distinct group of eight brainstem tumors that behave in a significantly different fashion from the typical infiltrating brainstem glioma (6, 15) (Fig. 1). Symptoms frequently began early in childhood and sometimes

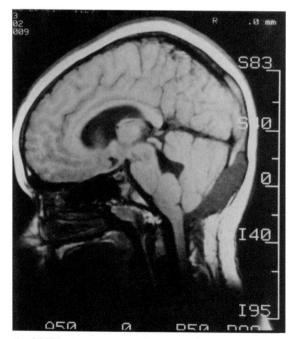

FIG. 1 T1 sagittal MRI, showing a dorsally exophytic tumor.

during infancy. In infants, the history tends to be one of intractable vomiting and failure to thrive, whereas in older children, signs of raised intracranial pressure, including papilledema, are frequently present. A long history can usually be elicited. These tumors protrude into and largely fill the fourth ventricle. They can extend into the cerebellar pontine angle, and they mushroom down over the dorsal surface of the cervical spinal cord. On CT scan they are hypodense and typically enhance brightly with the administration of contrast agent. These tumors are typically low-grade astrocytomas or gangliogliomas. Furthermore, these tumors are solid and not cystic in the vast majority. Subtotal surgical excision has been extremely successful.

In 1993 we reviewed the surgical treatment of these dorsally exo-phytic brainstem gliomas (12). Seventeen patients were alive at the conclusion of this study, with follow-up periods ranging from 33–212 months, with a mean of 110 months and a median of 113 months. One child who had stable disease postoperatively died of shunt malfunction at another institution 18 months after tumor excision. The two patients who received postoperative radiotherapy have no evidence of residual disease on follow-up imaging 61 and 135 months after surgery, respectively. Both children suffered radiation-induced alopecia, and one developed isolated growth hormone deficiency with resultant short stature.

Serial clinical and radiographic evaluations in the other 15 patients who were followed to the conclusion of the study have shown the complete disappearance of residual tumor in three children, stable residual disease in eight, and obvious tumor regrowth in four. In the latter four patients tumor enlargement was detected radiographically at 12, 28, 40, and 84 months, respectively, after surgery and was associated with recurrent symptoms in all but the one-third of patients in whom a large recurrence was detected (Fig. 2). In three patients the recurrent tumor contained a large cystic component.

Three patients underwent a second exploration for tumor excision when tumor growth was detected. The fourth child received radiotherapy at the time of the disease progression, although the solid component of the tumor diminished slightly in size on serial imaging studies. The patient became increasingly symptomatic from progressive enlargement of a multiloculated cystic component of the tumor and ultimately underwent repeat exploration. In each of the four patients the exophytic solid tumor component was relatively circumscribed from surrounding structures and was radically resected. In the three cystic tumors the exophytic portion of the cyst wall was excised, leaving intact the attachment of the cyst to the brainstem. As in the initial

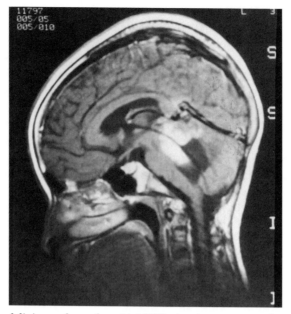

Fig. 2 T1 gadolinium-enhanced sagittal MRI, showing recurrent, dorsally exophytic tumor surrounding the implanted Lapras catheter.

operations no attempt was made to resect tumor growing within or directly upon the brainstem.

Both patients who received radiotherapy pre- or postoperatively at the time of tumor enlargement have shown a progressive decrease of tumor volume 28 and 65 months, respectively, after their second operations. The other two patients exhibited further regrowth 48 and 84 months, respectively, after their second operation and underwent a third tumor resection. One of these two patients received postoperative radiotherapy and has no evidence of residual disease 58 months after the third operation (165 months after the initial surgery). The other child has stable disease 27 months postoperatively (159 months after initial surgery). One of the three children who received radiotherapy for disease progression has subsequently manifested short stature as a result of growth hormone deficiency. No other radiation-related neuroendocrine deficits have been detected.

These tumors are approached in the same fashion as midline cerebellar neoplasms. The fourth ventricle is opened, and the tumor is debulked with the aid of the ultrasonic aspirator. If the child has hydrocephalus a Lapras catheter is passed through the aqueduct into the third ventricle and then down into the cisterna magna. Basically, the tumor is shaved flush with the surrounding floor of the fourth ventricle, and it is important not to go any deeper for fear of producing problems with the important cranial nerve nuclei.

DIFFUSE INTRINSIC ASTROCYTOMAS OF THE BRAINSTEM

The intrinsic astrocytomas which start in the pons and spread up into the midbrain and down into the medulla typically present with cranial nerve palsies and long tract signs (Fig. 3). Initially, the tumors show no enhancement and enlarge the brainstem. Subsequently, if they are treated with radiotherapy, the brainstem typically returns to a normal size; the children are well for a brief period; and then the tumor becomes enhancing, with nodular excrescences sticking out from the brainstem.

The patients with these diffuse intrinsic tumors rarely survive for more than 2 years despite aggressive therapy. At autopsy, these tumors are either malignant astrocytomas or glioblastoma multiforme. Furthermore, at autopsy there is frequently extensive leptomeningeal metastases.

No treatment has been shown to be effective in causing a significant survival in children with this type of tumor. Numerous surgeons have operated on these tumors with no effective results (4). Adjunctive therapy, including radiotherapy and chemotherapy, will palliate these

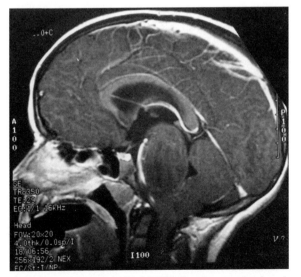

FIG. 3 T1 gadolinium-enhanced sagittal MRI, showing a nonenhancing, hypodense, diffuse intrinsic tumor.

patients, but eventually the tumor returns, and very few patients survive for more than 2 years.

FOCAL INTRINSIC BRAINSTEM ASTROCYTOMAS

Focal intrinsic gliomas make up about 20% of brainstem gliomas. They are common in the midbrain, but they can occur in the medulla and, rarely, in the pons itself. Depending on their location they can give rise to cranial nerve palsies and to long tract signs. They can be solid or cystic. After resection, 60% of patients require no further therapy, whereas 40% require adjunctive treatment because of recurrence.

The focal tumors can occur anywhere in the brainstem. The commonest group of focal tumors are the tumors in the midbrain. They usually involve a portion of the tegmentum (Figs. 4 and 5). I have found that one can elevate the temporal lobe, section the tentorium, and expose the side of the midbrain and make a horizontal incision in the midbrain exposing the tumor, which can then be debulked with the ultrasonic aspirator or the contact laser. The small tectal tumors can

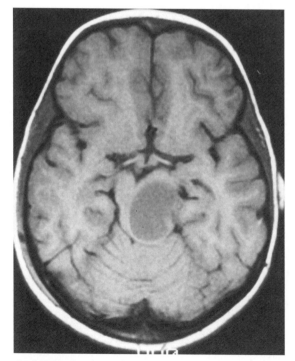

FIG. 4 T1 sagittal MRI, showing a focal tumor in the tegmentum of the midbrain.

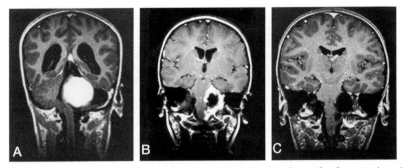

FIG. 5 (**A**) T1 gadolinium-enhanced coronal MRI, showing large focal tumor in mid-brain and pons. (**B**) T1 gadolinium-enhanced postoperative MRI, showing significant debulking of tumor. (**C**) T1 gadolinium-enhanced coronal MRI done 1 year after debulking, showing involution of residual tumor.

be very indolent and typically close off the aqueduct producing hydro-cephalus (Fig. 6). The hydrocephalus can be treated with a third ventriculostomy or a VP shunt. There is no need to resect these small indolent tectal gliomas (3, 10). However, one can get very large tectal gliomas that mimic pineal tumors. These tumors have to be explored and debulked (Fig. 6). The focal tumors in the pons are rare, and they are approached usually through a midline incision in the floor of the fourth ventricle.

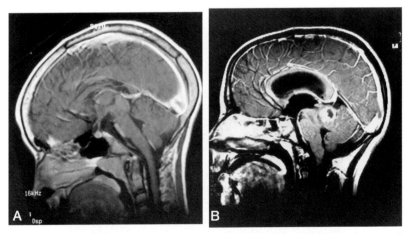

FIG. 6 (**A**) T1 gadolinium-enhanced sagittal MRI, showing a small tectal tumor that had not changed in size over a 4-year period. (**B**) T1 gadolinium-enhanced sagittal MRI, showing a large tectal tumor that was debulked.

The focal tumors in the medulla are approached through an incision in the midline or, when they bulge out laterally they can be approached from the external surface of the medulla (Fig. 7). In patients in whom resection is undertaken in the medulla it is important to keep those patients ventilated post operatively in the intensive care unit until one can be sure that breathing is effective and there is no evidence of CO_2 retention (1).

THE CRANIOCERVICAL BRAINSTEM ASTROCYTOMA

The craniocervical brainstem gliomas arise in the upper cervical cord and extend into the medulla (Fig. 8) (5). These patients typically present with long tract signs, and they may have lower cranial nerve signs as well. Laminotomy is a useful procedure. A midline myelotomy is made, and the tumor is debulked with the ultrasonic aspirator. The resection is carried rostrally to the level of the medulla, in which the resection becomes more conservative. The use of motor- and sensory-evoked potentials is essential.

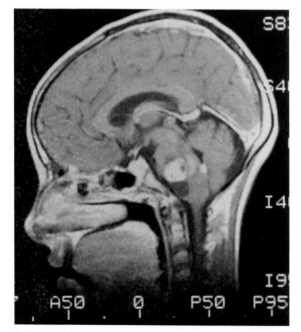

FIG. 7 T1 gadolinium-enhanced sagittal MRI, showing a focal tumor in medulla and pons.

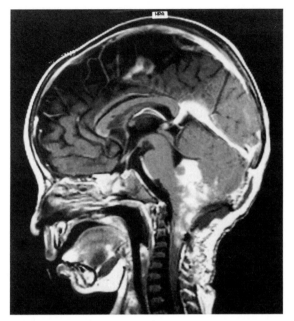

FIG. 8 T1 gadolinium-enhanced sagittal MRI, showing a craniocervical tumor.

CONCLUSIONS

Diffuse intrinsic brainstem tumors are malignant and do not benefit from any form of surgical intervention, including biopsy. The dorsally exophytic tumors, the focal tumors, and the craniocervical tumors are usually benign and benefit from surgical debulking, with some undergoing involution without the need of adjuvant therapy. The small tectal gliomas only need control of the hydrocephalus and observation. The large tectal gliomas can mimic a pineal tumor and should be explored and resected.

REFERENCES

1. Abbott R, Shiminske-Maher T, Wisoff JH, *et al.*: Intrinsic tumors of the medulla: Surgical complications. **Pediatr Neurosurg** 17:239, 1991 and 1992.
2. Bailey P, Buchanan DN, Bucy PC: *Intracranial Tumours of Infancy and Childhood.* Chicago, University Press, 1939, pp 188–241.
3. Chapman PH: Indolent gliomas of the midbrain tectum, in Marlin AE (ed): *Concepts in Pediatric Neurosurgery.* Basel, Karger, 1989, vol 10, pp 97–107.
4. Epstein F, McCleary EL: Intrinsic brainstem tumors of childhood: Surgical implications. **J Neurosurg** 64:11–15, 1986.

5. Epstein F, Wisoff J: Intra-axial tumours of the cervicomedullary junction. **J Neurosurg** 67:483–487, 1987.

6. Hoffman HJ, Becker L, Craven CMA: A clinically and pathologically distinct group of benign brain stem gliomas. **Neurosurgery** 7:243–248, 1980.

7. Koos WT, Miller MH: *Intracranial Tumors of Infants and Children*. Stuttgart, Georg Thieme Verlag, 1971, p 346.

8. Lassiter KRL, Alexander E Jr, Davis CH Jr, *et al.:* Surgical treatment of brain stem gliomas. **J Neurosurg** 34:719–725, 1971.

9. Matson DD: *Neurosurgery of Infancy and Childhood*. Springfield, IL, Charles C Thomas, 1969, pp 469–477.

10. May PL, Blaser SI, Hoffman HJ, *et al.:* Benign intrinsic tectal "tumors" in children. **J Neurosurg** 74:867, 1991.

11. Olivecrona H: *Handbuch der Neurochirurgie, Band 4, Teil 4*. Berlin, Springer-Verlag, 1967.

12. Pollack IF, Hoffmann HJ, Humphreys RP, *et al.:* The long-term outcome after surgical treatment of dorsally exophytic brainstem gliomas. **J. Neurosurg** 78:859–863, 1993.

13. Pool JL: Gliomas in the region of the brain stem. **J Neurosurg** 29:164–167, 1968.

14. Russell DS, Rubinstein LJ: **Pathology of Tumours of the Nervous System.** Baltimore, Williams & Wilkins, 1977, pp 181–182.

15. Stroink AR, Hoffman HJ, Hendrick EB, *et al.:* Transependymal benign dorsally exophytic brain stem gliomas of childhood: Diagnosis and treatment recommendations. **Neurosurgery** 20:439–444, 1987.

16. Vandertop WP, Hoffman HJ, Drake JM, *et al.:* Focal midbrain tumours in children. **Neurosurgery** 31:186–194, 1992.

17. Villani R, Gaini SM, Tomei G: Follow-up study of brain stem tumors in children. **Childs Brain** 1:126–135, 1975.

32

Ependymomas

ROBERT A. SANFORD, M.D., AND AMAR GAJJAR, M.D.

Ependymomas are glial neoplasms which differentiate along ependymal cell lines and are felt to arise from the lining of the cerebral ventricles, the central canal of the spinal cord, and filum terminale. When they occur in the cerebral hemisphere, they often are located within cerebral substance, rather than in the ventricles. The cells of origin are postulated to be ependymal rest cells.

Ependymomas account for 2–7.8% of all neoplasms of the central nervous system, with half presenting during the first two decades of life (1, 32, 36). Ependymomas represent 10–12% of pediatric central nervous system tumors (18). Seventy-five percent are benign, with 25% anaplastic and 50% occurring before 5 years of age. At present, the standard therapy is surgery followed by irradiation. With surgery alone, one can expect a 17–27% long-term survival (5, 9, 11, 29). None of these series had the benefit of modern neuroimaging to confirm the degree of resection. If following surgical resection radiation is added, survival statistics improve to 40–87% (2, 6, 20). The improved survival rate conferred by radiation is now a component of all modern series, although some experts question whether the efficacy of total resection should be restudied.

Review of the ependymoma literature reveals a number of clinical variables which seem to favor long-term survival: adult age group, hemisphere location, benign pathology, and total surgical resection. The unfavorable prognostic factors are young age (children, especially infants), posterior fossa location, anaplastic pathology, and subtotal resection. Our review will analyze these favorable and unfavorable prognostic clinical variables, including the series that support these accepted tenets.

RESULTS OF TREATMENT

Overall survival rates for intracranial ependymomas vary in the literature. Bloom's (2) historical review indicates the 5-year survival rate of 50% falling to 30% by 15 years. For children over 4 years of age, most recent reports indicate 5-year disease-free or progression-free survival rates from 45 to 60% (8, 21, 34).

HISTOLOGY

If we look at histology first, there are a number of articles in the literature that suggest a significant difference between the behavior of the benign ependymoma *versus* the malignant ependymoma (2, 4, 6, 8, 17, 21, 34). On the other hand, an equal number of series report that there is not a significant difference between the outcome in patients with benign *versus* malignant ependymomas (9, 22, 25, 27, 28, 30). Many of these series are limited by a small number of patients.

There is no doubt that some ependymomas recur in spite of conventional treatment and other children are apparently cured. Are there truly two or more varieties of ependymomas with different biological structures? If so, perhaps the confusion exists because conventional histology fails to accurately measure the variables that indicate malignancy, or perhaps the histologic features indicating malignancy in astrocytomas are different in ependymomas.

Foreman *et al.* (10) suggest that if there is importance to the histology, the difference should be based on cell density and the number of mitotic figures rather than the cellular pleomorphism, necrosis, and neovascularity associated with malignant biology in astrocytomas (10).

In two successive Pediatric Oncology Group protocols (POG 8532 and POG 9132) treating children with ependymomas, an independent review of the pathology revealed marked inconsistency in grading benign *versus* malignant tumors among academic institutions. Therefore, I must conclude that the histologic features used to label malignant *versus* benign ependymomas remain unproven. The clinician needs to be wary of predicting outcome in individual patients until the variables for benign *versus* malignant histology are confirmed with large numbers of patients.

SURGICAL RESECTION

There is no doubt from a review of an institutional series that the degree of surgical resection is important. A gross total resection confirmed by negative neuroimaging highly correlates with a favorable prognosis (14, 15, 24, 26, 31, 35). It is critical, however, that the gross total resection be confirmed by neuroimaging. No improvement in survival is noted with a 50–90% or even a >95% resection. A Pediatric Oncology Group study (POG 8532) begun in 1985 and completed in 1990 clearly demonstrated the importance of surgical resection, and in this series greater than 80% survival was achieved. However, these survival statistics are skewed by the fact that infant ependymomas were added during this period to a POG protocol for children less than 3 years of age with malignant tumors.

A new protocol POG-9132 was developed utilizing these data. Because previous studies indicated that subtotal resection resulted in a worse prognosis, this new study incorporated a more vigorous form of radiation (hyperfractionated dosage schedule) in an attempt to improve survival.

RADIOTHERAPY

There is still a debate regarding the appropriate radiation volume for intracranial ependymomas. The frequency of subarachnoid seeding is estimated at approximately 12% in several reviews compiling data from the last 4 decades (3, 18, 20, 33). Recent series indicate that overall neuraxis dissemination occurs in 3–16% of children, more often documented by cytology than by cranial and spinal imaging (13, 27, 31). Although historical data preceding the computed tomography (CT) era suggested a correlation between anaplastic posterior fossa ependymomas and subsequent seeding, more recent data fail to substantiate any apparent site or histologically specific relationship (3, 13, 19, 24, 27, 30). The incidence of neuraxis failure alone or combined with local recurrence is estimated at 12%. In most series, neuraxis failure is associated with simultaneous local recurrence 50% of the time. There is no evidence that prophylactic craniospinal irradiation reduced the occurrence of isolated or initial neuraxis failure. Disease control rates in contemporary series show no advantage of full cranial or craniospinal volumes compared to wide local fields based on moderate imaging (12, 19, 24, 27, 31). Therefore, standard local volumes for posterior fossa ependymomas should encompass the entire posterior fossa. For supratentorial ependymomas, wide local fields are defined as a preoperative tumor extent with margins of 2–3 cm. This should be extended to the 45-GY level. Boost doses of 55–65 GY have been recommended to be added directly to the small volumes of known disease residual.

AGE

Age is the most significant prognostic factor noted in all reported series. In an excellent modern pediatric series, less than 25% of children under 3 years of age had a 5-year survival rate (12, 14, 24, 27, 35). There are a number of factors that account for the poor results in infants. Radiation is so harmful to the developing brain that it is rarely given before 2 years of age, and the dosage is significantly reduced in the 3- or 4-year-old child which significantly decreases its efficacy. Most infant series have a small number of gross total resections.

Because gross total resection is the most important prognostic factor, its absence in infant series skews statistical analysis.

It is critical when analyzing ependymoma series that long-term follow-up is available. Ependymomas are unique in that they tend to recur until 5 years posttreatment, so that no series can be considered conclusive until all the patients are beyond the 5-year follow-up (27, 37).

This dismal prognosis was improved in a recent prospective series of infants (POG 8633). This was a cooperative study that treated young children with malignant brain tumors with chemotherapy, with the goal of preventing progressive disease until they reached 3 years of age when they could undergo radiotherapy (7). There were 198 children treated 47 of which had ependymomas. All were treated with cycles of two courses of cyclophosphamide and vincristine alternating with cisplatin and VP-16 with an attempt to delay radiation for 12 months in the 24- to 36-month age group and 24 months in the children less than 2 years of age. The most important prognostic variable noted in this series of children with malignant gliomas was the extent of surgery. In the overall group there was a marked difference between the children who had received a gross total resection *versus* any lesser resection. In the ependymoma group 19 infants received a gross total resection, as compared to 28 with incomplete resections. This multicenter study of aggressive surgery illustrates the difficulty of completely resecting infant tumors. A recent update of 5-year or greater follow-up reveals that the children who had a gross total resection have a 66% 5-year survival rate, whereas 25% of those with subtotal resection have a 5-year survival rate, which is equal to historical controls.

This group-wide study was piloted at St. Jude Research Hospital and brought to a group-wide multiinstitutional study in 1984. A second conclusion derived from this study is that infant ependymomas are sensitive to platinum and alkylating agents, demonstrating short-term disease control. One of the goals of the subsequent study (POG 9233) is an attempt to demonstrate the long-term efficacy of chemotherapy by further delay of radiation in children who complete chemotherapy with no evidence of tumor on neuroimaging. Chemotherapy for treatment of older children or adults with ependymomas remains investigational.

ST. JUDE RESEARCH HOSPITAL STUDY

Reviewing the ependymoma at St. Jude Research Hospital from 1985 through 1995, there were 49 patients, 18 years or less, with 26 (55%) less than 3 years of age. There were 13 supratentorial, 27 infratentorial, and 6 spinal cord ependymomas. In this cohort of patients, the 26 infants treated with aggressive surgery and chemotherapy, the survival rate was 60% at 4 years. Of the 23 children between the ages of 3 and 18 years the survival rate was 72% at 4 years, for an overall survival rate of 67%.

Cerebral hemisphere location is a favorable prognostic variable in most series probably because gross total resection is easier to achieve supratentorially than infratentorially. Again age, the most important variable, tends to skew this statistic. In our series, of the 27 children less than 3 years of age, only four were supratentorial. Twenty-three of the tumors were located in the posterior fossa, 12 arising in the fourth ventricle, and 11 in the cerebellopontine (CP) angle. Eight were also anaplastic (30%).

Infant tumors are usually quite large before becoming clinically apparent. Two factors account for this phenomenon. Initially the clinical signs of neurologic deficit, motor or cerebellar signs, are manifest by a delay in motor milestones and are overlooked because of the variability in normal development. Even signs of regression may be missed. The common symptom of increased intracranial pressure, headache, is manifested as irritability, as the infant is unable to verbalize. Vomiting is perceived as spitting up and is misdiagnosed as a feeding problem or gastric reflux or is diagnosed repetitively as viral gastroenteritis. Secondly, the infant accommodates the gradual increase in intracranial pressure by separation of the sutures and cranial enlargement, allowing the tumor to become quite large. Blockage of cerebrospinal fluid (CSF) may further increase the pressure, accelerating the diagnosis with the infant's rapid clinical deterioration.

A series by Ikezaki et al. (16) classified the anatomic origin of posterior fossa ependymomas. They divided them into three categories citing the origin as the roof of the fourth ventricle, the floor of the fourth ventricle, and lateral type (CP angle). Both the roof and floor ependymomas fill the fourth ventricle, but their site of origin impacts the degree of difficulty in achieving total surgical resection because removal of the tumor from the surface of the brainstem is hazardous. Ependymomas tend to recur at the site of origin, so complete excision is easier when the tumor arises from the roof of the fourth ventricle than when it arises from the floor. Commonly, the obex with its underlying medullary respiratory center is the site of attachment. Although the tumor can be shaved off of the brainstem, it is difficult to totally excise it from this location.

The lateral (CP angle) type is extremely difficult to excise completely because it usually extends the full length of the brainstem (mesencephalon, pons, medulla), encasing the cranial nerves V–XII unilaterally and the vertebral artery. The tumor also insinuates itself between the brainstem and basilar artery. The tumor grows slowly, and the perforating vessels from the basilar artery to the stem, typically less than 1 mm, may be elongated to greater than 1 cm in length. This variety of ependymoma is unique to the infant age group (16, 23).

Infant posterior fossa tumors usually grow quite large before becoming clinically apparent. The fourth ventricular ependymomas, both roof and floor type, typically do not produce symptoms until CSF flow is blocked, and the lateral type may grow to enormous size because the tumor begins in the CP angle, enlarges in the lateral space along the brainstem, and even may extend inferiorly into the spine. Symptoms often only result when the fourth ventricle component obstructs CSF or the tumor fills the posterior fossa.

In the infant, the smaller posterior fossa, limited blood volume, and large tumor bulk present a significant surgical challenge. If rapid or large transfusion is required, washed packed red blood cells or fresh whole blood must be used to avoid hyperkalemia and the coagulopathy of depleted clotting factors. Hyperthermia is problematic in length procedures as is maintaining the prone position in the infant.

Case 1

HP is a 2-year-old girl who presented with ataxia and daily emesis. Magnetic resonance imaging (MRI) demonstrated a large tumor filling the fourth ventricle (Fig. 1A and B). A gross total resection was achieved and confirmed by both visual observation and by immediate postoperative MRI (Fig. 1C and D). At the time of surgery the tumor arose from the right facial colliculus. A 1 mm thick × 5 mm tuft of tumor at the right facial colliculus (the site of origin) was coagulated vigorously. She awoke immediately postoperatively, with a right VIth and VIIth nerve palsy. On the 4th postoperative day she developed an acute infection of the abdomen secondary to gastric perforation in spite of H2 antagonists. Her postoperative course was complicated by *Pseudomonas* sepsis, pneumonia, and respiratory distress syndrome. She was treated with local posterior fossa irradiation 6 weeks postresection, and no chemotherapy was given. She eventually made an excellent functional recovery with clearing of her cranial nerve palsies, normal mentation, and mild ataxic gait. She had 1 year of unusual apneic episodes triggered by crying and agitation. For the next 3½ years the patient remained asymptomatic, and the MRI surveillance revealed no tumor recurrence. Four years and 9 months after surgical resection she developed symptoms of increased intracranial pressure, headache, and ataxia. MRI revealed a large tumor recurrence (Fig. 1E). She again underwent gross total resection (Fig. 1F); the site of origin appeared to be the original location, the floor of the fourth ventricle, at the level of the facial colliculus. She was given a stereo-

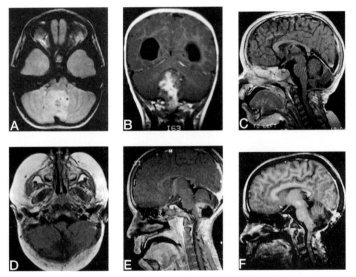

FIG. 1. (**A**) Axial T2 MRI demonstrates a large mass filling the fourth ventricle and compressing the medulla. (**B**) Coronal T1 MRI with gadolinium (Gd) enhancement of fourth ventricular tumor. (**C** and **D**) Sagittal and axial T1 MRI with Gd enhancement demonstrating no tumor. (**E**) Recurrence of tumor 4 years and 9 months after the initial resection. (**F**) Sagittal T1 MRI with Gd enhancement revealing no tumor.

taxic radiosurgical treatment at this location even though there was no visible residual tumor.

Case 1 illustrates the problem of tumor recurrence at the site of origin (floor of the fourth ventricle) and late recurrence (4½ years posttreatment), both common features of ependymoma.

Case 2

AH presented at LeBonheur Children's Hospital at 6 months of age. The family had noted a head tilt to the right, decrease in appetite, and occasional early morning vomiting. An MRI was obtained (Fig. 2A–C). She was begun on intravenous steroids and an H2 antagonist. Twelve hours after admission, she suddenly became decerebrate, requiring emergency ventriculostomy. She was taken to surgery in emergency fashion and underwent a gross total resection of her CP angle ependymoma. Postoperatively, she awoke immediately and recognized her mother. A left Vth, VIth, VIIth, IXth, and Xth cranial nerve deficit was noted. Her ventriculostomy was removed and a ventriculoperitoneal (VP) shunt was inserted. Feeding gastrostomy and tracheostomy were required. Follow-up MRI confirmed no residual tumor (Fig. 2D and E), with residual blood within the third ventricle and a small hemorrhagic

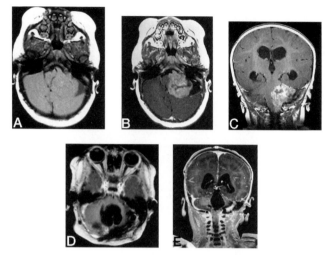

FIG. 2. (**A** and **B**) Axial T1 MRI with and without gadolinium (Gd) enhancement demonstrates a large lateral (CP angle) ependymoma compressing the medulla (**C**) Coronal T1 image demonstrates the longitudinal extent of the brainstem compression. (**D** and **E**) Axial and coronal T1 image with Gd enhancement reveals no residual tumor.

infarct in the distribution of the left middle cerebral artery. She was started on a chemotherapy protocol, using carboplatin, cyclophosphamide, and VP-16.

The CP angle ependymomas are the most difficult to remove surgically. The laterally placed tumors reach enormous size before they finally fill the fourth ventricle, producing hydrocephalus and increased intracranial pressure. None of our 11 infants with lateral tumors had cranial nerve deficit at presentation in spite of complete encasement of multiple nerves unilaterally. Two deteriorated with decerebrate posturing while awaiting surgery (case 2). Of the 11 infants, 8 had an initial gross total resection shortly after diagnosis. Three infants were operated on prior to referral to St. Jude Research Hospital; these were very limited resections. The three infants underwent three to five courses of chemotherapy, following which gross total resections were obtained with second operations. Chemotherapy was resumed followed by radiation at 3 years of age.

The average age was 17.91 months, and the average weight was 10.31 kilograms; 9 hours of surgery was required, with an average blood loss of 407 ml. Between the two groups, there was not a significant difference in the operating time of 9.1 hours *versus* 8.5 hours or the treatment with chemotherapy and delayed surgery, but there was a marked difference in the average blood loss. In the chemotherapy pretreated children, there was a 25.3 ml/kg blood loss *versus* 48 ml/kg, which represented 69% of the child's blood volume in the untreated infants. During surgery, the dissection was much simpler in the untreated children, inasmuch as the tumor was very soft and suckable with minimal adherence to the cranial nerves and vascular structures. The tumors were vascular so that constant blood loss occurred during the resection. In the infants pretreated with chemotherapy, the tumor was less vascular but was fibrous and more adherent to the cranial nerves, brainstem, and vertebral and basilar arteries.

The morbidity was high in both groups, with multiple unilateral cranial nerve deficits occurring in 9 of the 10 survivors. Nine children required tracheostomy and gastrostomy. Within 1 year six had normal swallowing ability with successful removal of tracheostomy and feeding appliances. The other cranial nerve deficits improved in 70–77% as well.

Of these 11 infants four deaths have occurred. One child had a VP shunt placed prior to referral which herniated upward within hours and presented with decerebrate posturing in the early morning. He was taken to surgery in an emergency fashion and underwent a gross total resection. When he did not improve immediately postoperatively and CT demonstrated midbrain hemorrhage, the parents elected to discontinue ventilatory support. One child died of progressive disease (the only anaplastic ependymoma in the series). One infant had an acute subdural hemorrhage after falling off a chair. This occurred during thrombocytopenia secondary to chemotherapy. At the time of death, he had no evidence of disease. Another infant, after having completed his chemotherapy and radiotherapy, died suddenly at home in Mexico City. MRI 1 month prior to death showed no evidence of tumor. It was suspected that his death was due to acute shunt malfunction. At present in this group of children with CP angle ependymomas with a 4-year average length of follow-up, we have six with no evidence of disease and one with a small nodule of tumor that has not progressed.

This is in keeping with our overall series of ependymomas in children less than 3 years of age, in which of the 26 children 10 have no evidence of disease, 7 have stable disease, 8 have died, and 1 has progressive disease. This 65% progression free survival rate is comparable to the result in the totally surgically resected group in the POG 8633 study of 66% (7).

CONCLUSIONS

In conclusion if you look critically at institutional series of ependymomas, the most important variable is age which overrides other variables. The children less than 3 years of age are very difficult to treat because they have large tumors arising in the posterior fossa, and the origin of the tumor is critical (16). Tumors arising from the floor of the fourth ventricle make total surgical resection extremely difficult. The ones arising in the CP angle involve multiple cranial nerves and are often, in most series, subtotally excised. Because the mainstay of treatment has been irradiation, these young children have not had the full benefit of therapy, until recent series using chemotherapy to delay irradiation.

An area of future investigation will be the use of a combination of radiotherapy and stereotaxic radiosurgery to give additional high-dose radiation to small areas of residual tumor. Also, it may be possible, using the new frameless stereotaxic systems, to accurately mark the area of origin of tumor for a radiosurgical or stereotaxic radiotherapy boost. Evaluation of chemotherapy is ongoing.

REFERENCES

1. Barone BM, Elvidge AR: Ependymomas: A clinical study. **J Neurosurg** 33:428–438, 1970.
2. Bloom HJG: Intracranial tumors: Response and resistance to therapeutic endeavors, 1970–1980. **Int J Radiat Oncol Biol Phys** 8:1083–1113, 1982.
3. Bloom JHG, Gless J, Bell J: The treatment and long-term prognosis of children with intracranial tumors. A study of 610 cases, 1950–1981. **Int J Radiat Oncol Biol Phys** 18:723–745, 1991.
4. Chin HW, Maruyama Y, Markesbery W, et al.: Intracranial ependymomas: Results of radiotherapy at the University of Kentucky. **Cancer** 49:2276–2280, 1982.
5. Cushing H: *Intracranial Tumors: Notes upon a Series of Two Thousand Verified Cases with Surgical-Mortality Percentages Pertaining Thereto.* Springfield, IL, Charles C Thomas, 1932, p 56.
6. Dohrmann GJ, Farwell JR, Flannery JT: Ependymomas and ependymoblastomas in children. **J Neurosurg** 45:273, 1976.
7. Duffner PK, Horowitz ME, Krischer JP, et al.: Postoperative chemotherapy and delayed radiation in children less than three years of age with malignant brain tumors. **N Engl J Med** 328(24):1725–1731, 1993.
8. Duncan JA, Hoffman HJ: Intracranial ependymomas, in Kaye AH, Laws ER Jr (eds): *Brain Tumors.* New York, Churchill Livingstone, 1996, pp 493–504.
9. Fokes EC Jr, Earle KM: Ependymomas: Clinical and pathological aspects. **J Neurosurg** 30:585–594, 1969.
10. Foreman NK, Love S, Thorne R: Intracranial ependymomas: Analysis of prognostic factors in a population-based series. **Pediatr Neurosurg** 24:119–125, 1996.
11. Gilles FH, Leviton A, Hedley-White ET, et al.: Childhood brain tumor update. **Hum Pathol** 14:834–845, 1987.
12. Goldwein JW, Corn BW, Finlay JL, et al.: Is craniospinal irradiation required to cure

children with malignant (anaplastic) intracranial ependymomas? **Cancer** 67:2766–2771, 1991.

13. Goldwein JW, Leahy JM, Packer RJ, *et al.*: Intracranial ependymomas in children. **Int J Radiat Oncol Biol Phys** 19:1497–1502, 1990.

14. Healey EA, Barnes PD, Kupsky WJ, *et al.*: The prognostic significance of postoperative residual tumor in ependymoma. **Neurosurgery** 28:666–672, 1991.

15. Hoppe-Hirsch E, Hirsch JF, Lellouch-Tubian A, *et al.*: Malignant hemisphere tumors in children. **Childs Nerv Syst** 9(3):131–135, 1993.

16. Ikezaki K, Matsushima T, Inoue T, *et al.*: Correlation of microanatomical localization with postoperative survival in posterior fossa ependymomas. **Neurosurgery** 32:38–44, 1993.

17. Kim YH, Fayos JV: Intracranial ependymomas. **Radiology** 0124:805–808, 1977.

18. Kun LE, Kovnar EH, Sanford RA: Ependymomas in children. **Pediatr Neurosci** 14:57–63, 1988.

19. Kovalic JJ, Flaris N, Grigsby PW, *et al.*: Intracranial ependymoma long term outcome, patterns of failure. **J Neurooncol** 15:125–131, 1993.

20. Liebel SA, Sheline GE: Radiation therapy of neoplasms of the brain. **J Neurosurg** 66:1–22, 1987.

21. Marsh WR Jr, Laws ER Jr: Intracranial ependymomas. **Prog Exp Tum Res** 30:175–180, 1987.

22. Mork SJ, Loken AC: Ependymoma. A follow up study of 101 cases. **Cancer** 40:907–915, 1977.

23. Nagib MH, O'Fallon MT: Posterior fossa lateral ependymomas in children. **Pediatr Neurosurg** 24:199–205, 1996.

24. Nazar GB, Hoffman HJ, Becker LE, *et al.*: Infratentorial ependymomas in childhood: Prognostic factors and treatment. **J Neurosurg** 72:408–417, 1990.

25. Oi S, Raimondi AJ: Ependymoma in children. In: *Pediatric Neurosurgery. Surgery of the Developing Nervous System.* New York, Grune & Stratton, 1982, pp 419–428.

26. Papadopoulos DP, Giri S, Evans RG: Prognostic factors and management of intracranial ependymomas. **Anticancer Res** 10:689–692, 1990.

27. Pollack IF, Gerszten PC, Martinez AJ, *et al.*: Intracranial ependymomas of childhood: Long-term outcome and prognostic factors. **Neurosurgery** 37:655–667, 1995.

28. Rawlings CE III, Giangaspero F, Burger PC, *et al.*: Ependymomas: A clinicopathologic study. **Surg Neurol** 29:271–281, 1988.

29. Ringertz N, Reymond A: Ependymomas and choroid plexus papillomas. **J Neuropathol Exp Neurol** 8:355–380, 1949.

30. Ross GW, Rubinstein LJ: Lack of histopathological correlation of malignant ependymomas with postoperative survival. **J Neurosurg** 70:31–36, 1989.

31. Rousseau P, Habrand JL, Sarrazin D, *et al.*: Treatment of intracranial ependymomas of children: Review of a 15-year experience. **Int J Radiat Oncol Biol Phys** 28:381–386, 1994.

32. Russell DS, Rubinstein LJ: Pathology of tumors of the nervous system. London, Arnold Press, 1977, ed 4, pp 203–226.

33. Salazar OM, Castro-Vita H, Van Houtie P, *et al.*: Improved survival in cases of ependymoma after radiation therapy: Late report and recommendations. **J Neurosurg** 59:652–659, 1983.

34. Shaw EG, Evans RG, Scheithauer BW, *et al.*: Postoperative radiotherapy of intracranial ependymoma in pediatric and adult patients. **Int J Radiat Oncol Biol Phys** 13:1457–1462, 1987.
35. Sutton LN, Goldwein G, Perilongo B, *et al.*: Prognostic factors in childhood ependymomas. **Pediatr Neurosurg** 16:57–65, 1990.
36. Svien HJ, Mabon RF, Kernohan JW, *et al.*: Ependymomas of the brain: Pathologic aspects. **Neurology** 3:1–15, 1953.
37. Tomita T, McLone DG, Lakshmi D, *et al.*: Benign ependymomas of the posterior fossa in childhood. **Pediatr Neurosci** 14:277–285, 1988.

33

Medulloblastoma

JAMES T. RUTKA, M.D., Ph.D.

Medulloblastoma is the most common malignant tumor in childhood. It accounts for approximately 25% of all pediatric brain tumors. Of interest, the incidence of medulloblastoma has recently been reported to be on the decline. In the past 10 years, the Japanese have reported that the incidence of medulloblastoma is 5–10% of childhood tumors. While detailed epidemiologic data are not currently available in North America, it is the author's impression that the number of patients with medulloblastoma is also decreasing slightly on our continent. This impression is based on our observed practice of intracranial tumors at The Hospital for Sick Children over the last 15 years. What is causing a potential decline in this tumor type, however, remains unknown.

CONTRIBUTIONS OF HARVEY CUSHING AND PERCIVAL BAILEY

We are deeply indebted to both Harvey Cushing and Percival Bailey for their classification of medulloblastoma as a separate tumor type. The nosology for this tumor was established in 1925. Although the choice of the term medulloblastoma is somewhat unfortunate in that there is no readily identifiable precursor cell type known as the "medulloblast," nevertheless, the distinctive histopathologic features of this tumor make it instantly recognizable and identifiable by pathologists throughout the world.

There perhaps is no better clinical description of patients who present with medulloblastoma than that written by Cushing (5). While the diagnosis of medulloblastoma can be made more swiftly today than in Cushing's time, largely because of advances in diagnostic imaging studies, the salient features of the presentation of a child with a rapidly growing posterior fossa tumor as described so knowingly by Cushing are germane to this day (Fig. 1A–E). By 1930, Cushing had operated on 61 patients with medulloblastoma. He was acutely aware of the tendency for these tumors to invade the brainstem and to metastasize. He was only cautiously optimistic about the child with a posterior fossa medulloblastoma at the end of his career. It was not

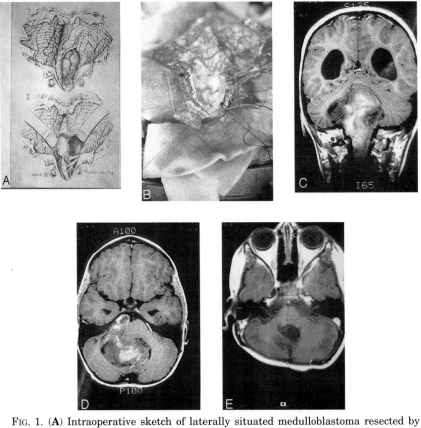

FIG. 1. (**A**) Intraoperative sketch of laterally situated medulloblastoma resected by Cushing. The tumor was completely excised through a paramedian cerebellar hemispheric incision. Once the tumor was removed, the lower cranial nerves were apparent. Surgical clips were used on the distal branches of the posteroinferior cerebellar artery to provide hemostasis. (Reproduced with permission from *Harvey Cushing: Selected Papers on Neurosurgery.* New Haven, CT, Yale University Press, 1969, p 164.) (**B**) Seventy years later, the author encountered a case almost identical to that depicted above. The tumor was a paramedian, desmoplastic medulloblastoma firmly adherent to the lower cranial nerves on the left side. A gross total resection of this tumor was achieved. (**C**) Gadolinium-enhanced coronal MRI through the posterior fossa showing a large tumor that extended through the foramen magnum into the upper cervical spinal cord. (**D**) Gadolinium-enhanced axial MRI of the same patient showing medulloblastoma extending through the left lateral foramina of Luschka to reside in part in front of the pons. (**E**) Postoperative axial MRI showing complete resection of medulloblastoma. The child has been well and free of disease for 4 years.

until the widespread acceptance and utilization of combined posterior fossa and craniospinal irradiation as initially described in 1953 by Patterson and Farr (12) that a new era was ushered in in terms of improved patient survival.

ETIOLOGY

No known direct cause has been found for human medulloblastoma. It is of interest, however, that certain genetic syndromes have been highly associated with the formation of medulloblastomas. They include the basal cell nevus syndrome, also known as Gorlin syndrome and Turcot's syndrome. The genetic basis for Gorlin and Turcot's syndromes is currently being mapped to precise chromosomal positions. Work from a number of laboratories has shown quite conclusively that the p53 gene is not mutated in human medulloblastomas (3, 15).

CLINICAL PRESENTATION

Today, the child with medulloblastoma typically presents with a short history. Symptoms and signs are usually of less than 2 months' duration. A syndrome of raised intracranial pressure characterized by headache, vomiting, and papilledema is most common. Cerebellar signs such as truncal ataxia, nystagmus, and impairment of rapid alternating movements are frequent observations. Occasionally, a child will have a facial nerve or bulbar palsies suggestive of brainstem invasion by a tumor. Rarely, a patient will present in extremis from an intratumoral hemorrhage which typically obstructs cerebrospinal fluid (CSF) pathways acutely. Finally, in less than 5% of cases, the presentation is one of symptomatic metastasis.

ADULT PATIENTS WITH MEDULLOBLASTOMA

The experience with adult patients with medulloblastoma is considerably smaller than that with children, but is nonetheless important to discuss here. In general, relapse and survival rates are similar to those in children. However, there are reports that suggest that adult patients with medulloblastoma relapse at distant sites in the neuraxis more frequently than at the primary site than do children (13). The overall survival rates for adult patients who can be classified into a low-risk category are similar to children. The experience with chemotherapy in adults is growing, and new protocols for adult patients will likely improve survival figures further.

IMAGING STUDY

In the computerized tomography (CT) era, an almost diagnostic feature for medulloblastoma on CT was a hyperdense posterior fossa lesion on a precontrast CT scan (Fig. 2). Following contrast administration, the tumor typically enhances boldly. There may be surrounding edema and occasionally calcification. Most medulloblastomas are located in the midline. However, it is clear that medulloblastomas can be found in the cerebellar hemisphere or in the cerebellopontine angle bordering the brainstem (Fig. 3). As such, medulloblastoma has often been called the great "masquerader" of tumors in the posterior fossa.

PATHOLOGY

The medulloblastoma typically fills the fourth ventricle arising from the cerebellar vermis (Fig. 4). The tumor is soft and friable. Frequently there are small intratumoral hemorrhages. Microscopically, the tumor is highly cellular. Homer-Wright rosettes are abundant (Fig. 5). Immunohistochemical analysis has revealed glial, neuronal, and ependymal differentiation. The demoplastic variant of medulloblastoma contains a stromal enriched portion. Recently, there has been a trend toward recognizing medulloblastoma as a primitive neuroectodermal tumor (PNET). Hart and Earle were the first to describe PNETs in the

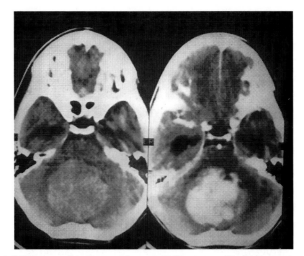

FIG. 2. Axial CT scan of patient with medulloblastoma. (**Left**) Precontrast axial scan through the posterior fossa shows a round, hyperdense lesion filling the fourth ventricle. Hyperdensity on precontrast CT usually implies a highly cellular tumor such as medulloblastoma. (**Right**) Following contrast administration, this medulloblastoma enhances brightly and heterogeneously.

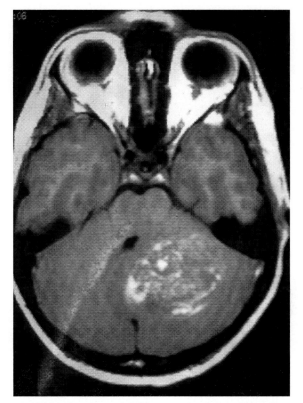

FIG. 3. Axial gadolinium-enhanced MRI scan of patient with left cerebellar hemispheric medulloblastoma. Medulloblastomas may arise in the vermis, the cerebellar hemisphere, the cerebellopontine angle, or rarely, the brainstem. As such, they may be construed as the great "masqueraders" of posterior fossa lesions.

supratentorial compartment (10). The nomenclature was formalized in 1978 by Rorke, Davis, and Becker. Interestingly, patients with supratentorial PNETs have had a far graver prognosis than those with medulloblastoma (7).

PUTATIVE PREDICTIVE MARKERS

Since the advent of immunohistochemistry, and, more recently, with the development of techniques in molecular biology, a number of putative predictive markers have been described for medulloblastoma (1, 2, 16, 18, 19). Immunohistochemical markers have included those for intermediate filaments such as glial fibrillary acidic protein (GFAP), and the neurofilaments (19) and nestin (18). Molecular markers have included isochromosome 17p and 17q deletions. Isochromosome 17q

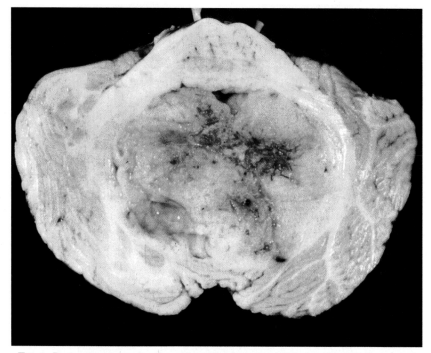

FIG. 4. Postmortem examination of medulloblastoma. Axial slice through the posterior fossa at the level of the pons. The tumor arises from the cerebellar vermis. It fills the fourth ventricle. Intratumoral hemorrhage is seen. The CSF pathway through the fourth ventricle is completely obstructed.

has been reported with high frequency (2). C-myc amplification has been found in 20% of medulloblastoma cell lines (1). Finally, the neurotrophin receptor trk C was recently found to predict better survival (16).

SURGERY

To Shunt or Not To Shunt

In the past, there was considerable controversy as to whether a patient should be shunted prior to posterior fossa surgery. This controversy has now been largely resolved. We do not recommend shunting a patient unless the patient is moribund from acute obstructive hydrocephalus. Most patients who are symptomatic from their mass lesions or from hydrocephalus will be symptomatically controlled on steroids until surgery is planned.

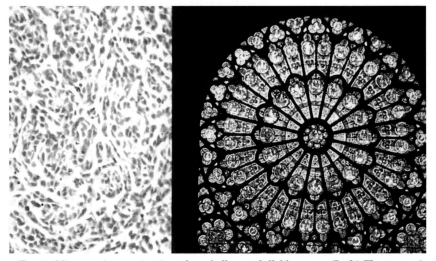

FIG. 5. Microscopic examination of cerebellar medulloblastoma. (**Left**) The tumor is typically comprised of small, blue cells with a prominent nucleus and scarce cytoplasm. The characteristic Homer-Wright rosettes are conspicuous in medulloblastoma. The medulloblastoma is a highly cellular tumor that frequently displays differentiation along neuronal, glial, or ependymal lines. H&E, ×150. (**Right**) The Alchemists' Rose Window depicting priests, prophets, and kings surrounding the virgin Mary from circa 1268 AD in Notre Dame cathedral, Paris, France. In many ways, the image of the rose window recapitulates the cytoarchitectural pattern of the medulloblastoma.

Patient Positioning

Patients are positioned prone on padded bolsters. Rigid head fixation in pins is preferred for children over age 4. For children aged 2–4 years, pin fixation can still be used, but with caution. Children under age 2 are placed on a padded horseshoe headrest. For lesions that reach the superior vermis and the tentorial hiatus, the concorde position as described by Sugita has been most helpful (Fig. 6) (17).

Exposure and Operative Approach

Midline cerebellar tumors such as medulloblastoma are best approached through a midline exposure. We are now performing a craniotomy using a high powered drill in most children. This enables a more anatomic closure of tissues at the end of the procedure. Upon opening the dura in a standard Y-shaped fashion, the tumor is often apparent between the cerebellar tonsils (Fig. 7). The inferior vermis is split. We use self-retaining retractors to help develop the plane between tumor and normal cerebellum. It must be stressed that retraction should be used sparingly, and the retractor blades should be

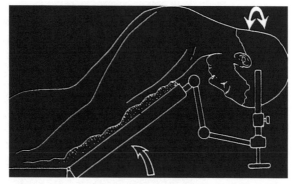

FIG. 6. Concorde position as described by Sugita (17). In this position, the patient's trunk is elevated while the head is flexed. This position enables an approach from below to the tentorial hiatus for medulloblastomas with a high rostral extent.

moved frequently to avoid retraction injury. The floor of the fourth ventricle is found early in the procedure. Cottonoids are used to protect the floor of the fourth ventricle at all times. The ultrasonic aspirator is used to resect the tumors expeditiously. For those tumors that do not invade the brainstem, a complete resection can be achieved (Fig. 8). It is important, before closing, to examine all margins for residual tumor. If the tumor is found to infiltrate the brainstem, no attempts are made to resect the tumor from within the brainstem. Serious neurological deficits will result if this is pursued.

STAGING: AN IMPORTANT ROLE IN THE CHILD WITH MEDULLOBLASTOMA

Whenever possible, we try to obtain a preoperative spinal magnetic resonance imaging (MRI) scan in children whose posterior fossa tumors are likely to be medulloblastoma. This obviates the need to wait 2 weeks after the procedure to allow for blood products to disappear on the MRI scan. Following surgery, we obtain an immediate postoperative MRI or CT scan to assess residual tumor. Some institutions still advocate the usefulness of CSF sampling 2 weeks after the surgical procedure.

BIOLOGICAL BEHAVIOR OF MEDULLOBLASTOMA

What clearly separates medulloblastoma from other posterior fossa tumors in children is its ability to spread throughout the CSF pathways. CSF dissemination has been found in 20–50% of cases. It has been our observation that CSF sampling from the cisterna magna even before any attempt to remove a tumor is performed leads to the iden-

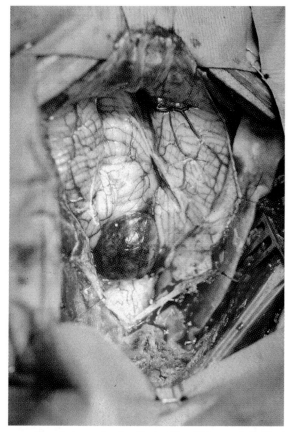

FIG. 7. Intraoperative photograph of patient with midline medulloblastoma. The dura has been opened. The tumor is readily seen descending below the cerebellar tonsils and closely applied to the floor of the fourth ventricle and upper cervical spinal cord. Removal of the tumor proceeds as the floor of the fourth ventricle is protected by carefully placed cottonoid patties.

tification of tumor cell fragments floating freely in the CSF (Fig. 9). The propensity of medulloblastoma to spread along CSF pathways can lead to gross deposits of tumor along the spinal axis. Approximately 40% of medulloblastomas will infiltrate the brainstem. Interestingly, this does not appear to affect overall prognosis. About 10% of medulloblastomas will show signs of systemic metastases to lung, lymph nodes, and bones. Although the posterior fossa is still the most common site of recurrence, relapse can be found outside the posterior fossa in the supratentorial compartment (Fig. 10).

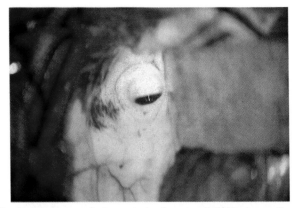

FIG. 8. Following the removal of a posterior fossa medulloblastoma, the neurosurgeon should inspect all margins for residual tumor. The aqueduct of Sylvius is directly visualized. If the tumor has invaded the brainstem, no attempt should be made to remove a small amount of residual tumor lest the patient awaken with serious neurologic deficits.

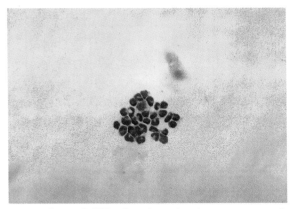

FIG. 9. Cytospin analysis of CSF taken from the cisterna magna of a patient with medulloblastoma before tumor removal. It is the author's experience that such samples frequently demonstrate medulloblastoma tumor micronodules. The significance of this finding is not clear. However, the metastatic potential of medulloblastoma can be appreciated by such CSF specimens.

POSTOPERATIVE PATIENT MANAGEMENT

Children recover quickly from posterior fossa surgery. Steroids are gradually tapered. Placement of perioperative external ventricular drains to manage hydrocephalus is still a frequently practiced and acceptable procedure. These days we do not typically place an external

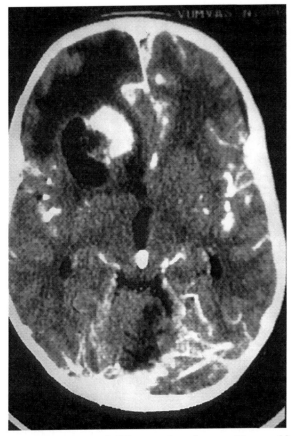

FIG. 10. Contrast-enhanced axial CT scan taken from an 11-year-old male 5 years after treatment for medulloblastoma. A right frontal metastatic tumor is seen. Late recurrence of medulloblastoma is seen, but is rare. Such patients frequently respond to intensive chemotherapy.

drain except in the very young child with marked enlargement of the ventricles. Approximately 25% of patients with medulloblastoma will ultimately go on to develop clinically significant hydrocephalus requiring VP shunt placement.

RISK SEGREGATION

Based on decades of clinical experience with medulloblastoma, patients in North America are categorized into either low- or high-risk groups. The low-risk group is characterized by children who are over age 3 in whom no residual tumor has been found on postoperative MRI or CT and in whom no distant metastases have been identified. In contrast, the high-risk group consists of children under age 3 in whom residual tumor is obvious on MRI or CT and in whom distant metastases have occurred.

SURVIVAL DATA

We reviewed our experience at The Hospital for Sick Children in the previous decade, 1980–1989. In this time period there were 50 patients with medulloblastoma. Twenty-six were low risk, and 24 were high risk. The 5-year survival rate for low-risk patients was 70%, and the 5-year survival for the high-risk group was 40%. These results compare favorably with reports from a similar time period. Based on these results, on our more favorable recent results with chemotherapy in the high-risk group, and on new results in the literature, the following treatment recommendations can be made.

TREATMENT RECOMMENDATION

Following gross total removal of a medulloblastoma, if the tumor has not disseminated based on imaging studies and if the patient is older than 3 years we recommend 3500 rads craniospinal radiation and 5500 rads to the posterior fossa. In those children in whom tumor dissemination is evident, we treat with preirradiation chemotherapy for two cycles, and this is followed by the same doses of craniospinal and posterior fossa radiation as described above over 6 weeks. Following this, eight cycles of postirradiation chemotherapy are given.

We are reluctant to irradiate the brain of a child under the age of 3 years. In this subset, we are using chemotherapy alone until such time that the child is of age to tolerate craniospinal irradiation.

ADVERSE EFFECTS OF RADIATION THERAPY ON THE CENTRAL NERVOUS SYSTEM

A number of adverse effects have been reported following irradiation of the developing brain. They include cognitive impairment, endocrinopathy, moyamoya syndrome, and the potential for a radiation-induced tumor (8, 11). Because of these adverse effects, attempts have been made to reduce craniospinal irradiation in low-risk patients. A study performed by the Pediatric Oncology Group and the Children's Cancer Study Group used a lower craniospinal dose (2340 rads *versus* 3500 rads) for low-risk patients. Unfortunately, the reduction in craniospinal irradiation was met with a rather rapid relapse in patients treated on this arm of the protocol (6). As such, the protocol was abandoned. At the present time, a reduction in the amount of craniospinal irradiation is not advised. However, ongoing cooperative studies will determine if the addition of intensive chemotherapy to irradiation will permit a lowering of the craniospinal radiation dose.

RECURRENT MEDULLOBLASTOMA

We have no good salvage therapy for the child with a recurrent medulloblastoma. However, intensive chemotherapy protocols are now leading to partial and complete tumor responses and prolonged survivals (Fig. 11). The chemotherapy protocol we are using at The Hospital for Sick Children for high-grade brain tumors such as medulloblastoma is "ICE" chemotherapy (iphosphamide, carboplatinum, and etoposide). The use of autologous bone marrow transplantation as advocated in several centers now may permit the use of higher doses of chemotherapy than are generally tolerated without transplantation (9).

IMPROVING PATIENT SURVIVAL

Prospects are brighter today than they were 20 years ago for children with medulloblastoma. Still, a significant number of children will succumb from their tumor. How can we improve patient survival? One option is to consider all patients with medulloblastoma as high risk. This concept is not new. Medulloblastoma is a cancer. It has the potential to metastasize. As such, we ought to treat it aggressively up

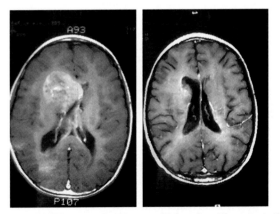

FIG. 11. (**Left**) Axial MRI scans of a 12-year-old female with metastatic medulloblastoma at relapse. A large right frontal metastatic tumor is seen in the right lateral ventricle. (**Right**) Following a trial of intensive chemotherapy, the patient had a complete tumor response and was well for 14 months before she showed signs of tumor progression and died. While there is no good salvage therapy for the child with a medulloblastoma, intensive chemotherapy as administered today can be more than palliative. Some durable clinical responses have been obtained and reported.

front. Therefore, a reasonable consideration would be to treat all patients with maximum radiation and chemotherapy. In this regard, the best reported survival statistics for patients with medulloblastoma have been reported by Cohen and Packer (4). In this study, 63 high-risk children were treated with cisplatinum, vincristine, and lomustine (CCNU). A progression-free survival at 5 years of 85% was found for the entire group. In those children in whom metastasis had been identified, the progression-free survival was 67% at 5 years. Interestingly, a 90% survival was found for children with local disease. It is hard to conceive of better results than these for medulloblastoma. Accordingly, all centers should strive to match these results.

FUTURE DIRECTIONS

We must continue to determine the optimum systemic therapy for medulloblastoma which will undoubtedly include refinements in chemotherapy. We must continue to identify and develop molecular markers involved in medulloblastoma progression. Finally, in the future, we may be in a position to test novel treatment strategies, such as gene therapy, especially for patients whose tumors have disseminated along CSF pathways (14).

REFERENCES

1. Bigner SH, Friedman HS, Vogelstein B: Amplification of the c-myc gene in human medulloblastoma cell lines and xenografts. **Cancer Res** 50:2347–2350, 1990.
2. Bigner SH, Mark J, Friedman HS, et al.: Structural chromosomal abnormalities in human medulloblastoma. **Cancer Genet Cytogenet** 30:91–101, 1988.
3. Cogen PH, Daneshvar L, Metzger AK: Deletion mapping of the medulloblastoma locus on chromosome 17p. **Genomics** 8:279–285, 1990.
4. Cohen BH, Packer RJ: Chemotherapy for medulloblastomas and primitive neuroectodermal tumors. **J Neurooncol** 29:55–68, 1996.
5. Cushing H: Experiences with cerebellar medulloblastomas: Critical review. **Acta Pathol Microbiol Scand** 1:1–86, 1930.
6. Deutch M, Thomas P, Boyett J, et al.: Low stage medulloblastoma: A children's cancer study group (CCSG) and paediatric oncology group (POG) randomized study of standard vs reduced neuraxis irradiation. **Proc Annu Meet Am Soc Clin Oncol** 10:A363, 1991.
7. Dirks PB, Harris L, Hoffman HJ, et al.: Supratentorial primitive neuroectodermal tumors in children. **J Neurooncol** 29:75–84, 1996.
8. Dirks PB, Jay V, Becker LE, et al.: Development of anaplastic changes in low-grade astrocytomas of childhood. **Neurosurgery** 34:68–78, 1994.
9. Dunkel IJ, Finlay JL: High dose chemotherapy with autologous stem cell rescue for patients with medulloblastoma. **J Neurooncol** 29:69–74, 1996.
10. Hart MN, Earle KM: Primitive neuroectodermal tumors of the brain in children. **Cancer** 32:890–897, 1973.

11. Kestle JRW, Hoffman HJ, Mock AR: Moyamoya phenomenon after radiation for optic glioma. **J Neurosurg** 79:32–35, 1993.

12. Patterson R, Farr RF: Cerebellar medulloblastomas: Treatment by irradiation of the whole central nervous system. **Acta Radiol** 39:323–326, 1953.

13. Peterson K, Walker RW: Medulloblastoma/primitive neuroectodermal tumor in 45 adults. **Neurology** 45:440–442, 1995.

14. Raffel C: Gene therapy for PNET. **J Neurooncol** 29:113–118, 1996.

15. Raffel C, Thomas GA, Tishler DM, et al.: Absence of p53 mutations in childhood central nervous system primitive neuroectodermal tumors. **Neurosurgery** 33:301–306, 1993.

16. Segal RA, Goumnerova LC, Kwon YK, et al.: Expression of the neurotrophin receptor Trk C is linked to a favorable outcome in medulloblastoma. **Proc Natl Acad Sci USA** 91:12867–12871, 1994.

17. Sugita K: Microneurosurgical atlas. Berlin, Springer-Verlag, 1985, pp 172–174.

18. Tohyama T, Lee VM-Y, Rorke LB, et al.: Nestin expression in embryonic human neuroepithelium and in human neuroepithelial tumor cells. **Lab Invest** 66:303–313, 1992.

19. Trojanowski JQ, Tohyama T, Lee VM-Y: Medulloblastomas and related primitive neuroectodermal brain tumors of childhood recapitulate molecular milestones in the maturation of neuroblasts. **Mol Chem Neuropathol** 17:121–135, 1992.

Index

Page numbers followed by *t* and *f* indicate tables and figures, respectively